e-Discovery

Healthcare Resource Guide to e-Discovery and Electronic Records

Kimberly A. Baldwin-Stried Reich, MBA, MJ, PBCI, RHIA, CPHQ, FAHIMA
Katherine L. Ball, MD, MSC
Michelle L. Dougherty, MA, RHIA, CHP
Ronald J. Hedges, JD

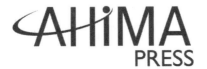
PRESS

ISBN: 978-1-58426-229-9
AHIMA Product No.: AB123109

AHIMA Staff:
Claire Blondeau, MBA, Senior Editor
Adrienne Cook, JD, Developmental Editor
Katie Greenock, MS, Editorial and Production Coordinator
Ashley Sullivan, Assistant Editor
Ken Zielske, Director of Publications

For more information about AHIMA Press publications, including updates, visit http://www.ahima.org/publications/updates.aspx

American Health Information Management Association
233 North Michigan Avenue, 21st Floor
Chicago, Illinois 60601-5809
ahima.org

Brief Contents

BRIEF CONTENTS

Contents

CHAPTER ONE   Overview   1

CHAPTER TWO   Foundation of Electronic
Discovery Rules   49

CONTENTS

CHAPTER THREE   e-Discovery in Practice   79

CHAPTER FOUR   Litigation Response Planning   183

**CHAPTER FIVE   Content and Records Management
and Electronic Discovery   237**

On the CD-ROM

Link to the Robert Williams 2006 Keynote Address at MER (Managing Electronic Records) Conference, including case law updates up to 2012 and continuing at the site
e-Discovery Glossary of Terms and Acronyms
e-Discovery Glossary of Websites
Update on State Discovery Rules

About the Authors

Kimberly A. Baldwin-Stried Reich, MBA, MJ, PBCI, RHIA, CPHQ, FAHIMA is a credentialed healthcare information management, quality management, case management, and compliance professional with over 25 years of experience in a variety of healthcare settings. She has been an active member of American Health Information Management Association (AHIMA) Working Groups since 2006 and is a national speaker and author on the topics of health information operations, e-discovery, and healthcare compliance. Since 2006, she has been an active member of the Health Level Seven (HL7) Working Group responsible for review and development of the Records Management and Evidentiary Support (RM-ES) profile for the design and development of the functional profile for electronic health record systems. In 2010, she was appointed to the AHIMA Quality Initiatives and Secondary Data Practice Council.

Ms. Reich was elected to the board of the Illinois Health Information Management Association (ILHIMA) in 2009 and currently serves as the second-year director of legislation and advocacy. In 2011, she was voted president-elect of ILHIMA. In addition to her ILHIMA volunteer activities, she also serves as the chairperson for the College of Lake County Health Information Technology Advisory Committee. She is an active member of The Sedona Conference Working Group I on Best Practices for Electronic Document Retention and Production, the Public Health Data Standards Consortium's Privacy, Security, and Data Sharing Committee, and the American Medical Informatics Association.

Ms. Reich holds a Master of Business Administration from the Lake Forest Graduate School of Management, a Master of Jurisprudence in health law and policy from the Loyola School of Law–Beazley Institute for Health Law and Policy in Chicago and a post-baccalaureate in clinical informatics from the Johns Hopkins School of Medicine. Ms. Reich is employed by Lake County Physicians' Association in Waukegan, IL, and lives in Lake Forest, IL, with her husband Joachim and their two cats, Rusty and Paris.

Katherine L. Ball, MD, MSc is the vice president and chief medical information officer for Mountain States Health Alliance of Johnson City, TN, as well as chief medical officer for Sycamore Shoals Hospital of Elizabethton, TN, and Johnson County Community Hospital of Mountain City, TN. She previously served as chief medical information officer at Holy Cross Hospital in Silver Springs, MD. She is board-certified in emergency medicine and internal medicine.

Michelle L. Dougherty, MA, RHIA, CHP, is a director of practice leadership for AHIMA. Dougherty provides professional expertise to AHIMA members and outside organizations on health information practice issues and develops written products aimed at furthering the art and science of health information management (HIM). She also serves as coordinator and project manager for AHIMA's Long Term Care Taskforce and Legal Health Record Taskforce, as well as co-chair of the Medical Records/Information Management technical committee for HL7. Ms. Dougherty is a frequent speaker on HIM and health-care industry topics. Prior to joining AHIMA in 1999, Ms. Dougherty served as an HIM consultant in the Post-Acute Consulting Services Group of Minneapolis-based Larson, Allen, Weishair & Co., LLP. As a consultant, she provided health information, documentation, survey, prospective payment system, and compliance consulting services to long-term care, home care, and subacute facilities. Ms. Dougherty holds a Bachelor of Arts degree in health information administration from the College of St. Scholastica in Duluth, MN.

Ronald J. Hedges, JD, is the principal of Ronald J. Hedges, LLC, in Hackensack, NJ. He has extensive experience in e-discovery and in management of complex civil litigation matters. Hedges was appointed in 1986 as a US Magistrate Judge in the US District Court for the District of New Jersey, where he served as the compliance judge for the Court Mediation Program, a member of the Lawyers Advisory Committee, and both a member and reporter for the Civil Justice Reform Act Advisory Committee. From 2001 to 2005 he was a member of the Advisory Group of Magistrate Judges. Hedges has also been an adjunct professor at Seton Hall University School of Law (1993–2007) and at Georgetown University Law Center since 2006. He is entering his second term as a visiting research collaborator with the Center for Information Technology Policy at Princeton University.

Dedication

Ruth Ann Withers was the wife of a prominent Baptist minister, the mother of three children, and a nursing educator in upstate New York who likely did not realize what a pioneer she was. She was one of a small cohort of medical professionals to study for an advanced degree in biomedical communications in the late 1960s, when the field was considered on the cutting edge of medical technology. She received her master's degree from Tulane University in 1968. She utilized the dominant communications medium of the time, producing and starring in a series of educational films aired on National Educational Television, the predecessor of today's Public Broadcasting Service. She advised hospitals in New York and New England on nursing education, specializing in the retraining of nurses who were returning to the workforce after raising families, and providing inservice education to medical professionals on "new" medical technologies.

But her training in biomedical communications was not limited to television production. It was the late 1960s, and digital technologies were just emerging. Her daughter recalls Ruth Ann talking about information coming out of NASA, which was utilizing the new technology to monitor the vital signs of astronauts in space and beaming the information in real time back to Earth. And her youngest son recalls Ruth Ann drafting a short paper that envisioned a computer terminal in every healthcare facility with direct links to the National Centers for Disease Control, Walter Reed Hospital, or any of several medical schools, which medical professionals could use to immediately access medical information on demand. The thesis of the paper was dismissed by her instructors as too visionary, as computers at that time were used to crunch financial numbers and not for collecting and distributing useful medical information.

The story may seem apocryphal, but it is true enough. The world of the late 1960s was just beginning to grasp the potential of digital information and computer-mediated communications. Ruth Ann Withers passed away unexpectedly in 1970 at the age of 44. She would not live to see the extent to which digital information technologies would permeate all aspects of healthcare. If her vision of at least one accessible computer terminal in every hospital was considered too advanced for 1968, the notion of medical professionals creating and managing patient records on handheld devices, networked worldwide, would have been astounding. But after the initial shock, Ruth Ann probably would have said, "let me try that." Yes, she was a pioneer, whether or not she realized it, and to her and many other unsung heroes of medical information technology, this book is dedicated.

Kenneth J. Withers
Director of Judicial Education and Content
The Sedona Conference

Acknowledgments

This book was written under the auspices of the American Health Information Management Association (AHIMA). AHIMA has had a longstanding interest in the laws surrounding medical record confidentiality, security, release of information, and discovery. The adoption of electronic health records (EHRs) and the establishment of a Nationwide Health Information Network (NHIN), along with the Federal Rules of Civil Procedure (FRCP) and the Uniform Rules of Evidence will unquestionably play a role in the redesign of the roles and responsibilities of HIM, legal, risk, and compliance professionals of the future.

Many thought leaders and experts have contributed to the publication of this book. Toward that end, the authors wish to thank and acknowledge Richard Braman, founder of The Sedona Conference, and Ken Withers, Director of Judicial Education and Content. Without their support and commitment to healthcare, this book would not have been possible. The dialogue and friendships that we have made through our involvement with The Sedona Conference are priceless. We would like to give a special thank you to Kevin Brady, Jonathan Redgrave, Sherry B. Harris, Thomas Y. Allman, Maura R. Grossman, Ariana J Tadler, Jeane A. Thomas, and Cecil Lynn for sharing their expertise and insights; and to Jason Baron, Director of Litigation at the National Archives and Records Administration in College Park, MD for his thoughts about the future usages of e-mail information including the storage and searching of same.

Thanks to Larry Center, Assistant Dean, Department of Academic Conferences and Continuing Legal Education, Georgetown University Law Center, and Robert Eisenberg, Program Co-Chair of the Advanced E-Discovery Institute of the Georgetown University Law Center and Chair of the Faculty of the Advisory Board of Georgetown Law's E-Discovery Training Academy. It was an honor and a privilege to participate in the November 2009 program; we appreciate your recognition as to the impact e-discovery will have on the healthcare industry.

Thank you to Judge Shira Scheindlin for your interest, support, and encouragement through The Sedona Conference for the adoption of electronic records in healthcare; the *Zubulake* decisions have established a good foundation for HIM and records management professionals everywhere in understanding the value and content of all relevant electronically stored information. Thank you to Judges Paul W. Grimm and John M. Facciola for your support and thoughts regarding the healthcare industry and the adoption of electronic health records.

Of special note, George L. Paul, a good friend and the author of two inspirational works used in the development of this work, *The Discovery Revolution: E-Discovery Amendments to the Federal Rules of Civil Procedure and Foundations of Digital Evidence*, thank you for making us push harder and try harder. You truly have challenged our thinking about "digital authenticity."

To Craig D. Ball, PC, the talk we shared about healthcare on the plane ride from California in 2008 will never be forgotten—it was a motivating factor as to why the authors wrote this book. Your statement, "The reality of electronic discovery is it starts off as the responsibility of those who don't understand the technology and ends up as the responsibility of those who don't understand the law" has never been more apropos than when applied to the context of today's developing healthcare technology. Here's hoping that one day soon, both technology and the law will intersect to improve care delivery while supporting the "just, speedy, and inexpensive determination of every action and proceeding."

To Mike Slovis, Esq. of Cunningham, Meyer & Vedrine, PC, the time and long hours you spent with the authors talking about your experiences and sharing your insights is truly appreciated. Thank you to Juanita Passyn, Esq., Kelly McLendon, RHIA, Reed Gelzer, MD, CHCC, and Beth Acker, RHIA, for your support of the authors' work.

Thanks to Harold Lehmann, MD, PhD, FACMI, FAAP, associate professor at the Johns Hopkins University School of Medicine and director of training and research for the Johns Hopkins Division of Health Sciences Informatics, for your undying commitment. Nancy Roderer, Patricia A. Abbott, PhD, RN, BC, FACMI, FAAN, Christoph Lehmann, MD, George Kim, MD, Anna Orlova, PhD, and Robert E. Miller, MD, from the Johns Hopkins Health Sciences Informatics program have provided the authors with solid informatics training and a quality education. A special thank you and recognition to the Office of the National Coordinator (ONC) for its support of this program and the IT education and training that was made possible to one of the authors.

To Mark Chudzinski, Esq., and Ivan Handler of the State of Illinois Office of Health Information Technology (OHIT), thank you for making the authors' practicum experience an invaluable one. The work being done by the OHIT today is establishing the health information exchange infrastructure of tomorrow and will be invaluable to the citizens of Illinois and surrounding states, and will establish the foundation for work to that will be done by HIM, legal, and compliance professionals in the future.

To the Lake County Physicians' Association (LCPA), Joe Liberatore, CPA, Karen Kness, MBA, MHA, Maya Zamir, RN, MA, CT, Cate McMahon, Teri Torkelson, Neil Puller, MD, Gerald Frank, MD, and Jai Nho, MD, words cannot express the debt of gratitude the authors have for all you have done to help make this publication a reality. Most importantly, thank you for your support in allowing LCPA to be a place in which these concepts and theories could be tested and put into practice.

To the Sunday morning coffee group at the Starbucks in Bannockburn, IL, thank you for putting up with me these past few years. Yes, "the book is finally done." And, yes, this was accomplished despite Joe Reich's prediction that changes in regulations the healthcare industry would cause the book to change scope and direction once again. I look forward to continuing to share in your friendship and intellectual conversations in the years to come.

To our families, without your love and support this project would not have been worthwhile. You are the reason we hope one day to make a positive difference in the lives of others; thank you for making all the difference in our lives.

Finally, a special debt of gratitude to Jessica S. Puller, MS, Claire Blondeau, MBA, Cynthia Douglas-Chernoff, and Adrienne Cook, JD, and all of the reviewers who worked hard to help produce this final work product. We sincerely appreciate your time and hard work and thank you as well. Without your technical expertise and excellent writing and editing skills, this publication would have not been accomplished.

Foreword

e-Discovery in Health Information Management

As electronic records have become increasingly pervasive within healthcare, so too have the medico-legal challenges. We live in a society where accountability, as manifested with complex, multitiered legal processes, is intertwined with relatively open access to medical information in order to facilitate patient safety and optimal care delivery. As an additional complicating factor, the transition from paper to electronic records coincides with a somewhat slower uptake of the US legal system migrating its rules and processes to address this record management evolution.

As this evolution from paper to electronic health records and the legal concepts surrounding legal record definition, discovery, and litigation response for these records are in a state of flux, it can be exceedingly difficult to find a text such as this that clearly articulates the many facets of both the law and record management that must be considered as strategies, policies, and potential litigation are articulated and put into practice.

The authors have gone to great lengths to codify and clarify a cogent approach to the wide subject matter associated with electronic health records, the nature of their data and metadata, and the judicial rules that guide their use in legal proceedings. This text is an advanced view of the subject of Federal Rules of Civil Procedure that drive the basis for e-discovery (discovery of electronic information that so vastly differs from paper-based documents), but with practical callouts that guide practitioners in formulating workable policies and operational guidelines. Examples of court decisions, standards, and other impacting regulations are also explained in detail.

This text is a natural companion to the book I recently authored for AHIMA, entitled *The Legal Health Record; Regulations, Policies, and Guidelines*, which lays the foundations and relatively simple methodology for defining your own legal health record sets. *e-Discovery: Healthcare Resource Guide to e-Discovery and Electronic Records* carries these ideas further, explaining how the medical record information can and will be used in various legal proceedings and courts, including, for example, how federal and state courts will differ in procedure and how to be ready for litigation.

This text is an invaluable as a reference for all health information managers, compliance officers, legal counsel, and medical informatics experts. Given the cost of not following the rules through increased liabilities and potential fines and sanctions, all professionals involved in electronic health records with an eye toward related legal processes should embrace and operationalize the concepts elucidated within these pages. Take your time understanding and using the information. Approach your use of this information with an organized, systematic program that is inclusive of the various stakeholders from your organization that have governance and impact on the preparations and processes to be established from the valuable information contained within these pages.

Kelly McLendon, RHIA
President, Health Information Xperts
and CompliancePro Solutions

Introduction

The inspiration for this book started on December 31, 1999, as the country was planning for Y2K. One of the authors inscribed the following on her organization's Y2K time capsule: *"In 100 years the medical record will be electronic and its data will be exchanged electronically."* As the healthcare industry prepares for adoption of electronic health records (EHRs) and ultimately the establishment of a Nationwide Health Information Network (NHIN), it will probably take far fewer than 100 years for the author's vision to be realized.

The publication of this book is actually the culmination of a four-year process in which the authors, all with diverse backgrounds and perspectives, collaborated in hopes of achieving two common goals:

1. To improve patient safety and healthcare quality through the establishment of systems and mechanisms that support the timely and appropriate capture of relevant information to support regulatory investigations and litigation
2. To support the spirit and intent of the FRCP 1, "to secure the just, speedy, and inexpensive determination of every action and proceeding"

The February 17, 2009, enactment of the Health Information Technology for Economic and Clinical Health (HITECH) Act actually changed the original scope and outline for this book. Today, there are incentives to adopt EHRs and penalties for failing to adopt them, which are rapidly advancing implementation and adoption. Additionally, electronic discovery and electronic evidence in healthcare have once again become hot topics for discussion and debate in the United States because of the unintended consequences and increased potential for exposure or liability that will result from the adoption of EHRs.

EHRs will dramatically change and redefine the legal process by which providers and legal counsel preserve, discover, and produce relevant information as evidence into a court of law. The purpose of this book is to lay the foundation for the evolving roles and responsibilities of health information professionals of the future as well as to serve as reference for compliance officers, legal counsel, and medical informatics experts.

The authors also hope the publication of this book will help to support and advance new legal systems and processes at the federal, state, and local court levels that support e-discovery and the widespread adoption of EHRs. It is the authors' collective desire to transfer the multidisciplinary knowledge that they have acquired through years of education and training in the law, medicine, clinical informatics, and health information management into this single resource. The book is neither designed nor intended to provide legal or other professional advice but is intended to serve as a reference tool and starting point for research and information.

While the authors acknowledge and respect that HIM professionals participate in a myriad of roles within their organizations, it is the legal, risk, and compliance departments along with the HIM department as well as those who develop and maintain information systems that will most likely benefit from this resource. The authors have divided the book into five chapters that focus on a variety of topics related to electronic discovery and important legal considerations for the HIM professional and others. In addition, a comprehensive glossary, which is included in the printed book, is intended to serve as a reference tool.

Although an understanding of the Health Insurance Portability and Accountability Act (HIPAA) and the legal aspects related to medical records are required competencies in the current Commission on Accreditation for Health Informatics and Information Management (CAHIIM) baccalaureate curriculum, chapters 1–3 focus on the legal process of discovery, relevant case law, the Federal Rules of Civil Procedure as well as the tools used to discover information. chapter 4 prepares organizations for litigation, while chapter 5 focuses on the adherence to sound content and record management principles future HIM professionals must know about in order to be prepared for the management of future e-discovery requests.

In 1999, the Institute of Medicine (IOM) concluded in its landmark report, *To Err is Human*, that thousands of Americans die each year from avoidable errors as a result of the healthcare they receive and hundreds of thousands of others are either harmed or injured. In 2001, in a follow-up report on the healthcare system, *Crossing the Quality Chasm*, the IOM further determined the ineffective use of technology, delayed translation of knowledge into practice, and inability to consistently deliver recommended care to be significant problems that were also impacting care delivery in the United States.

Today, just over a decade beyond the author's Y2K planning exercise, she often thinks about what she now would write in a Y2K time capsule if asked to repeat that same exercise today. Below is a summary:

> In 100 years, paper documents will be obsolete in the courtroom. All US courtrooms will be wired, and mechanisms will be in place to support the secure viewing and exchange of data in its native format. EHRs will become vital tools whose primary use is to help patients engage in their own care, prevent medical errors, and reduce data redundancy while improving provider timeliness and accessibility to the information securely contained within. The secondary uses of EHR data will include aiding in clinical research, promotion of public health, and quality initiatives, as well as to support regulatory investigations and the litigation process.

Technological advances, the widespread adoption of EHRs and the establishment of a NHIN, in which all healthcare information is captured and exchanged electronically, will revolutionize both the courtroom as well as the healthcare industry. It is incumbent upon HIM, IT, legal, risk, and compliance professionals to begin working collaboratively in the establishment of systems and processes to support the preservation and production of relevant information for e-discovery. All providers and healthcare organizations should have a plan in place describing the content of the EHR that is routinely released for disclosure purposes, how legal holds are established within the organization, and who is involved in the process.

One of the most important and evolving roles the HIM professional of the future will play will be in providing support to legal counsel with regard to the preservation, review, and production of EHR data needed for discovery. In order to do this, all HIM professionals must possess a working knowledge of their organization's EHR and information systems as well as the forms, format, and locations of all potentially relevant data within the organization. By doing so, the HIM manager will be an invaluable data steward who could potentially be called one day to testify as a 30(b)(6) witness for the organization.

Overview

Chapter Objectives

This chapter sets the stage for understanding the potential legal exposure for electronic health records, drivers for adoption of **electronic health records (EHRs)**, and electronic discovery (e-discovery) issues related to the health record. This chapter addresses unique aspects of electronic records that have an impact on e-discovery.

The objectives of this chapter are to:

- ➥ Define the potential legal exposure for EHR adoption
- ➥ Understand the key components of the **American Recovery and Reinvestment Act of 2009-Health Information Technology for Economic and Clinical Health Act (ARRA-HITECH)** and how it is driving adoption of EHRs in the United States
- ➥ Provide a foundational understanding of **e-HIM** and EHRs
- ➥ Identify the relationship between EHR implementation and e-discovery
- ➥ Understand the differences between EHRs and paper-based health records
- ➥ Define the legal EHR and related regulations, policies, and standards
- ➥ Identify new and emerging healthcare technologies that have a relationship to potential legal exposure

1.1 Overview

The healthcare industry is no stranger to government audit, investigation, and litigation, both civil and, on occasion, criminal. The electronic health record (EHR) will figure prominently in how healthcare providers respond to requests for information made by investigators and auditors and how healthcare providers respond to, prepare for, and participate in litigation.

This book provides a foundation for health information management (HIM) and information technology (IT) professionals in understanding e-discovery so they can assist legal counsel in the litigation process and prevent or reduce the exposure of healthcare organizations to unnecessary and expensive

1

litigation and associated losses due to HIM and IT issues. This book will inform the reader of how the EHR, broadly defined as it may be, is a part of the course of litigation. It will also explore the **Federal Rules of Civil Procedure (FRCP)** and what those rules, together with the case law interpreting the rules, require of healthcare providers.

Three cautions are in order. First, this book is not a detailed exploration of litigation. Instead, the reader will be presented with several frameworks by which the EHR can be considered for litigation purposes. Second, specific judicial decisions are discussed for illustrative purposes only. This book does not survey *every* decision that may bear on a particular issue. Specialized texts should be consulted for further research. Finally, the reader will learn that, effective December 1, 2006, the FRCP were amended to deal with e-discovery. References to these rules throughout this book will be, however, to the language of the rules as amended December 1, 2007, when they were restyled "to make them more easily understood and to make style and terminology consistent" (Advisory Committee Note Rule 1 and Rule 42). For our purposes, any changes in text from 2006 to 2007 are stylistic only. Moreover, throughout this book there are references to advisory committee notes. These notes constitute part of the history of the FRCP and guide the interpretation of those rules.

1.1.1 Managing Potential Legal Exposure Due to EHR

There are many significant reasons to research, evaluate, and describe potential legal exposure due to EHRs. Throughout this work, the authors hope to support the advancement and adoption of EHRs by demonstrating that they serve not only to improve safety and patient care but an EHR containing the necessary evidentiary support capabilities can also assist and defend both the provider and organization in any type of litigation or regulatory investigation. Additionally, the authors will discuss how organizations can manage risk by allocating resources in preparation for discovery.

We are at a time when reports of questionable **return on investment (ROI)** from EHRs are being discussed (Ash et al. 2007; Weiner et al. 2007; Hoffman and Podgurski 2008), and documented cases of increased legal exposure exist (Koppel and Kreda 2009; Korin and Quattrone 2007). Issues and factors such as these can ultimately reduce the adoption rate of clinical information technology and the EHR.

Due to recent changes in the law and ongoing advancements in technology, a unique opportunity exists to support improved practices in HIM. These improved practices can assure improved data and document integrity in production of **electronically stored information (ESI)** from healthcare IT applications. At present, the work procedures and processes of interdisciplinary healthcare teams responsible for litigation involving EHR systems have not been thoroughly discussed, nor has the functionality of EHR systems in supporting e-discovery been thoroughly addressed. Defining and incorporating these best practices into the operations of our healthcare system through new policies, procedures, and enhancements in IT may improve acceptance of EHR applications by various stakeholders. Finding solutions to these issues does not lend itself to precise analytical techniques, due to the complexity of healthcare and the law. Rather, it involves many subjective judgments.

Healthcare professional perspectives are beginning to focus on changes in the legal environment related to ESI. Healthcare lawyers with expertise in IT have had initial discussions on the significance of changes in e-discovery law at the organizational level (DeLoss and Shay 2007); however, the resulting reports have not thoroughly addressed how these and other changes to the law affect functionality requirements for nationwide interoperable EHR systems. Leaders in HIM, such as the **American Health Information Management Association (AHIMA)**, have taken notice of changes in discovery (AHIMA e-Discovery e-HIM Work Group 2006; Baldwin-Stried 2006; AHIMA e-Discovery Task Force 2008), and the best practice recommendations of **The Sedona Conference**, but still seek the strategic guidance for organizational solutions in navigating the complexities of the exceedingly regulated healthcare industry. Recognized standards development organizations (SDOs) are attempting to overcome obstacles by defining functional requirements for the legal EHR, but these SDOs do not have the capacity or the mandate to address the wide variety of legal and practical challenges caused by a fragmented vendor base and different state and federal legal systems (Dougherty 2008).

The legal community has been undergoing changes in the rules, practices, and standards related to ESI and its use in litigation. The changes will continue to impact healthcare in the same way other businesses are affected by the introduction of ESI to support their business operations. Healthcare organizations use a variety of computer-based applications and systems that may be relevant during litigation and e-discovery. The creation, maintenance, and use of healthcare records pose unique legal challenges in an EHR setting. One of the secondary uses for EHR data is for medico-legal purposes. These challenges originate in part due the fact that EHR data provide evidence of care provided, compliance with legislation, and competence of clinicians (HL7 RM-ES 2010). This book provides a foundation for addressing these medico-legal issues and the complexities of the EHR when intersecting with e-discovery and litigation.

The newest developments in authentication of electronic evidence and ESI are fundamentally shifting not only healthcare recordkeeping but also the healthcare industry itself. Given the disjointed environment of information management in the healthcare industry, a comprehensive review of the legal ramifications of this shift is needed. This book provides a foundation for further dialogue on these issues and their effects on the healthcare environment.

1.1.2 EHR Adoption in the United States

In 2004, leading experts in **health information technology (HIT)** systems reported that almost half of all US hospitals had implemented or were in the process of implementing an electronic medical record system (EMR) (Ball, Weaver, and Kiel 2004). The prevalence of adoption of EHRs in US hospitals is still quite low, however, despite earlier reports and an industry consensus that the use of HIT should lead to more efficient, safer, and higher-quality care. Only 1.5 percent of US hospitals have a comprehensive, fully integrated, enterprise-wide EHR system, and an additional 7.6 percent have a basic system in one or more clinical units. **Computerized provider order entry (CPOE)** for medications has had wider industry acceptance with implementation and use in 17 percent of hospitals (Jha et al. 2009).

1.1.2.1 ARRA and the Health Information Technology for Economic and Clinical Health Act

On January 8, 2009, in a speech at George Mason University, then-President-elect Barack Obama said this about HIT and the future of EHR (Change.gov 2009):

> To improve the quality of our health care while lowering its cost, we will make the immediate investments necessary to ensure that within five years, all of America's medical records are computerized. This will cut waste, eliminate red tape, and reduce the need to repeat expensive medical tests. But it just won't save billions of dollars and thousands of jobs—it will save lives by reducing the deadly but preventable medical errors that pervade our health care system.

Several weeks later, on February 17, 2009, President Obama signed the ARRA into law. An important component of ARRA is a piece of legislation called the HITECH Act. The HITECH Act was created to help save lives, lower costs, and improve the processes by which information is managed and communicated within the healthcare arena. The HITECH Act is comprised of four major goals (ARRA 2009):

1. For the federal government to take a leading role in developing standards to provide for the nationwide electronic exchange and use of health information to improve the quality and coordination of care
2. To appropriate $20 billion in investment by the federal government in a national health information infrastructure and provide Medicare and Medicaid incentives to encourage doctors and hospitals to use HIT to electronically share patients' health information
3. To save a projected $10 billion in governmental expenditures with additional savings realized throughout the healthcare industry through improvements in healthcare quality care coordination and reductions in duplicative services and medical errors
4. To strengthen federal privacy and security laws to protect identifiable health information from misuse as the healthcare sector increases use of health IT

Because many provisions of the HITECH Act will be established and rolled out over a five-year period, the exact form and format of the EHR is yet to be fully determined. It is incumbent upon legal, HIM, and IT professionals to be vigilant in their ongoing review and assessment of the HITECH Act and understanding its requirements and consequences (ONC 2009).

1.1.2.2 EHR Incentives and Meaningful Use

One of the primary goals of HITECH is to encourage the adoption of the EHR by providing for federal funding (grants and incentive payments). Section 1848 of the HITECH Act (HR 111-016) provides the foundation for the Medicare and Medicaid incentive payments for eligible professionals and providers. The Centers for Medicare and Medicaid Services (CMS) are charged with developing and administering the Medicare and Medicaid incentive program and requirements for "meaningful use." The requirements will ratchet up over time in stages until 2015 (HIT Policy Committee 2009). In order for a professional or provider to be eligible for the meaningful-use incentives, there must be successful demonstration to the Secretary of the Department of Health and Human Services of the following elements:

- Use of certified technology in a meaningful manner as determined to be appropriate by the Secretary
- Connection of the EHR in a manner that provides for the electronic exchange of information to improve the quality of care, such as the promotion of care coordination

- Establishment of mechanisms for reporting on clinical quality and other measures as determined by the Secretary

The exact details of each of these elements will depend on rules promulgated by the CMS through 2015. In general, the following types of requirements will be addressed in the EHR incentive payment and meaningful-use rules:

- The type of electronic exchange that will be required
- What clinical information will be required for use and reporting
- The extent of electronic prescribing to be required
- Guidance as to how providers may meet the requirement
- How much information is truly necessary for use and what type of EHR information is "meaningful"
- Stage 1 (2011–2012) objectives generally focus on requirements related to capturing data in coded format and beginning steps for exchanging data
- Stage 2 (2013–2014) objectives raise the bar by expanding the exchange of health information in the most structured format available
- Stage 3 (2015–2016) objectives achieve a goal of reporting quality for high-priority conditions, providing for patient self-management, and access to comprehensive data

1.1.2.3 EHR Standards and Certification

An explosion of primary and secondary use of data from health information systems is anticipated to occur, especially given the HITECH goal that US hospitals and professionals implement a certified EHR system by the year 2015. This explosion will change and redefine the landscape and standards for care delivery and the management of information within the United States (ONC 2009).

Healthcare industry leaders have articulated their vision of health and healthcare in the United States, as depicted in figure 1.1.

This vision includes the ability to measure and report healthcare quality measures electronically, with mechanisms for feedback to the provider and patient to effect real-time improvements in quality and safety. It also includes mechanisms to link and securely exchange the patient's **personal health record (PHR)** with a provider's EHR and facilitate timely access to clinical information for improved health maintenance and care coordination.

Figure 1.1   Vision of health and healthcare transformed

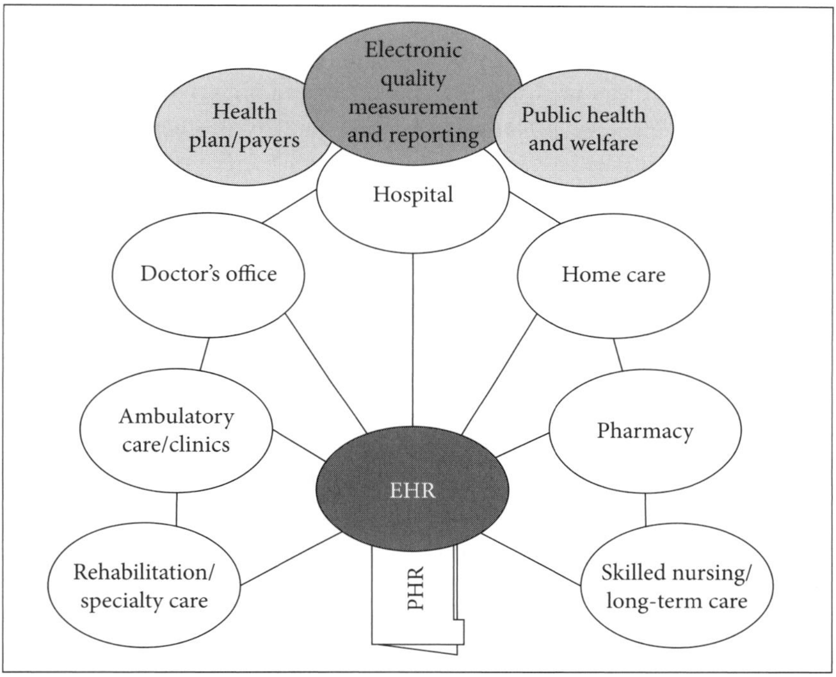

Source: © 2012 Kim Baldwin-Stried Reich.

To meet this vision and support EHR incentives for meaningful use, the **Office of the National Coordinator (ONC)** for Health Information Technology has and will continue to develop regulations identifying specific EHR and HIT standards. The requirements align with the meaningful-use objectives and stages to facilitate coordination and ensure that EHRs meet the goals and measures in the meaningful-use requirements.

The health IT standards promulgated by ONC to support meaningful-use objectives can be categorized into the following areas:

- Content exchange—standards used to exchange clinical information
- Vocabulary—standardized nomenclature and code sets
- Transport standards for HIE—communication protocols to allow exchange between systems
- Privacy and security—identification and implementation of standards to ensure privacy and security of electronic health information

To ensure that appropriate standards are incorporated into health IT and EHRs, the use of certified technologies is a component of the incentive program. ONC has developed rules for certification bodies and the certification process. The certification bodies and process play an important role by ensuring that products and applications incorporate standards in an acceptable way.

1.1.2.4 HITECH Expansion of HIPAA

Subtitle A of the HITECH Act established the ONC to promote adoption of HIT and ensure the security and protection of patients' health information while improving the quality of care and reducing healthcare costs. As a result, the HITECH Act expanded the original federal privacy and security rule—the **Health Insurance Portability and Accountability Act (HIPAA)**—to address the more contemporary issues in promoting adoption, secondary use of data, and exchange of electronic health information.

Subtitle D of the HITECH Act includes far-reaching provisions concerning the privacy and security of health information that will directly affect more entities, businesses, and individuals than ever before. Civil penalties for willful neglect will be increased under the HITECH Act. These penalties can extend up to $250,000, with repeat or uncorrected violations extending up to $1.5 million. Furthermore, the civil and criminal penalties that could be imposed upon providers under HIPAA have now been extended to business associates.

A summary of the HITECH Act privacy and security changes includes (AHIMA 2010a):

- Accounting of disclosures with EHR use—Covered entities using and disclosing PHI through an EHR are required to provide individuals with accounting, when requested, for the prior three years. Uses and disclosures of **protected health information (PHI)** through EHRs include treatment, payment, and healthcare operations.
- Access rights to electronic format—The HIPAA Privacy Rule is amended to give individuals the right to obtain access to their PHI in electronic format, if requested.
- Security breach notification—This imposes breach notifications for unauthorized users and disclosures of unsecured PHI. Covered entities, business associates, and others are affirmatively required to notify individuals and others of breaches of unsecured PHI.
- Healthcare operations—The definition of healthcare operations will be reviewed by the Secretary of HHS.

- Sale and marketing of PHI—Covered entities and business associates are prohibited from directly or indirectly receiving any remuneration in exchange for any PHI of an individual unless a valid authorization is obtained from the individual, except in a very limited number of circumstances. Greater restrictions have been placed on the use health information for marketing purposes.

1.2 e-HIM Initiative

At AHIMA's 74th Annual Meeting in September 2002, Chief Executive Officer, Linda Kloss, announced the e-HIM initiative. AHIMA's e-HIM initiative was established to support HIM professionals and the healthcare industry (AHIMA 2003). The e-HIM initiative was comprised of three major goals:

1. Accelerate the migration from paper to an electronic health information infrastructure
2. Reinvent how HIM professionals manage records and information, from creation through use
3. Deliver measurable cost and quality results from improved information management

The e-HIM initiative has proven to be a pioneering effort, especially when measured against a governmental goal for the adoption of a certified EHR by 2015. Since its inception, the HIM initiative has not only advanced the HIM profession, but it also provided a basis for a variety of HIT projects and collaborative efforts related to the management of health information. Through the e-HIM initiative, AHIMA has collaborated with governmental agencies and other professional organizations on the adoption and advancement of HIT technology. Now, an assessment of the e-HIM goals affirms the significant role and impact the e-HIM initiative has had in helping to shape and redefine the role and use of health information and technology in healthcare.

It is incumbent upon providers of care, HIM professionals, IT specialists, and legal professionals to work collaboratively with state and local policy makers to establish e-HIM initiatives to support the adoption of the EHR systems while maintaining strong privacy and security laws.

Irrespective of what form or forms the EHR eventually takes, certainly the process for discovery of electronic information, the management of e-HIM, and the discovery approach will require collaboration among a team of legal, HIM, and health IT professionals, as depicted in figure 1.2.

Figure 1.2 The management of e-HIM and e-discovery requires collaboration

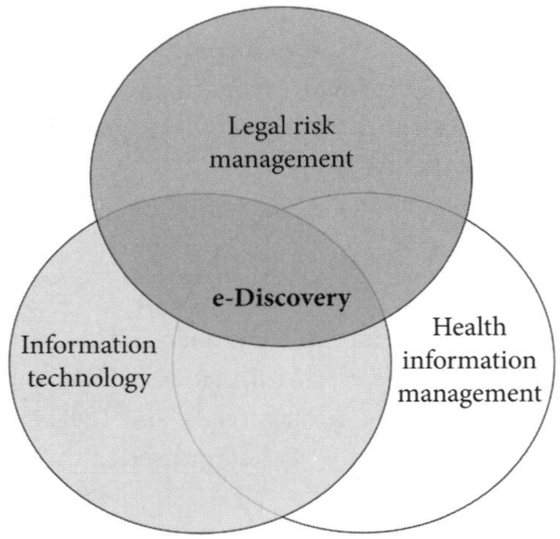

An effective and defensible approach to discovery involves integration and collaboration in the approach to the management of e-HIM.

Source: © 2012 Kim Baldwin-Stried Reich.

1.2.1 EHR Implementation and e-Discovery

The digital age brings about unlimited possibilities for EHR applications regarding the handling, dissemination, and exchange of patient health information. Whether individual patient information is stored in computers and shared with others on closed networks or through the Internet, there are virtually countless ways in which the storage and management of patient health information using computers and networks can impact a patient's care.

Digital recordkeeping through EHR systems is rapidly replacing paper-based recordkeeping systems as the most common form of media in which patient health information is stored and maintained. As a result of these advances in technology, enactment of the FRCP in 2006 and recognition by the courts of the importance of electronically stored information in civil litigation, the legal process of discovery is evolving and changing as rapidly as today's electronic record systems are themselves.

The discovery of electronically stored patient health information along with implementation of EHRs presents a new set of opportunities and challenges to legal counsel and the court system. Traditionally, the paper-based process of discovery was relatively static and straightforward. In the paper realm, a typical medical malpractice lawsuit might evolve as follows:

1. Occurrence of sentinel/untoward event—Patient death occurs in the operating room due to anesthesia complication.
2. Quality review and investigation—An internal peer/quality review is conducted. Risk management and/or legal counsel diary file and establish reserves.
3. Legal notice—In advance of a legal complaint, a subpoena or a subpoena *duces tecum* is sent to the director of the HIM department as the official custodian or keeper of the medical record. The Health Information Management Department notifies the risk management department. The subpoena is evaluated to verify that it is valid. Valid subpoenas are processed by the HIM department in accordance with the department's requirements. The paper medical records are copied, numbered sequentially, and produced to the requesting party and the HIM department director or a designee prepares an affidavit to attest that the medical records are true and correct copies of the original record.
4. Records secured—Legal counsel will generally make the determination as to which original paper records must be secured. This decision may or may not happen in advance of a legal notice. Immediately upon receipt of a legal notice in which the organization is a party to litigation, the original paper medical records must be sequestered and filed into a separate locked file or vault until the outcome of litigation. Generally, the HIM department manually monitors and controls access to the original paper record throughout the time it is sequestered.
5. Discovery process—Legal counsel from both parties will review and investigate the facts and circumstances of the case in detail. The standard as to what forms of information and records can be discovered is broad; quite simply, any information in any form that is relevant to the case is discoverable. Adoption of the 2006 FRCP made it clear that ESI is treated is equivalent to paper. Various devices used in the FRCP include:
   - **Complaint**—A written document generally filed with the clerk of a court to allege facts and claims relevant to a lawsuit. The complaint is served on the defendant.
   - **Subpoena**—A document requiring an appearance at a certain time and place, most commonly used to compel an appearance of an individual for trial or deposition.

- **Subpoena *duces tecum*** —A specific form of subpoena that commands a person to appear and produce certain documents or other materials. In lieu of an appearance, counsel may choose to accept an affidavit attesting that attached copies are true and correct copies of originals. This affidavit may be signed by the HIM director as official custodian of the record.
- **Interrogatories** —A set of written questions that the opposing party in litigation must answer under penalty of perjury.
- Document production requests—A request for the opposing party in litigation to produce documents or other information.
- Deposition—Out-of-court testimony made under oath and recorded for later use in court.
- Records inspection requests—Uncommonly granted in private litigation, most public and governmental organizations have well-defined policies, procedures, and forms by which records may be inspected and copied.
- Requests for admissions—A process by which one party asks the other to admit or deny key facts in litigation.

6. Disposition of the case—At any time, a case may be dismissed by the plaintiff, dismissed by the court, or settled. Alternatively, following the discovery phase, the case may proceed to trial. In healthcare litigation, as in all other litigation, most cases are disposed of before trial.

Prior to the digital era, all business documents were stored and maintained in a single format—paper. It did not matter if the document was a business contract, financial record, or the patient's medical record; it was created, stored, and maintained in a single, static media source: paper.

Whether the organization was involved in an audit, a governmental investigation, and/or litigation, legal counsel would simply request and read through paper documents. The paper-based discovery process was a labor-intensive, time-consuming, tedious process, but it also was a straightforward one.

The process of e-discovery is vastly different from paper discovery. With ARRA in its early stages, and without a uniform standard for EHR systems and the exchange of health information, the approaches and methods to discover relevant information now and into the foreseeable future are anything but straightforward. Not only do the techniques and methods used to discover relevant information rely on the aid of computers, but as landmark e-discovery cases such as *Zubulake v. UBS Warburg LLC*, 220 F.R.D. 212 (S.D.N.Y. 2003) have shown, legal counsel will now have a professional responsibility for understanding how information is managed within the organization.

In today's healthcare industry, paper documents, including printouts from EHR applications, by far continue to serve as the most common media for document production in discovery. Despite enactment of the FRCP and other state and local laws governing e-discovery, overall, the industry is slow to deploy new approaches to the discovery of ESI.

The reasons for slow implementation of new approaches to the discovery of ESI within healthcare are various, but include cost, functional design limitations of EHR systems, lack of a uniform approach to electronically exchanged health information, lack of uniform state and local discovery laws, and resistance to change among legal, HIM, and HIT professionals. Perhaps one of the biggest obstacles to e-discovery in healthcare are beliefs by physicians and other healthcare providers that e-discovery will reveal too much information about the case and make it harder for the healthcare providers to defend themselves. In reality, the opposite may be true, as case law and practical work experience have demonstrated. Providers and organizations that plan for discovery and establish appropriate policies, procedures, and mechanisms to preserve and maintain potentially relevant information, all will end up ahead of the discovery curve, rather than toppled by it. A well-constructed plan that describes how information is managed within the organization, along with the structure to support it, will result in a more efficient, less costly discovery process and, most importantly, one in which legal counsel can more easily evaluate the case to defend it.

The EHR plays a crucial role as the basis for planning and communication of patient care, and now, as the healthcare industry transforms, it will soon become the tool used to measure and assess healthcare quality and safety. In this way, the EHR can also become the provider's and the organization's best defense in litigation.

To effectively function in the digital age, all healthcare professionals must be able to adapt to changing business requirements and develop new skill sets associated with managing patient care and the information associated with it. There are many differences between care delivery that is documented and conducted in the digital age versus care delivery documented and conducted in the paper realm. Table 1.1 provides a synopsis of some these unique differences.

Table 1.1   Synopsis of differences between paper and e-HIM

Difference	Description
1. Volume and Reproducibility Issues	• e-HIM exists in substantially greater volumes • Automated replication of electronic information • Paper does not need device such as computer to be read • e-HIM HIPAA standards for transmission of PHI
2. Dynamic Content and Nature of Electronic Data	• e-HIM easier to change than paper • Content of electronic information can change without human intervention • Transmission and transfer of e-HIM not fixed in final form
3. Metadata	• e-HIM contains metadata—paper does not • System, application, and/or user metadata not readily apparent • Metadata adds new set of retention and preservation obligations
4. Lifespan/Persistence of Electronic Data	• e-HIM much harder to dispose of—paper can be shredded • Electronic data not easily deleted
5. e-HIM Environment	• e-HIM may be incomprehensible when separated from its environment • Legacy systems and migration of e-HIM—differs significantly from imaging
6. Search and Retrieval of Electronic Data	• e-HIM may reside in numerous locations • Paper documents consolidated and maintained in single file folder • e-HIM environment may obscure origin, completeness, or accuracy of information
e-HIM is evidence which must be authenticated and reviewed prior to submission into a court of law. HIM and IT professionals must begin working with legal counsel early on in litigation.	

Source: © 2012 Kim Baldwin-Stried Reich.

A comprehensive understanding of the effects of the new discovery laws on the forms of data production, form of report and document outputs, **metadata**, and handling of legacy data in EHR systems demands further dialogue and research involving domain experts across several disciplines.

The knowledge and organizational expertise necessary to contribute to an efficient discovery process varies. The health information professional must be well informed about the forms, formats, and locations of all business and medical records maintained by the organization. IT professionals must be expert in the operation, architecture, and technical engineering of the organization's information systems, for they will be increasingly called upon to testify to about operations, integrity, and effectiveness of the organization's information systems while HIM professionals will be expected to knowledgeably describe organizational policies and practices with regard to the management of information within the organization, and assimilate and produce relevant information requested. Organizations ill-equipped to effectively manage and maintain their records could be subject to sanctions and penalties.

The healthcare records discovery processes are undergoing drastic changes as a result of the 2006 amendments to the FRCP. These changes, coupled with an ever-increasing scrutiny of compliance with federal and state rules, have mandated the healthcare industry seek organizational solutions.

1.2.2 Evidence and Discovery of Health Records

Health records, like other business records, are admitted into evidence as an exception to the hearsay rule. The same exception applies to computer-based records. To satisfy hearsay objections, the **Federal Rules of Evidence (FRE)** require that business, medical, and computer-based records

> (1) were made in the regular course of business at or about the time of the act, condition, or event recorded
> (2) the circumstances of their creation demonstrate that the records are trustworthy and
> (3) the sources of information and circumstances of their preparation were such as to indicate their trustworthiness. (AHIMA e-HIM Work Group on the Legal Health Record 2005)

Healthcare organizations face a variety of litigation—employment, contract, malpractice, and others. In a medical malpractice case, the lawsuit is often brought by a patient or family member, and the health record is a prominent source of information because it allows the plaintiff attorney to investigate what happened during the treatment, and the record provides information about what the physician and treating clinicians knew and when they knew it.

Most of today's healthcare organizations maintain a dual system for health records: a hybrid record that includes conventional paper charts and computer-based records in the EHRs. Both paper and electronic forms of health records are discoverable. Therefore, discovery requests must include both paper and electronic records. Attorneys are advised to obtain the records in both forms without assuming that the forms are identical because hard copy and electronic forms of the same document are not necessarily equivalent. This is particularly relevant with computer printouts from EHR systems—printouts are not an exact replica of how the clinician saw or entered data into the EHR and the full printout does not contain all of the potentially relevant information within the EHR. A Washington, DC Circuit Court ruling recognized this issue and stated that printouts were not exact copies of a computer record unless the "paper versions included all significant material contained in the electronic records" (Marchand 2001). The court analogized that the two documents were more like kissing cousins as opposed to identical twins. As a result, healthcare organizations and attorneys need to plan for discovery requests for the relevant paper-based records (whether they are handwritten or printouts from the EHR system), as well as access and review of the ESI.

1.3 Electronically Stored Information (ESI) in Healthcare

ESI consists of files or other data that are stored on computers, file servers, disks, tape, or other devices or media. In healthcare, a wealth of ESI can accumulate about a patient. It must be noted that other types of electronic files can provide a rich source of information in healthcare:

- Electronic calendars (evidence regarding meetings and patient appointments)
- Personal digital assistants (PDAs) and handheld devices
- Home computers
- Laptops
- Databases such as word-processing and accounting programs
- E-mail and instant messaging systems
- Voice-mail systems
- Backup tapes and files
- Audit trails or audit logs (chronological sequence of audit records with evidence of business processes or system functions)

To understand the unique challenges of ESI, it is helpful to clarify and understand the key differences between paper and electronic evidence (Logan et al. 2005):

- Destructibility—Electronic evidence is harder to destroy than paper evidence because it is easier to disseminate and has metadata stored with it.
- Accessibility—There are three categories of accessible data: active online, near-online, and offline archives. Inaccessible data include data on backup tapes that have been erased, fragmented, or damaged (also known as residual data).

- **Metadata**—One significant difference between paper and electronic records is that all electronic files have metadata associated with them. Metadata includes systems of origin, audit trails, author and date information, version information, format information, and other types of stored information.
- Content—People express ideas in e-mail and instant messages that they would never dream of committing to paper. More than half of the evidence presented in US trials is in the form of e-mail.
- Volume—Microsoft Word, PowerPoint, and Outlook have made prolific authors of everyone. Storage is inexpensive, it is easier to save than paper, and it takes up less floor space.
- Versions—Multiple versions of documents exist, and the changes to them are often revealing. This is different from paper where many multiple copies may exist, but not many versions.

To successfully manage litigation involving ESI, healthcare organizations must understand the inherent differences between paper-based and electronic information, and establish a records management program and governance for both.

1.3.1 How Are Electronic Health Records Different from Paper?

As mentioned earlier in this chapter, medical records have traditionally been maintained on paper—a single, static source of information. Portions of many EHR systems are inherently different because they are not document-based word processing systems. Most EHR systems are transactional processing systems, built on database platforms with underlying tables and field attributes. The database structure provides many advantages in capturing clinical events or actions, such as maintaining consistency in data by updating the table once and using the data in multiple locations.

One of the challenges of a transactional database system for health records is its use as a recordkeeping system. The transaction records retained in an EHR provide a historical picture of clinical events and actions, but often lack the requirements for maintaining business records, such as capturing and retaining all of the required metadata to create complete, reliable, and authentic records. Because health records have many secondary uses beyond patient care (such as payment, regulatory compliance, quality reporting, and litigation), organizations must have the ability to create and maintain legally valid health records over long periods of time to meet multiple business needs.

For the EHRs to be authentic digital business records, they must contain attributes for the following (Paul 2008):

- ▪ Integrity—The record has not been changed in an unknowable way. Amendments, corrections, or changes are made in a transparent way or identified through the metadata.
- ▪ Identity—Who created, attested, edited, and transmitted the record is known.
- ▪ Time—The date and time of when the record was created, received, edited, transmitted are known.
- ▪ Other attributes—Other attributes are noted such as printing or viewing.

The healthcare community is impacted by the shift to e-discovery for litigation as a result of the 2006 FRCP. In the past, litigation and malpractice cases utilizing health records primarily relied on paper records or printouts. With e-discovery, ESI and EHRs are increasingly requested. Questions about the authenticity and integrity of the EHR is beginning to be raised by the courts. As a result, health IT standards, early adopters of EHRs, and savvy EHR vendors are beginning to recognize and understand the need for addressing the issues of digital record authenticity and recordkeeping.

1.3.2 Structured vs. Unstructured Data in Healthcare

Today's EHR systems are designed with both structured and unstructured data as described in the system data model. A **data model** is an abstract model that describes how data are represented and accessed. Data models define data elements and relationships among data elements for an area of interest. A data model that explicitly establishes the meaning of data (values that a computer can process) is known as **structured data** (LaTour and Eichenwald-Maki 2010). A structured data file is described as a container or template and defines how the data within the files are arranged so that a computer can use them efficiently. Structured data allow various technologies to query and report against predetermined data types by computer-understood relationships. Note that this does not necessarily imply that the computer user can use a structured data file more efficiently.

Examples of structured files are database files characteristic of modern clinical software systems:

1) computer template–driven clinical documentation forms are an example of structured data, or
2) clinical flow sheets that allow specific data elements to be entered by the user in a clinical context to the field of entry; for example, an Ins and Outs (I and O's) interactive flow sheet.

These template tools frequently use structured text entry and outputs of standard clinical terminology or conventional medical phrases.

Additional structured health data examples include: "data elements in a patient's automated laboratory order, result, or demographic and financial information system are coded and alphanumeric. Their fields are predefined and limited. In other words, the type of data is discrete, and the format of these data is structured. Consequently, when a healthcare professional searches a database for one or more coded, discrete data elements based on the search parameters, the engine can easily find, retrieve, and manipulate the element" (AHIMA e-HIM Work Group on the Legal Health Record 2005).

An **unstructured data** file lacks this container or template, and thus is an efficient organization of data for the computer user (Schuler et al. 2009; The Sedona Conference 2007). Examples of unstructured data files used for clinical documentation include word processing documents, such as dictations, or other free-text entry clinical documentation, and copy-and-paste entries, flow sheets, ordering tools derived from spreadsheets, and even imported e-mails. Unstructured data are different from information or data stored in fielded form in databases or annotated (semantically tagged) in documents (Schuler et al. 2009). These files are not apparently unorganized to the clinician, but are difficult for the computer to read.

The CMS rulemakers for meaningful use anticipate redefining their objectives in advancing stages 1–3 (defined earlier in this chapter) to include not only the capturing of data in electronic format but also the exchange (both transmission and receipt) of that data in increasingly structured formats (42 CFR 412, 413, 422).

> *Stage 2:* Our goals for the Stage 2 meaningful-use criteria, consistent with other provisions of Medicare and Medicaid law, expand upon the Stage 1 criteria to encourage the use of health IT for continuous quality improvement at the point of care and the exchange of information in the most structured format possible, such as the electronic transmission of orders entered using computerized provider order entry (CPOE) and the electronic transmission of diagnostic test results (such as blood tests, microbiology, urinalysis, pathology tests, radiology, cardiac imaging, nuclear medicine tests, pulmonary function tests, genetic tests, genomic tests and other such data needed to diagnose and treat disease). For the final rule, we elaborate on our plans for Stage 2.

Data mining is routinely utilized for establishing new knowledge for clinical operations. Examples of data mining include query use for quality metric

Figure 1.3   Examples of structured and unstructured data in EHRs

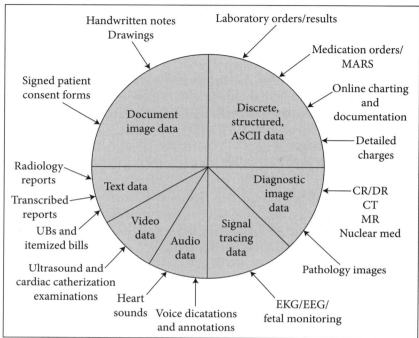

reporting. Data mining is more difficult when using unstructured data than structured data sources. It is easy to surmise that analyzing unstructured data for e-discovery purposes is also more difficult than analysis from unstructured clinical sources. E-discovery experts have described how e-discovery researchers (Baron and Thompson 2007) associated with the **Text Retrieval Conference (TREC) Legal Track** (Baron et al. 2009) are using information retrieval and artificial intelligence research to tackle some of the many challenges of efficiently conducting searches for relevant documents in large, heterogeneous electronic data sets, for the purpose of litigation response.

Many of the data entered in today's EHR systems are unstructured, and thus have necessitated clinical system designers to allow integration of the unstructured data sets within data warehousing supporting such HIT applications. HIM and informatics professionals must have an awareness of the characteristics of both the structured and unstructured data components that comprise the clinical documentation systems they manage.

ESI in unstructured data may actually be semi-structured. Even in a Microsoft Word-generated document, for example, there is an underlying structure found in the **bits** and **bytes**. The necessity of understanding these underlying metadata is described in chapter 3.

For healthcare discovery purposes, much information for litigation purposes is buried in unstructured data. Discovery of this information requires health information professionals to work collaboratively to understand their HIT systems' functionalities to effectively interpret unstructured data and to articulate that unstructured data are linked with the structured information maintained in the clinical software.

For e-discovery and litigation purposes, health information leaders must bridge the chasm between structured and unstructured knowledge contained not only within the clinical systems they manage, but within all the organization's information systems—clinical, administrative, or otherwise. To achieve these complex actions in healthcare, information management requires a strategic and global approach toward the governance of information at the organizational level. The concept of information governance and enterprise content records management concepts and principles are discussed in detail in chapter 5.

1.4 What Is the Legal EHR?

The term **legal EHR** has held different meanings depending on one's professional perspective. The legal EHR is an umbrella term made up of multiple concepts that have a relationship or direct impact on e-discovery and the EHR (Dougherty 2010):

- **Governance**—Because of the distributed nature of health IT systems that contain or comprise the record of care, healthcare organizations must establish a governance process that includes record management policies, retention schedules, destruction procedures, privacy and security practices, and custodianship/stewardship roles and functions.
- Defining the record of care—Technically part of governance, but critically important with EHRs, defining the record of care involves declaring in organizational policy the data and information in the EHR system that constitutes the record of care for an episode of care to ensure compliance and meet business needs for the medical records (in HIM this is also called defining the legal record). Declaring the record is an important step with EHRs, which have been developed on database platforms, and which are not document based. Records must be defined in the system and then locked to ensure an accurate historical picture for an encounter or episode of care.

- Record management functionality to support integrity and authenticity—The EHR system must have appropriate record management and evidentiary support functionality to ensure the integrity of the record through its lifecycle.
- Documentation quality—The EHR system contains documentation that reflects the healthcare actions, services, and condition—it "tells the story" accurately and completely.
- Disclosure management—The record of care must be in a form and format that can be disclosed for a multitude of requirements and business purposes. There are complex rules and requirements governing disclosure that must be administered by HIM. Also critically important is the need to get adequate reports or outputs from EHR systems that are useable, concise, and accurate to meet the disclosure requirements.
- **Compliance**—There are regulations governing medical records regardless of the form and format (paper or electronic) as well as laws, payer policies, standards, and generally accepted practices. Healthcare organizations must be aware of the compliance requirements related to medical records (both the content and management) to ensure that EHR systems where appropriate, are supported through governance and system functionality.

1.4.1 The Legal Record in Healthcare

Healthcare organizations gather information on patients for a variety of purposes—clinical, financial, and administrative. As a result, there is a need to define the official business record or the legal record to ensure compliance with regulations and professional standards, and to identify the subset of the health information that comprises the official health record.

Defining the legal health record in a digital environment poses challenges ideally suited for multidisciplinary teams. The typical healthcare organization encompasses a multitude of separate systems to manage including reports, images, documents, web delivery systems, e-mail archival data, and custom applications and IT tools to support the content of the comprehensive legal EHR.

AHIMA, through expertise of e-HIM workgroups, has shaped the concept of the legal health record and legal EHR. Three foundational principles embody the legal EHR:

- Maintaining a legally sound and compliant health record (paper or electronic)—This concept incorporates governance, business rules, and system functionality to support a record that has integrity and can support both the clinical and business needs of the organization.

■ Defining the legal record—A healthcare organization collects a variety of information on individuals (clinical, financial, and administrative). Organizations must identify and declare, in policy, the content of the formal health record that will be the official representation of a stay, encounter, or episode of care, and disclosed upon request.

■ Using the health record and health information for secondary uses: litigation, payment, quality reporting, and public-health reporting—The health record and information are used in support of many business processes beyond patient care. EHR systems, organizational governance, and processes must align with the requirements for use and disclosure of the records and information.

These foundational principles are further explored in the practice briefs found in the appendices of this book.

1.4.2 Regulations and Accreditation Standards for Health Records

By regulation and standards of practice, healthcare organizations are required to maintain medical records. Compliance with applicable regulations and standards may become relevant when litigation involves health records. State and federal regulations, as well as healthcare accreditation organizations, define requirements for maintaining medical records and also establish expectations for electronic records. The CMS Conditions of Participation for Hospitals Section 482.24 defines the standards and requirements for medical records regardless of whether they are paper or electronic:

■ A medical record must be maintained for each patient.
■ A medical record must be properly filed and retained to ensure prompt retrieval.
■ A medical record must be accessible.
■ The medial record system must ensure that medical record entries are not lost, stolen, destroyed, altered, or reproduced in an unauthorized manner.
■ Locations where medical records are stored or maintained must ensure the integrity, security, and protection of the records.
■ All entries in the medical record must be timed, dated, and authenticated, and a method established to identify the author.

The federal and state regulations and accreditation standards for health records may be a factor in litigation. At a foundational level, medical record systems, either paper-based or electronic, should comply with applicable regulations, laws, and standards.

In addition to requirements for maintaining a medical record, there are requirements for the content of the medical record. The requirements may be defined in federal and/or state regulations for a care setting as well as accreditation standards. The regulations, laws, and standards are important for establishing the baseline content for the legal health record.

The CMS Conditions of Participation for Hospitals require the following content in the medical record:

- Written documentation, computerized information, radiology film/ scans, and lab reports
- Documentation and assessments to justify continued stay
  - To support the diagnosis
  - To describe the patient's progress
  - To describe the patient's response to medications, interventions, and services
- Documents planning for a patient's care and the decisions made on the provision of care

Healthcare organizations may voluntarily choose to participate in accreditation processes. The most common accreditation organization for healthcare providers is the Joint Commission. CMS may grant accrediting organizations like the Joint Commission deeming authority if their standards meet or exceed the Medicare and Medicaid certification requirements. Deemed status options are available for:

- Ambulatory surgical centers
- Clinical laboratories
- Critical access hospitals
- Durable medical equipment, prosthetics, orthotics, and supplies
- Home health
- Hospices
- Hospitals

Providers of these healthcare services would have the option of seeking deemed status through the accreditation body and undergo an accreditation survey rather than one conducted by a state agency on behalf of CMS (the Joint Commission 2011).

The Joint Commission accreditation standards include requirements for health records and these standards are applied to paper-based, electronic, and hybrid (part paper, part electronic) health records. The 2011 hospital and ambulatory accreditation manuals provide an excellent foundation for the requirements of the standards. The Record of Care, of Treatment, and Services chapters contain a wealth of information about the components of a complete medical record. A highly detailed document when seen in its entirety, the record of care comprises all data and information gathered about a patient from the moment he or she enters the hospital to the moment of discharge or transfer. As such, the record of care functions not only as a historical record of a patient's episode(s) of care, but also as a method of communication between practitioners and staff that can facilitate the continuity of care and aid in clinical decision making. Whether the hospital or physician practice keeps paper records, electronic records, or both, the contents of the record remain the same. Special care should be taken, however, by hospitals and clinics that are transitioning from paper to electronic systems, as the period of transition can present increased opportunity for errors in record-keeping that can affect the delivery of quality care. Following is a summary of the high-level requirements from the 2011 Joint Commission Manuals for clinical records as outlined in the Record of Care (RC) section of the hospital and ambulatory manuals:

- RC.01.01.01: The organization maintains complete and accurate clinical records.
- RC.01.02.01: Entries in the clinical record are authenticated.
- RC.01.03.01: Documentation in the clinical record is entered in a timely manner.
- RC.01.04.01: The organization audits its clinical records.
- RC.01.05.01: The organization retains its clinical records.
- RC.02.01.01: The clinical record contains information that reflects the patient's care, treatment, and services.
- RC.02.01.03: The clinical record documents operative or other high-risk procedures and the use of moderate or deep sedation or anesthesia.
- RC.02.01.05: The clinical record documents of the use of restraint (and/or seclusion for hospitals).
- RC.02.01.07: The clinical record contains a summary list for each patient who receives continuing ambulatory care services.
- RC.02.03.07: Qualified staff receive and record verbal orders.

Each RC standard has additional, detailed subcomponents, which can be found in the accreditation manual. The requirements vary depending on the care setting. The accreditation standards may be applicable during litigation if compliance, performance, quality of care, or content of the record are relevant to the case. These requirements also help inform organizational policy and governance to ensure maintenance of a compliant health record and when declaring the content of the legal record.

1.4.3 Declaring the Official Health Record in Policy

Because EHR systems gather vast amounts of information in the database(s) for clinical, financial, and administrative purposes, it is necessary to declare (define in policy) the reports, screen shots, scans, video, photos, standard flow sheet views, and other content that comprise the official (legal) health record. Applicable regulations, laws, and accreditation standards as outlined in the previous sections provide the foundation for the content. Unfortunately, in healthcare today, there is not one common definition of the content of the medical record—it is different depending on the care setting (hospital, physician practice, long-term care), the applicable regulations, the reimbursement rules, the unique organizational policies, documentation processes, and capabilities of the EHR system. These factors require each healthcare organization to define in policy the formal content of the health record that officially represents a stay or encounter. Because health records may be paper or electronic, best practices recommend identifying the content, whether the content is paper or electronic, and if electronic, where in the system it is located.

The best way to define routinely released LHR documents is to create a tailored LHR definition for disclosure by building upon and updating existing paper records, policies, procedures, and principles (McLendon and Lowe 2011). McLendon and Lowe (2011) describe:

> The first task to be accomplished, after identifying of your stakeholders and project structure, is to request a list of all clinical information EHR systems. These may be referred to as clinical EHR modules or source systems. The list should include not just the names of these systems but additional data fields such as the resident system expert, vendor name, data format, and others listed in table 1.2. Formulating and maintaining a list of other organization record custodians and their corresponding record sets is advised. Be sure to delineate who responds to subpoenas and other appropriate legal requests for diagnostic imaging studies (films

Table 1.2   Health record legal source legend

Documents Defined as the LHR			Location of System	HQ Site Name of System	Vendor Application Name	Responsible Department	LHR Custodian	Business Owner/Source System Custodian	IT Primary Contact	Media and Storage (P) Paper (E) Electronic	Data Format(s)	Retention Period
Document Name Data Set Report Name	Source System	Comments										

Source: McLendon and Lowe 2011.

and images) and patient accounts records, as well as any other records for which there are additional custodians. Adding IT and EHR support staff to these lists is recommended as well.

The next task is to create a list, called a document matrix, of all documents and data that comprise your current LHR utilized for routine disclosure. This may actually be a list or simply point to the master document table within an electronic document management system (EDMS). This typically comprises a list of hundreds of documents and can become unwieldy. Therefore, it is recommended that you create a list of chapters (or sometimes known as index tabs) that are *included* in your paper or hybrid medical record and begin a spreadsheet-based matrix to manage these data. It is a good idea to create a single spreadsheet-based workbook (using Microsoft Excel or a comparable program) and to have these lists of source systems and LHR data and documents on separate worksheets within the workbook.

It is important to bear in mind the reason for creating your document matrix as a part of your LHR definition. The record custodian has the responsibility to not only determine what business records, or components of these records, he or she will release upon legal request, but also determine which records actually fulfill the content of the record request as stated in the request document. See table 1.3.

1.4.4 HIPAA/HITECH Compliance, Protected Health Information, and the Legal Record

A major consideration for maintaining a legal record is compliance with existing regulations, standards, and laws for medical (health) records as discussed in the previous section. The HIPAA provides an important foundation for privacy and security practices, which also shape compliance requirements of the legal health record.

HIPAA provides a baseline of privacy and security requirements for a healthcare organization that is a covered entity and required to comply with the act. The privacy and security requirements in the act govern PHI, which is individually identifiable information (oral or recorded) that is created or received by a healthcare provider. PHI includes the content of the health record, so privacy and security practices are a critical component of the legal health record.

Table 1.3   Document matrix for documents, data, and reports to be defined as included in or excluded from an LHR according to facility-specific decisions and guidelines

Facility: _____

Document Name Data Set Report Name	EHR or Hybrid	Source System	Comments
To Be Determined for LHR and Routine Disclosure			
Exterrnal or other provider medical record copies (that were received and accepted before or during the patient visit)			
Exterrnal or other provider medical record copies (that were received after the patient visit)			
Audio files			
Diagnostic or clinical still pictures			
E-mail			
Diagnostic video			
Internal EHR messaging			
Alerts, reminders, pop-up clinical reminders			
Personal health record			
Portal documents			
Previous versions of documents, data, and reports			
Snapshots of data within the EHR			
Interface reconciliation records			
MPI merge records			
Aggregate data that contain PHI			
Back-up data			
Downtime recovery paper documents			
Original source files for EHR data (contained within various EHR modules)			
Use to catalog your documents, data, and reports to be determined for inclusion in your defined LHR.			

Source: McLendon and Lowe 2011, 36.

The security components of HIPAA are critical for maintaining a legally sound EHR system. The following requirements are critically important for securing **electronic PHI (e-PHI)** within EHR systems:

- Data encryption
- Virus protection
- Technical safeguards to protect e-PHI (access controls, audit controls, authentication of users and entities, transmission security)
- Monitoring of access to e-PHI

EHR systems may also support the privacy requirements of HIPAA and the policies of the organization. For example, the HIPAA Privacy Rule allows for access to PHI by the individual. EHR systems can provide a mechanism to authenticate the individual as a user to allow access in support of this requirement. HIPAA requires an accounting of disclosures. The EHR system can assist the healthcare organization in complying with this requirement by building in a mechanism to track export, printing, or disclosures of PHI and records from the system.

Another component of HIPAA is the concept of the designated record set, which overlaps with the legal health record. According to the HIPAA rule, the designated record set includes a group of records maintained by a covered entity that includes medical and billing records, case management records, and information used in whole or in part to make care-related decisions. Individuals have a right to request access to the designated record set, which includes more than the medical record. Most requests for information are related to the subset of content for the legal health record (as identified in policy). Figure 1.4 displays the breakdown of different types of materials available.

1.4.5 EHR Standards for Records Management and Evidentiary Support

Discussion about the EHR standard for record management and evidentiary support impacts a number of e-discovery practice issues in this book. As healthcare increasingly implements automated, electronic systems and applications, HIT standards are established to improve interoperability, content, efficiency, and functionality. A number of standards organizations have tackled specific issues that support a legally sound electronic health record system. **Health Level Seven (HL7)**, a healthcare IT standards organization, has developed one of the most comprehensive standards called the **records**

Figure 1.4   Relationship of the designated record set to the legal health record

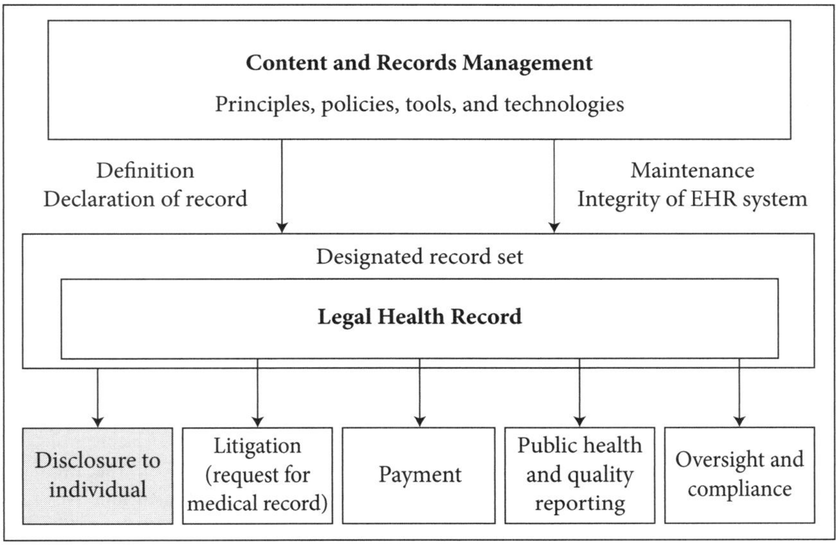

```
┌─────────────────────────────────────────────────────────────────────┐
│  ┌───────────────────────────────────────────────────────────────┐  │
│  │              Content and Records Management                     │  │
│  │          Principles, policies, tools, and technologies          │  │
│  └───────────────────────────────────────────────────────────────┘  │
│                                                                       │
│        Definition                            Maintenance             │
│   Declaration of record                  Integrity of EHR system     │
│                    │                            │                     │
│                    ▼                            ▼                     │
│  ┌───────────────────────────────────────────────────────────────┐  │
│  │                   Designated record set                         │  │
│  │  ┌─────────────────────────────────────────────────────────┐  │  │
│  │  │                 Legal Health Record                      │  │  │
│  │  └─────────────────────────────────────────────────────────┘  │  │
│  └───────────────────────────────────────────────────────────────┘  │
│         │         │          │           │            │              │
│         ▼         ▼          ▼           ▼            ▼              │
│  ┌─────────┐ ┌─────────┐ ┌───────┐ ┌──────────┐ ┌────────────┐     │
│  │Disclosure│ │Litigation│ │Payment│ │Public health│ │Oversight and│  │
│  │   to     │ │(request │ │       │ │and quality │ │ compliance │     │
│  │individual│ │  for    │ │       │ │ reporting  │ │            │     │
│  │          │ │medical  │ │       │ │            │ │            │     │
│  │          │ │record)  │ │       │ │            │ │            │     │
│  └─────────┘ └─────────┘ └───────┘ └──────────┘ └────────────┘     │
└─────────────────────────────────────────────────────────────────────┘
```

Source: AHIMA.

management and evidentiary support profile (RM-ES profile) related to EHR systems. The HL7 standard provides a framework of functions and conformance criteria for EHR systems as a mechanism to support an organization in maintaining a legally sound health record (HL7 RM-ES 2010).

The RM-ES standard is based on the premise that an EHR system must be able to create, receive, maintain, use, and manage the disposition of records for evidentiary purposes related to business activities and transactions for an organization. Because legal validity is at stake for uses of electronic records for evidentiary purposes, including admissibility of medical records, the RM-ES profile is important to healthcare operations and to interoperability (HL7 RM-ES 2010).

The RM-ES profile identifies EHR system functions as critical for maintaining a legally sound health record. Tables 1.4 through 1.6 provide a description of each function and its legal rationale.

The HL7 RM-ES standard for EHR systems can be used by vendors in developing and refining their systems, or by healthcare providers to evaluate their current system functionality in support of a legal EHR or in procuring new systems.

Table 1.4   Security functions

ID and Name	Function Description	Legal Rationale
IN.1.1 Authentication	Authenticate EHR-S users and/or entities before allowing access to an EHR-S. Examples of authentication include: • Username/Password • Digital certificate • Secure token • Biometrics	Authentication is a critical component to maintain the legal integrity of the health record contained within the EHR-S. One of the foundational underpinnings of the validity of the record is identification of the users and assurances that they are accurately identified. As a result, the method used by the organization is very important. One of the most common and cost-effective methods of authentication is user ID and password. Other methods of authentication are considered stronger than user ID and password. Over time, as legal standards evolve, it is anticipated that the bar will be raised and stronger methods of authentication will need to be utilized by healthcare organizations to assure that their users are accurately identified in the system.
IN.1.2 Authorization	Manage the sets of access-control permissions granted to entities that use an EHR-S (users). Enable EHR-S security administrators to grant authorizations to users, for roles, and within contexts.	The authorization process is important legally because it provides the system rules and context for actions recorded within the EHR system. The actions and individuals may be called into question retrospectively. Authorization functionality is also important to constrain users to the system rules such as limiting printing or output capability. This is important legally to maintain controls on the location of outputs from the system.
IN.1.3 Entity Access Control	Verify and enforce access control to all EHR-S components, EHR information and functions for end users, applications, sites, etc., to prevent unauthorized use.	Controls to limit access to only authorized users are important for supporting the authenticity and trustworthiness of the electronic health record.

ID and Name	Function Description	Legal Rationale
IN.1.4 Patient Access Management	Enable a healthcare delivery organization to allow and manage a patient's access to the patient's personal health information.	Similar to above, access controls, including patient access, are important for maintaining the electronic health record's integrity and trustworthiness.
IN.1.5 Nonrepudiation	Limit an EHR-S user's ability to deny (repudiate) the origination, receipt, or authorization of a data exchange by that user.	Nonrepudiation is a critical function in support of a legally sound record. System functionality must support the integrity of the data and record and prevent against denial of origination or receipt.
IN.1.6 Secure Data Exchange	Secure all modes of EHR data exchange.	It is important that the information received and used for patient care comes from a trusted source and that standards/protocols are in place to ensure that the data sent are the same as the data received.
IN.1.7 Secure Data Routing	Route electronically exchanged EHR data only to/from known, registered, and authenticated destinations/ sources (according to applicable healthcare-specific rules and relevant standards).	It is important that the information exchanged is from a trusted and authenticated source and is securely transported.
IN.1.8 Information Attestation	Manage electronic attestation of information including the retention of the signature of attestation (or certificate of authenticity) associated with incoming or outgoing information.	Legally it is critical that the author of an entry (including all contributors or co-authors) be accurately identified and that every entry has an author who is responsible for the content. Over time it is anticipated that the bar will be raised and that stronger authentication/attestation processes will be required to prevent someone from refuting that they were the author.
IN.1.9 Patient Privacy and Confidentiality	Enable the enforcement of the applicable jurisdictional and organizational patient privacy rules as they apply to various parts of an EHR-S through the implementation of security mechanisms.	Organizational practices related to privacy and security jurisdictional laws (e.g., HIPAA) could be called into question during a legal proceeding. Adherence to applicable laws supports the credibility and trustworthiness of the organization.

Source: Dougherty 2008.

Table 1.5   Health record information and management functions

ID and Name	Function Description	Legal Rationale
IN.2.1 Data Retention, Availability, and Destruction	Retain, ensure availability, and destroy health record information according to scope of practice, organizational policy, or jurisdictional law.	Adherence to organizational retention and destruction policies that comply with jurisdictional law is critical in legal proceedings to prevent accusations of spoliation of evidence and establish that the organization destroyed records as part of their good faith practices. Organizations must develop a policy that defines their official medical record for official disclosure purposes (reimbursement, litigation, regulatory, etc.). The EHR-S must be able to support the retrieval of the elements the organization considers part of their legal medical record. This includes business context data (such as metadata) retained by the system, which may provide context of when a record was created, by whom, etc.
IN.2.1.1 Record Preservation	Preserve data from normal destruction practices including a duty to preserve material evidence when the organization reasonably should know that the evidence (health record information) may be relevant to anticipated litigation.	Organizations have a duty to preserve information that is or could be relevant to a legal proceeding whether litigation is threatened (the potential for) or impending. Systems must provide the ability for users to place a legal hold on electronic health information (suspend their normal destruction practices for all potentially relevant information) and prevent from loss, destruction, alteration, or unauthorized use.
IN.2.2 Auditable Records	Provide audit capabilities for system access and usage indicating the author, the modification (where pertinent), and the date and time at which a record was created, modified, viewed, extracted, or deleted. Auditable records extend to information exchange, to audit of consent status management, and to entity authentication attempts. Audit functionality includes the ability to generate audit reports and to interactively view change history for individual health records or for an EHR-S.	The audit functionality provides traceability to show the activities "behind the scenes." With traceability comes trustworthiness in the electronic records to be used in legal proceedings.

ID and Name	Function Description	Legal Rationale
IN.2.2.1 Metadata (Point of Record, System and Software Application)	Metadata is an inextricable part of electronic records management and is utilized for a variety of functions and purposes. In a legal setting, metadata may be used to authenticate the evidentiary value of electronic information and/or describe contextual processing of a record. Metadata at the point of patient record capture includes information about the context of record creation, the business context, the agents involved, and metadata about the content, appearance, structure, and technical attributes of the record itself. System metadata is information about the physical structure of the EHR system itself. This function includes defining, collecting, and storing important data to describe the EHR architecture, hardware/physical systems, and the infrastructure in use over a definable time range. Software application metadata is information about the software/ applications used in the EHR. This function includes defining, collecting, and storing important data to describe the EHR software, its components, and their evolution over time.	Metadata (data about data) can validate and quantify the authenticity, reliability, usability, and integrity of information over time and enable the management and understanding of electronic information (physical, analogue, or digital). The metadata collected and retained may vary by organization and within jurisdictions according to: • Business needs • Jurisdictional regulatory environment • Risks affecting business operations Effective utilization of metadata requires appropriate management of metadata information. All EHR applications must adhere to established standards, which enable the creation, registration, classification, access, preservation, and disposition of records through time and within and across information systems. Metadata supports the interoperability strategies by enabling the authoritative capture of records created in diverse technical and business environments and is sustained for as long as required (ISO 23081).
IN.2.4 Extraction of Health Record Information	Manage data extraction in accordance with analysis and reporting requirements. The extracted data may require use of more than one application and it may be preprocessed (for example, by being de-identified) before transmission. Data extractions may be used to exchange data and provide reports for primary and ancillary purposes.	Extraction may be needed in response to a request from the court or an opposing party.

(continued)

Table 1.5   Health record information and management functions *(continued)*

ID and Name	Function Description	Legal Rationale
IN.2.5 Store and Manage Health Record Information	Store and manage health record information as structured and unstructured data.	Organizational policies on creation, capture, storage, and maintenance of health record information may be called into question during legal proceedings. Adherence to organizational policy, standards of practice, and jurisdictional law will be critical.
IN.2.5.3 Manage Record States: • Pending State • Amended, Corrected, and Augmented State • Document Succession Management and Version Control • Retracted State	Manage health record information during the various states of completion. Health record information may be started, updated, but not completed. The records, although not complete, can represent an important piece of healthcare information particularly if viewed for patient care purposes. Updates to health record information made after finalization (or the signature event) will be handled as an amendment, correction, or augmentation. A system shall retain previous versions of a document and manage document succession. A system shall provide the ability to remove (retract) a document from view if it is deemed erroneous and cite the reason	Health record information may reside in various states that must be managed. An important underlying principle for managing record states is the need to retain health information records that have been viewed for patient care purposes even if the record has not been completed or attested, was created or placed in error, was in a previous version, or has been amended. This principle has important legal impact because it provides a record of what the provider relied on for clinical decision making. Proper amendment and correction procedures are just as important in electronic systems as they were in paper-based record systems. When changes are made they should be transparent—a user or reviewer should be able to access the original entry and determine when and by whom amendments and corrections were made. The trustworthiness and integrity of the record can be called into question or placed under suspicion when previous entries are destroyed.
IN.2.5.4 Redaction	Remove from view (redact) for disclosure or reporting purposes portions of an EHR (at either the data or record level) and cite the authority for doing so.	Systems must provide the ability to redact information at the data level or at the record level, provide a mechanism to capture the reason for redaction, and retain a copy of the redacted records that were disclosed. Redaction may be used for a variety of purposes such as protecting certain types of confidential or privileged information from being disclosed including disclosure for litigation purposes.
IN.2.5.5 Health Record Completeness	Support the ability to identify a report or record as complete and identify the status as defined by the organization.	Prior to disclosure for legal proceedings or other official purposes, an organization analyzes the health record for completeness. EHR systems must provide the ability to define a minimum set of content to be analyzed for timeliness and completeness and provide a report of the status.

ID and Name	Function Description	Legal Rationale
IN.2.5.6 Chronology of Events	Support the ability to view and disclose the patient care events that happened over a range of time in chronological order.	Functionality to support chronology of events allows the organization to display or disclose the patient care events in the sequence that they occurred. This view provides a beneficial retrospective look at the unfolding of events and timing of decision making, which is important in the audit and review process and legal process.
IN.2.5.7 Replication of Views	Support the ability to replicate or recreate a view (both read and write) to the extent possible from metadata.	Replication of views may be required for litigation to see information the way a clinician would have viewed, entered, or used it at a given time. Those handling litigation might expect the EHR system to capture a "snapshot" of every EHR action taken by the clinician to diagnose and treat each given patient. The ability to produce a replicated view is not guaranteed and is limited to audit and metadata. Best practice for replication of view approaches will evolve over time.
IN.2.5.8 Downtime Procedures, Storage, and Back-Up	Provide mechanisms for reliable and consistent availability of the system and data.	EHRs and/or data transmitted and retained in an interoperable HIT system must be stored and be secure from access by unauthorized and unidentified persons or users. This applies to all data regardless of storage location. Records must be retained—unaltered, readable, and retrievable—and record retention must comply with all applicable laws and regulations. Regardless of the physical location where the EHR is stored, the EHR must at all times be actually available, by legal process or as otherwise authorized by law, to patients, governmental and private payers, and law enforcement.
S. 2.2 Report Generation and Health Record Output	Support the export of data or access to data necessary for report generation and ad hoc analysis. Support the definition of the formal health record, a partial record for referral purposes, or sets of records for other necessary disclosure purposes.	Report generation functionality is important to provide an output of relevant information from EHR systems for legal proceedings. Reports are not limited to the formal medical record, but may include any kind of system. Systems should also have the ability to provide a report of audit record and metadata for disclosure if required for litigation.

Source: Dougherty 2008.

Table 1.6   Business rules and workflow management

ID and Name	Function Description	Legal Rationale
IN.6 Business Rules Management	Manage the ability to create, update, delete, view, and version business rules including institutional preferences. Apply business rules from necessary points within an EHR-S to control system behavior. An EHR-S audits changes made to business rules, as well as compliance to and overrides of applied business rules.	The care delivery and documentation process captured within an EHR-S is based on system business rules. These rules will likely be called into question during a legal proceeding to understand the organization's good faith practices and when practices deviated from the norm.
IN.7 Workflow Management	Support workflow management functions including both the management and set up of work queues, personnel lists, and system interfaces as well as the implementation functions that use workflow-related business rules to direct the flow of work assignments.	The workflow processes that support care delivery and documentation captured within an EHR-S will likely be called into question during a legal proceeding to understand the organization's good faith practices and when practices deviated from the norm.

1.5 New Technologies: Cloud Computing and Web 2.0

Even as this text goes to print, new technologies introduce technical and legal issues that must be addressed within existing precedent for ESI and EHRs in healthcare organizations. Two such technologies are "the Cloud" (or "**cloud computing**") and **Web 2.0**. Figure 1.5 shows a vision of health and healthcare in an era of cloud computing.

In essence, the Cloud consists of electronic information and applications hosted on the Internet by a variety of third parties (similar to Application Service Providers—ASPs, ASP, or Software as a Service—SAAS). Many organizations are choosing this technical approach for their EHR systems and applications. Web 2.0 is a set of technologies that combines user-provided content and automated networking applications to create interactive information (such as social networking, video sharing, wikis, and blogs). The two technologies are distinct in theory and overlap in practice. Healthcare organizations are impacted by Web 2.0 technologies as well—functionality could be embedded within current applications, used on organization intranets, or on the public Internet. In addition, staff could engage in social networking or blogs and disclose confidential or inappropriate information about the organization or patients.

Figure 1.5   A vision of health and healthcare in an era of cloud computing

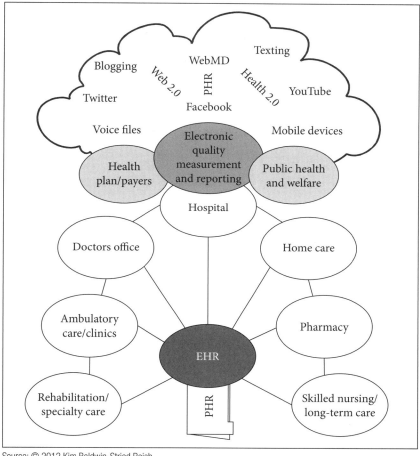

What issues arise from the Cloud and Web 2.0? As organizations evaluate and implement new technologies for their EHR and business operations, the following questions should be considered to help assess record management that may potentially have an impact on litigation:

- Do the Cloud and Web 2.0 create new sources of ESI that must be preserved and produced in litigation?
- Is there a duty to preserve information in the Cloud or on a Web 2.0 technology that may be ephemeral or transitory in nature?
- Do statutes or regulations create a duty to retain or preserve the information?

- What of the relationship between a party and a third party hosting the former's information over the Internet—what contractual provisions will afford reasonable protections for the party as well as the third party?
- What happens to the information if the third party goes out of business?
- What rights of access does the party have to the information? And what is the cost of out-of-the-ordinary access, say, for litigation needs?
- How will records retention policies govern information maintained in the Cloud or on a Web 2.0 technology?
- What will possession, custody, or control mean when information is in the Cloud or on Web 2.0 technology?
- How will information in the Cloud or on an interactive Web 2.0 application be safeguarded and who should be responsible for security breaches?

These few questions suggest that organizations must undertake cost/benefit analyses in reaching a decision to use the Cloud or a Web 2.0 technology—and that costs and benefits may not always be apparent.

Similarly, legal decisions will stem from existing law. That may involve the creation and enforcement of contracts, the relationship and duties of principal and agent, and litigation-related obligations imposed by the FRCP, related state laws and rules, and the common law.

1.6 EHR Systems, Coding Systems, Secondary Uses, Testing, and Sampling

Healthcare organizations and EHR systems utilize medical coding systems for a variety of purposes. It is important to understand what they are and how they may impact litigation. The coding and classification of diagnostic procedures dates back to seventeenth-century England through a system called the London Bills of Mortality. In 1937, the London Bills of Mortality evolved into the International List of Causes of Death (ICD). In 1948, the World Health Organization (WHO) published a statistical list that was used to track both morbidity and mortality. This listing, known as the International Classification of Diseases (ICD), is the system that led the way for the text currently used internationally for the coding and classification of health-related conditions and procedures, known as the International Classification of Diseases, Ninth Revision (ICD-9).

The ninth revision of ICD, published in 1977, attained wide recognition internationally. This prompted the US National Center for Health Statistics

(NCHS) to modify statistical analysis with clinical information. These clinical modifications provided a way to classify morbidity data for indexing of medical records, medical case reviews, and ambulatory and other medical care programs, as well as for basic health statistics. The result was the **International Classification of Diseases, Ninth Revision, Clinical Modification (ICD-9-CM)**, commonly referred to as ICD-9. This version precisely delineates the clinical picture of each patient, providing exact information beyond that needed for statistical groupings and analysis of healthcare trends.

Today's current Acute Care Prospective Payment System for Medicare reimbursement of inpatients is based upon correct ICD-9-CM and **diagnosis-related group (DRG)** assignment. The DRG system was developed by a Yale University group at the request of Congress. Initially, the DRG system was established as a way to monitor the utilization of resources and monitor the quality of healthcare services; then, a short time later, the New Jersey Department of Health experimented with the DRG classification system as a mechanism for reimbursement. In 1982, Congress passed the Tax Equity and Fiscal Responsibility Act (TEFRA), which mandated the implementation of the DRG classification system by the end of 1983.

In 1988, Congress passed the Medicare Catastrophic Coverage Act, and ICD-9 coding took on new importance. Although this act was later repealed, the mandate requiring use of ICD-9 codes on claims submitted by physicians was upheld. This mandate became effective on April 1, 1989. Basic guidelines regarding the use of ICD-9 codes were published by the CMS and put into effect by each state. The CMS provides specific guidelines to aid in standardizing coding practices across the United States. The failure to use or correctly use ICD-9 codes can lead to severe repercussions, including fines, sanctions, loss of participation in the Medicare program, and even jail time.

Efforts are underway today to establish a new healthcare coding system to support the transition to EHRs and the ultimate development of a Nationwide Health Information Network (NHIN), in which all health data will be coded, captured, and exchanged electronically. Therefore, the quality and integrity of coded health data has become increasing important as it is vital to the measurement and reporting of healthcare quality efforts, research, and public health. The quality and integrity of coded data will become equally important to the litigation process as well, especially once litigators become more sophisticated in data testing and sampling techniques.

The CMS and the Centers for Diseases Control and Prevention (CDC), have created a general equivalence mapping (GEM) system to help prepare the industry for the transition to the ICD-10-CM/PCS coding systems and to assist with the translation of legacy data between ICD-9-CM and ICD-10-CM/PCS (CMS 2010a).

The ICD-10 coding system is important to the litigation processes because ICD-10 coded data will provide much more specific diagnostic and procedural coding information, and will provide better information for measuring healthcare quality, safety, and utilization. Healthcare providers and health plans have until October 2013 to adopt the new ICD-10 healthcare coding and classification system. Industry experts believe that not only will ICD-10 codes provide more accurate reimbursement, the ICD-10 system will provide "much needed clarity and accuracy in the health care system" (Bureau of National Affairs 2009).

1.6.1 Differences between ICD-9-CM and ICD-10-CM

Table 1.7 outlines some of the major differences between ICD-9-CM and ICD-10-CM. Specifics of the code sets will be discussed in the sections that follow.

Table 1.7   Comparing ICD-9-CM and ICD-10-CM

ICD-10-CM differs from ICD-9-CM in its organization and structure, code composition, and level of detail.	
ICD-9-CM	**ICD-10-CM**
• Consists of three to five characters • First digit is numeric or alpha (E or V) • Second, third, fourth, and fifth digits are numeric • Always at least three digits • Decimal placed after the first three characters	• Consists of three to seven characters • First digit is alpha • All letters used except U • Second and third digits are numeric • Fourth, fifth, sixth, and seventh digits can be alpha or numeric • Decimal placed after the first three characters
Code Structure of ICD-10-CM versus ICD-9-CM ICD-10-CM codes may consist of up to seven digits, with the seventh digit extensions representing visit encounter or sequelae for injuries and external causes.	
ICD-9-CM Code Format	**ICD-10-CM Code Format**
X X X . X X category etiology, anatomic site, manifestation	X X X . X X X X category etiology, anatomic site, severity extension

Source: Barta et al. 2008.

1.6.1.1 ICD-9-CM

The ICD-9-CM is based upon the WHO ICD-9. ICD-9-CM is a three-volume classification system that serves as the official system for the assignment of diagnoses and procedures associated with hospital utilization in the United States and to code and classify mortality data from death certificates (CDC 2010a).

ICD-9-CM has been in use since 1983 as the basic input for assigning diagnosis-related groups for Medicare's Inpatient Prospective Payment System. ICD-9-CM volumes 1 and 2 and ICD-9-CM volume 3 were adopted as HIPAA code sets in 2000 for reporting diagnoses, injuries, impairments, and other health problems and their manifestations, and causes of injury, disease, impairment, or other health problems in standard transactions, respectively (45 CFR 162).

The ICD-9-CM classification system is comprised of (CDC 2010a):

- A tabular list containing a numerical list of the disease code numbers
- An alphabetical index to the disease entries
- A classification system for surgical, diagnostic, and therapeutic procedures (alphabetic index and tabular list)

The NCHS and CMS are responsible for overseeing all changes and modifications to ICD-9-CM.

1.6.1.2 ICD-10-CM

The **International Classification of Diseases, Tenth Revision, Clinical Modification (ICD-10-CM)** is based upon the WHO Tenth Revision, International Classification of Diseases (ICD-10). ICD-10-CM is the planned replacement for ICD-9-CM, volumes 1 and 2. ICD-10-CM is owned and copyrighted by the WHO and was developed following extensive evaluation by a technical advisory panel with additional review and consultation by physician groups, clinical coders, and others to assure clinical accuracy (CDC 2010b).

The ICD-10-CM classification system is comprised of:

- Index to diseases and injuries
- Draft official guidelines
- Tabular list of diseases and injuries

1.6.1.3 Comparison of ICD-9-CM and ICD-10-CM

The ICD-9-CM and ICD-10-CM coding and classification systems share a number of similarities. For example, ICD-10-CM is comprised of the same hierarchical structure as ICD-9-CM and shares many of the same conventions, instructional notes, and guidelines (Bowman 2004).

Although the two systems share many of the same characteristics and are structured somewhat similarly, a number of notable differences exist between the two systems including (Bowman 2004):

- ICD-10-CM is entirely alphanumeric (all letters except U are used).
- ICD-10-CM codes may be up to seven characters in length.
- Some chapters have been restructured in ICD-10-CM.
- Some diseases have been reclassified in ICD-10-CM.
- New features have been added to ICD-10-CM.

The transition from ICD-9-CM to ICD-10-CM allows for greater specificity, detail, and further expansion of the classification system than was possible with ICD-9-CM. Specific improvements to ICD-10-CM include (CDC 2010a):

- The addition of information relevant to ambulatory and managed care encounters
- Expanded injury codes
- The creation of combination diagnosis/symptom codes to reduce the number of codes needed to fully describe a condition
- The addition of sixth and seventh characters; incorporation of common fourth and fifth digit subclassifications
- Laterality
- Greater specificity in code assignment

1.6.1.4 ICD-10-PCS

The International Classification of Diseases, Tenth Revision, Procedure Coding System (ICD-10-PCS) is the official procedure coding system developed by CMS that will be used to collect data, determine payment, and support the EHR for all inpatient procedures performed in the United States. In the ICD-9-CM classification system, these procedures were coded using ICD-9-CM Volume 3. The ICD-10-PCS uses seven alpha or numeric digits while the ICD-9-CM coding system uses three or four numeric digits. Table 1.8 describes these structural differences.

Table 1.8   Basic differences between ICD-9-CM, volume 3, and ICD-10-PCS

ICD-9-CM Volume 3	ICD-10-PCS
Follows ICD structure (designed for diagnosis coding)	Designed and developed to meet healthcare needs for a procedure code system
Codes available as a fixed or finite set in list form	Codes constructed from flexible code components (values) using tables
Codes are numeric	Codes are alphanumeric
Codes are three or four digits long	All codes are seven characters long

Source: CMS 2010b, 1.5.

1.6.1.5 ICD-10's Potential Impact

The implementation of ICD-10 will also have significant impact on the litigation process. Through the testing, sampling, and review of claims and clinical data, the ICD-10 coding and classification system and provider databases will give a much more detailed and clearer picture of the quality of care and outcomes. As litigators become more knowledgeable about HIT and sophisticated in their approaches to discover and analyze electronically stored clinical databases, it is predicted that the discovery and review of medical databases in cases such as *Youle v. Ryan, MD and Sarah Bush Lincoln Health Center and Kevin M.,* Ill. App. 3d 377, 380, 811 N.E.2d 1281, 1283 (2004) will become commonplace in the courts.

References

45 CFR 162: Administrative requirements. 2009.

42 CFR 412, 413, 422: Electronic health record incentive program. 2010.

Advisory Committee Note to 2007 Amendment to Rule 1 and Rule 42.

AHIMA e-Discovery e-HIM Work Group. 2006. The new electronic discovery civil rule. Journal of AHIMA 77(8):68A–68H.

AHIMA e-Discovery Task Force. 2008. Litigation response planning and policies for e-discovery. Journal of AHIMA 79(2):69–75.

AHIMA e-HIM Work Group on the Legal Health Record. 2005. Update: Guidelines for defining the legal health record for disclosure purposes. Journal of AHIMA 76(8):64A–G. http://www.healthit.nd.gov/files/2010/07/hit_legal_health_record_considerations.pdf.

AHIMA. 2003 (February). AHIMA mobilizes to meet the e-HIM call. AHIMA Advantage 7:1.

AHIMA. 2010a. Overview of the Proposed Rule: Modifications to the HIPAA Privacy, Security, and Enforcement Rules Under the Health Information Technology for Economic and Clinical Health Act. http://ahima.org/downloads/pdfs/advocacy/Analysis%20of%20Privacy%20Rule%20Fule%20Content%20fin%20.pdf.

AHIMA. 2010b. Practice brief: Managing the transition from paper to EHRs. Appendix A: Legal Source Legend (Updated 2010).

American Recovery and Reinvestment Act of 2009. Public Law 111-5. http://thomas.loc.gov/cgi-bin/query/z?c111:H.R.1.enr:.

Ash, J.S., D.F. Sittig, E.G. Poon, K. Guappone, E. Campbell, and R.H. Dykstra. 2007. The extent and importance of unintended consequences related to computerized provider order entry. Journal of AHIMA 14(4):415–423.

Baldwin-Stried, K. 2006. e-Discovery and HIM. Journal of AHIMA. 77(9):58, 60, 63, 65 passim; quiz 71–72.

Ball, M., C. Weaver, and J. Kiel, eds. 2004. Healthcare Information Management Systems, 3rd ed. New York: Springer-Verlag.

Baron, J., and P. Thompson. 2007. The search problem posed by large heterogeneous data sets in litigation: Possible future approaches to research. Paper presented at the Eleventh International Conference on Artificial Intelligence and Law.

Baron, J., B. Hedin, D.W. Oard, and S. Tomlinson. 2009. Overview of the TREC 2009 Legal Track. Paper presented at the Eighteenth Text Retrieval Conference. http://trec-legal.umiacs.umd.edu.

Barta, A., et al. 2008. ICD-10-CM primer. Journal of AHIMA. 79(5):4–66.

Bowman, S. 2004. Preparing for the ICD-10 journey. Journal of AHIMA 75(3): 60–62.

Bureau of National Affairs. 2009. Federal News 15(16).

Centers for Disease Control and Prevention. 2010a. International Classification of Diseases, Ninth Revision, Clinical Modification (ICD-9-CM). http://www.cdc.gov/nchs/icd/icd9cm.htm.

Centers for Disease Control and Prevention. 2010b. International Classification of Diseases, Tenth Revision, Clinical Modification (ICD-10-CM). http://www.cdc.gov/nchs/icd/icd10cm.htm.

Change.gov. The Office of the President-Elect. 2009 (January). Press Release: President-elect speaks on the need for urgent action on an American Recovery and Reinvestment Plan. http://change.gov/newsroom/entry/president-elect_obama_speaks_on_the_need_for_urgent_action_on_an_american_r/.

DeLoss, G.E., and E.F. Shay. 2007. Electronic discovery and electronic health records: The impact of "e-discovery" involving "EHR" upon healthcare entities. Health Lawyers News 11(5):4.

Dougherty, M. 2008. How legal is your EHR? Identifying key functions that support a legal record. Journal of AHIMA 79(2):24–28, 30.

Dougherty, M. 2010. Still seeking the legal EHR. Journal of AHIMA 81(2):43.

HHS-Centers for Medicare and Medicaid Services. 2006. Conditions of Participation for Hospitals Section 482.24: Medical Record Services. https://www.cms.gov/CFCsAndCoPs/downloads/finalpatientrightsrule.pdf.

HHS-Centers for Medicare and Medicaid Services. 2010a. General equivalence mapping files. http://www.cms.gov/ICD10.

HHS-Centers for Medicare and Medicaid Services. 2010b. ICD-10-PCS Reference Manual. http://www.cms.gov/ICD10/11b_2011_ICD10PCS.asp.

HIT Policy Committee. 2009. Final Meaningful Use Objectives and Measures 2011-2013-2015. http://healthit.hhs.gov/portal/server.pt?open=512&objID=1325&&PageID=16490&mode=2&in_hi_userid=11113&cached=true.

HL7 RM-ES. 2010. HL7 EHR Records Management and Evidentiary Support Functional Profile Release 1. https://www.hl7.org/store/index.cfm?ref=nav.

Hoffman, S., and A. Podgurski. 2008. Finding a cure: The case for regulation and oversight of electronic health record systems. Harvard Journal Law and Technolology 22(1):1–63.

Jha, A.K., C.M. DesRoches, E.G. Campbell, K. Donelan, S.R. Rao, T.G. Ferris, A. Shields, S. Rosenbaum, and D. Blumenthal. 2009. Use of electronic health records in US hospitals. The New England Journal of Medicine 360(16):1628–1638.

The Joint Commission. 2011. Record of Care, Treatment, and Services (RC) section from the 2011 Joint Commission Accreditation Manual for Hospitals and Joint Commission Manual for Ambulatory Care.

Koppel, R., and D. Kreda. 2009. Health care information technology vendors' "hold harmless" clause: Implications for patients and clinicians. The Journal of the American Medical Association 301(12):1276–1278.

Korin, J.B., and M.S. Quattrone. 2007. Litigation in the decade of electronic health records. New Jersey Law Journal 188(11):183.

LaTour, K., and S. Eichenwald-Maki. 2010. Health Information Management: Concepts, Principles, and Practices, 3rd ed. Chicago: AHIMA.

Logan, D., J. Bace, and M. Gilbert. 2005. Understanding e-Discovery Technology. Report for Gartner Research.

Marchand, L. 2001. Discovery of electronic medical records. Paper presented at American Trial Lawyers Association Annual Convention.

McLendon, William Kelly, and Michael R. Lowe. 2011. The Legal Health Record: Regulations, Policies, and Guidance, 2nd ed. Chicago: AHIMA.

Office of the National Coordinator for Health Information Technology. 2009. Notice and request for comments. Federal Register. 74(101):25550–25552. http://edocket.access.gpo.gov/2009/pdf/E9-12419.pdf.

Paul, G.L. 2008. Foundations of Digital Evidence. Chicago: ABA Publishing.

Schuler, K., C.P. Peterson, É. Vincze, and D. Benton. 2009. e-Discovery: Creating and Managing an Enterprisewide Program: A Technical Guide to Digital Investigation and Litigation Support. Burlington, MA: Syngress Publishing.

The Sedona Conference. 2007. The Sedona Conference Glossary: e-Discovery & Digital Information Management, 2nd ed.

Weiner, J.P., T. Kfuri, K. Chan, and J.B. Fowles. 2007. "E-iatrogenesis": The most critical unintended consequence of CPOE and other HIT. Journal of the American Medical Informatics Association. 14(3):387–388; discussion 389.

Youle v. Raymond Ryan, MD and Sarah Bush Lincoln Health Center and Kevin M., Ill. App. 3d 377, 380, 811 N.E.2d 1281, 1283 (2004).

Zubulake v. UBS Warburg LLC, 220 F.R.D. 212 (S.D.N.Y. 2003).

Foundation of Electronic Discovery Rules

Chapter Objectives

The purpose of this chapter is to provide a description of the rules governing electronic discovery, the legal process, and how the electronic discovery rules are applied in the courts. Readers will also be introduced to the legal process and the concept of cooperation between parties in litigation.

The objectives of this chapter are to:

- Define discovery and electronic discovery
- Provide a foundation for understanding the Federal Rules of Civil Procedure (FRCP) and how they are applied in a court of law
- Compare and contrast state, local and uniform rules for electronic discovery
- Provide direction to e-discovery resources and best practice guidance in electronic discovery
- Discuss the implementation of the HITECH Act and the advent of electronic discovery in healthcare
- Review and discuss court decisions involving the application of the FRCP and The Sedona Conference Cooperation Proclamation

At the conclusion of this chapter a series of questions are put forth to help HIM and IT professionals evaluate how processes will change through the advent of electronic discovery.

2.1 Overview

In one sense, there no longer is electronic discovery. Electronically stored information (ESI) is everywhere. When we speak of electronic discovery we create an unwarranted distinction between information, wherever and however it may reside, and the means by which that information is created and maintained. Nevertheless, electronic discovery as a term is ubiquitous and so this book will continue to use that term. This chapter provides the foundation for e-discovery and chapter 3 delves into the details of the rules as they apply to healthcare.

As apparent from chapter 1, any discussion of electronic discovery begins with the FRCP, which were amended effective December 1, 2006, to address electronic discovery and to, among other things, remove any doubt that ESI was discoverable. A number of states have also addressed electronic discovery by statute or rule. Given the various ways in which the states have done so, however, this book will provide only a broad overview. Importantly, the reader must understand that rules and statutes, both federal and state, are subject to interpretation and explanation by courts. This book will provide examples of how courts have dealt with ESI. Before that, however, some introduction to the world of ESI and electronic discovery is appropriate.

2.1.1 What Is Electronic Discovery?

Reduced down to its essentials, electronic discovery is simply the preservation, collection, review, and production of information relevant to a particular issue or issues in litigation and that is in electronic form. That information, or ESI, can reside in many locations and be in many forms. For example, ESI can be found in mainframe computers, servers, desktops, personal data assistants (PDAs), and smart phones. ESI can exist as native data (in other words, in the manner in which it resides in the normal course of use), as a tagged image file format (TIFF) image, or as a portable document format (PDF) file. ESI can also include what can be best described as hidden data, that is, data not apparent on the face of an electronic document but which can be retrieved with varying amounts of difficulty. ESI can be voluminous, dispersed, mutable (or changeable), and sometimes difficult to find. It is also maintained in complex systems.

2.2 The Rules

The FRCP are promulgated by the US Supreme Court and approved by Congress. A description of the structure and general content of the FRCP is summarized in table 2.1.

2.2.1 Federal Rules

The FRCP are the starting point for understanding electronic discovery (FRCP 2007). As noted above, the FRCP were amended effective December 1, 2006, after a long process of public notice, comment, and revision, to address electronic discovery. This book will address specific FRCP and case

Table 2.1   Federal Rules of Civil Procedure

Category	Category Description	Rules in Category	General Content in Category
I	Scope	1 and 2	Category I describes the purpose of the rules and their role in governing civil action in federal district courts.
II	Commencement of civil suits	3 to 6	Category II contains the rules that provide for the commencement of a civil suit, including the filing, summons, and service of process (legal notice).
III	Pleadings and motions	7 to 16	Category III provides for civil suit pleadings, motions, defenses, and counterclaims. The complaint is the plaintiff's pleading. The answer is the defendant's pleading.
IV	Parties	17 to 25	Category IV describes the capacities in which a party or parties can be sued. It maintains the provisions describing the mechanisms for the filing of countersuits, joinder claims, class action lawsuits, and other actions.
V	Discovery	26 to 37	Category V contains the rules governing discovery (e-discovery included). In general, discovery rules help ensure that neither party is subjected to surprises at trial. In many states discovery can occur only through formal request. In contrast, the FRCP requires parties to divulge certain information without a formal discovery request.
VI	Trial	38 to 53	Category VI provides for the plaintiff's right to a trial by jury or by the court. Additionally, this category contains the rules that describe how cases are assigned for trial, how actions are dismissed, and how subpoenas are handled. On December 1, 2006, FRCP 45 (subpoenas) was amended to conform to the e-discovery rules.
VII	Judgment	54 to 63	Category VII maintains the provisions governing legal judgment and costs. Judgment is the decree and any other order from which an appeal lies. Category VII judgment rules maintain provisions for establishing new trials, amending judgments, and the enforcement of judgments.

(continued)

Table 2.1   Federal Rules of Civil Procedure *(continued)*

Category	Category Description	Rules in Category	General Content in Category
VIII	Provisional and final remedies and special proceedings	64 to 71	Category VIII contains the series of rules that provide for the final provision or remedy of a case. The rules covered in this category include seizure of property, injunctions, offers of judgment, and execution of judgments.
IX	Special proceedings	72 to 76	Category IX contains the rules governing special civil action proceedings, such as condemnation of real and personal property, magistrate judges, and pretrial orders.
X	District courts and clerks	77 to 80	Category X provides direction concerning the business and operations of the district courts. The rules covered in this category include hours of operation, filing of pleadings and orders, trials and hearings, orders in chambers, procedures for books and records maintained by the clerk, the role of stenographers, and transcripts as evidence.
XI	General provisions	81 to 86	Category XI explains to which proceedings the rules apply (US district courts vs. state courts) and provides direction on their general applicability, jurisdiction and venue, local rules applications, and judges' directives.

law in subsequent chapters but, for the purpose of this chapter, simply note the following:

- Rule 26(a)(1) requires parties to disclose certain information at the outset of litigation.
- Rule 26(f) requires parties to meet and confer before any initial scheduling conference and, prior to that conference, submit a discovery plan to the presiding judge.
- Rule 16(b) authorizes the judge to issue scheduling orders.
- Rule 26(b)(2)(B) establishes two tiers of ESI, distinguishing between accessible and not reasonably accessible ESI.
- Rule 26(b)(2)(C) is the proportionality rule.

- Rule 34(a) allows parties to inspect, copy, test, or sample an adversary's ESI.
- Rule 34(b) addresses the form or forms in which ESI may be requested and produced.
- Rule 37(e), the so-called safe harbor, is intended to protect a party from sanctions when ESI is lost through the routine operation of a computer system.
- Rule 45 governs subpoenas to nonparties and, among other things, adopts the two-tiered standard of Rule 26(b)(2)(B).

The FRCP are not the whole story of electronic discovery. First, there are the Federal Rules of Evidence (FRE), which govern the admissibility of ESI on dispositive motions and trials. Second, there is newly enacted Federal Rule of Evidence 502, which addresses waiver of attorney-client privilege and work product protection.

Third, the US district courts and bankruptcy courts—which are the trial-level federal courts—are permitted, by law, to adopt local rules that supplement the FRCP. Many of these courts have done so or, in the alternative, have created protocols that address electronic discovery. This book will not describe in detail any local rules or protocols. Bear in mind, however, that these vary from court to court and may impose obligations on parties far beyond the FRCP themselves.

Finally, there is the inherent authority of the court. Courts are held to possess power to, among other things, impose sanctions, which are not based on any particular Rule. This authority resides in federal courts and, unless limited by law, state courts. Federal rule, local rule, evidence rule, and inherent authority all operate to regulate electronic discovery.

2.2.2 State and Local Rules

Each state has its own unique rules of civil procedure. Those rules are often largely based on the FRCP and the federal courts' applications of them. The amendments to the federal rules have prompted a number of states to address electronic discovery. Additionally, a number of local e-discovery rules exist within the states. Since enactment of the FRCP, the states have, generally speaking, addressed e-discovery in three ways:

1. Several have adopted the December 1, 2006, amendments to the FRCP.
2. Some have adopted one or more of the amendments. Idaho, for example, adopted the language of Rule 34.

3. Others have gone their own way and created unique rules. For example, Texas adopted Rule 196.4, which shifts the cost of production of ESI from the producing to the requesting party. (This reverses the presumption in federal courts that producing parties bear their own costs).

Other commentators have suggested that "few state discovery regimes place as much mandatory emphasis on electronic discovery as the federal rules now do" and that "state courts are viewed as the forum where electronic discovery tends to be less extensive and less burdensome" (Allman 2010). States continue to adopt statutes or rules that address electronic discovery (such as California and New York have recently done) and electronic disputes certainly are found there.

2.2.2.1 Establishing Uniformity in State and Local Rules

After months of evaluation and discussion, in September 2005, the Judicial Conference Committee on Rules of Practice and Procedure suggested that adoption of the 2006 Federal Amendments would help to bring about uniformity of practice within the federal court system as well as to forestall the ever increasing numbers of diverse local e-discovery rules (JCCRPP 2005).

The Judicial Conference Committee further stated, "Without national rules adequate to address the issues raised by electronic discovery, a patchwork of rules and requirements is likely to develop," and will result in "uncertainty, expense, delays and burdens" that would ultimately be imposed upon both small organizations and litigants as well as upon larger public and private organizations (JCCRPP 2005).

2.2.2.2 The Uniform Rules Relating to the Discovery of Electronically Stored Information

Concurrent with the drafting of the federal amendments by the Civil Rules Advisory Committee, another national law group known as the **Uniform Law Commission (ULC)**'s **National Conference of Commissioners on Uniform State Laws (NCCUSL)** was also discussing and drafting a separate set of rules for the discovery of electronically stored information and possible enactment at the state level. Following years of study and discussion by ULC, on June 17, 2005, then Chairman Rex Blackburn, in his role as chairman of the NCCUSL Study Committee, said this about e-discovery rules at the state level: "The adoption of . . . uniform rules would provide the benefit of decisional law of other jurisdictions whose courts have considered a particular issue" (Allman 2010).

Two years later, on August 2, 2007, at the 116th meeting of the ULC, the NCCUSL approved this independent set of rules for electronic discovery known today as **Uniform Rules Relating to the Discovery of Electronically Stored Information** (NCCUSL 2007). The intent of the enactment of the Uniform Rules was to provide the states with a set of rules regarding mandatory conferences and reporting, rules governing scope and form of discovery, limitations on sanctions, rules covering claims of privilege, and rules for discovery directed at third parties. The Uniform Rules mirror the spirit, direction, and language of the 2006 amendments to the FRCP and today, many states consider them to be a significant influence and resource to guide and help bridge the gap between the FRCP mandates and state-specific requirements for their own state rules. State governments as well as the District of Columbia, Puerto Rico, and the US Virgin Islands have been appointed independent commissioners to research, draft, advise, and promote enactment of uniform state laws in areas where uniformity is desirable and practical.

2.2.2.3 Additional Resources for State and Local Courts and Judges

There are other well-known resources that also currently serve as references and educational resourses for state and local courts and judges in the discovery of electronically stored information:

- US Conference of Chief Justices—Guidelines for State Trial Courts re Discovery of Electronically-Stored Information—These guidelines were developed to help reduce uncertainty in state court litigation and stimulate the thinking of state rules revision committees. The Guidelines are also used to help identify the issues and factors that may be considered by trial judges faced with a dispute over e-discovery. They are not intended to be treated as model rules for incorporation into a state's procedural scheme; rather, they were developed only to offer guidance to those faced with addressing the practical problems of the digital age.
- *Managing Discovery of Electronically Stored Information: A Pocket Guide for Judges*—This pocket guide was developed to help judges manage the discovery of ESI. It covers issues unique to the discovery of ESI, including its scope, allocation of costs, form of production, waiver of privilege and work product protection, preservation of data, and spoliation.
- Best practice organizations—Legal think tanks and industry standards groups commonly referenced and cited by judges and the legal profession with regard to electronic discovery practice and standards:
  - **The Sedona Conference**—A 501(c)(3) research and educational institute comprised of academics, industry experts, lawyers, and

judges dedicated to the advancement of law and policy in the areas of antitrust law, intellectual property rights, and complex litigation.

- American Bar Association: Science and Technology Section—The Electronic Discovery and Digital Evidence Committee (EDDE) of the Section of Science and Technology Law of the American Bar Association brings together practitioners, technologists, and prominent judges to discuss and publish ideas about electronic discovery and digital evidence.

- Seventh Circuit Electronic Discovery Pilot Program—A multi-year, multiphase project initiated on October 1, 2009, to reduce the burden and cost of electronic discovery in litigation pending in the federal district courts of Illinois, Indiana, and Wisconsin (SCEDC 2009). The purpose of this pilot program was to establish a "process to develop, implement, evaluate, and improve pretrial litigation procedures that would provide fairness and justice to all parties while seeking to reduce the cost and burden of electronic discovery consistent with Rule 1 of the Federal Rules of Civil Procedure." Phase one of the pilot program was completed on May 1, 2010; phase two of the program ran from July 1, 2010, until May 1, 2011 (SCEDC 2009, 2010).

■ In addition to the best practice organizations named above, there are other organizations that benchmark and evaluate the process by which electronic discovery is accomplished and the technologies used to support it. A summary of these benchmarking organizations is outlined below.

- **The Electronic Discovery Reference Model (EDRM)**—An industry group to develop and establish practical guidelines and standards for electronic discovery. The EDRM was established in 2005 as a result of the identification in 2003 and 2004 that there was a lack of standards and guidelines for legal technologies used in discovery.

- Socha-Gelbmann Electronic Discovery Survey—An independent electronic discovery survey, conducted annually, which examines the size, scope, and growth of the electronic discovery market (Socha and Gelbmann 2004).

2.2.2.4 Status of Adoption of e-Discovery Rules by the States

Now, years later, roughly two-thirds of the states have established e-discovery provisions, in one form or another, in their state or local civil procedures or codes. Recent developments in the states such as the June 29, 2009, enactment the Electronic Discovery Act (EDA) by the state of California (2009) and the petition filed with the state supreme court by the Wisconsin Judicial Council proposing amendments to state statutes based upon (or consistent with) the 2006 amendments suggest that the acceptance of the Federal Amendments is being achieved within state courts and there will be further efforts among the remaining states to adopt e-discovery rules based upon the 2006 Federal Amendments and/or the Uniform Rules or some combination thereof.

The great majority of litigation in the United States is conducted in state or local courts and not in federal court. Therefore, for now, the primary focus of this book is on electronic discovery in federal courts because of the comprehensive approach to electronic discovery articulated by the rules and case law and because, but for local rules, electronic discovery is somewhat uniform across the federal courts.

2.3 Legal Process

In US district courts, an action begins with the filing of a complaint, which is then served on the defendant or defendants. As will be discussed later, service may be the event that triggers an obligation on a defendant to preserve relevant ESI—as well as paper. Plainly, a plaintiff's obligation to preserve—which is not often discussed—arises earlier than the filing of the complaint.

All litigation proceeds through stages, as depicted in figure 2.1. A defendant may choose to answer a complaint served on it or may move to dismiss the complaint for any one of a number of reasons described in Rule 12(b). Should it move, discovery may or may not be stayed (that is, either no or only limited discovery may be conducted until the motion is decided). At some point, parties will be required under Rule 26(f) to meet and confer and to submit a discovery plan to the judge who will preside over discovery, either a US magistrate judge or a US district judge. Disclosures will be made by the parties under Rule 26(a)(1). The presiding judge will issue a scheduling order, which will, among other things, control the timing and scope of discovery, be it electronic in nature or otherwise. Discovery may also extend to the production of expert reports for use at trial. Summary judgment motions may be made at some point and, in absence an award of summary judgment or settlement, the action will proceed to trial.

This description of the course of litigation is, of course, simplified. It is important to note, however, that ESI is likely to be central to each phase of litigation. Attorneys must consult with their clients before filing a complaint on the client's behalf and ESI relevant to the decision to file and the allegations of the

Figure 2.1   Stages of litigation

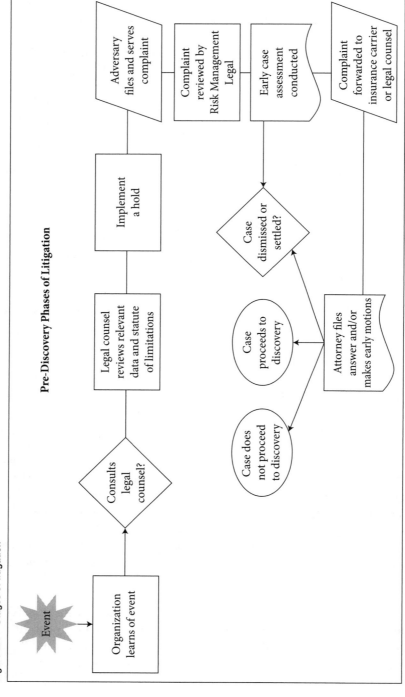

Pre-Discovery Phases of Litigation

complaint must be reviewed by the attorney. The same holds true when an answer to the complaint is filed or a motion to dismiss is made.

Rule 26(a)(1) disclosures may include ESI. Topics to be discussed at the meet and confer and at scheduling conferences will most likely include ESI and electronic discovery, along with expert reports and disclosures. ESI may be used for and against dispositive motions and at trials. Thus, electronic discovery, which includes the preservation, collection, review, and use of ESI, pervades litigation from before its start until the end.

2.3.1 Preservation vs. Production

There is one fundamental point to be made with regard to electronic discovery and discovery in general: The duty to *preserve* relevant information is distinct from the duty to *produce* that information, and the former is likely to encompass more information than the latter. Why?

Once a decision is made by a plaintiff to file a complaint or service of process is made on a defendant, that party has an obligation to preserve relevant information. The determination of the scope of that duty (in other words, how much information must be preserved) is usually made unilaterally, that is, there are no discussions about scope made in the first instance between parties. Absent some agreement, and given the attorney's concern to protect his or her client, scope may be interpreted broadly. The scope of preservation is one of the topics that should be addressed at the initial Rule 26(f) meet and confer and, unless agreed to by the parties, presented to the presiding judge at the earliest opportunity.

That being said, a party may preserve information that is relevant to the issues raised by a particular litigation *but* that need not be produced. The distinction must be borne in mind.

2.3.2 Impact of the Rules Relating to Discovery of ESI

The FRCP did not specifically address electronic discovery before December 1, 2006. Nevertheless, before that date, parties routinely requested and produced ESI and fought over electronic discovery. Indeed, a number of important decisions on electronic discovery preceded December 1, 2006, the most well-known being a series of decisions written by Judge Shira A. Scheindlin of the US District Court for the Southern District of New York in the *Zubulake v. UBS Warburg*, 220 F.R.D. 212 (S.D.N.Y. 2010) litigation.

In any event, we operate under the FRCP today. These, together with local rules, evidence rules, inherent authority, and case law, provide the framework within which parties engage in electronic discovery. After a look at the implications of electronic discovery for healthcare professionals, we turn to discussion of this framework in some detail. Remember, however, that the discussion will be general, that no legal advice is intended to be given, and that the reader should consult with his or her attorneys for that advice.

2.4 Advent of e-Discovery in Healthcare

The United States spends 16 percent of the gross domestic product (GDP) on healthcare, compared with 8 to 10 percent in most major industrialized nations. In September 2010, the Office of the Actuary in the Centers for Medicare and Medicaid Services (CMS) released a revised forecast of the annual projections of healthcare spending in the United States following the passage of the Patient Protection and Affordable Care Act (PPACA, Affordable Care Act). The purpose of these revised projections was to isolate the impact of healthcare reform and the necessary legislative and regulatory changes that occurred subsequent to CMS's publication of the initial 2009–2019 projections.

Outlined in the following paragraphs is an adaptation from the CMS Office of the Actuary forecast of National Health Expenditure Projections in the United States from 2009–2019 (CMS 2010).

2.4.1 National US Health Expenditure Projections 2009–2019

Growth in national health expenditures (NHE) in the United States over the coming decade is expected to be slightly higher as a result of the implementation of the Affordable Care Act, as well as other relevant legislative and regulatory changes. Average annual growth in NHE for 2009 through 2019 is expected to be 6.3 percent, 0.2 percent faster than pre-reform estimates. NHE as a share of GDP is expected to be 19.6 percent by 2019, or 0.3 percentage points higher than projected before the enactment of healthcare reform. Projected growth in NHE for 2010 is higher than previously estimated by 1.2 percent for a total of 5.1 percent. Conversely, growth in NHE for 2011 is projected to be 4.2 percent, or 1.0 percent slower than the previous estimate.

Because many of the major Affordable Care Act provisions will go into effect in 2014, substantive differences in projected growth of NHE compared to estimates made pre-reform are anticipated. An expansion of Medicaid coverage (to all persons under age 65 in households with incomes less than 138 percent of the federal poverty level), combined with the advent of state-level health insurance exchanges, is expected to result in NHE growth of 9.2 percent in 2014 (2.6 percent higher than projected before reform was passed). Over the latter stages of the projection period (2015 through 2019), the impact of the Affordable Care Act on health coverage is anticipated to continue as more people acquire, or shift, into new or different coverage. By 2019, 92.7 percent of the US population is expected to have health insurance (an increase of 10 percent) driven, in part, by growth in Medicaid, which when combined with the Children's Health Insurance Program (CHIP), is projected to cover 82 million persons. Also by 2019, 30.6 million people are expected to be enrolled in Health Insurance Exchange plans.

In 2014, private health insurance (PHI) expenditure growth is projected to reach 12.8 percent, 6.1 percent higher than the pre-Affordable Care Act estimate, as a projected 16 million people sign up for coverage through the state-level health insurance exchange plans. For 2015 through 2019, PHI spending is expected to average 6.6 percent, or 0.3 percent faster than was projected before health reform was enacted, in part due to the continued transition of many into the exchange plans who were previously uninsured. In 2014, out-of-pocket (OOP) spending is projected to decline by 1.1 percent as the major provisions of the Affordable Care Act are implemented and millions of people, many of whom were previously uninsured, attain health coverage through Medicaid or the health insurance exchanges. Prior to passage of the Affordable Care Act, OOP spending growth was expected to be 6.4 percent.

By 2018, OOP spending growth is expected to accelerate to 9.6 percent, about 4 percent higher than that expected before reform was passed. The relatively higher growth in OOP expenditures in 2018 reflects greater cost-sharing as employers are expected to scale back the generosity of the coverage they offer to minimize their exposure to the excise tax applicable to high-cost insurance plans.

Principally due to the expansion of Medicaid eligibility and additional CHIP funding in 2014, Medicaid and CHIP enrollment is expected to increase by 21.8 million people with total spending projected to grow 17.4 percent (11.1 percent faster than the pre-reform projection). The federal government is expected to finance most of the care for the new Medicaid beneficiaries through a 100-percent Federal Medical Assistance Percentage, which will phase down to 90 percent in 2020 and thereafter.

Beginning December 1, 2010, there was a 23 percent reduction in Medicare physician payment rates.

Provisions of the Affordable Care Act are projected to result in a lower average annual Medicare spending growth rate for 2012 through 2019 (6.2 percent), 1.3 percent lower than pre-reform estimates. The relatively lower projected Medicare expenditure growth rate reflects reduced annual payment updates for most Medicare services, substantial reductions to managed care plan payments, and the creation of the Independent Payment Advisory Board.

In addition to the passage of the PPACA, wide variations in cost and quality across the United States underlie these national trends, indicating opportunities to increase efficiency. On June 15, 2009, six months following his January 8, 2009 speech at George Mason University, President Obama addressed the American Medical Association in Chicago, President Obama spoke once again about the future of healthcare and the investment in electronic health records (Obama 2009). Some of his comments are provided in figure 2.2.

Before ESI, under common law, the traditional, paper-based document discovery process was considered to be rather uncomplicated; yet, the relative straightforwardness of the traditional discovery procedural obligations in a paper world did not imply a scarcity of resources required to complete the process. Still, the costs of discovery will not be reduced as a result of the federal amendments and technology, but rather are projected to continue to increase (Socha and Gelbmann 2009a).

The authors predict the trend for growth in the e-discovery marketplace will continue to grow and evolve dramatically through 2014, especially within the healthcare sector. The impact of the Health Information Technology for Economic and Clinical Health Act (HITECH) is going to continue to drive the adoption of EHRs and the establishment of HIEs. Regulatory compliance initiatives will remain in the forefront of the healthcare industry through ongoing recovery audit contractor (RAC) audits and other compliance initiatives such as Stark compliance reviews. The industry's migration from the ICD-9 to ICD-10 coding system will cause healthcare providers to update their current information systems in preparation for a major overhaul in the way in which healthcare claims are coded and processed. Finally, beginning in 2014, according to CMS estimates, the United States will experience a 9.2 percent growth in NHEs while private health insurance growth is projected to be 12.8 percent when an estimated 16 million people are expected to sign up for healthcare coverage through the state-level health insurance exchange plans.

Figure 2.2   Healthcare reform

Components of President Obama's Speech to American Medical Association (AMA)—Chicago, June 15, 2009

"[W]e are spending over $2 trillion a year on health care—almost 50 percent more per person than the next most costly nation. And yet, for all this spending, more of our citizens are uninsured; the quality of our care is often lower; and we aren't any healthier. In fact, citizens in some countries that spend less than we do are actually living longer than we do. . . .

Health care reform is the single most important thing we can do for America's long-term fiscal health. . . . If we fail to act, one out of every five dollars we earn will be spent on health care within a decade. And in 30 years, it will be about one out of every three. . . .

First, we need to upgrade our medical records by switching from a paper to an electronic system of record keeping. And we have already begun to do this with an investment we made as part of our Recovery Act. . . .

But as important as they are, investments in electronic records and preventive care are just preliminary steps. . . .

We've put about $950 billion on the table—and that doesn't count some of the long-term savings that we think will come about from reform—from medical IT, for example, or increased investment in prevention."

The advantage of electronic information, although a more costly and complicated process when it comes to litigation, is that evolving technologies support modern business practices in healthcare, which parallel other industries. The information tools used for production, preservation, and storage of routine business records increasingly include ESI, which, in turn, provide the basis for modern documents.

2.4.2 The e-Discovery Process within Healthcare

How will the e-discovery process impact the healthcare industry? The answer begins with defining exactly what information is discoverable. The Federal Rules define a document as, "any designated documents or electronically stored information—including writings, drawings, graphs, charts, photographs, sound recordings, images and other data compilations—stored in any medium from which information can be obtained either directly or, if necessary, after translation by the responding party into reasonably usable form" (FRCP 2008).

The FRCP definition of a document coupled with the increasing development and adoption of electronic health records through the passage of the American

Recovery and Reinvestment Act (ARRA) and HITECH Act require that health-care organizations think beyond the traditional definitions of an electronic record or document and consider the entire range of digital information as the potential subject of a discovery order. Simply put, any information in any form that is relevant to the case is potentially discoverable. Does this mean that the healthcare organization is not required to establish a mechanism to retain all electronic information because it is potentially discoverable?

The answer as to when the duty to preserve relevant information begins can be found in *Zubulake v. UBS Warburg*, 220 F.R.D. 212, (S.D.N.Y. 2003). In this decision, the court held that the duty to preserve relevant information begins "at the time the organization knew or should have known that litigation could be reasonably anticipated". In this case, the duty began at the latest when Laura Zubulake filed her Equal Employment Opportunity Commission (EEOC) charge, but through discovery (e-mails and testimony) the court held that there were relevant people at UBS who anticipated litigation in April 2001, and therefore, the duty to preserve evidence essentially began at that time.

Judge Scheindlin revisited *Zubulake* in *Pension Committee of the University of Montreal Pension Plan et al. v. Banc of America Securities LLC*, 2010 WL 184312 (S.D.N.Y. 2010). Finding that a number of plaintiffs had been negligent or grossly negligent in their preservation and collection efforts, the judge imposed a range of sanctions, including adverse inferences. In so doing, Judge Scheindlin provided a detailed review of her holdings in *Zubulake* and explored the relationship between culpability ("state of mind") and burdens of proof. She also criticized parties for their failure to issue written litigation hold notices and cautioned against self-collection by custodians.

Compare and contrast *Pension Committee* to *Rimkus Consulting Group v. Cammarata*, 2010 US Dist. LEXIS (S.D. Tex. 2010). In this major decision, Judge Lee Rosenthal (who was in large part responsible for the 2006 amendments to the Federal Rules of Civil Procedure) imposed sanctions against the defendants for *intentional* destruction of ESI. Judge Rosenthal canvassed the different approaches taken to sanctions among the federal appellate courts regarding the state of mind required for the imposition of sanctions and crafted an adverse inference instruction different from that of Judge Scheindlin in *Pension Committee*.

2.4.2.1 The Scope of Preservation of the Evidence

In the healthcare industry, there are inherently higher risks than those of most other industries. Therefore, the question often arises whether a healthcare provider must establish policies that require every piece or paper or e-mail be retained because of the inherently higher risk of litigation as opposed to other industries. Generally, in the healthcare industry, as is the case of other industries, a party is under duty to preserve information in accordance with federal and state regulations, and also when it knows, or reasonably should know that it is in possession of information relevant to an action. The same goes for information that is reasonably calculated to lead to the discovery of admissible evidence and is likely to be requested during discovery, and/or is the subject of a pending discovery request (see *Zubulake*).

Today's EHR is undergoing a period of rapid transformation and along with it so are the responsibilities of the legal, HIM, and IT professionals. Traditionally, the HIM department served as the custodian or keeper of the record and was responsible for the release of information within the organization (production of copies of paper-based medical records), while the IT department was responsible for maintenance of the technical infrastructure of the organization and generally did not become too involved in discovery and/or the release of information. In today's digital realm, however, e-mail messages, voice files, mobile device messages, server log files, HL7 message codes, and other types of data (such as metadata) are also targets of legal investigations.

As a result of efforts to overhaul the healthcare system and the rising costs of EDD, the process of discovery within the healthcare industry will soon change drastically. These changes the healthcare industry will undergo will result not only from the overhaul of the US healthcare system, but also as a result of the enactment of FRCP amendments, increasing adoption of e-discovery rules at the state and local levels, and the advancements that will be realized in the development of electronic health records. These changes, coupled with requirements that healthcare organizations comply with an ever-growing list of regulatory compliance demands and federal and state rules, will cause the healthcare industry to seek organizational solutions to compliance requirements. Healthcare organizations will change and are being challenged to revisit their care delivery methodologies and the way in which they manage and store information. Legal counsel and health information professionals must begin discussions focused on ESI that directly relates to healthcare delivery (for example, integrated electronic health record systems, patient-physician communications, voice mail, employee and patient tracking tools, as well as routine organizational information stored electronically, organizational e-mail, and document management tools).

2.5 Cooperation in Discovery

The FRCP, coupled with the ever increasing adoption of state and local rules governing e-discovery, provide the foundation for the electronic discovery process. But in order to be effective the e-discovery rules will only go so far—another factor equally important as the FRCP is the communication that occurs between legal counsel and the judiciary. On October 7, 2008, after conducting a multiyear, multipronged effort designed to establish a set of guidelines for the promotion of greater cooperation in e-discovery, The Sedona Conference officially released a five-page, groundbreaking document known as the Cooperation Proclamation. This simple and concise document is one of the most important pieces of guidance established on the subject of discovery, with a purpose of assisting the courts in securing the just, speedy, and inexpensive determination of civil cases, and to promote whenever possible, the early resolution of disputes regarding the discovery of electronically stored information. The Cooperation Proclamation has been endorsed by judiciaries across the country and has become a national call "to promote open and forthright information sharing, dialogue (internal and external), and training and development of practical tools to facilitate cooperative, collaborative, transparent discovery" (The Sedona Conference 2008). Since its release, the Cooperation Proclamation has been cited in at least a dozen judicial opinions, and the courts appear to be sending strong messages to legal counsel that when it comes to e-discovery, legal counsel must:

1. Remain cognizant of the scope and intent of Federal Rule of Civil Procedure 1—". . . the just, speedy, and inexpensive determination of every action and proceeding."
2. Take measures to carefully preserve relevant information.
3. Tailor the e-discovery request to the matter at hand, after conducting careful research in advance.
4. Provide a factual basis for objections.
5. Communicate and cooperate with opposing counsel.

Summarized below are recent and notable opinions in which the judiciary has cited the Cooperation Proclamation:

1. *Mancia v. Mayflower Textile Services Co.*, 2008 WL 4595275 (D. Md. Oct. 15, 2008)—A collective action filed by six laundry employees for payment of wages under the Fair Labor Standards Act of 1938 and Maryland state law that involves an e-discovery dispute, which arose because the plaintiffs served extensive discovery requests on the defendants, while the defendants responded to a number of the requests with "boilerplate objections."

   • Judge Paul Grimm handed down this groundbreaking opinion shortly after the official release of The Sedona Conference's Cooperation Proclamation and his opinion provides broad principles, which are applicable to any discovery process. Judge Grimm held that the defendants failed to sufficiently specify to the court the grounds on which they objected to the discovery requests as required by FRCP 33(b)(2). Further, the court noted that FRCP 26(g)(1) requires counsel to cooperate in e-discovery and that failure to do so can be construed as a violation of the duty of reasonable inquiry prior to certifying demands or responses. The court held that the defendants were most likely in violation of FRCP 26(g)(1) by failing to specify the grounds for their objections.

   • The court expressed concern over the extensive nature of the plaintiffs' discovery request and ordered the parties to meet and confer to determine a discovery budget reflective of what was at stake in the case. Judge Grimm reminded legal counsel that the FRCP impose a duty upon counsel to "behave responsibly during discovery, and to ensure that it is conducted in a way that is consistent 'with the spirit and purposes' of the discovery rules . . ." Counsel were advised to consider the cost and the burden of its discovery requests as well as offer a factual basis for objections. Judge Grimm also reminded legal counsel that the court has the ability to impose sanctions on counsel for violating the rules without justification. The court encourages attorneys to meet early on in discovery in accordance with Rule 26(b)(2)(C) to "discuss the amount and type of discovery and what the amount in controversy is, and how much, what type, and in what sequence, discovery should be conducted so that its cost-to all parties-is proportional to what is at stake in the litigation."

2. *Newman v. Borders*, 257 F.R.D. 1, 3 (D.D.C. April 6, 2009)—A racial profiling case brought by plaintiff Ronald Newman, involving a number of e-discovery disputes, including the cost of attorney's fees that arose because the defendants were not knowledgeable about company policy regarding the retention of e-mail documents. In a motion to compel, the plaintiff sought an additional 30(b)(6) deposition, after the

defendant's representative Lisa Morrow testified that she did not know what "e-mails were searched, what search terms were used, whose e-mails were searched, whether received mail was searched in addition to sent mail or e-mail." The court held that rather than allow a second 30(b)(6) deposition to be taken, the court directed the defendant to file an affidavit with responses to specific questions posed by the court.

- Judge John M. Facciola ordered the defendant to file an affidavit from a knowledgeable Borders representative who could provide adequate responses to the following questions:
  1. What kind of e-mail system does Borders have (such as Outlook, Lotus Notes, or proprietary)?
  2. Is that system programmed to delete e-mails automatically that have been in existence for a certain period of time? If the answer is yes, what is the period of time and was that system shut off or kept on after the incident involving the plaintiff?
  3. Does Borders have a policy that requires either the retention or deletion of e-mails and, if so, what is the policy and is it in writing? If it is in writing, it will be appended to the affidavit.
  4. Was it necessary to make efforts to prevent the deletion of e-mails after the incident involving plaintiff, and, if so, what efforts were made?
  5. Is Borders aware of the deletion of any e-mails pertaining to the incident involving the plaintiff?
  6. Who was responsible for searching for any e-mails pertaining to the incident involving the plaintiff?
  7. How did this person or these persons conduct the search? What receptacles of electronically stored information were searched? Network servers, individual hard drives?
  8. If individual hard drives were searched, whose were they?
  9. Did the search involve the use of keywords and, if so, what were they?

In *Newman v. Borders*, the court made specific commentary about the scope and intent of FRCP 1. On April 6, 2009, as he handed down his opinion on the plaintiff's request for an additional 30(b)(6) deposition, Judge Facciola said:

I also have the unquestioned right (if not the duty) to bring discovery disputes to a just and inexpensive conclusion. Fed. R. Civ. P. 1. I am stunned by how much time and effort has been spent on discovery in a case that involves confrontation between plaintiff and a store detective that could not have taken that much time. I am well past being convinced that the potential legal fees in this case, thanks to the many discovery disputes, will dwarf the potential recovery, if there is one. The time has come (it may have come and gone) for me to bring this particular controversy about e-mail to a quick and merciful end without another costly deposition.

The *Newman v. Borders* case provides a good example of how litigation costs can spiral out of control when no attempt is made to discuss and manage costs early on in the litigation process. Relying upon FRCP 1, Judge Facciola reminded legal counsel of its ethical obligation to abide by the scope and intent of the FRCP and was able to limit some of the costs of discovery, even though under 42 U.S.C. §1988, civil rights litigation attorneys can recover their fees.

Although the court relied upon Rule 1 to limit the scope and costs of discovery in a relatively straightforward matter, legal counsel should not overlook the important roles FRCP 26(b)(2)(B) and 26(b)(2)(C) play in discovery, as Rule 26(b)(2)(B) provides a mechanism by which a party may not provide discovery of ESI from sources the party identifies as "not reasonably accessible because of undue burden or cost," while Rule 26(b)(2)(C) authorizes the court to limit the extent of discovery otherwise allowed.

2.6 Case Analysis and the Complexities of the e-Discovery Rule Applied

At this time there are very few cases involving e-discovery and EHRs. For healthcare to gain insights into the rule applied and the thought process of the court, it is useful to understand non-healthcare cases and the issues that arose. To help illustrate the application of the e-discovery rule, we will examine the case *Capitol Records, Inc. et al. v. MP3tunes, LLC*, 2009 WL 2568431 (S.D.N.Y. 2009) and explore not only what the court has to say about cooperation in discovery, but also analyze the court's application of Rule 26(b)(2)(B), screening for relevancy, custodianship, privilege, information systems infrastructure, e-discovery software applications, and the burden and costs of production of paper records in the future.

1. *Capitol Records, Inc. et al. v. MP3tunes, LLC*, 2009 WL 2568431 (S.D.N.Y August 13, 2009)—A music copyright infringement filed by five entities (the EMI Labels) that contends defendant MP3tunes infringed their music copyrights through the operation of two websites, www.sideload.com and www.mp3tunes.com. The cases involve

several e-discovery disputes that arose because the plaintiffs initially produced a discovery request, which the defendants argued was "overbroad and unduly burdensome." The initial request from plaintiffs' counsel is summarized as follows:

- All documents concerning the functionality, development, and operation of MP3tunes' storage of user files; sideload feature; and streaming, play, download, and locker-sync features
- All communications involving MP3tunes' principal and three other persons concerning the "functionality, structure, operations, or source of MP3tunes"

At a pretrial conference on February 18, 2009, Judge Frank Maas concluded that the plaintiffs' reference to the "operation" of the MP3tunes' website made this request overly broad and urged the parties to "develop agreed search terms which would focus on the macro level of MP3tunes' software by requiring MP3tunes to produce documents relating to the design of its site" (*Capitol Records v. MP3tunes* (S.D.N.Y. 2009)).

At the pretrial conference counsel for MP3tunes expressed agreement with a proposed course of action for search terms and stated to Judge Maas, "We are fine with developing search terms for e-mails if we strike the word operation, just about the design and development of the . . . software" (*Capitol Records v. MP3tunes* (S.D.N.Y. 2009)).

Subsequently, however, rather than sitting down with the plaintiffs' counsel to agree on the scope of the e-discovery search parameters and terms, MP3tunes' counsel unilaterally directed his client to conduct a search of MP3tunes' e-mails in April 2009 using the word "design" as the only search term (*Capitol Records v. MP3tunes* (S.D.N.Y. 2009)).

- Judge Maas questioned the wisdom of the decision of MP3tunes' legal counsel and held a telephone conference on June 15, 2009, to discuss this approach and scope of the e-discovery request. Defendants' legal counsel told Judge Maas that, "he actually considered this one-word search to be 'overly broad.'"
- Judge Maas stated that after he "observed that MP3tunes' unilateral decision regarding its search reflected a failure to heed Magistrate Judge Andrew Peck's recent 'wake-up call' regarding the need for cooperation concerning e-discovery" (Judge Maas cited *William A. Gross Constr. Assocs, Inc. v. American Mfrs. Mut. Ins. Co.*, 256 F.R.D. 134 [S.D.N.Y. 2009] and The Sedona Conference's Cooperation Proclamation).

MP3tunes' counsel apologized for not having also used the word 'development' as a search term.

- Following his telephone conversation with the defendant's attorney, Judge Maas directed counsel to confer further with plaintiffs' counsel in an attempt to reach agreement on search terms, which "would elicit e-mails concerning the design and development of MP3tunes' software." Judge Maas directed the parties to confer and then submit to him a list of their agreed and disputed search terms.

- Following their meet and confer, Judge Maas noted that the parties were able to agree upon 9 search terms, while an additional 30 terms remained in dispute. MP3tunes argued "that many of the additional search terms sought by the plaintiffs (such as stream or download) were so integral to their business that they would generate 'thousands upon thousands' of responsive e-mails."

- MP3tunes ultimately entered an objection on relevance and burden grounds in that the plaintiffs were "improperly seeking to increase the number of e-mail custodians whose files had to be searched from seven to 13 and requested to add six low-level employees who had no control over software design or development" (*Capitol Records v. MP3tunes* (S.D.N.Y. 2009)).

The *Capitol Records v. MP3tunes* case provides an excellent example of how important it is for parties to meet and confer throughout the process. Had the parties focused their attention on discussing their differences, rather than drafting dueling epistles for submission to the court, MP3tunes undoubtedly would have realized that the EMI Labels were not asking to be provided with a transaction history for each search term, so long as they received assurances that the search methodology that MP3tunes employed would lead to the production of all responsive e-mails. As noted above, now that that has been clarified, MP3tunes no longer argues that the mere task of conducting the searches sought by the EMI Labels is unduly burdensome. Nevertheless, MP3tunes apparently adheres to its claims that the 30 disputed search terms will not lead to discovery of admissible evidence, and that they should not be required to search the files of six low-level employees who were not architects of the MP3tunes software development program.

2. Application of Rule 26(b)(2)(B)—Unlike MP3tunes, the EMI Labels continue to suggest that the discovery sought by their adversary is unduly burdensome. Rule 26(b)(2)(B) of the Federal Rules of Civil Procedure states that a "party need not provide discovery of [ESI] for sources that the party identifies as not reasonably accessible because

of undue burden or cost." Pursuant to the rule, when an adverse party seeks to compel the production of such material, the party resisting discovery must show that the material sought is "not reasonably accessible because of undue burden or cost." If that showing is made, the burden shifts to the requesting party to show good cause for the production of not-reasonably accessible ESI. In deciding whether the requisite showing has been made, the FRCP require the court to consider—as it must in any discovery dispute—whether (i) "the discovery sought is unreasonably cumulative or duplicative, or can be obtained from some other source that is more convenient, less burdensome, or less expensive," (ii) "the party seeking discovery has had ample opportunity to obtain the information by discovery in the action," or (iii) "the burden or expense of proposed discovery outweighs its likely benefit, considering the needs of the case, the amount in controversy, the parties' resources, the importance of the issues at stake in the action, and the importance of the discovery in resolving the issues."

3. Relevancy and custodianship—It may well be, as MP3tunes argues, that only the more senior present or former MP3tunes employees sent or received e-mails that are relevant to the issues in this case. By the same token, however, it also may be true that employees at that level took care not to say anything incriminating and that lower-level employees were less guarded in their e-mail communications. Although EMI Labels may have increased the size of the group that they are asking to have searched, MP3tunes has not shown that the production of all of the requested employees' e-mail communications would be unduly burdensome or that a search of their files would not potentially yield relevant information. MP3tunes is therefore directed to search the files of each of the custodians identified by the plaintiffs.

4. Privilege—Finally, turning to the privilege argument, it obviously is correct that at some point in most civil suits the focus of the principals' discussions shifts from the acts or omissions giving rise to the claims to the prosecution or defense of the lawsuit. Here, that transition certainly would have taken place by the time this action was filed, but arguably may have occurred earlier since the parties had a prior skirmish in California. Therefore, to minimize the burden on MP3tunes, the court will not require it to record on its privilege log any attorney-client communications or work product documents created after the date the California declaratory judgment action was filed. This same privilege log cutoff date will also apply to the EMI Labels' e-mail production.

5. Information systems infrastructure: e-Discovery software and production of paper records in the future—The EMI Labels, which employ approximately 120 people in the global infrastructure services, filed and "probably have [two] terabytes" of data on their servers, host no e-discovery software on their servers, and apparently are unable to conduct centralized e-mail searches of groups of users without downloading them to a separate file and relying on the services of an outside vendor. The day undoubtedly will come when burden arguments based on a large organization's lack of internal e-discovery software will be received about as well as the contention that a party should be spared from retrieving paper documents because it had filed them sequentially, but in no apparent groupings, in an effort to avoid the added expense of file folders or indices. Nonetheless, at this stage of development of e-discovery case law, the court cannot say that the EMI Labels' failure to acquire such software and to configure its systems to permit centralized e-mail searches means that its burdensomeness arguments should be disregarded. I therefore conclude that the EMI Labels' e-mail files that MP3tunes seeks to search are not reasonably accessible within the meaning of Rule 26(b)(2)(B).

The *Capitol Records v. MP3tunes* case provides not only an excellent example of how important it is for the parties to meet and confer early on and throughout the course of litigation, but also provides notice to EHR vendors and information management professionals about the role and future direction of litigation involving the EHR.

2.7 Considerations and Questions for Healthcare Information Professionals

Capitol Records v. MP3tunes (S.D.N.Y. 2009) provides a glimpse into the roles and expectations of legal counsel and HIM and IT professionals in the future. The definition of the records custodian or keeper of the record is changing and the HITECH Act will forever change the way in which health information is managed and exchanged. The paper-based medical record will soon become obsolete and expensive to maintain and it is inconceivable to think that one day the paper-based medical record may not meet FRE 1002 (the best evidence rule) because most of today's medical records are hybrid in nature (combination of paper and electronic forms) and one could argue that it is the not true original record as it resides in a form both static and dynamic in nature.

Today's paper-based record, when entered into evidence, can and will tell a very different story than does the EHR. To illustrate, the paper-based medical record contains handwritten entries (often illegible), which are timed and dated by the author, while the EHR is comprised of entries both human text and machine-readable text. The EHR contains a wealth of apparent and non-apparent information (such as metadata) that can more easily and efficiently be searched, which theoretically can portray a more accurate picture of who knew what when than that of the paper-based medical record. The time and date signatures of the authors of the EHR can much more easily be verified and authenticated than the handwritten signatures of authors in the paper-based medical record. Although there has been very little case law to date that has challenged the authenticity and admissibility of the EHR, those concepts and case law will be discussed in chapter 3.

HIM professionals have an important role to play in the future EHR environment and the litigation process—they will become the key in helping legal counsel understand how information is managed within the organization and where to cull and search for relevant information. The e-HIM initiative is helping to pave the way and the changes in the management of health records should not be feared, but embraced. The HIM professional of the future will be an information manager rather than the records custodian or keeper of the records. In the e-discovery realm, the HIM professional should be called upon early on in the litigation process to help legal counsel better understand the information infrastructure and location, source, and types of relevant information. This allows legal counsel to meet and confer with opposing counsel to establish a discovery plan versus being served with a subpoena for the production of records.

IT professionals will have an equally important role to play in the future EHR environment and the litigation process—they will also be key in helping legal counsel understand how information is managed within the organization, but from a perspective different than that of HIM. The IT professional will be responsible for ensuring compliance with the organization's information system infrastructure and operational requirements. The IT professional will be the expert knowledgeable in how the systems operate, how electronic data are maintained, and the costs and burdens associated with the location and production of information from the systems. HIM and IT professionals should possess complementary skills and both should work collaboratively with legal counsel in the development of discovery plans.

As is demonstrated by the Seventh Circuit Pilot Program, there is growing recognition among the judiciary for the adoption principles, guidelines, and/

or rules regarding the discovery of electronically stored information. To date, over half of the states have established their own sets of rules, many based in whole or in part on the FRCP.

During the next decade, the healthcare industry will realize some of its biggest changes and challenges with regard to the discovery of electronically stored information. Through HITECH, $36 billion of funding has been authorized to put in place an electronic HIT infrastructure and the US Department of Health and Human Services (HHS) has been granted statutory authority for HIT initiatives. The legislation authorizes funds for administrative structures and processes for developing interoperable systems, as well as funding and incentives to deploy the electronic infrastructure and encourage its adoption. As the healthcare delivery landscape changes and evolves, so too will its technological systems. In a sense, healthcare is now experiencing "a rise of the 'information ecosystem'" (Paul 2008). Efforts are increasing both nationally and within the court system for the discovery of electronically stored information to become a straightforward routine way of life, rather than the exception that it currently is.

Key Questions/Considerations

1. In addition to the FRCP, what state and local rules are in place that govern the discovery of ESI?
2. Have any of the judges within the jurisdiction established their own set of principles, rules, or orders for the discovery of ESI?
3. How well do legal counsel (internal and external) communicate and cooperate with one another?
4. What is legal counsel's working relationship with IT and HIM?
5. Is the information management plan current, and if requested by opposing counsel legal counsel, will it assist good faith operations?
6. What requirements will or should be placed upon the EHR vendor to provide functionality that will support e-discovery?
   a. Does our EHR have the capability to do a legal hold and if so, who is responsible for monitoring and managing the legal hold?
7. What e-mail system(s) are in place within the organization?
   a. What are the retention policies for e-mail?
   b. To what degree is the organization's e-mail system used for differing purposes (for example, personal communication, forwarding business documents, patient care communication that may become part of the medical record)?

c. Who and how will we perform the search and retrieval function of our e-mail systems?

d. To what extent is PHI sent via e-mail and if so, what mechanisms are in place to ensure it is secure?

8. How are our employees educated and trained on the organization's information management policies and procedures?

a. Does staff have awareness about the organization's retention policies and procedures?

9. Is the organization's information management current and can legal counsel defend good faith operations?

10. To what extent will physicians need to be educated on the organization's e-mail and information management policies and procedures?

11. Do the physicians have an awareness of e-discovery?

References

Allman, T. 2010. Personal notes as role of observer to the drafting committee led by Dean Carroll.

Capitol Records, Inc. et al. v. MP3tunes, LLC, 2009 WL 2568431 (S.D.N.Y. 2009).

Centers for Medicare and Medicaid Services. 2010. Office of the Actuary, national health expenditure projections, 2009–2019. https://www.cms.gov/NationalHealth ExpendData/03_NationalHealthAccountsProjected.asp.

Federal Rules of Civil Procedure. 2007. http://www.uscourts.gov/rules/civil2007.pdf.

Federal Rules of Civil Procedure. 2008. http://www.uscourts.gov/rules/CV2008.pdf.

Federal Rule of Civil Procedure 34(a)(1)(A).

Judicial Conference Committee on Rules of Practice and Procedure. 2005. Summary of the Report of the Judicial Conference Committee on Rules of Practice and Procedure. http://www.uscourts.gov/uscourts/rulesandpolicies/rules/Reports/ST09-2005.pdf.

Keehan, S., A. Sisko, C. Truffer, S. Smith, C. Cowan, J. Poisal, and M.K. Clemens. 2008 (Feb. 21). Health spending projections through 2017. Health Affairs—Web Exclusive. W146. http://content.healthaffairs.org/content/27/2/w145.full?sid=7dee5b3f-6f4d-4588-9ae8-6fdfdfe26008.

Mancia v. Mayflower Textile Services Co., 2008 WL 4595275 (D. Md. 2008). Memorandum Opinion. http://www.law.ufl.edu/news/events/ediscovery/documents/mancia_mayflower_abridged.pdf.

National Conference of Commissioners on Uniform State Laws. 2007. Uniform Rules Relating to the Discovery of Electronically Stored Information. http://www.law.upenn.edu/bll/archives/ulc/udoera/2007_final.htm.

Newman v. Borders, 257 F.R.D. 1, 3 (D.D.C. 2009). Memorandum Opinion. https://ecf.dcd.uscourts.gov/cgi-bin/show_public_doc?2007cv0492-68/.

Obama, B. 2009 (June 15). Remarks by the President to the Annual Conference of the American Medical Association. Chicago. http://www.whitehouse.gov/the_press_office/Remarks-by-the-President-to-the-Annual-Conference-of-the-American-Medical-Association/.

Paul, G.L. 2008. Foundations of Digital Evidence. Chicago: ABA Publishing.

Pension Committee of the University of Montreal Pension Plan et al. v. Banc of America Securities, LLC, 2010 WL 184312 (S.D.N.Y. 2010).

Rimkus Consulting Grp. v. Cammarata, 2010 US Dist. LEXIS (S.D. Tex. 2010).

The Sedona Conference. 2008. The Sedona Conference Cooperation Proclamation. http://www.thesedonaconference.org/content/tsc_cooperation_proclamation/proclamation.pdf.

Seventh Circuit Electronic Discovery Committee. 2009. Seventh Circuit Electronic Discovery Pilot Program: Statement of Purpose and Preparation of Principles. http://www.ilcd.uscourts.gov/Statement%20-%20Phase%20One.pdf.

Seventh Circuit Electronic Discovery Committee. 2010. Seventh Circuit Electronic Discovery Pilot Program: Report on Phase One. http://www.du.edu/legalinstitute/pdf/Chicago.pdf.

Socha Consulting LLC and Gelbmann & Associates. 2004. Socha-Gelbmann Electronic Discovery Survey. http://www.sochaconsulting.com/Publications/LawTechnologyNews%20Article%208.04.pdf.

Socha, G. and T. Gelbmann. 2009a (Aug. 11). A look at the 2008 Socha-Gelbmann survey. Law Technology News—Web Exclusive. http://www.law.com/jsp/lawtechnologynews/PubArticleLTN.jsp?id=1202423646479&slreturn=1&hbxlogin=1.

Socha, G. and T. Gelbmann. 2009b (Aug. 1). Strange times. Law Technology News. http://www.law.com/jsp/PubArticle.jsp?id=1202435558482.

State of California. 2009. Electronic Discovery Act. http://www.leginfo.ca.gov/pub/09-10/bill/asm/ab_0001-0050/ab_5_bill_20090629_chaptered.pdf.

Zubulake v. UBS Warburg LLC, 220 F.R.D. 212 (S.D.N.Y. 2003).

e-Discovery in Practice

Chapter Objectives

The purpose of this chapter is to identify and provide an understanding of key components of e-discovery that may impact healthcare organizations and their successful support for the process. To help provide an understanding of e-discovery issues, related record management issues and concepts, and illustrative cases are discussed and electronic health record (EHR) standards referenced.

The objectives of this chapter are to:

➡ Understand the importance of retention obligations and how they relate to litigation holds and preservation of electronically stored information
➡ Distinguish the difference between disclosure and discovery
➡ Discuss key aspects of how discovery is conducted and rules that guide decision making
➡ Understand the various forms and forms of production for electronically stored information in EHRs
➡ Explain the concept of privilege
➡ Discuss subpoenas and different court considerations
➡ Evaluate admissibility of healthcare data, custodianship and chain of custody authentication issues, and other evidentiary challenges for the EHR

3.1 Record Retention, the Litigation Hold, and Preservation

There is an interrelationship between records retention policies, the implementation of a litigation hold, and the preservation of electronic and other information pursuant to a hold. Policies allow electronic information to be created and maintained in a manner that suits an organization's business needs. Policies should also include a mechanism to hold, or preserve, information when necessary to comply with litigation obligations.

3.1.1 Records Retention Policies

Every organization must have a records retention policy. Records retention policies further important organizational goals. Among other things, policies enable the organization to:

- Comply with requirements established by statute or regulation for the retention of records
- Maintain business records for operational purposes logically and in a manner suited to the organization's business needs
- Comply with obligations imposed on it to preserve information when required to do so for investigatory, regulatory, or litigation purposes
- Destroy information once that information need no longer be maintained

Records retention policies must have, at the least, these features:

- Consistent application to avoid an inference that particular records were not destroyed due to the ordinary course of business but instead to avoid some legal obligation
- A review mechanism to attempt to ensure that an organization follows its particular policy
- An "off" switch by which destruction can be suspended when necessary

A reasoned and consistently applied retention policy is the first line of defense when an organization finds itself in litigation and is challenged over its retention or destruction of information.

3.1.2 Retention Obligations

A distinction should be drawn between retention and preservation of information. The former arises from duties by statutes or regulations. The latter is a creation of litigation. Examples of obligations for healthcare information retention that are independent of litigation and are defined by jurisdictional and compliance rules are discussed in chapter 5.

Statutes and regulations create obligations to retain certain information for specific periods of time. These obligations should be recognized by, and incorporated into, records retention policies. It should be noted, however, that these obligations may be trumped by the need to preserve information for the purposes of litigation.

3.1.3 EHR Records Management and Evidentiary Support (RM-ES) Standard—Retention and Destruction

As healthcare organizations implement and maintain EHR systems for their medical records, the system must have the capability to address record retention needs and requirements. As initially introduced in chapter 1, the HL7 RM-ES (2010) standard for EHR systems requires retention and destruction record management functions.

> IN.2.1—Data Retention, Availability and Destruction: Retain, ensure availability, and destroy health record information according to scope of practice, organizational policy, or jurisdictional law. This includes retaining all EHR-S data and clinical documents for the time period designated by policy or legal requirement; retaining inbound documents as originally received (unaltered), ensuring availability of information for the legally prescribed period of time to users and patients; and providing the ability to destroy EHR data/records in a systematic way according to policy and after the legally prescribed retention period.

As discussed above, the ability to adhere to organizational retention and destruction policies that comply with jurisdictional law is critical for regulatory compliance and legal proceedings to prevent false appearances or accusations of spoliation of evidence and to establish that when records were destroyed it was part of established good faith practices. An EHR system must also allow an organization to identify data/records to be destroyed and review and approve destruction before it occurs. In such cases, it should provide record destruction date information along with existing data when providing records to another entity. The following criteria from the RM-ES standard may be used to evaluate whether an EHR system has basic functionality for retention and destruction:

- The EHR system shall provide the ability to store and retrieve health record data and clinical documents for the legally prescribed time or organizational policy.
- The EHR system shall provide the ability to identify specific EHR data/records for destruction review and confirm destruction before it occurs.
- The EHR system shall provide the ability to destroy EHR data/records so that data are not retrievable in a reasonably accessible and usable format according to policy and legal retentions periods.
- The EHR system should pass along record destruction date information (if any) along with existing data when providing records to another entity/organization. (HL7 2010)

On the surface, retention and destruction appear to be straightforward processes. However, as many healthcare organizations transition to EHRs, the record retention and destruction process will no longer be a simple and straightforward endeavor. Currently, it is common for organizations to create a hard copy report, electronic print, or an image of their legal record from the native source EHR applications, then destroy these copies in the required time frame and not destroy content in the source application data. Healthcare organizations must have policies that address retention and destruction of content in various clinical applications and the EHR system.

3.1.4 The Litigation Hold

An organization has an obligation to preserve or hold information relevant to the litigation at the time it becomes aware of the litigation or reasonably anticipates that such litigation will commence. This event is known as the "trigger."

On its face, the litigation hold concept is simple and straightforward. Once the organization reasonably anticipates litigation, all relevant information must be preserved (The Sedona Conference Working Group Series 2007). As illustrated in figure 3.1, however, the process involved in establishing the legal hold is anything but simple.

Figure 3.1 exemplifies the complexity of decision making and process flow for a legal hold. An organization is responsible for formulating the policies and establishing the processes necessary for identifying the triggers and communicating and auditing an effective legal hold. For more discussions on litigation response planning, refer to chapter 4. Once litigation is reasonably anticipated, by identification of a trigger, the organization should establish a legal (litigation) hold, and reasonable measures should be taken to identify and preserve all information relevant to the claim. For example, when an individual or an organization is named in and/or served with a complaint, subpoena, or subpoena *duces tecum*, or receives notice of a governmental investigation, litigation can be reasonably anticipated.

The advent of electronically stored information (ESI) in healthcare and e-HIM challenge the traditional practices and mechanisms by which the organization's legal counsel and health information managers respond to litigation. In the paper realm, the process of legal hold was reasonably clear cut; relevant paper records were secured and sequestered in a locked file with securely controlled access. In the digital realm, the challenge for legal, risk, health information management (HIM), informatics, and information technology (IT) professionals lies not only in the dynamic nature of the information, but also

Figure 3.1.   The legal hold: simple concept—complex process

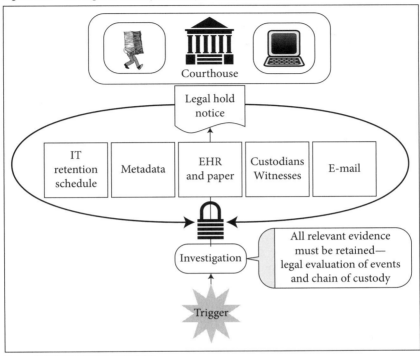

in knowing when, what, where, and how to secure the relevant electronic information. Many of today's EHR systems lack the capacity to establish a basic legal hold. Additionally, relevant information exists in various electronic forms and formats. These varied forms of ESI may or may not be within the control of the organization. Examples of ESI contained within EHRs that are not within full control of the healthcare organization include ESI maintained by application service provider (ASP) applications or other remote hosting suppliers, ESI within health information exchanges (HIEs), or patient-maintained personal health records.

Healthcare organizations must begin identifying litigation triggers for the organization and take appropriate action. A few categories and examples of healthcare litigation triggers include:

- **Adverse events**—Untoward, undesirable events, such as improper administration of medication or the unanticipated death of a patient, an employee, or a visitor

- **Serious injuries**—Accidents or falls occurring on the property resulting in serious physical or psychological injury or harm to a patient, employee, or visitor
- **Sentinel events**—Process variations that require immediate investigation and response because the event carried significant risk of death or serious physical or psychological injury
- Birth injuries—Newborns suffering from injuries or disfigurement as a result of complications from delivery
- Labor/employment disputes—Any legal notice from the Department of Labor or the Equal Employment Opportunity Commission (EEOC)
- Medical device injury or harm—Malpractice or medical errors that can occur in regard to medical devices

Figure 3.2 provides a general depiction of the processes involved in a legal hold process. Determining the risk and evaluating the scope of pending litigation require collaborative, organizational pre-litigation planning. The duty to preserve and the need to establish a legal hold could arise well before an official legal notice is served. Making a determination as to when to establish a legal hold is not a rote decision. In August 2007, The Sedona Conference published commentary on the establishment of legal holds and outlined a series of guidelines for organizations to follow whether the initiator or the target of litigation.

When faced with the prospect of potential litigation, the organization litigation response team will evaluate the situation and weigh a number of factors, including:

- The potential risk of litigation (type, source, and credibility of threat) to the organization
- The potential risk to the organization if a legal hold is not established
- Identification of any and all individuals who may be named in the litigation and who are the custodians of any potentially relevant information
- Assessment of the sources and level of knowledge an individual(s) has about the matter and where the information relevant to the claim is located
- Organizational policy and procedure for communication of the legal hold within the organization
- The timeframe for the review of the legal hold
- Organizational policy and procedure for lifting the legal hold and communication of same within the organization

Figure 3.2.   General process flow of a legal hold

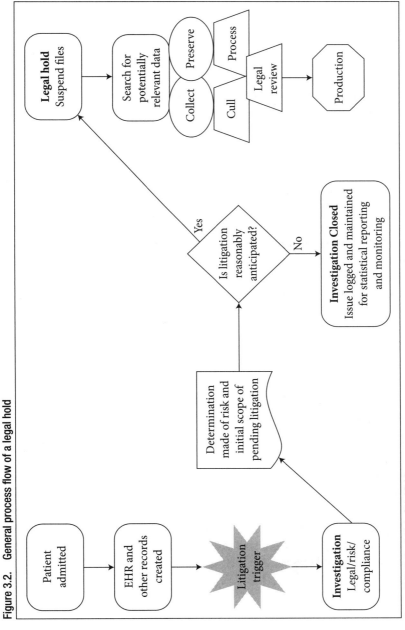

Source: © 2012 Kim Baldwin-Stried Reich.

There is no rule that addresses or defines the triggers for an organization. Instead, courts often are required to engage in fact-intensive inquiries to determine when a duty to preserve arises in a particular litigation. HIM experience, best practices, and healthcare industry standards, however, should be considered in determination of triggers and organizational thresholds. As external drivers, including legislation and regulation, are becoming more prescriptive of what defines quality in healthcare, it is anticipated that new categories of triggers may arise. For example, as connections to cost and quality are tied to implementation of EHR functionalities such as decision alerting tools and compliant use, do data on outlier physician system use or behavior increase justification for action? In addition, comparative quality data of clinical staff may become the source of triggers. Particular attention should be paid to the concern that, if there is a dispute, "years after the fact, a court will judge whether you preserved enough documents, whether they came from the right sources, and whether you adequately started preserving documents when you should have known that it was reasonably likely that litigation would occur" (Lender 2006).

A key concept to preservation is the notion of reasonableness. As stated in Sedona Principle 5 (2007), "[t]he obligation to preserve . . . [ESI] requires reasonable and good faith efforts to retain information. . . . However, it is unreasonable to expect parties to take every conceivable step to preserve all potentially relevant . . . [ESI]."

3.1.5 EHR Records Management and Evidentiary Support (RM-ES) Standard—Record Preservation

The HL7 EHR system standard for records management and evidentiary support recognized the importance of the legal hold function and the need to preserve data and communicate a preservation notice. This function is not typically found in EHR systems today because litigation involving the EHR is still in the early phases. When evaluating EHR systems currently in place or to be implemented, it is critical that a record preservation function be requested from the vendor to support future needs to support the litigation process. The RM-ES standard describes the record preservation function in the following way (HL7 2010):

> IN.2.1.1—Record Preservation: EHR systems must support a need to preserve data from normal destruction practices. Organizations may have a need to preserve certain types of health information for business purposes (for example, select face sheet, diagnostic, or discharge information). Organizations may also have a duty to preserve information that is or could be relevant to a legal proceeding whether litigation is threatened or impending. Systems must provide the ability for users to preserve select information from destruction or place a legal hold on electronic

health information (suspend their normal destruction practices for all potentially relevant information) and prevent from loss, destruction, alteration or unauthorized use.

Even though the record preservation function is not limited to litigation, there are aspects unique to e-discovery that require attention. The following criteria from the RM-ES standard can be used to evaluate whether an EHR system has basic functionality for retention and destruction (HL7 2010):

- The system should provide the ability to secure data/records from un-auditable alteration or unauthorized use for preservation purpose such as a legal hold.
- The system shall have the ability to preserve records beyond normal retention practices.
- The system should provide the ability to identify the reason for preserving records beyond the normal retention practices.
- The system may map medical record elements to the metadata to provide the business context.
- The system should provide the ability to generate a legal hold notice identifying who to contact for questions when a user attempts to alter a record on legal hold or an unauthorized user attempts to access a record on legal hold.

Healthcare organizations must establish organizational policy with respect to legal holds and communication of such, including how a hold would be applied to EHR content and all source applications—for example, lab, pharmacy, radiology applications—integrated with the EHR. In the absence of such functionality, a work-around will be necessary. Some organizations address this issue by planning to make a mirror image of the EHR database at the time that a litigation hold is triggered. Many organizations use an electronic document management system (EDMS) to house the legal record for the long term. This approach works for providing access to just one form of the official medical record, however, attorneys for the plaintiff may also request access to the source applications. Ultimately, organizations will need to work with their system vendors to establish a long-term approach to preservation of select information within the source EHR application along with the relevant metadata.

3.1.6 Demand Letters

The scope of a litigation hold may not be clear at the time of a trigger or formal onset of litigation. A party may well need to make unilateral decisions concerning how much ESI should be preserved. Conversely, if a party is a defendant, it may be served by a plaintiff with a preservation demand letter even before litigation is commenced and that may purport to require the defendant to maintain ESI from defined sources and in a particular form or format. When faced with such a demand, the defendant can concede, refuse, or open up negotiations as to scope. Judicial assistance in defining the scope of preservation, generally speaking, is unavailable *before* litigation actually commences.

An example of an imaginative attempt to secure pre-litigation judicial assistance was made in *State of Texas v. City of Frisco*, 2008 WL 828055 (E.D. Tex. 2008). In that action, a Texas municipality demanded that the Texas Department of Transportation preserve all data associated with planning a highway project. The demand also stated that a "potential exists for litigation" over the project. The state, in response, commenced an action in the US district court, seeking a declaration by the court as to its preservation obligations. The court held that a mere threat of litigation was "insufficiently immediate to establish an actual controversy," and dismissed the action. *State of Texas v. City of Frisco* (E.D. Tex. 2008) illustrates that pre-litigation assistance is unlikely.

Cache La Poudre Feed, LLC v. Land O' Lakes Inc., 244 F.R.D. 614 (D. Colo. 2007), is another example of how a court may address a preservation demand. In *Cache La Poudre*, the plaintiff sought sanctions against the defendant, arguing that the defendant's implementation of a litigation hold was untimely. The plaintiff had served pre-litigation preservation demands on the defendant, which, the court concluded, were equivocal on whether litigation would be commenced. Holding that the demands did not make litigation reasonably foreseeable, the court declined to impose sanctions.

In summary, interpreting preservation demands poses difficulties and judicial assistance is unlikely. Parties must gauge the demand, determine whether the demand makes litigation reasonably foreseeable, and formulate an appropriate response. Note, in this regard, that there are circumstances under which a demand may give rise to a duty to preserve to allow appropriate analysis.

3.1.6.1 Demand Letters in Healthcare

Reacting to a demand letter in healthcare is easier said than done. Many demand letters are related to issues other than medical malfeasance such as displacement of a grieving response, financial, or credit implications of healthcare bills, or lack of satisfaction of service rather than quality of medical care. The scope of litigation may extend into areas including compliance variances such as clinical trial billing, or non-party involvement in workers' compensation or auto injury. Regardless of the source of a demand, it is essential for healthcare organizations to establish collection tactics to assure that data from health information technology (HIT) systems and their associated policies are securely stored and preserved prior to further processing, review, and production.

The collection methodologies and technologies used for preservation will vary greatly depending on organizational resources, HIT system functionalities, and pre-defined processes and policies for data retention. It is recommended that an e-discovery expert be involved in these early information management decisions for litigation-prone industries such as healthcare.

3.1.7 Preservation Hold Notices

Once a preservation hold is triggered, an organization has an obligation to communicate that hold to appropriate custodians of ESI. This is commonly known as a preservation hold notice. Before any such notice is given, the organization must make a preliminary determination of what information must be preserved and who should be advised to undertake the preservation effort. One way to accomplish this, as suggested in the leading decision of *Zubulake v. UBS Warburg LLC,* 220 F.R.D. 212 (S.D.N.Y. 2003) would be to identify so-called key players or persons holding relevant ESI, advise them of the duty to preserve, and collect or duplicate ESI from them.

What should the preservation hold notice contain? There is no simple—or complete—answer. At a minimum, however, the notice should presumably state that:

- Certain litigation has commenced or is reasonably anticipated.
- The litigation addresses certain issues.
- Information relevant to those issues must be preserved.
- The operation of any record retention (destruction) policies affecting the relevant information should be suspended.
- There will be consequences for anyone who does not comply.

Not only should the hold be communicated, but it should be periodically reissued *and* the hold should also be monitored to ensure compliance and effectiveness.

Preservation of relevant information is the key to a successful hold. For example, in *Cache La Poudre* (D. Colo. 2007), the defendant was found to have violated the duty to preserve when it failed to interview ex-employees to determine to whether they had possession of relevant ESI. In other words, exit interviews might include as a subject whether the interviewee had information subject to a hold so that such information might be collected and preserved.

A preservation hold notice may become a subject of dispute. This possibility arises when a party seeks to prove that its adversary violated its duty to preserve. Preservation notices, if issued by or at the direction of an attorney, may be protected from discovery because such notices are subject to the **attorney-client privilege** or entitled to work product protection. This was the case in the holding of *In re Ebay Seller Antitrust Litigation*, WL 2852364 (N.D. Ca. Oct. 2, 2007). However, that court, while protecting the notice itself, allowed an inquiry into what employees did to implement the notice issued in that litigation and which employees received the notice.

The preservation hold notice is crucial for any organization involved in litigation. Specific language or semantics contained in a hold notice are important. Its circulation to appropriate personnel is also important—and to whom it should be circulated should be a subject of review and revision, as should the scope of the hold instituted by the notice as a particular litigation proceeds. Lastly, a decision should be made as to whether to cloak the notice with privilege or whether the notice should be transparent or available.

Ethical questions arise in healthcare around the degree of transparency required for preservation hold notices. For example, if circumstances around a defect in a clinical information system are known to have the potential to cause patient harm or actual harm itself, would it be better to cloak the hold notice or be transparent? What if the EHR system was not part of the complaint? What obligations would health service organizations have if the circumstances of harm were around potential medical device liability? What about off-label use medications supported by the organization? Characteristics and protections of the data and the preservation notice may be important for other reasons, such as vendor contract hold harmless clauses or work product in preparation for peer review.

3.1.8 Preservation of Ephemeral Information

In *Convolve, Inc. v. Compaq Computer Corp.*, 223 F.R.D. 162 (S.D.N.Y. 2004), decided before the 2006 amendments to the Federal Rules of Civil Procedure (FRCP), the court held that a party was not obligated to preserve wave readings on an oscilloscope, concluding that those readings were ephemeral in nature, not being recorded in the normal course of the party's operations. This led to the concept of ephemeral electronic information, which was assumed by many not to fall within any duty to preserve. This assumption was changed by *Columbia Pictures, Inc. v. Bunnell,* 245 F.R.D. 443 (C.D. Cal. 2007).

At issue in *Columbia Pictures, Inc.* (CD Cal. May 29, 2007) among other things, was the preservation of server log data. The plaintiffs, essentially the motion picture and television industries, brought suit against a website for facilitating the illegal distribution of movies and TV shows over the Internet and sought the preservation of the data, which they alleged would reveal the Internet protocol (IP) addresses of visitors to the website and what they had accessed. A defendant objected, arguing that the server log data were contained within the random access memory (RAM) of the defendant's servers, that the RAM resided on servers for only seconds, and that the RAM was ephemeral.

This argument was rejected by the presiding judge, who concluded that the RAM constituted electronically *stored* information within the meaning of the FRCP because it was fixed on the defendant's servers, however briefly, and because the RAM was capable of being preserved. The court also held that the RAM sought was highly relevant to the plaintiffs' claims. This holding was affirmed at *Columbia Pictures, Indus. v. Bunnell,* 2007 U.S. Dist. LEXIS 63620 (C.D. Cal. Aug. 24, 2007).

Columbia Pictures, Indus. created somewhat of a sensation when it was decided. Organizations feared that there were no limits to what should be preserved. However, with the passage of time, that fear has apparently dissipated. Concern became focused on the nature of the ESI that might be subject to preservation and its relevance.

For example, in *Arista Records, LLC v. Usenet.com Inc.,* 2009 WL 185992 (S.D.N.Y. Jan. 26, 2009), the plaintiffs brought suit against Usenet, contending that Usenet had allowed its subscribers to illegally load copyrighted musical works onto its servers. The plaintiffs argued that the defendants failed to preserve relevant ESI, including user data and the music itself. The court, on a motion for sanctions, concluded that the lost ESI, although transitory, should have been preserved, and that, "once defendants had actual notice that plaintiffs were requesting the data, defendants had an obligation to preserve it, if possible, or at least negotiate in good faith what data they could produce."

Arista Records demonstrates that, as with any ESI, *relevance* is a key to preservation. Moreover, *Arista Records* and *Columbia Pictures, Indus.* demonstrate that another key to preservation of transitory information may be a request for it by an adversary.

3.1.9 Relevance of Clinical Decision Support and Ephemeral Data in Litigation

Requirements for **clinical decision support (CDS)** are incorporated in the Health Information Technology for Economic and Clinical Health (HITECH) portion of the American Recovery and Reinvestment Act (ARRA). To achieve the maximum incentive, clinicians must have had a qualifying EHR system put into "meaningful use" by 2011. The ONC HIT Policy Committee Workgroup *meaningful use preamble* states, "the specific use of information technology that will enable the desired outcomes, and our ability to monitor them. For example, demonstrating improved performance . . . will require a host of new care processes for many outpatient providers (for example, monitoring medication adherence, use of evidence-based order sets, clinical decision support tools at the point of care, patient outreach and reminders)" (ONC HIT Policy Committee 2009). HITECH itself, however, does afford a glimpse into what is considered a qualified EHR. A qualified EHR is capable of **e-prescribing**; includes demographics and clinical health information; provides clinical decision support; captures and allows querying of quality measures; and can exchange a certain level of data with other EHRs. The incentives decrease year after year, with initiation of increasing financial penalties for nondeployment or nonmeaningful use of HIT starting in 2015.

On January 13, 2010, the ONC released the criteria in an interim final rule (IFR) in the *Federal Register*, 45 CFR Part 170, entitled "Health Information Technology: Initial Set of Standards, Implementation Specifications, and Certification Criteria for Electronic Health Record Technology." The IFR described, in the first of the three proposed stages, the following: "The Stage 1 meaningful use criteria focuses on electronically capturing health information in a coded format [and defines] the requirement for implementing clinical decision support tools to facilitate disease and medication management; and reporting clinical quality measures and public health information." The evolving definition of meaningful use is anticipated to recommend increased usage of CDS within HIT systems, therefore the importance of the ESI in CDS toward future healthcare litigation should not be underestimated.

Systematic review of the literature by medical informatics experts demonstrates a potentially beneficial effect of computerized provider order entry (CPOE) when coupled with CDS (Chaudhry et al. 2006). A complementary research study funded by the Commonwealth Foundation suggests that although other forms of HIT are beneficial, CDS within HIT applications is associated with the greatest cost savings and outcome improvements

(Amarasingham et al. 2006). One caveat is that high alert frequency can lead to alert fatigue, resulting in decreased user responsiveness to alerts (Koppel et al. 2005). There are other fallibilities of computerized provider order entry (CPOE) as well (Wagner and Kenreigh 2005), which have been summarized and published, categorizing CPOE error types such as software causing unintended adverse consequences (Campbell et al. 2006) and describing 22 types of medication error risks (Koppel et al. 2005). Another study has indicated that tiered alerting by severity (such as, the most critical alerts are not overwritable) was associated with higher compliance rates of drug-drug interaction alerts in the inpatient setting, and lack of tiering was associated with a high override rate of even severe alerts (Paterno et al. 2009).

Decision support tools usually fall into two general categories to assist clinicians in determining *what is true* about the patient or *what to do* for the patient (Shortliffe and Cimino 2006). Interpretation of the codified rules of HITECH suggest policy makers are most interested in HIT supporting physicians and other healthcare providers in the latter task. The two main models of decision support include the *consulting model*, where decision support serves as an advisor, and the *critiquing model*, which informs clinicians about the appropriateness of their proposed patient management plan. The majority of decision support tools found in current HIT industry products follow the consulting model for CDS, such as drug-drug interactions, drug-allergy interactions, drug-disease interactions (for example, dosage adjustments for renal insufficiency), dose-range indicators, and weight- and age-based calculations (Jenders et al. 2007). Intelligent filtering including pop-ups, alerts and reminders, clinical guidelines, order sets, dashboards, documentation templates, and the like are varieties of CDS and also contain relevant ESI. CDS assists clinicians in what to do for a patient and is potentially relied upon as system-generated medical advice. Refer to section 3.9. for further discussion of legal issues surrounding the distinction between system-generated and system-stored information.

CDS may be provided in an *active* or a *passive* format. The active format requires either acceptance or nonacceptance of the proposed recommendation. The passive format (for example, information buttons, virtual Post-it notes, transitory pop-ups) does not mandate that the provider perform an action related to the recommendation or computer-generated advice. It is difficult, if not impossible, to adequately measure a nonaction in computerized systems. The salutary health outcomes and operational improvements expected from CDS are directly reliant on the quality and validity of the knowledge and logic embedded in the underlying decision support system, reliability of the clinical software system, and the methods for enhancing the knowledge base driving the CDS functions.

3.1.10 CDS and Significance to e-Discovery

The obligation to preserve ephemeral ESI is dependent upon the *relevance* of the ESI. Healthcare information professionals must consider the ephemeral nature of many clinical decision support solutions in a manner analogous to the RAM of *Columbia Pictures* or the transitory *Arista Records* server data. Many of the CDS systems used in EHRs today are delivered or communicated to the clinician as ephemeral data. The meaningful use definition requires EHR systems to "automatically and electronically generate and indicate in real-time, alerts and care suggestions based upon clinical decision support rules and evidence grade" (45 CFR Part 170). The occurrence of a CDS alert may not be captured, and the output, formerly known as the chart, may not capture acceptance or nonacceptance of the actual recommendation, which was made by a prompt, pop-up, or clinical alert in the EHR output. Little dispute should arise about the importance of capturing CDS data in the evidentiary record or in the routine business records of the medical practice. The final 45 CFR Part 170 does suggest that alert statistics be captured stating that eligible providers must "automatically and electronically track, record, and generate reports on the number of alerts responded to by a user." This criterion falls short of capturing what advice was actually provided by the clinical information system itself.

Issues of negligence and product liability related to ESI from EHR need to be considered. If the reasonable person or community standard of care is for a clinician to use an EHR system equipped with CDS, does the failure to act in accordance with the computer advice support a claim of negligence in a medical malpractice allegation when an adverse outcome occurs? Conversely, what assurances does the clinician have from the vendors and the organizations that actually implemented the EHR (and might have modified the alert logic) as to the reliability of the embedded rules and logic to provide reasonable medical evidence standards? One healthcare legal scholar writes, "although the law usually permits industries and professions to set their own practice standards, courts have also ruled that entire industries and professions can be negligent by failing to adopt new technologies, especially those that are inexpensive and effective, and that judges and juries must ultimately determine what is reasonable" (Annas 2006). System reliability discussions are expected to arise more often in litigation proceedings as the amount of informatics evaluation research and scholarly law writings (Paul 2008) amplify concerning the trustworthiness of computer-generated data. Refer to section 3.9 of this chapter on admissibility for more on system reliability of computer-generated information.

EHR systems may not have the potential to retain CDS-related ESI. Even if such a function exists, information managers might not recognize its importance in operations or litigation of CDS-related ESI retention or preservation. An access audit trail does not typically contain the metadata necessary to reconstruct a notice or warning to the provider, namely, information seen on the screen from the CDS relevant to their decision making.

In addition to auditing and reporting issues related to the ephemeral nature of CDS, the following critical questions arise for those professionals responsible for managing health information systems for evidentiary purposes:

- Is the acceptance or nonacceptance visible in the clinical documentation and/or the metadata?
- Have you observed any potential problems or errors in decision support that might have an effect on patient safety?
- Are statistics on decision support acceptance or nonacceptance covered under privileged peer review policies or deliberations?
- Does your EHR system allow setting thresholds for or disabling of clinical decision support pop-ups, prompts, and alerts? If yes, who (vendor, organization, provider, or other) determines this and what rationale is used to determine the threshold?
- Does your EHR vendor or HIT team support timely clinical and administrative content changes (for example, Food and Drug Administration [FDA] warnings, Joint Commission recommendations, Centers for Medicare and Medicaid Services [CMS] quality measures, national patient safety goals)?
- Does your EHR vendor contract specifically exclude liability for clinical outcomes or the practice of medicine, including CDS performance?

AHIMA considers the technical and operational issues of health data management in detail, but there are further sociotechnical complications that merit additional consideration as well, due to legal implications.

As an example, significant debate in medical literature has recently arisen related to the validity of the concept of the learned intermediary (Koppel and Kreda 2009) as an IT vendor's defense for software defects and malfunctions. Others have effectively argued that the previous FDA draft decision exempting clinical software from regulatory oversight on the basis of the "competent human intervention exemption" (Hoffman and Podgurski 2008) must be reconsidered. Safe and effective transition to computerized medical records cannot be achieved without federal regulation, especially in the face of a rapidly expanding mandate for HIT use and an increased role in mediating medical care decisions for this technology. The HIT industry mitigates liability by reliance on the legal doctrine known as learned intermediary that holds physicians, nurses, and allied healthcare providers responsible for HIT system errors because these professionals are presumed to have the ability to intervene between the application and the patient by identifying and remedying medical mistakes generated by software defects. The ephemeral or non-ephemeral data may indeed show that the concept of learned intermediary is unreasonable in that no human being, learned or otherwise, could have recognized erroneous information that resulted in an adverse outcome.

The FDA (Bierman and Buenafe 2009) and the Joint Commission (Joint Commission 2008) appear to have an increased interest in HIT safety. The FDA considers EHR systems, including those with CDS capabilities, within its jurisdiction for regulatory scrutiny. Jeffrey Shuren, MD, JD, director of the FDA's Center for Devices and Radiological Health, testified that "given the FDA's regulatory authorities and analytical tools, [the FDA] could potentially, at a minimum, play an important role in preventing and addressing HIT-related safety issues, thereby helping to foster confidence in these devices" (Shuren 2010). The FDA, however, has not aggressively pursued these intentions to date. Thus, many of the applications identified as "qualified" may be required to undergo pre-market approval and post-market surveillance by the FDA in the future. The same holds for pharmaceuticals and medical devices. The Joint Commission's suitably named Sentinel Events Alert on HIT describes organizational accreditation responsibilities and suggested actions to mitigate risks related to HIT systems.

A national working group in Sweden prepared a guidance report to assist compliance with the medical device regulation in the European Union, with goals to improve patient safety. The summary report was initiated from a number of serious incidents involving HIT systems at a time when the manufacturer's responsibilities were considered vague (Medical Products Agency Working Group on Medical Information Systems 2009).

In summary, lawyers faced with the possibility of e-iatrogenesis (patient harm caused by the application of HIT) (Weiner et al. 2007; Campbell 2007) caused by EHRs should consult with informatics staff, HIM managers, and IT staff to determine the retention and preservation processes of ESI within CDS and review the information prior to responding to any discovery request. Counsel should have an intimate familiarity with the potential ephemeral nature of CDS-related ESI and its associated metadata in future litigation preparation.

3.1.10.1 EHR Records Management and Evidentiary Support (RM-ES) Standard—Business Rules including Clinical Decision Support

The HL7 EHR system standard includes the use of clinical decision support and other types of embedded business rules. There are two areas in the standard utilizing decision support and business rule capabilities—in the infrastructure of the system for management of the rules, and in the direct delivery of care and documentation such as medication ordering. From a record management perspective, the management of business and clinical decision support rules is critical for litigation to understand the organization's protocols and practices for the period in question. The RM-ES standard requires the following functionality for EHR systems (HL7 2010):

> IN.6—Business Rules: EHR systems need to manage the ability to create, update, delete, view, and version business rules including institutional preferences. EHR systems need to apply business rules from necessary points within an EHR-S to control system behavior. An EHR-S audits changes made to business rules, as well as compliance to and overrides of applied business rules. EHR-S business rule implementation functions include decision support, diagnostic support, workflow control, and access privileges, as well as system and user defaults and preferences.

> An EHR-S should support the ability of providers and institutions to customize decision support components such as triggers, rules, or algorithms, as well as the wording of alerts and advice to meet realm specific requirements and preferences.

The care delivery and documentation process captured within an EHR system may be based on system business rules. These rules are likely to be called into question during a legal proceeding to understand the organization's good faith practices and when practices deviate from the norm. The system should be able to provide an export of the business rules for a given time to inform participants in the litigation process of the rules in place at a specific time. The export could be a printout or other type of report. The specific criteria for evaluating an EHR system's management of business and decision support rules include the following (HL7 2010):

- The system shall provide the ability to manage business rules.
- The system should provide the ability to create, import, or access decision support and workflow control rules to guide system behavior.

- If the system uses decision support and workflow control rules, then the system shall provide the ability to update decision support and workflow control rules.
- If the system uses decision support and workflow control rules, then the system shall provide the ability to customize decision support and workflow control rules and their components.
- If the system uses decision support and workflow control rules, then the system shall provide the ability to inactivate those rules and archive inactivated rules per retention period as designated by organizational policy and jurisdictional law.
- If the system uses decision support and workflow control rules, then the system shall provide the ability to destroy the decision support rules per retention period as designated by organizational policy and jurisdictional law.
- The system should provide the ability to create access privilege rules to guide system behavior.
- The system shall support the ability to selectively export business rules.

Many of today's EHR systems do not have the capability to manage business and decision support rules as they change over time. Some healthcare organizations are using a separate content management system to maintain and retain versions of the rules in place over time.

3.2 Cooperation in Discovery

Cooperation in discovery. Is this an oxymoron? Our popular culture certainly paints a picture of attorneys as gladiators who routinely flout any rules (The Sedona Conference Cooperation Proclamation 2008a). This landmark proclamation promotes cooperation by all parties to the discovery process or a "just, speedy, and inexpensive determination of every action" (FRCP 1 1938).

Notwithstanding this popular misconception, the FRCP encourages and, indeed, mandates some level of cooperation. These specific rules should be borne in mind when preparing for and engaging in litigation. "The overriding theme of recent amendments to the discovery rules has been open and forthright sharing of information by all parties . . . with the aim of expediting case progress, minimizing burden and expense, and removing contentiousness as much as practicable. . . . If counsel fails in this responsibility—willfully or not—these principles of an open discovery process are undermined, coextensively inhibiting the courts' ability to objectively resolve their clients' disputes and the credibility of its resolution" (*Board of Regents v. BASF Corp.,* 2007 WL 3342423 [D. Neb. Nov. 5, 2007]).

"The costs associated with adversarial conduct in pretrial discovery have become a serious burden to the American judicial system. *The burden has risen significantly in the face of the discovery of electronically stored information.* In addition to rising monetary costs, courts have seen escalating motion practice, overreaching, obstruction, and extensive, but unproductive discovery disputes—in some cases precluding adjudication on the merits altogether—when parties treat the discovery process in an adversarial manner. Neither law nor logic compels these outcomes" (The Sedona Conference 2007a, emphasis added by author). The FRCP provides a viable means to avoid these outcomes. Additional case analysis and discussion on cooperation in e-discovery can be found in chapter 2.

3.2.1 The Initial Meet and Confer

Rule 26(f) requires parties in most proceedings to confer before their first appearance in court. It also requires that certain subjects be considered at this "meet and confer." Among the topics are several that pertain to electronic discovery:

- Preserving discoverable information, Rule 26(f)(2)
- Any issues about disclosure or discovery of electronically stored information, including the forms or forms in which it is to be produced, Rule 26(f)(3)(C)
- Any issues about claims of privilege or protection as trial-preparation materials, including whether the parties agree on a procedure to assert these claims after production and whether to ask the court to include their agreement in an order, Rule 26(f)(3)(D)

Once the meet and confer is completed, the parties are obligated to prepare a discovery plan or report for the court.

E-discovery, especially in complex litigation, is evolving into a process in the initial meet and confer. First, the meet and confer is becoming iterative: parties make inquiries of their adversaries about the latter's ESI and then reconvene after a period of time to continue formulation of a plan. Second, for better or worse, consultants are becoming involved in the meet and confer process to assist their clients in dealing with electronic discovery issues. Third, as noted above, individual US district courts are creating local rules or policies to expand the ESI-related topics that parties must address at the meet and confer. For example, the District of New Jersey requires parties to consider whether "restoration of deleted digital information may be necessary; whether back up or historic legacy data is within the scope of discovery and the media, format, and procedures for producing digital information" (*D.N.J. L. Civ. R.* 26.1(d)(3)(a)).

Rule 26(f) gives parties the opportunity to agree on the outline of the litigation in which they are involved and, as importantly, agree on what they *disagree* on. Their disputes can then be presented to the presiding judge for resolution at the onset of litigation.

Care must be taken, however, before entering into agreements with adversaries. Illustrative of this admonition is the admittedly extreme decision of *In re Fannie May Securities Litigation,* 2009 WL 21528 (D.C. Cir. Jan. 6, 2009), in which an appellate court affirmed a contempt citation against a government agency. Agency attorneys had entered into an agreement with a party that sought certain records and, in attempting to review the records it agreed to produce, the agency retained 50 contract attorneys and expended more than 9 percent of its budget. Nevertheless, the agency could not meet court-ordered deadlines and found itself in contempt. The moral of *Fannie Mae* is to enter into agreements *only after* confirming that the agreement makes sense.

3.2.2 Subsequent Meet and Confers

Rule 26(f) speaks of an *initial* meet and confer before the parties appear before the presiding judge at an *initial* scheduling conference under Rule 16(b), at which the judge issues an *initial* scheduling order and presumably addresses the disputes presented by the parties. However, proceedings often have a number of scheduling conferences and the practice has developed in various US district courts for parties to meet and confer in advance of these subsequent conferences. Moreover, Rule 37 (a)(1) requires that, before any motion to compel discovery is made in a US district court, the moving party certify that it has "in good faith conferred or attempted to confer with the person or party failing to make . . . discovery in an effort to obtain it without court action." Thus, the rules embody cooperation—or at least encourage it.

3.2.3 Failure to Cooperate

Case law is developing, which enforces the obligation to meet and confer. For example, parties have been barred from raising disputes if they have not been the subject of a meet and confer. See, for example, *RLI Ins. Co. v. Indian River School Dist.,* 2007 WL 3112417 (D. Del. Oct. 23, 2007). In a memorable decision for *Peskoff v. Faber,* 244 F.R.D. 54 (D.D.C. 2007), the court admonished parties to "play nice" or they would be required to confer in its presence!

Moreover, courts are interpreting other rules to require cooperation. Rule 26(g) requires that "every discovery request, response, or objection must be signed" and, by signing, "an attorney or party certifies that to the best of the person's knowledge, information, and belief formed after a reasonable inquiry," the discovery request or response is appropriate.

In *Mancia v. Mayflower Textile Servs. Co.,* 253 F.R.D. 354 (D. Md. 2008), the court held that boilerplate objections to discovery requests violated Rule 26(g), that discovery should not be a "tactical battlefield," and that the parties should meet and confer to develop a discovery plan proportionate to the issues involved in the litigation. Thus, Rule 26(g) furnishes another basis for appropriate cooperation between adversaries.

3.3 Disclosure vs. Discovery

At the outset, parties to federal proceedings must distinguish between disclosures and discovery. These concepts are fundamentally different and distinguishable.

3.3.1 The Obligation to Disclose

In 1993, the FRCP were amended to require parties to disclose, without a discovery request, certain information. Today, absent some exemption, a party must disclose within 14 days of the initial Rule 26(f) discovery conference "unless a different time is set by stipulation or court order, or unless a party objects. . . ," the following information that the party "may use in support of its claims or defenses":

- The name and, if known, the address and telephone number of each individual likely to have discoverable information—along with the subjects of that information, Rule 26(a)(1)(A)(i)
- A copy—or a description by category and location—of all documents, electronically stored information, and tangible things that the disclosing party has in its possession, custody, or control, Rule 26(a)(1)(A)(ii)

A party must also disclose "a computation of each category of damages claimed" and the existence of any relevant insurance, Rule 26(a)(1)(A)(iii, iv). Failure to make timely disclosures, or to amend disclosures as necessary, may result in sanctions, Rule 37(c)(1).

Thus, ESI may be subject to disclosure at the earliest stage of litigation. This obligation should be one more topic for the parties to address at the initial meet and confer under Rule 26(f).

Refer to section 3.9.2.7, Data Source Mapping for Litigation, to better understand differences of requirements of data mapping for healthcare operations compared to litigation purposes.

3.4 Discovery in General

Rules 26 through 37 generally speaking, govern discovery in the US district courts. Previous sections have already discussed Rules 26(a)(1), 26(f), 26(g) and, to some degree, Rules 37(a) and (c). Didactic attention now turns to the *means* by which discovery is conducted and the *scope* of discovery.

3.4.1 How Discovery Is Conducted

Unless authorized by an order, discovery does not commence until parties have engaged in the initial Rule 26(f) meet and confer. Indeed, among the topics for the meet and confer are "the subjects on which discovery may be needed, when discovery should be completed, and whether discovery should be conducted in phases or be limited to or focused on particular issues," Rule 26(f)(3)(B).

Discovery is conducted through written interrogatories (Rule 33), requests to produce (Rule 34), oral and written depositions (Rules 30 and 31), physical and mental examinations (Rule 35), and requests for admissions (Rule 36). Moreover, discovery encompasses the production of experts' reports and disclosures as well as expert depositions, Rule 26(b)(4). Not surprisingly, the timing and scope of discovery are subject to the discretion of the presiding judge.

Judges are vested with considerable discretion in controlling discovery (*Crawford-El v. Britton,* 523 U.S. 574, 598 [1996]). For example, in *Regan-Touhy v. Walgreen Co.,* 526 F.3d 641 (10th Cir. 2008), the plaintiff, who had brought suit against the defendant for alleged wrongful disclosure of medical information, appealed from a grant of summary judgment against her. One of her arguments on appeal was that the presiding judge had denied her discovery of computerized log files and e-mail. The court of appeals affirmed the award of summary judgment, concluding that the judge had properly exercised his discretion in denying the plaintiff's overly broad discovery requests, which amounted to a "kitchen sink." The court of appeals also observed that discovery disputes should not displace trial on the merits as the focus of the parties' attention. As the following sections will demonstrate, there is ample room for that exercise under the rules.

3.4.1.1 Managing Excessive Discovery Requests in Healthcare

Healthcare organizations rarely understand the implications of pre-litigation preparation requirements, or how to address these expectations in a timely, cost-effective manner for the Rule 26(f) meet and confer and beyond. Organizations must be able to define and explain the location of both paper and electronic data to meet litigation requirements. Counsel and HIM must rapidly triage and stratify data for relevancy to the case. These mapping efforts are the first steps necessary to fully understand the merits of a pending lawsuit. Strategic decisions must be made in a very short time, usually in less than a hundred days, which will impact the entire course of the litigation. Health service organizations must balance the resources needed for ongoing operational needs with those needed to inform outside counsel about their complex health information systems. Simultaneously, internal risk management and counsel that may have been complacent or otherwise uninvolved during clinical systems implementation may also require reallocation of already scarce operational resources for internal litigation preparation and education. Additionally, inside counsel, HIM, and IT resources rarely have the capacity to manage the technical and volume challenges of ESI stored in EHR systems.

To deliver what and when the court expects, a key strategy to approaching the 26(f) rule is to include a representation of the entire HIT infrastructure. This must be a portrayal of all data repositories, clinical, financial, and otherwise as well as associated data retention policies, as a comprehensive data map. This chapter later discusses data mapping and the differences of mapping approaches for litigation compared to operational purposes. For information on data source mapping for litigation and pre-litigation preparedness teams, refer to the chapter 4 section titled Developing the Litigation Response Plan.

3.4.2 The Scope of Discovery

Under Rule 26(b)(1), "[p]arties may obtain discovery regarding any non-privileged matter that is *relevant* to any party's claim or defense." Moreover, "[f]or good cause shown, the court may order discovery of any matter relevant to the subject matter involved in the action." Note that, "[r]elevant information need not be admissible at the trial if the discovery appears reasonably calculated to lead to the discovery of admissible evidence."

This distinction is often difficult to grasp. "The dividing line between information relevant to the claims and defenses and that relevant only to the subject matter of the action cannot be defined with precision" (*Advisory Committee Note to 2000 Amendment to Rule 26(b)(1)*). For the purposes of this book, it is sufficient to note that liberal discovery is contemplated in federal litigation absent party agreement, court order, or rule. That brings us to a fundamental distinction between discovery of paper records and ESI.

3.4.3 Not Reasonably Accessible ESI

Rule 26(b)(2)(B) places specific limitations on discovery of ESI. It provides that, "[a] party need not provide discovery of . . . [ESI] from sources that the party identifies as not reasonably accessible because of undue burden or cost." If the parties cannot resolve the matter among themselves, the party from whom discovery is sought must prove undue burden or cost. However, even if that party proves that the source or sources are not reasonably accessible, the court may order discovery "if the requesting party shows good cause, considering the limitations of Rule 26(b)(2)(C)."

What does this mean? Among other things, as described in the Advisory Committee Note to the 2006 Amendment to Rule 26(b)(2)(B):

- The rule recognizes that "[i]t is not possible to define . . . the different types of technological features that may affect the burdens and costs of accessing" ESI.
- Rule 26(b)(2)(B) "does not relieve the party of its . . . duties to preserve evidence."
- Parties must confer before bringing any motion with regard to ESI that is asserted to reside on a source that is not reasonably accessible.
- The requesting party may need discovery to test any assertion that ESI resides on such a source, thus leading to so-called satellite discovery or discovery about discovery.

- Even if the producing party meets its burden of establishing undue burden or cost, discovery can proceed if the requesting party can establish that "its need for the discovery outweighs the burdens and costs of locating, retrieving, and producing the information."
- Limitations under Rule 26(b)(2)(C) can be placed on any discovery of not reasonably accessible information that a court might allow.

3.4.4 Decisions Illustrating Not Reasonably Accessible ESI

Not surprisingly, there are a number of decisions that address not reasonably accessible ESI. It is impossible to describe or catalog all of these; however, some examples are appropriate.

In *Knifesource LLC v. Wachovia Bank, N.A.,* 2007 US Dist. LEXIS 58829 (D.S.C. Aug. 10, 2007), the defendant bank argued that it could not produce a former employee's statements because it did not maintain physical copies and the bank would be required to create the statements from computer records. The court held that, inasmuch as the bank did not demonstrate that the source of the computer records was not reasonably accessible, the bank was obligated to produce the statements. Thus, mere creation of a computer record—or conversion of information from one medium (paper) to another—does not lead to the ESI being not reasonably accessible.

Palgut v. City of Colorado Springs, 2007 WL 4277564 (D. Colo. Dec. 3, 2007) addressed a hardware question. The court there found that the defendant's backup tapes were not reasonably accessible because the defendant lacked the necessary hardware to access the tapes.

Determination of whether a source is not reasonably accessible is inherently fact-sensitive. The mere assertion of not reasonably accessible will not satisfy a requesting party's burden of proof. Moreover, as noted above, discovery may nevertheless be allowed.

3.4.4.1 Not Reasonably Accessible ESI in Healthcare

Many factors come into play in determining if information will be perceived within an organization as not reasonably accessible. However, common declarations such as lack of records management processes or resources are not usually acceptable to the requesting party. For more information on building a business case for enterprise content management (ECM) for litigation purposes, refer to chapter 5.

A recent investigation (Ball 2008) surveyed healthcare counsel and information professionals and asked experts to describe how they might determine the cost and resource burdens for production of ESI contained in backup data and legacy system(s) in their legal EHR. Their responses as to organizational preparedness to address not reasonably assessable data are as follows:

- Predict future costs from previous litigation experiences
- Estimate costs by a modeling a business case scenario to assess potential resource burdens
- Adjust future estimates by analyzing a gap analysis of forecasted costs to true costs of litigation
- Estimate costs with respect to state legislative restrictions on production by allowable charges per page
- Evaluate cost estimates from e-discovery vendors
- Evaluate cost using information from industry publications
- Address lack of the development of a plan and process to determine the costs associated with not reasonably accessible data
- Do not establish estimates, just absorb costs as they occur during the litigation process (Ball 2008)

Besides legacy data, other ESI from HIT systems may be controlled by vendors and may not be readily available for operational needs let alone litigation purposes such as the ability to query quality measures (Grossman 2007). Many documents and data on system reliability reside in the control of HIT suppliers, for example, identified errors related to patient safety by other vendor system clients. Contract and intellectual property implications may prevent other vendor's clients from revealing such information. Issues related to third parties and discovery are discussed in more detail later in this chapter.

3.4.5 Proportionality

A long history exists in law fundamental to the concept of **proportionality**. In 1938, the FRCP were adopted to provide for "the just, speedy, and inexpensive determination of every action." The Advisory Committee Note to 1983 Amendment to Rule 26(b) noted that the amendments were intended to "guard against redundant or disproportionate discovery by giving the court authority to reduce the amount of discovery that may be directed to matters that are otherwise proper subjects of inquiry." The 1993 amendments began to explicitly address "the information explosion of recent decades" and increases in discovery costs (*Advisory Committee Note to 1993 Amendment to Rule 26(b)*).

"All discovery is subject to the limitations imposed by Rule 26(b)(2)(C)." As referred to above, Rule 26(b)(2)(B) also refers to (C) should a court decide that there is good cause for discovery of ESI that is on a not reasonably accessible source.

Rule 26(b)(2)(C) is the proportionality rule. It provides that, either in response to a motion made by a party *or on its own*, a court must limit discovery if it finds that:

- The discovery sought is "unreasonably cumulative or duplicative, or can be obtained from some other source that is more convenient, less burdensome, or less expensive," Rule 26(b)(2)(C)(i)
- "The party seeking discovery has had ample opportunity to obtain the information by discovery in the action," Rule 26(b)(2)(C)(ii)
- "The burden or expense of the proposed discovery outweighs its likely benefit, considering the needs of the case, the amount in controversy, the parties' resources, the importance of the issues at stake in the action, and the importance of the discovery in resolving the issues," Rule 26(b)(2)(C)(iii)

Illustrative of a proportionality analysis is *Spieker v. Quest Cherokee, LLC,* 2008 WL 4758604 (D. Kan. Oct. 30, 2008). *Spieker* was brought by individual plaintiffs on behalf of a class that had not yet been certified or approved by a court. The claims of the individual plaintiffs did not exceed $100,000, yet they sought discovery of 32 gigabytes of data or an estimated 1.4 million pages of documents. The defendant refused to incur the expected production costs and the plaintiffs refused to narrow their requests. The court refused to allow the discovery as sought by the plaintiffs to proceed, noting that the class had not been certified, the plaintiffs' individual claims were limited, and the discovery was not relevant to class certification issues. Thus, the discovery costs were disproportionate to the amount at issue at the time. However, the court did note that the discovery might become appropriate should a class be certified.

Also illustrative of proportionality is *American Society for the Prevention of Cruelty to Animals v. Ringling Bros. and Barnum & Bailey Circus,* civil action no. 03-2006 (D.D.C. Aug. 5, 2008). In a hotly contested action between animal rights activists against circus operators, the defendants had deposed the plaintiffs' star witness for days over his management and preservation of ESI. The court declined to allow the deposition to proceed, finding that, "any further discovery pertaining to his [the witness'] alleged spoliation [or destruction] of e-mails or documents in light of the production of so many e-mails and other documents . . . would be unreasonably cumulative or duplicative."

Proportionality underlies all discovery in federal proceedings. It also underlies discovery of ESI from sources that are found to be not reasonably accessible. Courts have wide discretion under Rule 26(b)(2)(C) to limit or impose conditions on electronic (or other) discovery. "The conditions may take the form of limits on the amount, type, or sources of information required to be accessed and produced" (*Advisory Committee Note to 2006 Amendment to Rule 26(b)(2)(B)*). That discretion encompasses cost-shifting, that is, imposing the costs of discovery, in whole or in part, on the party requesting, rather than producing, discovery.

3.4.6 Cost-Shifting

Cost-shifting is one of the devices available to a judge under Rule 26(b)(2)(C). "The conditions [for discovery] may also include payment by the requesting party of part or all of the reasonable costs of obtaining information from sources that are not reasonably accessible" (*Advisory Committee Note to 2006 Amendment to Rule 26(b)(2)(C)*). Moreover, the Advisory Committee Note brings cost-shifting into the determination of whether good cause exists to allow discovery of ESI from sources that are not reasonably accessible: "A requesting party's willingness to share or bear the access costs may be weighed by the court in determining whether there is good cause." Thus, cost-shifting is considered to be a *possible* condition for discovery under the rules.

Three caveats are in order. First, there is case law for the proposition that cost-shifting is available *only* for not reasonably accessible information. For example, see *Peskoff v. Faber,* 240 F.R.D. 26 (D.D.C. 2007); *Zubulake v. UBS Warburg LLC,* 217 F.R.D. 309 (S.D.N.Y. 2003) (pre-2006 amendment decision using the word inaccessible). Second, as outlined in the 2006 federal Advisory Committee notes, "[T]he producing party's burdens in reviewing the information for relevance and privilege may weigh against permitting the requested discovery." Those costs that may be shifted are generally those associated with collection and production, and *not* those borne by the producing party in reviewing information for relevance or privilege (*Advisory Committee Note to 2006 Amendment to Rule 26(b)(2)(B)*). Third, at least one court has held that any application to shift costs must be made before any costs are incurred (*Cason-Merenda v. Detroit Med. Ctr.,* 2008 WL 2714239 [E.D. Mich. July 7, 2008]).

Courts have evolved tests for determining whether to shift costs. For example, in *Zubulake,* the court articulated a seven-part test, which has been widely followed by other courts in 217 F.R.D. at 322–23:

1. The extent to which the request is specifically tailored to discover relevant information
2. The availability of such information from other sources
3. The total cost of production, compared to the amount in controversy
4. The total cost of production, compared to the resources available to each party
5. The relative ability of each party to control costs and its incentive to do so
6. The importance of the issues at stake in the litigation
7. The relative benefits to the parties of obtaining the information

Cost-shifting does take place; however, the reader should understand that it happens *rarely.* There are alternatives to cost-shifting, including *sampling.* Before turning to sampling, however, some discussion of the concept of inspection of an adversary's ESI is warranted.

3.4.7 Inspection or Direct Access

Rule 34(a) was amended in 2006 "to confirm that discovery of . . . [ESI] stands on equal footing with discovery of paper documents" (*Advisory Committee Note to 2006 Amendment of Rule 34(a)*). Among other things, Rule 34(a) permits a party to request that it be allowed to "inspect, copy, test, or sample . . . items in the responding party's possession, custody or control," including ESI "stored in any medium from which information can be obtained either directly or, if necessary, after translation by the responding party into a reasonably useable form."

On its face, Rule 34(a) *might* be read to suggest that a requesting party can have direct access to an adversary's ESI. That is not, however, the intent of the rule. "Inspection or testing of certain types of . . . [ESI] or of a responding party's electronic information system may raise issues of confidentiality or privacy. The addition of testing and sampling to Rule 34(a) . . . is not meant to create a routine right of direct access to a party's electronic information system, although such access may be justified in some circumstances" (*Advisory Committee Note to 2006 Amendment to Rule 34(a)*). This is consistent with case law both before and after the 2006 amendments.

In *John B. v. Goetz*, 531 F.3d 448 (6th Cir. 2008), the court of appeals reserved an order issued by the judge presiding over a protracted action arising out of the alleged failure of the state of Tennessee to provide proper care for children enrolled in a state program. The order allowed the plaintiffs' computer expert, under the supervision of an appointed monitor and with the assistance of a US marshal, to inspect the hard drives of state agencies and some 50 state employees and to visit the latter's homes to do so. In reversing, the court of appeals emphasized that it was the responsibility of the producing party to provide discovery to its adversary and that, "mere skepticism that an opposing party has not produced all relevant information is not sufficient to warrant drastic electronic discovery measures."

Admittedly, the facts of *John B.* are extreme. Nevertheless, *John B.* demonstrates that something other than suspicion must be shown to allow direct access. On the other hand, *In re Honeywell Int'l, Inc.*, 2003 US Dist. LEXIS 20602 (S.D.N.Y. Nov. 18, 2003) demonstrates when direct access may be warranted—the court allowed access to a nonparty's audit work papers after it found that the nonparty had not provided "adequate means to decipher how the documents are kept" in electronic form.

In other words, a party to litigation need not accept its adversary's kind invitation to bring the adversary's expert into the party's workplace and inspect or image the party's ESI. Of course, as with all else, there might be discussion of direct access at a Rule 26(f) meet and confer and of circumstances under which a party *might* allow some measure of access. We know of very few cases in which the courts or counsel allowed adversary's access to native clinical applications. Not the least among the numerous reasons for this is the potential risk to an organization (such as a HIPAA violation) that could result by allowing an adversary online real-time access to the organization EHR or clinical applications. The complexities of the systems, version, local processes, and configuration and jurisdictional regulations suggest these permutations contribute to the industry philosophy that no two clinical information systems are alike even at similar healthcare organizations using the same vendor. More consideration of access to native ESI is discussed later in the section titled Discovery—Form or Forms of Production.

3.4.8 Sampling

How might sampling be used to avoid undue burden or expense? *McPeek v. Ashcroft*, 202 F.R.D. 31 (D.D.C. 2001), provides a leading example.

The plaintiff in *McPeek* brought a retaliation claim against federal officials and, to prove his claim, sought discovery of ESI from backup tapes. Rather than order the restoration and search of *all* backup tapes, the court adopted the economic principle of marginal utility and decided to take "small steps and perform, as it were, a test run." The court ordered the restoration of ESI from backup tapes for a limited period as a "convenient and rational starting point to search for evidence of retaliation."

During the test run, it was learned that only certain backup tapes were available. Rather than allow *all* the backup tapes to be restored and searched, the court observed that, "[t]he likelihood of finding relevant data has to be a function of the application of the common sense principle that people generate data referring to an event, whether e-mail or word processing documents, contemporaneous with that event, using the word 'contemporaneous' as a rough guide." Applying that principle, the court allowed the restoration and search of *one* backup tape for *one* date in *McPeek*.

McPeek demonstrates that sampling is often an iterative process, dependent on the willingness of the presiding judge to control that process. The iterative nature of sampling and of e-discovery in general is also demonstrated by *Haka v. Lincoln County,* 246 F.R.D. 577 (W.D. Wisc. 2007). *Haka* was brought by a plaintiff who represented himself and also alleged retaliation by his employer, the defendant. The ESI sought by the plaintiff totaled some four tetrabytes stored on various media. The court noted that neither party had deep pockets and ordered the parties to "proceed incrementally" with limited searches on accessible ESI stored on hard drives. The parties were also directed to share the costs of a neutral party who would undertake the searches.

In a sense, *Haka* squares the circle between sampling and cost-shifting. The court ordered an iterative approach to the discovery of a potentially enormous volume of ESI and also split the cost of that approach.

3.5 Discovery Form or Forms of Production

How, or in what form or forms, ESI may be requested or produced is governed by Rule 34(b). This seemingly simple rule has lead to an explosion of case law on the interpretation of its language. After consideration of the rule itself, our discussion will focus on some of this language.

3.5.1 Rule 34(b)

Recall that Rule 34(a) permits a party to request that another party produce ESI. Rule 34(b)(1)(C) permits the requesting party to "specify the form or forms in which . . . [ESI] is to be produced." Rule 34(b)(2)(D) addresses responses to requests: "The response may state an objection to a requested form for producing . . . [ESI]. If the responding party objects to a requested form—or if no form was specified in the request—the party must state the form or forms it intends to use."

Rule 34(b)(2)(E) describes procedures that apply to production if ESI, "[u]nless otherwise stipulated or ordered by the court":

(i)   A party must produce documents as they are kept in the usual course of business or must organize and label them to correspond to the categories in the request

(ii)   If the request does not specify a form for producing . . . [ESI], a party must produce it in a form or forms in which it is ordinarily maintained or in a reasonably useable form or forms

(iii)   A party need not produce the same . . . [ESI] in more than one form

Detailed reference to the Advisory Committee Note to the 2006 amendment to Rule 34(b) is in order:

- The production of . . . [ESI] should be subject to comparable requirements [to produce documents as kept in the "usual course of business" or to organize and label the documents] to protect against deliberate or inadvertent production in ways that raise unnecessary obstacles for the requesting party.

- The form of production is more important to the exchange of . . . [ESI] than of hard-copy materials, although a party might specify hard copy as the requested form. Specification of the desired form or forms may facilitate the orderly, efficient, and cost-effective discovery of . . . [ESI].

- The rule recognizes that different types of production may be appropriate for different types of . . . [ESI]. Using current technology, for example, a party might be called upon to produce word processing documents, e-mail messages, electronic spreadsheets, different image or sound files, and material from a database. Requiring that such diverse types of . . . [ESI] all be produced in the same form could prove impossible, and even if possible could increase the cost and burdens of producing and using the information. The rule therefore provides that the requesting party may ask for different types of production for different types of . . . [ESI].

- A party that responds to a discovery request by simply producing . . . [ESI] in a form of its choice, without identifying the form in advance of the production in the response required by Rule 34(b), runs a risk that the requesting party can show that the produced form is not reasonably usable and that it is entitled to production of some or all of the information in an additional form.

- [T]he option to produce in a reasonably usable form does not mean that a responding party is free to convert . . . [ESI] from the form in which it is ordinarily maintained to a different form that makes it more difficult or burdensome for the requesting party to use the information efficiently in the litigation. If the responding party ordinarily maintains the information it is producing in a way that makes it searchable by electronic means, the information should not be produced in a form that removes or significantly degrades this feature. (Advisory Committee Note to 2006 Amendment to Rule 34(b)).

In other words, ESI exists in many forms. Parties may request and produce ESI in more than one form. Parties that maintain ESI should not take steps to downgrade ESI to make the ESI harder to search by an adversary. And, while not quoted above, the Advisory Committee note explicitly references the need for parties to meet and confer before they bring any dispute about form of production to a court. The note also reminds parties that ESI may be maintained in a form that is "not reasonably usable" and gives as an example " 'legacy' data that can be used only by superseded systems." In such circumstances, Rule 26(b)(2)(B) controls.

3.5.1.1 Forms and Formats in EHR ESI

The following definitions are provided to assist the reader concerning the form of preservation and production of ESI relevant to e-discovery. (Please refer to the comprehensive glossary to aid in a further understanding of the semantics of e-discovery, HIT, and HIM.)

The word "form" is used in the same context routinely discussed for legal discovery to describe the form of preservation or form of production of electronic data or documents. Form is specifically used to describe any combination of the following:

- Data format—The electronic version of data (for example, native file or static images)
- Output—The EHR version available for routine business use by end users. The output may be a version of:
  - The human-computer interface (HCI)
  - Reports—Standard structured data reports produced from the legal EHR (for example, Crystal Reports, Business Objects, SQL reports)
- Metadata:
  - Information embedded in a native file that is not ordinarily viewable or printable from the application that generated, edited, or modified it

- Information generated automatically by the operation of a computer or other IT system when a native file is created, modified, transmitted, deleted, or otherwise manipulated by a user of such system. Metadata is a subset of ESI.
- **Native file(s)**—ESI in the electronic format of the application in which such ESI is normally created, viewed, and/or modified. Native files are a subset of ESI.
- Static image(s)—A representation of ESI produced by converting a native file into a standard image format capable of being viewed and printed on standard computer systems. For example, a static image could be provided in either tagged image file format (TIFF, or .TIF) or **portable document format (PDF)**.

3.5.1.1.1 Various Forms and Formats of the Legal EHR

Until recently, the production of healthcare clinical documents in a discovery request assumed only one form, paper. That paper was indexed and organized for counsel, resembling the routine business record order. In the era of manila folders as the solitary container of the medical record, HIM professionals had sardonically declared, "that everything on the right side of the folder is discoverable and everything on the left was not relevant" (Dougherty 2007). Production of these types of records in the electronic form would have been considered an exercise of expensive scanning and useless to opposing counsel who would most likely have converted these electronic documents back to paper for litigation purposes.

In only a few sectors of the economy are the highest-level professionals responsible for the majority of the production, customer service, and clerical work as mandated in healthcare. The comprehensive health record started as a note to oneself or fellow clinical colleagues, likened to a laboratory entry of an intellectual scientist making notations of the day's work, and the (medical) decision-making processes. The clinical record has morphed into a menu of communications for government, third-party payers, regulators, lawyers, policy makers, and beyond. Satisfying the clinical, administrative, and regulatory requirements of data entry for each clinical encounter is daunting, no matter in what medium, paper or electronic.

How we balance structured and unstructured data, while adopting standards of excellence for care processes, has not been determined. Defining this balance is even more pressing an issue as the Stage 2 criteria (IFR 45 CFR part 170, 2010) of "meaningful use" in order "to encourage the use of health IT for continuous quality improvement at the point of care and the exchange of information in the most structured format possible," including clinical summaries, such as clinical care documents (CCD) or clinical care records (CCR), is required in the not too distant future.

In the present era of increased adoption of EHRs, the expectation is that counsel will encounter a greater number of form-of-production disputes. These disputes will involve not only paper versus electronic form, but disputes about different types of electronic production. Presently, the minority of documents produced for discovery from HIT systems are in an electronic form, the exception being radiological images. Most health record electronic production usually mimics paper document production. The electronic files may be just an image that is converted from the native file format into a static image and essentially serves as a photocopy of the electronic version of the document. At a glance, this type of electronic reproduction may appear more satisfactory than early, more primitive EHR systems that were essentially clinical word processors or basic documentation templates. The production of these document-centric systems in an electronic form simply involved a copy, as it would appear on a screen or in a paper printout.

The more complex, integrated EHRs systems make it more problematic for healthcare organizations to make decisions regarding the form of production. The chart in many modern EHRs is a summation of a variety of note types that may be derived from different native electronic media. The spectrum spans from simple, scanned paper and note entries on Microsoft Word–like templates to a sophisticated multimillion-dollar proprietary vendor software system composed of transactional databases. Chapter 1 provides a primer on the advantages of these types of transactional systems for clinical purposes and shares some of the challenges for HIM professionals.

Figure 3.3 provides examples of the various forms of EHRs with a focus on clinical elements of a typical IP encounter. These examples should not be considered a comprehensive list related to form or format of ESI in EHRs. Many of the problems also apply to the form of administrative data usually considered a part of the evidentiary health record; however, this book's focus is on records from clinical software systems. The intent is to illustrate the complexities of what has previously been described as a simple discovery rule related to form and the associated challenges for litigation decision makers about the use of integrated HIT systems.

Certain FRCP Rule 34 considerations are exemplified with the above-mentioned subset of clinically relevant components of an EHR system.

Figure 3.3.   Examples of potential available forms from a single inpatient encounter

---

Emergency department notes: Structured data entry and database output

- General information: Standalone emergency department (ED); system interfaced with a hospital HIT system
- Forms from originating ED system
  1. XML: contains every keystroke of data entry into the system and all metadata for both the system and application
  2. PDF printout with author/creator, time/data stamp metadata
  3. Print screen or screen capture from human-computer interface
- Forms from ED encounter available in the main hospital system
  1. TIFF file: Static image imported though interface, no metadata
  2. Print screen or screen capture from human-computer interface

History and physical: Transcription from dictation

1. Original digital voice file of dictation, electronic media
2. Printed transcription that has been reviewed and validated

Daily progress notes

1. Free text note, printed
2. Structured template note, database output report
3. Handwritten note, back-end scanned into EHR system

Consultant note: Uploaded from homegrown template carried on peripheral device (for example, a USB drive)

1. Cut and paste upload; no metadata
2. Original copy on consultant's peripheral device in standard Word format, with embedded metadata

Anesthesia notes: Paper and scanned by HIM

1. Original paper
2. Scanned image of paper, PDF, or paper

Nurse notes: Structured template note, database output report

1. Printed report
2. Print screen or screen capture from human-computer interface
3. Nursing flow sheet (used in the normal course of business, requires access to proprietary system)

Laboratory data

1. EHR review tab windows: metadata contains time of order (used in the normal course of business, requires access to proprietary system)
2. EHR lab flow sheets: metadata contains time of order, time results were reviewed (used in the normal course of business, requires access to proprietary system)
3. Laboratory information system (CLIA subpart K standards of retention): metadata, time of order, time of collection, time of results, time-critical results called to provider

---

Medication administration record (e-MAR)

- Nurse, physician, and/or pharmacists screen views (used in the normal course of business, required access to proprietary system)
    1. No printing function available
    2. Report writer from separate database, export potential to Excel format
    3. Print screen or screen capture from human-computer interface

Radiology images/reports

1. An electronic copy of certain components of the record (does not contain wet readings)
2. Access to proprietary system (contains wet readings)
3. Printed copy of final reports and addenda (does not contain wet readings)

Biomedical data

- Cardiac rhythm strips interfaced with EHR
    1. Comprehensive data maintained in system until patient discharged (not usually kept in normal course of business)
    2. Imported strips in EHR
- Smart infusion pump data
    1. Data maintained in pump for limited number of encounters unless output exported to another medium, usually printed output (not usually kept in normal course of business)

Various forms exist for production from each component that makes up the legal EHR. The form satisfying the best evidence rule may be difficult to determine due to HIT system limitations and the lack of organizational litigation-readiness team involvement in early system decision making. As expectations of health communications and health information exchange add new types of ESI that must be managed—including but not limited to provider-patient e-mail, personal health records (PHRs), other medical device data (for example, insulin pumps), and home device data (for example, electronic scales, gluco-meter readings)—difficulties will arise in defining the boundaries of the complete record components. Expect an increase in dissention among parties concerning best forms for production and completeness of relevant ESI in future healthcare legal proceedings involving clinical applications.

In litigation, designated forms of production must satisfy specific requests. Contrary to popular belief among many stakeholders, including non-HIM laypersons, public policy makers, and many legal experts, there is not a universal "print" button for HIT applications to support the comprehensive data and documents optimal for litigation purposes. The courts which are still very document-centric in their understanding of the medical record, and will sooner rather than later begin to recognize the need to reevaluate previous assumptions as more difficult cases are heard involving e-discovery and modern clinical software systems.

Discussions focus on hospital-based clinical software systems. The concepts also are common to many ambulatory systems as well. As previously discussed, printing may be in an electronic or paper form from the original EHR system. Many controversial reasons exist as to why printing may be less than adequate for both clinical and litigation purposes.

Industry experiences and informatics research have described significant problems with printed output from EHRs. Printing problems include, but are not limited to (Rollins 2007; Ball et al. 2008):

- Inadequate quality testing of printing in pre- and post-implementation planning
- Inability to print portions of the encounter
- Report logic and writer/scripting that does not contain all the relevant data
- Printed reports that contain data duplications
- Printed reports that contain discrepancies in data elements
- Format of output not reasonably usable by counsel
- Format of output not reasonably searchable by counsel
- Lengthy printouts, not categorized as maintained in normal course of business
- Printouts with unclear meaning of data
- Lack of minimal necessary metadata in printed reports (for example, identifying originating author/creator, and time/date stamp)
- Lack of assurances of data quality and integrity
- Discrepancies over time of printed output due to system or report writer/scripting changes

Presently, medical litigators usually receive paper copies of essential clinical documentation and administrative data (Shay 2007). Rarely, some clinical documentation is reproducible from EHRs in an electronic media such as a standard PDF. PDFs are files that are highly portable across many computer platforms. Metadata limitations should be taken into consideration when printing to paper or electronic files. Health records are rarely produced in native format.

The reasons for such heavy reliance on print copies are straightforward. First, the developers and vendors did not take into account clinical software requirements for basic evidentiary purposes. Second, EHR functionalities were initially implemented to assist in the communication across the continuum of care delivery to support operational outcomes with little regard to business records retention regulations or litigation rules. Some experts suggest that vendors may have ignored evidentiary record and patient safety concerns under contract provisions perceived as shielding (Koppel and Kreda 2009). This self-protection has been described by informatics experts as a reflection of a larger problem where vendors have an inappropriate overconfidence of the HIT industry itself (Silverstein 2009).

King and Bunsen (2009) provide of an industry leading-edge medical malpractice case in regard to forms of production from EHR systems. The actual case name and citation was not revealed due to the ongoing active medical malpractice case. This case provides an example of a court order for production of EHRs in native format and highlights future considerations for counsel and vendors. In a complaint alleging failure to recognize in a timely manner and prevent complications of sepsis, a court compelled NorthShore University Health System to produce medical records in their native form from Epic software. NorthShore, the defendant, disclosed paper printouts of a 63-day inpatient stay; however, the plaintiff requested access to the Epic record and filed a motion to compel production of the record in its native format. The plaintiff's attorney described lack of easy or usable paper records in determining author and date stamps of entries from the paper output. The plaintiff's attorney obtained a court order for an on-site review of the medical record in Epic, claiming they wanted to see what the physicians saw. Despite an affidavit filed on NorthShore's behalf defining their legal electronic record, the court ordered both parties to coordinate a solution.

NorthShore's information system and legal teams developed a read-only legal medical record. A HIM nurse auditor developed read-only legal medical records and performed integrity audits. The developed electronic version prevented changes such as deletions or additions. NorthShore counsel reviewed the read-only record to ensure compliance with the court order. Interestingly, the court ordered the vendor to split the cost of creating the read-only version of the electronic records.

Changes are imminent in both vendors' and the healthcare organizations' sophistication in future interpretations of Rules 36(b), 26(f), and 45(d)(1)(C) and organizational consideration for forms and formats produced in litigation.

Another concern arises as health organizations are becoming more reliant on third-party vendors to maintain their ESI. For example, web-based ASP models have become more commonplace. Details of Rule 45 and third parties are discussed in greater detail in the Rule 45 section later in this chapter.

Litigation requirements for an evidentiary record from clinical documentation software are a late addition to EHR systems and explain part of the difficulty in defining completeness of the record and HIM and counsels' ability to manage data effectively for legal purposes. The authors' experiences reveal that the HIT industry standard does not afford the functionality for litigators to produce EHR data in a form compatible with that used in the usual course of business, except where required by regulations as discussed in more detail.

3.5.1.1.2 EHR Records Management and Evidentiary Support Standard— Health Record Output

The HL7 RM-ES standard addresses the output from EHR systems. More work needs to be done to bridge the gap for usable, concise reports and output for medical records. One of the challenges is the healthcare industry's slowness to recognize the importance of the output from the EHR systems. At the core is a perception that the move to EHRs means there should not be paper printouts, reports, or other types of output. Unfortunately, that position does not reflect the reality of how health records are used and shared for many different purposes. The RM-ES standard describes the following functionality for EHR systems (HL7 2010):

> S.2.2.1—Health Record Output: EHR systems must support the definition of the formal health record, a partial record for referral purposes, or sets of records for other necessary disclosure purposes. The system must provide hardcopy and electronic output that fully chronicles the healthcare process, supports selection of specific sections of the health record, and allows healthcare organizations to define the report and/or documents that will comprise the formal health record for disclosure purposes. Systems should support the ability to view and disclose the patient care events over a range of time in chronological order.

> The formal health record, also called the legal health record, is the official representation of an episode of care. Organizations identify and declare in policy data and records that comprise the health record. This health record defined by the organization is the version disclosed upon request. A mechanism should be provided for both chronological and specified record-element output.

An auditable record of these requests and associated exports may be maintained by the system. This record could be implemented in any way that would allow the who, what, why, and when of a request and export to be recoverable for review. The system has the capability of providing a report or accounting of disclosures by patient that is in accordance with scope of practice, organizational policy, and jurisdictional law.

To support the disclosure process, systems may provide functionality to redact reports prior to view or disclosure. Redaction is the process of obscuring or removing from view data in a report or document to prevent the receiver from seeing that data. This may be necessary in responding to litigation requests in which a portion of report must be disclosed, but some data elements may not (HL7 2010).

The report process (whether the health record or other reports from the EHR system) is required to support the litigation process and the requirement to provide relevant information and records. EHR systems should be able to perform the following minimum criteria related to reporting health record output (HL7 2010):

- The system shall provide the ability to generate reports consisting of all or part of an individual patient's record.
- The system shall provide the ability to define the records or reports that are considered the formal health record for a specified disclosure or disclosure purposes.
- The system shall provide the ability to generate reports in both chronological and specified record-elements order.
- The system shall provide the ability to create hardcopy and electronic report summary information (procedures, medications, labs, immunizations, allergies, and vital signs).
- The system should provide the ability to specify or define reporting groups (such as print sets) for specific types of disclosure or information sharing.
- The system shall provide the ability to include patient-identifying information on each page of reports generated.
- The system shall provide the ability to customize reports to match mandated formats.
- The system shall provide the ability to generate a report that includes record metadata for disclosure.
- The system should provide the ability to redact (remove from view and/or output) data elements or portions of a report to prevent the recipient from seeing certain data.
- The system may provide the ability to cite the reasons for redaction.
- The system may provide the ability to reproduce a copy of the redacted document/record.

- The system should provide the ability to sort/configure patient care events by date and time ranges and data/record type.
- The system should provide the ability to maintain a record of disclosure/release that includes the recipient and outbound content.

Even with robust reporting processes, the input process and the output processes are different for EHR systems. This has been a sticking point for litigation involving EHRs because record output looks different than the screen inputs. This is a reflection of the database design of EHRs and the variability of the input, queries, and outputs. HIM professionals must work with their organizations to define their legal health record policy and with their EHR system/vendor to improve functionality, usability, and comprehensiveness of the health record output.

3.5.1.1.3 Issues of Evidence and e-Discovery and EHR Databases

The complexities in defining just what *is* a record from a database are not unique to healthcare. A brief discussion of the topic and its relevance to e-evidence and e-discovery follows.

One of the most evident issues related to e-discovery is experts' dialogues on the form of preservation and production of the legal EHR. The FRCP required that issues related to production of form responsive records be discussed early and often. A major problem with disclosure of records, in the form of queries or outputs from database reports, is their very dynamic nature. Database information is constantly changing and being updated, and has implications across the discovery process from form of production to authentication.

Regulatory precedence exists in healthcare related to dynamic database outputs and business records retention and production needs. The Clinical Laboratory Improvement Amendments (CLIA), subpart K, specifically states a requirement that laboratories must retain or be able to produce an *exact duplicate* of each testing laboratory's report; this is *not* a PDF or tiff/jpeg scan of the original report, but rather the report as it was originally available for clinical purposes (CLIA subpart K, 817 Section 493.1291: Test report).

(i) If a laboratory refers patient specimens for testing—

(i)(1) The referring laboratory must not revise results or information directly related to the interpretation of results provided by the testing laboratory.

Interpretive Guidelines Section 493.1291(h)(i)(1):

> If these standards are imposed on EHRs for clinical documentation, obvious difficulties must be considered for those managing HIT databases. Archived data must be independent of hardware and software. Management of legacy systems becomes a very difficult and significant consideration of e-evidence, metadata, and authentication, and admissibility must be taken into account in lifecycle decision making. Data must remain unchanged once it is archived. Archiving requires metadata to be meaningful and contain the minimal metadata to prove the data is unchanged.

As exemplified by the experiences of the financial industry, *In re Vee Vinhnee,* 336 B.R. 437 (9th Cir. BAP 2005) summary reports from databases, preserved statements, and reports generated from transaction data are not adequate because those who may scrutinize data integrity understand that the outputs are partial, aggregate reports of a larger conglomerate of data.

The CLIA subpart K regulation sheds light and provides precedence for some of the evidentiary issues related to EHR query reports that are ordinarily maintained for routine business, especially if those reports have a tendency to change due to structural and data element changes of dynamic databases. The differences between the original and later disclosed outputs may be related to the "now phenomenon" of relational databases (for example, updates in persons' address or allergies), logic (for example, logic calculations for present age based on date of birth even if patient is deceased), or artificial intelligence (for example, decision support systems), or system version releases (for example, upgrades and service packs.)

3.5.1.1.4 CLIA, Health Information Exchange, and Electronic Health Records

The CLIA Revised Interpretive Guideline (CMS 2010) redefines certain CLIA interpretive guidelines related to the transmission of laboratory results in the era of health information exchange. This represents the beginning of what CMS expects to be a series of memoranda in support of the electronic exchange of laboratory information.

The new interpretive guidelines appear to allow for the potential to diminish the standards of laboratory information systems (LIS) data integrity. This is done in order to encourage the ease of HIT adoption and HIE and lessen the burden that LIS must retain or be able to produce an exact duplicate of an output that contains information that provides an accurate, complete, and easily understood *display* of previously reported data retained or retrieved from the laboratory's record system. The interpretation of these CLIA changes may allow potential new latitudes in LIS output for health information exchange and unlock unintended discussions about data integrity and system reliability concerns with electronic evidentiary legal experts.

3.5.1.1.5 Forms and Access to Non-Party Proprietary Systems

Many applied informatics professionals, clinicians, and providers argue that the best method for reproducing a patient encounter is by displaying relevant clinical data through direct viewing on proprietary systems. Navigating the actual systems may be the only manner to simulate who knew "what" and "when" related to the medical decision-making process. Counsel may have innumerable reasons and rationale for why the opposing teams should not be afforded such an open invitation, including risk to data integrity; security and privacy risks; intellectual property clauses in vendors' contacts; vendor claims of "non-party"; and training requirements.

Adequate training to pilot many modern EHR systems takes weeks to months, a time frame neither party is willing to entertain. Although clinical systems experts are available, configuration, customization, and local processes are usually determined at the health facility level. As stated by an experienced healthcare attorney, "if you know one EHR, you know one EHR" (Shay 2007).

3.5.1.1.6 Mitigating Risks to Data Integrity

Risks to data integrity may potentially be mitigated if parties have the ability to access a view-only status of the data, a security capability common in roles-based systems, or alternatively, for certain downtime views of many systems. Non-healthcare industry case law may give us some insight into the courts' rulings about a vendor's non-party claims to Rule 34 and non-party claims of privilege of proprietary systems. In *In re Honeywell International, Inc.* (S.D.N.Y. 2003), a securities class action, the plaintiffs served PriceWaterhouseCoopers (PWC) a non-party subpoena. In response, PWC produced 63,500 hard-copy pages. The plaintiff moved to compel production in electronic form, claiming that the data as produced were neither in business record order nor labeled to correspond to the categories of the request as required by Rule 34. Plaintiffs complained that the manner in which the papers were produced made it impossible to establish which data elements, documents, or attachments belonged to a particular work paper.

The case is further summarized by respected e-discovery expert Kenneth Withers (2006):

> The court acknowledged that PWC had produced paper versions but stated it was "insufficient because they were not produced as kept in the usual course of business." The court required that PWC produce the data in electronic form and said that PWC could avoid the $30,000 expense by also producing the proprietary software to access the data. The court noted that the plaintiffs were not competitors and a confidentiality order was already in place, so PWC's trade-secret interests in the electronic form would be adequately protected. (*In re Honeywell International, Inc.* (2003)).

In re Honeywell International, Inc. opens up challenging discussions for attorneys involved in EHRs and the 34(b) rule including quality and usability of paper reports from custom-built clinical software and issues of the status of the proprietary nature of non-parties' systems. Frontline HIM, informatics, and risk management professionals are aware that many of the hard copies of EHRs may be considered "papers with hieroglyphic indices that render the[m] . . . essentially incomprehensible" (*In re Honeywell International, Inc.* (2003)).

3.5.1.1.7 EHR Records Management and Evidentiary Support Standard—Entity Authentication, Entity Authorization, and Entity Access Control

Because EHR software is not readily available in off-the-shelf form for plaintiff parties to use in accessing native files, performing data manipulations, and review, healthcare organizations may find it necessary to provide access to the EHR system, such as through remote access or on-site review, if negotiated. The following system security functions will be critical if allowing a plaintiff's attorney access to the EHR application. The HL7 RM-ES standard describes the following functionality (HL7 2010):

> IN.1.1—Entity Authentication: Authenticate EHR-S users and/or entities before allowing access to an EHR-S.

> IN.1.2—Entity Authorization: Manage the sets of access-control permissions granted to entities that use an EHR-S (EHR-S users).

> IN.1.3—Entity Access Control: Verify and enforce access control to all EHR-S components and EHR information and functions for end-users, applications, and sites to prevent unauthorized use of a resource.

If healthcare organizations need to provide access to the EHR system, the plaintiff attorney(s) should be authenticated as a unique user(s) with permissions and access limited to only the relevant record(s) and time frames.

3.5.2 Illustrative Case Law

This book is intended to be an introduction to e-discovery. Accordingly, rather than attempt to review the many decisions that have addressed form of production, several have been chosen and summarized in this section.

3.5.2.1 Possession, Custody, or Control

What does it mean to have possession, custody, or control over ESI? This question becomes especially important for organizations that rely on third-party vendors to maintain the organizations' ESI. The answer to the question of control dictates whether a party may request production of such ESI in a Rule 34 request or must subpoena a non-party.

In *Tomlinson v. El Paso Corp.,* 254 F.R.D. 474 (D. Colo. 2007), the plaintiffs sought production by the defendant of electronic pension plan records held by a non-party pension plan administrator. The court found that the records were within the possession, custody, or control of the defendant because it had a statutory obligation to maintain the data.

Healthcare organizations are required by law to maintain vast amounts of ESI. Consistent with *Tomlinson,* it would appear that such ESI is within an organization's control and need be produced in discovery by the organization in response to a discovery request. Moreover, should an organization attempt to argue that it does not have control over ESI in the possession of a third-party vendor, the organization should expect that any contract with the vendor would be discoverable.

3.5.2.2 Usual Course of Business

What does it mean to produce ESI in the usual course of business? Several decisions demonstrate what that phrase does *not* mean.

In *Ak-Chin Indian Community v. United States,* 85 Fed. Cl. 397 (Ct. Ct. 2009), electronic documents sought by the plaintiff tribe had been transferred to an agency, which used an off-the-shelf commercial software package to index the documents. The court found that, "[o]nce . . . disassembled . . . and reorganized to comport with the filing system," the documents were no longer kept in the usual course of business. The agency was ordered to organize and label the documents to correspond with the tribe's requests.

Similarly, in *SEC v. Collins & Aikman Corp.*, 2009 U.S. Dist. LEXIS 3367 (S.D.N.Y. Jan. 13, 2009), a defendant objected to the manner in which the SEC responded to requests to produce. The SEC had turned over some 1.7 million documents, but had not categorized these in a manner consistent with the defendant's requests. The court found that the documents were not kept by the plaintiff agency in the usual course of business as these were gathered as a result of the agency's investigation into possible securities fraud and ordered the agency undertake the categorization.

Ak-Chin and *SEC* demonstrate that the usual course of business is just that: a party may avail itself this option to produce electronic records only if these are created and maintained on a regular basis. Manipulation of ESI is not usual.

3.5.2.2.1 EHR Form in the Usual Course of Business

In many modern sophisticated HIT systems, providers are usually less familiar with accessing an archival document-centric repository or a paper print version of reports for routine care encounters. Normally, providers utilize various types of relevant retrieval review, sort, and filter functions directly accessed from the EHR. This manner of navigation is how providers using EHRs routinely behave in clinical practice and are most familiar for retrieving pertinent patient information to formulate a synopsis of a care encounter in their usual course of business. Dilemmas may arise at the time of the deposition related to data translations from printed outputs unfamiliar to the provider now serving as a witness.

So the question arises, is the only real record maintained in normal course of business the actual integrated EHR system itself? Is counsel willing to allow witnesses and opposing litigating teams to have access and manipulate their organization's EHR systems?

Clinical notes in the electronic world take on many forms and formats, and the ability to reproduce these adequately for discovery depends on the how, what, and where the data were initially entered and retrieved; embedded computer logic; scripting language/logic allowing extraction from databases; and the ability to "freeze" data. Regardless of the infrastructure of modern EHR systems, HIT developers and vendors have chosen essentially two paths to managing and maintaining clinical records for routine business purposes' disclosure and discovery: either to maintain the final completed, validated, and attested document in a static format (with or without metadata), maintained in a central, and usually separate, archival repository; or, alternatively, to be satisfied with a dynamic database structure without accounting for the risks of producing different outputs during disclosure. At a glance, this spectrum of extremes may appear an oversimplification, but it is presently the harsh reality of the review process in EHRs. The latter is more common to the industry as it moves to large transactional database systems.

The dynamic nature of these federated and interfaced databases systems makes it difficult and expensive to take a snapshot for litigation. Some vendors, however, have begun to retain parallel database environments that retain a significant portion of transactional data. The existence of these repositories is not always disclosed during litigation.

Other questions related to privilege may arise if these repositories are used in the normal course of business for operational purposes such as quality reporting and peer review. In *Youle v. Ryan*, 349 Ill. App. 3d 377, 380, 811 N.E.2d 1281, 1283 (2004), Youle sued Ryan, a physician, for negligence in the removal of her gallbladder. Youle requested production of Ryan's surgical database. Ryan refused and argued the database contained all of Ryan's other patient histories, including his past gallbladder surgeries. Youle claimed that the past surgeries were relevant in proving her negligence claim because the database might show a pattern of negligence. The trial court granted Youle's motion, and Ryan appealed. Ryan claimed that the contents of the database were protected and would not lead to any discoverable information. The appellate court reversed with instructions, ruling that the trial court should examine the database **in camera**, and determine whether the database contains discoverable information. The appellate court ruled that the trial court should have taken this action before granting the motion to compel because the database may have contained no discoverable information.

3.5.2.3 Downgrading ESI

What does it mean to downgrade ESI? *In re Classicstar Mare Lease Litigation*, 2009 WL 250954 (E.D. Kan. Feb. 2, 2009) offers an example of what downgrading does *not* mean. In *Classicstar*, a party converted ESI into TIFF images without embedded metadata. The production order did not specify form. The court found that the defendant did not downgrade data by this conversion under the circumstances but that, based on an agreement between counsel, production in native format (for example, with metadata intact) was required.

3.5.2.3.1 Downgrading EHR ESI

Metadata has become extremely important in assessing reliability and dependability of healthcare information for legal, clinical, regulatory, and research needs. While metadata plays an important role in assessing the integrity of the components of legal EHR systems, do existing EHR software applications have the ability to preserve the minimum metadata necessary for assurance of non-repudiation of the health record?

Industry experience has suggested that paper output from EHRs may lack critical data elements including metadata. Despite describing evidentiary elements in the EHR metadata, only a quarter of the experts in one investigation reported that the ability existed to print metadata from the components of the legal EHR (Ball 2008). Fewer than 5 percent of experts indicated that legal EHR systems had the ability to capture an alert or decision-support information so it could be displayed to counsel in the format in which the original user visualized it.

3.5.2.4 Metadata

According to The Sedona Conference Working Group Series 2007, "A large amount of . . . [ESI], unlike paper, is associated with or contains information that is not readily apparent on the screen view of the file. This additional information is usually known as 'metadata.'" A spreadsheet is a simple example of metadata. On its face, the spreadsheet consists of numbers in cells. Where do those numbers come from? The number in each cell is generated from a formula into which raw numbers are inserted, and neither the raw numbers nor the formulas are apparent on the spreadsheet. Plainly, when the information on the spreadsheet is relevant, the formula and the raw numbers are relevant too. Only the formula and the raw numbers allow the information on the spreadsheet to be tested and challenged.

Is metadata subject to discovery? The answer, not surprisingly, is that it depends. Is the metadata relevant? *Aguilar v. ICE Div.,* 2008 WL 5062700 (S.D.N.Y. Nov. 21, 2008) is a nuanced and extensive exploration of metadata. The plaintiffs in this civil rights class action requested the production of metadata from e-mail and electronic documents as well as the production of spreadsheets and databases in native format. The defendants offered to produce ESI in text-searchable TIFF format. Metadata had not been the subject of a Rule 26(f) meet and confer and had been mentioned by the attorneys only in passing.

Aguilar showed that, if requested in a timely manner, courts grant access to metadata and direct that production be in native format. However, absent a timely request, such results were unlikely as the producing party would have to make a second production. Production of metadata or native format would be ordered only if doing so would produce relevant ESI or materially aid the search for relevant ESI. The court found that metadata would be, at best, marginally relevant to the plaintiffs' claims and would not materially aid their search of the ESI already provided. Thus, it would allow production only if the plaintiffs bore the costs. The court did, however, order the production of spreadsheets in native format.

The authors provide more discussions on metadata under challenges to data integrity discussions and admissibility in the section on Admissibility later in this chapter.

3.5.2.4.1 EHR Metadata

The basic questions that HIM and litigation preparedness teams should entertain in formulation of approaches to metadata and forms for discovery may include the following:

- Does the form of the legal EHR produced at discovery routinely contain metadata?
- Do the organization's routine custodians of health records have the ability to access metadata associated with legal EHR?
- Do the components comprising the EHR system support user-friendly outputs of the metadata for transmission, printing, or export?
- What is the ordinary retention cycle for the organization's legal EHR system metadata?
- If the legal EHR output does not contain metadata, would lack of this information in the output downgrade the usability of the ESI for discovery purposes?
- Does the date/time/user stamp for each clinical entry at the data-element level entered appear in the metadata?
- If an expert were needed to analyze metadata for the legal EHR for counsel, who would your organization provide for this expertise?
- Are you aware if the time clock of each component computer system that comprises your organization's legal EHR is synchronized in some manner?
- Does your system allow for differentiation of date/time/user stamps indicating when patient care is delivered versus when patient care is documented?

As discussed briefly in chapter 1, the standards community is beginning to tackle specific issues that support a legally sound EHR system. The HL7 standard provides a framework of functions and conformance criteria for EHR systems as a mechanism to support an organization in maintaining a legally sound health record (Dougherty 2007).

3.5.2.4.2 Electronic Super-Record Model

The electronic superrecord (Ball 2008), or e-super record, is an ideal form of the comprehensive electronic business record. Essential elements in defining the e-super record follow. The e-super record is:

- Ordinarily maintained for routine business and transactional purposes
- Adapted specifically to an organization's business needs
- Meant to contain predetermined and known data sources
- Finite in size, although it may be large
- Set up to contain only the minimum necessary metadata sets
- Manageable for general business and evidentiary needs
- Capable of being safely destroyed when no longer considered an organizational asset

3.5.2.4.3 The Minimum Necessary Metadata Set

The **minimum necessary** metadata set is a subcategory of the e-super record and includes both system logic metadata and component-user metadata (Ball 2008). These types of metadata are distinguished by changes based on the input of people (application metadata), metadata reflecting changes from the computer system itself (system metadata), and programming logic. The minimum set is all that is needed to prove that e-evidence is authentic.

In legal EHR e-discovery, the minimum metadata set must identify who accessed the record, what they did to or with the record, and when they accessed it, thus establishing authorship, access, creation, amendments addenda, and electronic printing or copying. E-evidence experts describe metadata in terms in terms of an electronic chain of evidence. Metadata, if considered relevant, is discoverable evidence that healthcare information professionals are obliged to preserve and produce in litigation. Relevance of metadata should be taken into consideration in regard to forms produced and the associated evidentiary significance.

3.5.2.4.4 EHR Records Management and Evidentiary Support Standard—Minimum Metadata Set and Retention

EHR systems collect a vast amount of audit data for security and system and application function. The HL7 RM-ES standard identifies a subset of audit data (metadata) that supports the electronic medical records authenticity and integrity. The RM-ES standard called this specific type of audit data the point of record minimum metadata set (HL7 2010).

> IN.2.1.1—Point of Record Minimum Metadata Set: Metadata provides electronic evidence that describes record characteristics such as the origin, usage, and modification. EHR-S information must maintain a minimum set of metadata on medical record information for the legally prescribed timeframe in accordance with organizational policy to retain legal validity of the record. EHR-S information and records that are part of the organization's formal medical record must include a minimum set of metadata (audit record data) retained over the lifespan of the record/information. This concept is similar to the requirements for paper documents in which a minimum set of data elements is retained for the life of the document. These elements indicate who created a document, when, the modifications made, and information related to document access. Metadata helps to validate the authenticity, reliability, usability, and integrity of electronic information over time and enables the management and understanding of electronic information (physical, analogue, or digital).
>
> The capture and retention of select pieces of metadata provides support for the validity of the record and is necessary to establish the trust of a receiving party in data that is being exchanged. Metadata also supports internal audit processes within a healthcare organization.

Metadata provides evidence that supports the authenticity and trustworthiness of electronic records and information used in legal proceedings. The RM-ES standard includes the following criteria to evaluate a system's compliance (HL7 2010):

- The system shall note and record identifiers for the author(s) of record/information.
- The system shall capture and retain the time stamp for object or data creation, modification, view, and deletion.
- The system shall capture and record identifiers for viewers of the organization's electronic medical record.
- The system shall capture and record identifiers of author(s) of changes in a record.
- The system shall capture and retain the change history of a record.

- The system may produce metadata that identifies the source of non-originated data (for example, pre-positioned, templated, copied, duplicated, boilerplate, and such).
- The system shall retain the medical record metadata in accordance with the legally prescribed timeframe or organizational policy.
- The system should have the ability to include the minimum metadata set for medical record data upon exchange or release of EHR data/records.
- The system may provide the ability to include the minimum metadata information on the health record output (for example, a report).

3.6 Privilege

One basic premise of litigation is that information subject to the attorney-client privilege or entitled to work product protection (hereinafter referred to as privilege) should be protected from disclosure. E-discovery, which can involve enormous volumes of ESI in different forms, poses particular problems for the protection of privilege: "The risk of privilege waiver, and the work necessary to avoid it, add to the costs and delay of discovery. When the review is of . . . [ESI], the risk of waiver, and the time and effort required to avoid it, can increase substantially because of the volume of the . . . [ESI] and the difficulty in ensuring that all information produced has in fact been reviewed" (*Advisory Committee Note to 2006 Amendment to Rule 26(b)(5)*).

We will not describe the *nature* of the privilege here. We will, however, discuss the rules that address the assertion and protection of privilege as well as illustrative case law.

3.6.1 Rule 26(b)(5)(A)

Rule 26(b)(5)(A) deals with assertion of privilege. "When a party withholds information otherwise discoverable by claiming that the information is privileged . . . , it must:

(i) Expressly make the claim [of privilege]
(ii) Describe the nature of the documents . . . not produced or disclosed—and do so in a manner that, without revealing information itself privileged or protected, will enable parties to assess the claim."

This rule, which existed prior to the 2006 FRCP amendments, requires the preparation and disclosure of a privilege log. The adequacy of privilege logs is the frequent subject of dispute in litigation.

Two points should be made here about privilege logs. First, privilege logs are often subject to in camera review by courts or by court-appointed special masters. This can lead to delay in litigation and, if a special master is appointed, additional cost. Second, courts are divided on how e-mail message threads should be identified on a log. Recently, one court held that individual items in a thread need not be logged (*Muro v. Target Corp.,* 2007 WL 3254463 [N.D. Ill. Nov. 2, 2007]). Another held that individual items must be logged (*Rhoads Industries, Inc. v. Building Materials Corp.,* 2008 WL 96404 [E.D. Pa. Nov. 26, 2008]). This uncertainty, as well as possible cost and delay, mandate that privilege issues be discussed as early as possible at the initial Rule 26(f) meet and confer.

3.6.2 Rule 26(b)(5)(B)

Rule 26(b)(5)(B) was adopted in 2006. It established a uniform procedure across US courts for claiming privilege over information inadvertently produced in discovery. "[T]he party making the claim may notify any party that received the information of the claim and the basis for it." The receiving party, on being notified, "must promptly return, sequester, or destroy the specified information and any copies it has; must not use or disclose the information until the claim is resolved; must take reasonable steps to retrieve the information if the party disclosed it before being notified; and may promptly present the information to the court for a determination of the claim."

Rule 26(b)(5)(B) does not establish any substantive law governing the waiver (or loss) of privilege. "The courts have developed principles to determine whether, and under what circumstances, waiver results from inadvertent production of privileged information. Rule 26(b)(5) provides a procedure for presenting and addressing these issues" (*Advisory Committee Note to 2006 Amendment to Rule 26(b)(5)*). However, the rule "works in tandem with Rule 26(f), which is amended to direct the parties to discuss privilege issues in preparing their discovery plan, and which, with amended Rule 16(b), allows the parties to ask the court to include in an order any agreements the parties reach regarding issues of privilege . . ." (*Advisory Committee Note to 2006 Amendment to Rule 26(b)(5)*). We will turn to a new substantive law later in the chapter. Before we do so, however, we should discuss so-called non-waiver agreements between parties and a possible consequence of entering into these.

3.6.3 Non-Waiver Agreements and Privilege Review

Recall that under Rule 26(b)(1), "[p]arties may obtain discovery regarding any unprivileged matter." Parties must collect relevant information, including ESI, responsive to a discovery request and review that information to determine whether anything is subject to privilege and *not* discoverable. The costs associated with privilege review may be enormous.

Parties have attempted to deal with cost and the risk of waiver by entering into clawback or quick peek agreements. Under the former, parties agree that information produced inadvertently *after* a privilege review will be returned to the producing party. Under a quick peek agreement, parties agree to forgo or limit a privilege review and return any privileged information that is made available for inspection.

Illustrative of the *need* for some agreement is *SubAir Systems, LLC v. Precision-Aire Systems, Inc.,* civil action no. 06-2620 (D.S.C. Feb. 19, 2009). In *SubAir,* a party allowed its adversary to inspect documents on site and designate certain documents for copying. The party then objected to the copying of several of the designated documents, contending that they were privileged. The court concluded that the party had waived its privilege by failing to supervise the adversary's attorney during the inspection process and by having failed to object to the adversary's designation sooner. Presumably, a quick peek agreement would have avoided this result.

Disputes can arise between parties under either a clawback or a quick peek agreement. One party may object to another's designation of particular information as being subject to privilege. However, "[a]greements reached . . . and orders including such agreements . . . may be considered when a court determines whether a waiver has occurred. Such agreements and orders ordinarily control if they adopt procedures different from those in Rule 26(b)(5)(B)" (*Advisory Committee Note to Rule 26(b)(5)*). This again emphasizes the importance of the initial Rule 26(f) conference to minimize disputes and streamline any review process.

Increasingly, given the cost and volume of privilege review of ESI, parties are turning to automated tools to replace, or at least reduce, review by attorneys. *Victor Stanley, Inc. v. CreativePipe, Inc.,* 250 F.R.D. 251 (D. Md. 2008) demonstrates the possible consequence of *not* entering into a non-waiver agreement. In *Victor Stanley,* the defendant sought the return of a number of privileged electronic documents that it had inadvertently produced to the plaintiff (165 out of some 9,000 documents). The plaintiff objected and sought an order from the court that the defendant had waived privilege. The court agreed, finding that the automated privilege search conducted by the defendant was unreasonable. There were too many false positives and false negatives and the defendant did not audit the search results. "Rather, it appears . . . that they simply turned over . . . all the text-searchable ESI files that were identified by the keyword search . . . as non-privileged." The court also noted on more than one occasion that, had the defendant entered into a non-waiver agreement with the plaintiff, there might have been a different outcome.

Victor Stanley emphasizes the importance of party agreement on privilege review and waiver. It also emphasizes the need for a party to use a reasonable, that is, explainable and defensible, privilege review mechanism. Paradoxically, *Victor Stanley* may also lead to an increase in litigation cost.

Attorneys and judges are laypeople when it comes to understanding and explaining how automated search tools work. This reality leads to the possibility that expert opinion and testimony may be necessary to assist the judge in deciding whether a particular search mechanism produced reliable results. In *Equity Analytics, LLC v. Lundin*, 248 F.R.D. 331 (D.D.C. 2008) and *United States v. O'Keefe*, 2008 WL 44972 (D.D.C. Feb. 18, 2008), the court discussed the need for expert opinion on the selection of search terms. Absent agreement, and depending on what type of expert opinion a court expects to receive, discovery costs could increase substantially (Thomas and Hedges 2010).

3.6.4 Federal Rule of Evidence 502

Federal Rule of Evidence 502 was enacted into law in September 2008. It is intended to reduce the cost of privilege review, provide guidance on the law of waiver, protect against broad waiver of privilege, and make non-waiver orders effective. We will summarize the rule, focusing on the last purpose.

Federal Rule of Evidence 502(a) addresses the intentional disclosure of privileged information in judicial proceedings or to federal agencies. It provides that such a disclosure gives rise to a waiver of privilege with respect to the information disclosed and to any other information on the same subject matter that "ought in fairness be considered together." This subsection is particularly relevant to the healthcare industry, members of which may often be the subject of government investigation and must decide whether otherwise privileged information should be shared.

Federal Rule of Evidence 502(b) is the substantive counterpart to FRCP 26(b)(5)(B), discussed above in section 3.6.2. Subsection (b) addresses inadvertent disclosure in federal proceedings. It operates in the absence of party agreement and provides that a disclosure is not a waiver when it was made inadvertently, the disclosing party "took reasonable steps to prevent disclosure," and that party "promptly took reasonable steps to rectify the error, including (if applicable) following . . . [Rule] 26(b)(5)(B)." Federal Rule of Evidence 502 applies to waiver arguments made in federal or state proceedings.

Subsection (b) has been interpreted by some courts. For example, in *Rhoads Industries, Inc. v. Building Materials Corp.* (WL 4916026 2008), the court used a five-part test developed before the rule was enacted to determine what reasonableness meant under the rule. Subsection (b) promises to be a fertile ground for judicial interpretation as courts consider what reasonable means and, perhaps as happened in *Rhoads,* apply preexisting tests to do so.

Federal Rule of Evidence 502(c) speaks to disclosures made in state proceedings. Subsection (c) provides that such disclosures will not give rise to a waiver in a federal proceeding if the disclosure "is not the subject of a state-court order concerning waiver," and either "would not be waiver . . . if it had been made in a federal proceeding" or "is not a waiver under the law of the State where the disclosure occurred."

Subsection (e) addresses the effect of agreements between parties: "An agreement on the effect of disclosure in a federal proceeding is binding only on the parties to the agreement, unless it is incorporated into a court order." Federal Rule of Evidence 502 created a hierarchy of privilege and waiver. First, subsections (b) and (c) operate absent party agreement. Subsection (e) addresses party agreement. The heart of the rule is 502(d), which deals with the effect of court orders.

Subsection (d) is worth quoting in full: "A federal court may order that the privilege or protection is not waived by disclosure connected with the litigation pending before the court—in which event the disclosure is also not a waiver in any other federal or state proceeding."

Federal Rule of Evidence 502(d) is intended to resolve the so-called third-party problem, which arises when parties to a particular litigation enter into a non-waiver agreement and exchange information. When they do so, and if privileged information is disclosed, a non-party could argue that, by disclosing the privileged information to an adversary, the producing party waives any privilege. This problem was presented in *Hopson v. City of Baltimore*, 232 F.R.D. 228 (D. Md. 2005). In *Hopson,* the court suggested that, if the parties before it engaged in a meet and confer and presented a non-waiver agreement to the court for inclusion in an order, the order would constitute judicial compulsion and any disclosures made under it would not give rise to a third-party waiver. FRE 502(d) removes any doubt as to the effect of such an order.

Subsection 502(d) raises a number of interesting questions that, no doubt, will be considered by courts in the future, including whether a court could or should order a quick peek or clawback without party agreement. One immediate question, however, is whether a party should forgo or limit a privilege review in reliance on subsection (d).

Judge John Facciola summarized the following in regard to some of the ethical considerations of FRE 502 (Facciola 2010):

> In my view, a lawyer cannot inform his client adequately without a thorough explanation of how the remedies provided by FRCP 26(b)(2) and FRE 502 operate and what may be gained by their use. Lawyers should remember the famous sign on a bar in the Bowery: "Free Lunch—5 cents." The lawyer must also point out any possible dangers that might arise in terms of potential waiver or forfeiture of the privilege and the consequences of that waiver or forfeiture in present and future litigation. For example, the lawyer should emphasize that there is an argument that FRE 502 is unconstitutional and, should that argument prevail, the validity of agreements made in reliance upon it may be in jeopardy. Resistance by state court judges to enforcing agreements made in federal courts also has to be taken into account. The lawyer is bound to be as candid and frank as possible in helping the client weigh what is to be gained and what may be lost by the course of action the lawyer is recommending to the client.

3.7 Sanctions

Sanctions figure prominently in any discussion of e-discovery. The permutations and possibilities for legal practice errors to occur and courts to impose sanctions are vast and arise from many sources. Sanctions can be monetary and, if warranted, case-dispositive. **Scienter**, having the requisite knowledge of the wrongness or illegality of an act or conduct, or intent, is also a factor in the imposition of sanctions. Moreover, the test for the imposition of sanctions varies among courts.

In the area of spoliation (Hedges 2007),

> [C]ase law generally holds that the "punishment must fit the crime," and that extreme sanctions are appropriate only in extreme circumstances. While language is used loosely in this area, there is a distinction between a finding of spoliation and a finding that the specific act of spoliation justifies the extreme sanction . . . . There may be a finding that spoliation occurred (that is, that potential evidence has been destroyed), but under

circumstances in which the appropriate sanction is additional discovery with shifting of costs and a monetary sanction.

3.7.1 Authority to Impose Sanctions

Federal courts derive their authority to impose sanctions for electronic discovery abuse from various sources. These include:

- Rule 16(f)(1)(C), for failure to "obey a scheduling or other pretrial order"
- Rule 26(g)(3), which provides that, "[i]f a certification violates this rule without substantial justification, the court, on motion or on its own, must impose an appropriate sanction on the signer, the party on whose behalf the signer was acting, or both . . . "
- Rule 37, which authorizes the award of sanctions for, among other things, failure to comply with a discovery order
- Rule 45(e), for failure fail to obey a subpoena "without adequate excuse"
- 28 U.S.C. Sec. 1927, which states that, "[a]ny attorney . . . who so multiplies the proceedings in any case unreasonably and vexatiously may be required by the court to satisfy personally the excess costs, expenses, and attorneys' fees reasonably incurred because of such conduct"

Courts also have inherent authority to impose sanctions for spoliation and may hold a party in contempt for failure to comply with an order, as happened in *In re Fannie Mae* (D.C. Cir. 2009).

3.7.2 Illustrative Decisions

Discussion of decisions imposing or declining to impose sanctions could consume this entire book. Rather than doing so, several recent decisions are noted.

Bray & Gillespie Management LLC v. Lexington Ins. Co., civil action no. 07-222-Orl-35KRS (M.D. Fl. 2009), was an action to recover insurance proceeds for hurricane damage. The plaintiff downloaded ESI from native format to TIFF images and failed to capture relevant metadata. The defendants objected and sought to compel production in native format. The court found that the production was not in the form requested by the defendants, ESI produced was not reasonably usable, and that the plaintiff and its attorneys concealed information and made material misrepresentations. The court found that the plaintiff, "as the client, has the obligation to supervise its lawyers," that an inside counsel cannot blindly rely on outside counsel, and that the latter had acted in bad faith. The court imposed monetary and other sanctions and advised that it would issue an order to show cause why one attorney should not be personally sanctioned.

In *Cumberland Truck Equip. v. Detroit Diesel Corp.*, 2008 WL 511194 (E.D. Mich. Dec. 2, 2008), an antitrust action, the defendants sought spoliation sanctions, arguing that the plaintiffs failed to preserve certain ESI. The court denied the motion as premature. The defendants had shown only a suspicion of prejudice, there was showing of intent, and this was "not a situation where one party had access to the evidence and derived an advantage therefrom while denying the opposing party access. . . ."

In *Hawaiian Airlines, Inc. v. Mesa Air Group, Inc.*, 2007 WL 3172642 (Bankr.D. Haw. Oct. 30, 2007), an officer of the defendant airline destroyed files from laptops after receiving a legal hold notice. Rejecting the officer's contention that he was wiping adult content, the court imposed an adverse inference on the defendant and made a finding that the defendant improperly obtained and used the plaintiff's trade secrets. All this resulted from a finding that the officer's conduct was intentional and in bad faith, and that the defendant was culpable for having failed to back up the officer's hard drives.

Wachtel v. Health Net, Inc., 239 F.R.D. 81 (D.N.J. Dec. 6, 2006) was an action brought by Employee Retirement Income Security Act (ERISA) beneficiaries against healthcare insurance providers. The defendants were found to have ignored their preservation obligations, had delayed searches for e-mail until the e-mail had been destroyed, failed to advise outside counsel of the existence of relevant ESI, and ignored orders. Sanctions were imposed, including the striking of summary judgment filings and other pleadings, and the appointment of a special master at the defendants' expense. The court also considered the imposition of personal sanctions on an attorney.

These decisions demonstrate that wrongful conduct has consequences. The severity of the consequence is dependent on the party's intent, the materiality of the information lost, and the prejudice to the party who requested the lost information.

3.7.3 The Safe Harbor of Rule 37(e)

Rule 37(e) was adopted in 2006 (and was then numbered 37(f)). It reads: "Absent exceptional circumstances, a court may not impose sanctions under these rules on a party for failing to preserve . . . [ESI] lost as a result of the routine good-faith operation of an electronic system." As explained in the 2006

Advisory Committee Note, "routine operation refers to the "the ways in which such systems are generally designed, programmed, and implemented to meet the party's technical and business needs." Moreover, good faith "may involve a party's intervention to modify or suspend certain features of that routine operation to prevent the loss of information" (*Advisory Committee Note to 2006 Amendment to Rule 37*). In other words, a litigation hold may "trump" Rule 37(e).

Rule 37(e) was originally called a safe harbor for parties who lost ESI in the normal operation of electronic information systems. It was then called a lighthouse, pointing the way for parties to protect against any sanctions. It has also been called an uncharted minefield. We will not discuss Rule 37(e) further, except to note *ex rel. Edmondson v. Tyson Foods, Inc.,* 2007 WL 1498973 (N. D. Okla. May 17, 2007), which warned parties "to be very cautious in relying on any 'safe harbor' doctrine."

3.8 Subpoenas

3.8.1 General Overview

A **subpoena** is a legal document served upon an individual and commands the person appear and give testimony to a court or other tribunal, such as an administrative agency. In many states, the subpoena will be served upon the organization and command that the official custodian of the record appear and bring organizational records and/or other documents to court or a designated place. This type of subpoena is called a **subpoena** *duces tecum*, which literally means "command and bring."

In the healthcare industry, historically, the processing of subpoenas has been a function of the HIM department with the director of the HIM department named as the official custodian or keeper of the record.

In both federal and state courts, there are specific procedures that must be followed to object to the validity, scope, and appropriateness of a subpoena. Failure to respond to a valid subpoena without an appropriate reason may subject the party or the organization to a finding of contempt by the court.

Depending upon the type of subpoena, state, and venue, there may be specific elements of information and conditions for appropriate service of the subpoena in order for it to be valid. Therefore, all organizations should establish and maintain a policy that specifically outlines who is designated to accept subpoenas on behalf of the organization. Although the elements of a subpoena and conditions for service of the subpoena may vary by state, in general a subpoena will contain the following:

- Location of court or identification of administrative agency
- Names of parties to litigation (plaintiff and defendant)
- Name, address, and phone number of attorney issuing the subpoena
- Docket number
- Court seal
- Proper witness and mileage fees
- Date, time, and place of appearance or production

A subpoena *duces tecum* may require the HIM director appear in court to testify as to authenticity of the record. More commonly, in lieu of an appearance, the subpoena will stipulate that the records may be sent to the requesting attorney or a designated location.

3.8.1.1 State Courts

The procedures for service of a subpoena varies by state and the location of the court. In general, a state court subpoena is issued by the clerk of the court where the action is pending and is valid throughout the state. State law dictates how a subpoena can be served upon the organization, therefore, each organization should be knowledgeable about state-specific procedures.

3.8.1.2 Federal Courts

Federal court subpoenas are issued by the district court where the trial or hearing is to be held, or where the deposition, or production, or inspection of records will occur. Rule 45 governs the issuance of subpoenas for federal cases. That rule was amended in 2006 to parallel other e-discovery-related amendments to the rules. Moreover, it has been interpreted in some judicial decisions to afford a greater opportunity to shift costs in favor of non-parties who must respond to subpoenas. Although not discussed further, note that, at least on receipt of a subpoena, a non-party has an obligation to preserve information relevant to the scope of the subpoena. For example, see *In re Napster, Inc. Copyright Litigation,* 2006 WL 3050864, *9 (N.D. Ca. Oct. 25, 2006).

3.8.2 Rule 45 in General

Rule 45 was amended in 2006 to explicitly address ESI. Rule 45(a)(1)(C) provides that, "[a] command to produce . . . [ESI] may be included in a subpoena commanding attendance at a deposition, hearing, or trial, or may be set out in a separate subpoena." The rule also provides that, "[a] subpoena may specify the form or forms in which . . . [ESI] is to be produced." Rule 45(a)(1)(D) provides that, "[a] command in a subpoena to produce . . . [ESI] requires the responding party to permit inspection, copying, testing, or sampling of the materials."

Rule 45(d)(1) prescribes procedures for the production of ESI. Rule 45(d)(1)(A) provides that, "[a] person responding to a subpoena to produce documents must produce them in the ordinary course of business or must organize and label them to correspond to the categories in the demand." Rule 45(d)(1)(B) provides that, "[i]f a subpoena does not specify a form for producing . . . [ESI], the person responding must produce it in a form or forms in which it is ordinarily maintained or in a reasonably useable form or forms." Rule 45(d)(1)(C) provides that ESI need not be produced in more than one form.

Rule 45(d)(1)(D) tracks in almost identical language the provisions of Rule 26(b)(2)(B), which created the concept of not reasonably accessible ESI. As with a party under the latter rule, a subpoenaed non-party need not produce ESI from such sources, but may be required to prove that the sources are in fact not reasonably accessible due to undue burden or cost. Should the non-party meet that burden, it may nevertheless be required to produce the ESI on a showing of good cause, subject to the proportionality analysis of Rule 26(b)(2)(C).

These amendments were intended to "conform to the provisions for subpoenas to changes in other discovery rules, largely related to discovery of . . . [ESI]" (*Advisory Committee Note to 2006 Amendment to Rule 45*).

3.8.3 Protection under Rule 45 of Those Subpoenaed Protection of Those Subpoenaed under Rule 45

Rule 45 recognizes that subpoenas may impose a hardship on non-parties. Rule 45(c)(1) states that, "[a] party or attorney for issuing and serving a subpoena must take reasonable steps to avoid imposing undue burden or expense on a person subject to a subpoena." It also states that, "[t]he issuing court must enforce this duty and impose an appropriate sanction—which may include . . . reasonable attorney's fees—on a party or attorney who fails to comply."

Objections to a subpoena must be served "before the earlier of the time specified for compliance or 14 days after the subpoena is served," per Rule 45(c)(2)(B).

If compliance with a subpoena is ordered after objection, "the order must protect a person . . . from significant expense resulting from compliance," per Rule 45(c)(2)(B)(ii). This language suggests that cost-shifting may be more readily available to *non-parties* who are subpoenaed than to *parties* who are served with discovery requests. See *The Sedona Conference Commentary on Non-Party Production & Rule 45 Subpoenas* at 3–4 (The Sedona Conference 2008b).

The Advisory Committee Note to 2006 Amendment to Rule 45 also cautioned with respect to Rule 45(a)(1)(D), which was amended to allow testing and sampling together with inspection and copying: "Because testing or sampling may present particular issues of burden or intrusion for the person served with the subpoena, . . . the protective provisions of Rule 45(c) should be enforced with vigilance when such demands are made. Inspection or testing of certain types of . . . [ESI] or of a person's electronic information system may raise issues of confidentiality or privacy. The addition of sampling and testing to Rule 45 . . . is not meant to create a routine right of access . . . , although such access might be justified in some circumstances. Courts should guard against undue intrusiveness resulting from inspecting or testing such systems."

There is limited case law that interprets Rule 45 as it relates to ESI. However, given the many parallels between it and Rule 34, case law interpreting the latter should guide in the interpretation of Rule 45.

3.8.4 Rule 45 and Assertion of Privilege

Rule 45 was also amended to parallel the 2006 creation of Rule 26(b)(5)(B), which established a uniform procedure for asserting claims of privilege and work product protection. Rule 45(d)(2) mirrors the latter rule.

3.9 Admissibility

Admissibility is not about discovery. Admissibility is the means by which information produced in discovery (among other things) is introduced into evidence on a dispositive motion or at trial. Admissibility is governed by the evidence rules. These make no explicit reference to the admissibility of ESI. However, the concepts incorporated in the evidence rules do encompass it.

The leading decision on admissibility of ESI is *Lorraine v. Markel Am. Ins. Co.,* 241 F.R.D. 534 (D. Md. 2007). In *Lorraine,* the plaintiff and the defendant had both moved for summary judgment. The court dismissed the motions because "neither party to this dispute complied with the requirements of [the summary judgment rule] . . . that they support their motion with admissible evidence." The court then proceeded to undertake an exhaustive analysis of the admission of ESI under the evidence rules.

3.9.1 Steps to Admissibility

Evidence Rule 104(a) provides that, "[p]reliminary questions concerning . . . the admissibility of evidence shall be determined by the court, subject to the provisions of subsection (b)." Evidence Rule 104(b) provides that, "[w]hen the *relevancy* of evidence depends upon the fulfillment of a condition of fact, the court shall admit it upon, or subject to, the introduction of evidence sufficient to support its finding of the fulfillment of the condition." In other words, the judge makes threshold determinations on admissibility and the jury determines whether admitted evidence is what the proponent of the evidence claims it to be.

The first hurdle to admission is relevance. Evidence Rule 401 requires that the information have a tendency to make some relevant fact more or less probable than it otherwise would be. If it does, absent some basis for exclusion, and unless its probative value is substantially outweighed by undue prejudice, the information is admissible under Evidence Rule 403. The next hurdle is authenticity under Evidence Rules 901 and 902. Authenticity "is satisfied by evidence sufficient to support a finding that the matter in question is what the proponent claims." For example, testimony by someone familiar with it that a document is what it purports to be, may be sufficient to establish authenticity. The third hurdle: is the evidence hearsay? **Hearsay** is an out-of-court statement offered to prove the truth of the matter asserted. If the statement is not hearsay, it is admissible. If it is hearsay, the statement may nevertheless be admissible under one of several exceptions to the hearsay rule: Evidence Rules 803, 804, and 807. One hearsay exception, Evidence Rule 803(6), is for business records. Electronic information is often admitted through the circumstances that qualify it as a business record. Lastly, the information must satisfy the original writing rule. Evidence Rules 1001–1008 are intended to ensure that only the best evidence is admitted.

It must be emphasized that the presiding judge functions as a gatekeeper at trial. The judge's obligation is to ensure evidence meets the minimal threshold determination of admissibility. The finder-of-fact at trial, usually a jury, determines the weight to be given to evidence once admitted by the judge.

Parties may lose sight of the need to ensure that ESI produced in discovery will be admissible on a dispositive motion or at trial. Care should be taken in receiving ESI from another party or a subpoenaed non-party to establish the facts necessary to show relevance and authenticity, deal with any hearsay objection, and satisfy the most fitting evidence rule. Organizations should also recognize that, no matter the volume of e-discovery, only a relative handful of records are likely to be admitted into evidence. Moreover, e-discovery cannot be counted on to eliminate doubts about evidence. For example, in *Fox Cable Networks, Inc. v. Goen Technologies Corp.*, 2008 WL 2165179 (D.N.J. May 20, 2008), the court denied a plaintiff's motion for summary judgment, finding that a cryptic and unclear e-mail exchange was insufficient to establish as a matter of law that a contract had been formed between the parties. That and other related questions were left for a jury.

3.9.1.1 Considerations for Healthcare

Brady (2007) describes a story given that prior to *Lorraine v. Markel Am. Ins. Co.* (2007), "very little [had] been written about what is required to ensure that ESI obtained during discovery is admissible into evidence at trial" (The Sedona Conference 2008c). Judge Paul W. Grimm's *Lorraine* opinion is extremely important for HIM professionals' understanding of their significance to healthcare litigation response teams (The Sedona Conference 2008c):

> Considering the significant costs associated with discovery of ESI, it makes little sense to go to the bother and expense to get electronic information only to have it excluded from evidence or rejected from consideration during summary judgment because the proponent cannot lay a sufficient foundation to get it admitted.

In summary, Judge Grimm, in *Lorraine*, described five evidentiary hurdles that must be addressed whenever ESI is offered as evidence (Brady and Grimm 2007):

1. Is the ESI relevant?
2. If relevant, is it authentic?
3. Is it offered as truth, hearsay, or applicable exemption?
   a. Business records exemption
   b. Health information exemption
4. What is the form of the ESI?
   a. Original or duplicate, original writing rule
   b. Admissible secondary evidence to prove content of the ESI
5. Is the probative value of the ESI greater than the uncertain dangers of introduction (for example, risk of unfair prejudice)?

Figure 3.4. Whose perspective of the ESI?

Perspective / Determination	Court	Proponent of ESI	Fact Finder (Jury)	HIM/HIT Best Practices
Admissibility	✓			Education Early preparation Risk mitigation
Authentication		Methods Authenticate		Education Early preparation Risk mitigation
Authenticity	✓ Threshold		✓	Education Early preparation Risk mitigation

Figure 3.4 offers a simple schema of the terms of admissibility, authentication, and authenticity and determination by perspective in the case. Admissibility is a determination by the court. Authentication provides a means for the proponent (usually, an attorney for one of the parties) to demonstrate that the evidence is what the proponent claims it to be. Various methodologies are commonly used to satisfy authentication. The courts have outlined steps to provide guidance on authentication determination. Authenticity is a factual determination by the fact finder, a role usually filled by the jury. The facts considered in making the determination of authenticity must be admissible evidence. A spectrum of experts on legal EHR systems might be required to provide evidence of the integrity and trustworthiness (accuracy) of the media and computer systems they used to generate the computer output of an EHR.

Legal experts have described the methods of authentication most appropriate for computerized records under the Federal Rules of Evidence.

Distinguishing among computer-generated records and computer-stored records patterns in the courts to date is described in detail by legal scholar George Paul (2008) and summarized herein.

In *In re Vee Vinhnee* (9th Cir. BAP 2005), the court adopted 11 steps for consideration for authenticating electronic business records. These indicators of authentication include (The Sedona Conference 2008):

1. The business uses a computer.
2. The computer is reliable.

3. The business has developed a procedure for inserting data into the computer.
4. The procedure has built-in safeguards to ensure accuracy and identify errors.
5. The business keeps the computer in a good state of repair.
6. The witness had the computer readout certain data.
7. The witness used the proper procedures to obtain the readout.
8. The computer was in working order at the time the witness obtained the readout.
9. The witness recognizes the exhibit as the readout.
10. The witness explains how he or she recognizes the readout.
11. If the readout contains strange symbols or terms, the witness explains the meaning of the symbols or terms for the trier of fact.

One should anticipate a vigorous debate when counsel engages frontline health information professionals in pretrial preparations addressing the ability to satisfy these authentication methods. Spirited discussions with HIT, HIM, and counsel stem from the reality that many integrated health records systems were not designed with a specific eye towards compliance or litigation needs. Healthcare legal experts ask provoking questions of health information professionals such as, "Are [hospitals] using authentication under the FRE as a surrogate for record retention decision purposes or alternatively as a surrogate for compliance with a federal or state records maintenance standard," such as HIPAA or Medicare Conditions of Participation (CoP) (Herrin 2008)?

HIPAA and Medicare CoP mandate independent authentication obligations, and one should distinguish between authentication requirements for litigation and the courts described in the next section.

3.9.1.2 Authentication

In the legal system, authentication is a process of handling and certifying records for submission to a court. With health records, the term **authentication** is defined as the process by which the healthcare providers (physicians and/or other practitioners) sign entries into the medical record to attest to the information (authenticating the *data*). To complicate matters, security practices with EHRs use the term authentication to validate the identity and allow access to the system (authenticating the *user*). Summarized below is the portion of the HIPAA Security Rule related to user authentication.

Summary under the HIPAA Security Rule—Emphasis on authentication—
Knowledge of who is accessing, making entries in, and modifying the
data set:

- 45 CFR 164.312(a)(1)—implement technical procedures to allow
  access only to those persons or programs that have been granted
  access rights
- 45 CFR 164.312(d)—implement procedures to verify that a person
  or entity seeking access to e-PHI is the person claimed (that is, who
  he or she purports to be)
- 45 CFR 164.312(b)—implement mechanisms that record and examine activity in information systems that contain or use e-PHI

Related to medical records, there are various methods to legally authenticate
an entry, the most common being handwritten, digital, and rubber stamp signatures. Summarized below is a description of the federal regulation governing
authentication of records for hospitals:

Authentication under Medicare Conditions of Participation—Medicare
CoPs focus on health providers' active and actionable ability to accept
responsibility for authenticating each entry in the medical record:
A-0450 (HHS/CMS 2008).

- §482.24(c)(1): All patient medical record entries must be legible,
  complete, dated, timed, and authenticated in written or electronic
  form by the person responsible for providing or evaluating the service provided, consistent with hospital policies and procedures.

Interpretive Guidelines §482.24(c)(1): All entries in the medical record must be legible. Orders, progress notes, nursing notes,
or other entries in the medical record that are not legible may be
misread or misinterpreted and may lead to medical errors or other
adverse patient events.

All entries in the medical record must be complete. A medical
record is considered complete if it contains sufficient information
to identify the patient; support the diagnosis/condition; justify the
care, treatment, and services; document the course and results of
care, treatment, and services; and promote continuity of care among
providers. With these criteria in mind, an individual entry into the
medical record must contain sufficient information on the matter
that is the subject of the entry to permit the medical record to satisfy
the completeness standard.

All entries in the medical record must be dated, timed, and authenticated, in written or electronic form, by the person responsible for providing or evaluating the service provided.

— The time and date of each entry (orders, reports, notes, and such) must be accurately documented. Timing establishes when an order was given, when an activity happened, or when an activity is to take place. Timing and dating entries is necessary for patient safety and quality of care. Timing and dating of entries establishes a baseline for future actions or assessments and establishes a timeline of events. Many patient interventions or assessments are based on time intervals or time lines of various signs, symptoms, or events (42 CFR 482.24 2006).

— The hospital must have a method to establish the identity of the author of each entry. This would include verification of the author of faxed orders/entries or computer entries.

— The hospital must have a method to require that each author takes a specific action to verify that the entry being authenticated is his/her entry or that he/she is responsible for the entry, and that the entry is accurate.

The requirements for dating and timing do not apply to orders or prescriptions that are generated outside of the hospital until they are presented to the hospital at the time of service. Once the hospital begins processing such an order or prescription, it is responsible for ensuring that date and time of the implementation of the order or prescription are promptly noted in the patient's medical record.

If a practitioner writes orders or uses a preprinted form, the physician must sign, date, and time each page.

Authentication of medical record entries may include written signatures, initials, computer key, or other code. For authentication, in written or electronic form, a method must be established to identify the author. When rubber stamps or electronic authorizations are used for authentication, the hospital must have policies and procedures to ensure that such stamps or authorizations are used only by the individuals whose signature they represent. There shall be no delegation to another individual.

Where an electronic medical record is in use, the hospital must demonstrate how it prevents alterations of record entries after they have been authenticated. Information needed to review an electronic medical record, including pertinent codes and security features, must be readily available to accreditation surveyors to permit their review of sampled medical records.

Any entries in the medical record made by residents or non-physicians that require countersignature by supervisory or attending medical staff members must be defined in the medical staff rules and regulations.

A system of auto-authentication in which a physician or other practitioner authenticates an entry that he or she cannot review—for example, because it has not yet been transcribed, or the electronic entry cannot be displayed—is not consistent with these requirements. There must be a method of determining that the practitioner did, in fact, authenticate the entry after it was created. In addition, failure to disapprove an entry within a specific time period is not acceptable as authentication.

The practitioner must separately date and time his or her signature, even though there may already be a date and time on the document. Where the date and time that the physician reviewed the electronic transcription are automatically printed on the document, the requirements of this section would be satisfied. However, if the e-generated document only prints the date and time that an event *occurred* (for example, EKG printouts, lab results, etc.) and does not print the date and time that the practitioner actually *reviewed* the document, then the practitioner must either authenticate the date and time on the document itself or incorporate an acknowledgment that the document was reviewed into another document (such as the history and physical, a progress note, etc.), which would then be authenticated, dated, and timed by the practitioner.

3.9.1.2.1 EHR Records Management and Evidentiary Support (RM-ES) Standard—Information Attestation

To better differentiate the use of the term authenticate, the HL7 standard uses authentication in reference to the security process of granting access of a user to the system (user authentication) and the term attestation for signing and taking responsibility for an entry or record (data authentication). The functionality related to information attestation also encompasses the electronic signature capability within the EHR system. The RM-ES standard describes information attestation as the following (HL7 2010):

> IN.1.8—Information Attestation: The EHR system must manage electronic attestation of information including the retention of the signature of attestation (or certificate of authenticity) associated with incoming or outgoing information. The purpose of attestation is to show: 1) authorship and assign responsibility for an act, event, condition, opinion, or diagnosis; and 2) lock an entry, which requires amendment or correction procedures, to prevent inadvertent changes. Every entry in the health record must be identified with the author and should not be made or signed by someone other than the author unless they have authority to do so.
>
> - **Author**—All users who create or contribute content and have a role in the development of an entry. Some entries may be created by an author whose role is student, transcriber, or scribe.
> - Attester—A user who takes legal authority for the content of the entry. The attester is often the same as the author, but they may also be an individual with authority to take responsibility for the content of the entry created in whole or in part by another author(s) (for example, student, scribe, or transcriber).
>
> Attestation is required for (paper or electronic) entries such as narrative or progress notes, assessments, flow sheets, and orders. Electronic signatures (for example, ESIGN, biometrics, use of a PIN, or action to attest an entry) may be used to implement document attestation. For an incoming document, the record of attestation must be retained. Attestation functionality must meet applicable legal, regulatory, and other applicable standards or requirements.

Systems must be able to accommodate complex attestation scenarios. This includes entries with multiple authors or contributors and the ability to link the content to the originating author. Another scenario includes identification of an author (one who created the content) and an attester (one who formally takes responsibility for the entry). An example of an author and attester includes an intern or student and the individual responsible for his or her work.

It is critical that the author of an entry (including all contributors or co-authors) be accurately identified and that every entry has an author who is responsible for the content. Over time it is anticipated that stronger authentication/attestation processes will be required to prevent someone from refuting that they were the author. The RM-ES standard identifies the following criteria to evaluate information attestation functionality in EHRs (HL7 2010):

- The system shall provide the ability to associate any attestable content added to or changed in an EHR with the content's author.
- The system shall provide the ability for attestation of EHR content by the content's author or authors.
- The system shall indicate the status of attestable data, which has not been attested.
- If the attester is different from the author(s), then the system shall provide the ability for attestation as allowed by users' scope of practice, organizational policy, or jurisdictional law.
- If more than one author contributed to the EHR content, then the system shall provide the ability to associate and maintain all authors/contributors with their content.
- If EHR content was attested by someone other than the author, then the system shall indicate both the author(s) and attester.
- If EHR content was attested by someone other than the author, then the system shall provide the ability to present (for example, view, report, display, and access) the author(s) and attester.
- If a record is completed by multiple authors, then the system shall allow for multiple attestations linking the content completed to the appropriate author.
- The system shall provide the ability to display the name and credential of the author on outputs (for example, display, reports, and such).
- The system should provide the ability to use digital signatures as the means for attestation

3.9.1.3 Admissibility of the Medical Record

In general, medical records are considered hearsay, or out-of-court declarations. The method for medical record admissibility is spelled out in the FRE in the business records exemption and the health information exemption.

3.9.1.3.1 Business Records Exemption, FRE 803(6)

Records of regularly-conducted activity:

A memorandum, report, record, or data compilation, in any form, of acts, events, conditions, opinions, or diagnoses, made at or near the time by, or from information transmitted by, a person with knowledge, if kept in the course of a regularly conducted business activity, and if it was the regular practice of that business activity to make the memorandum, report, record or data compilation, all as shown by the testimony of the custodian or other qualified witness, or by certification that complies with

Rule 902(11), Rule 902(12), or a statute permitting certification, unless the source of information or the method or circumstances of preparation indicate lack of trustworthiness.

- Rule 902(11) Certified domestic records of regularly conducted business under FRE 803(6)
- Rule 902(12) Certified foreign records of regularly conducted business under FRE 803(6)

3.9.1.3.2 Health Information Exemption, FRE 803(4)

Statements for purposes of medical diagnosis or treatment:

Statements made for purposes of medical diagnosis or treatment and describing medical history, or past or present symptoms, pain, or sensations, or the inception, or general character of the cause or external source thereof insofar as reasonably pertinent to diagnosis or treatment.

3.9.1.4 Authentication and Authenticity of EHR and e-Evidentiary Issues

Evidentiary issues surrounding ESI in systems generating healthcare records are a cornerstone to the authentication process. Various types of legal EHR and ESI require different approaches to the authentication process, whether scanned paper copies, patient-physician e-mails, computer-stored records, or databases and associated reports. The court cannot consider unauthenticated documents from EHR systems.

3.9.1.5 Basic Evidentiary Challenges for Legal EHR and ESI

In anticipating new ESI evidentiary issues, The Sedona Conference has defined some general challenges for ESI.

1. Determining the owner
2. Identifying qualified custodians for testimony
3. Threats of data integrity
4. Limits of technology in authentication
5. Volume overload

Armed with HIM and informatics expertise, the authors shall selectively confront these challenges as they appear to relate to ESI contained within the legal EHR. Special consideration shall be taken concerning issues of EHR system reliability and accuracy of information generated from a computer versus information stored in a computer.

3.9.1.6 Owner of ESI

Identifying the contemporary owner of the information components that comprise the medical record is the first challenge. As a general rule, a provider or healthcare facility owns a patient record subject to the patient's interest in the information. Business-to-business agreements usually further define responsibilities for software, hardware, and other equipment acquisition and data lifecycle and storage. Many states' statutes provide that the records are the property of the organization or provider that maintains or possesses the records. The Privacy Rule in HIPAA only provides that individuals have a right to assert interest over their PHI and e-PHI including access and request for amendments. Neither federal nor state law, however, directly extends property rights to patients (Hall and Schulman 2009). The patient might have a proprietary interest in information contained in the medical record; however, there is no independent constitutional right to the information (Roach and AHIMA 2006).

3.9.1.7 Data Source Mapping for Litigation

Differences in data source mapping details are evident when comparing HIT operational and litigation perspectives in mapping. Most health service organizations have some level of data mapping of their health information technologies and documents supporting application inventories for operational and clinical systems. The spectrum of this type of operational topology data source mapping typically identifies accountable business owners, technical support person(s), and technical details of the data population, application version, operating system, platform, migration, and server.

The assigned business owner may or may not have the knowledge or the accountability of maintaining data content integrity and is less likely to serve as the organization's custodian for a particular software application. Commonly for clinical applications, the accountable business owner is not an actual expert user of the application or even a licensed healthcare provider. The business owner's lack of requisite system knowledge may lead counsel to realize that the business owner is not prepared to respond to typical questions that may arise during litigation.

Obscurities arise between the difference in HIT and legal perspectives of the granularity that is needed in data mapping for routine operational requirements compared to litigation needs (Mitchell 2007). In developing a topology of data system infrastructure to support litigation, some general principles apply. The total number of applications used by a hospital system to support its business record and the legal health record may vary greatly. Data source maps for litigation purposes routinely identify expert users, not just where the data are located (Mitchell 2007).

Data maps may vary for litigation, depending on the nature of the claim and type of dispute. Initial mapping is usually a starting point, and additional information relationships and sources should be expected throughout the litigation process. Conner Crowley, a litigator and expert advisor on e-discovery, describes the two approaches for preparing a data map for litigation purposes (Crowley 2010):

1. A data map prepared without specific litigation in mind and which identifies the software, systems, and sources of ESI considered most likely to be relevant to current and future litigation matters; and,
2. A data map that focuses on the software, systems, and sources of ESI implicated by the information flow relevant to specific claims or defenses. Although the former has the advantage of being reusable, it is likely to contain much information that is simply not relevant to particular matters and can quickly become out-of-date. A data map prepared for a specific matter may not be usable in other matters but, if properly prepared, can provide a useful level of detail with respect to the information flow in a specific matter and may be less likely to contain information that should not be shared with opposing counsel. Such a data map should also aid in the identification of systems whose ongoing operations is likely, without intervention, to result in the loss or destruction of potentially relevant information.

Health record systems may be based on "best of breed," specialty clinical applications potentially extensively interfaced with a central record archive or repository. The repository becomes the proxy for truth for retrieval of clinical care data, but not necessarily for litigation response. As the industry trends toward more complexly integrated and more complete EHR transactional systems, a vendor suite of systems may eliminate these repository systems for clinical maneuvering but potentially retain it for litigation purposes.

3.9.1.8 Creator of ESI

Determining the creator of the record at a glance is assumed to be fairly straightforward; however, creator determination might not be so clear cut. The legal EHR is usually a compilation of record types and component system data elements. These records may be created by a single person, an aggregate of information gathered from multiple authors or, alternatively, a summation of data compiled by HIT system logic, such as summary outputs or reports from several databases.

Examples of the legal EHR components containing ESI with a single creator include dictations, scanned handwritten notes, and individual clinician progress notes, history, and physicals. Alternatively, the modern electronic record, used and maintained in the normal course of business, may be an aggregate from interoperable structured data entry sources. For example, it may consist of the output viewed on the computer screen; human-computer interface; or the printed report (usually a summary query of data elements from multiple providers). Additional examples of aggregate clinical records are ICU flow sheets or clinical dashboards and daily rounding summaries that typically pull data from several different sources. Many HIT systems do not contain the ability to export ESI of aggregate data views used routinely in medical decision making into either an electronic or paper format. Additionally, summary reports often allow a physician to review and attest to data derived from nursing, other allied health providers, or pre-populated data such as those contained in a continuing care record (CCR) or another creator's last charted value. These types of summary outputs derived from disparate electronic sources may not contain essential metadata to determine the original creator of the individual data elements. The system, organizational policies, or both may not support retention of the metadata necessary for identifying the minimal metadata set at the time of litigation.

System-created information may be directly relevant to the litigation dispute and, if retained, may be found buried in the software source code that is rarely manipulated by anyone other than EHR software designers. Types of ESI based on EHR software configuration and system operation may include:

- Logic and threshold determination for clinical decision support tools and safety alerts
- Systems functionality for auto-archiving and printing allowing override of previous versions of the business record
- Software system versions such as upgrades or service packs

Refer to the section Doctrine of Hearsay of Computer-Generated Records and System Reliability for a discussion of system-created information in clinical information systems.

3.9.1.9 Qualified Custodian

Identifying a qualified custodian or other qualified witness to testify about sources of information, business circumstances around the record's creation, or regular organizational business practices may not be as easy as in the paper medical record world. The circumstances around the ESI in EHRs usually involve a multitude of clinical applications, each involving its own group of custodial and system control factors. Determining who is the best to represent an organization at a 30(b)(6) conference meet and confer under FRCP 26(f), or simply to provide a record affidavit, becomes a series of complex decisions with regard to present day HIT systems. E-discovery experts recommend identification of these variables and determination of the individuals who may be involved, which requires extensive work long before litigation arises (Brady et al. 2008). Qualified information professionals, such as health informatics, health information, and HIT managers, must work collaboratively with counsel for comprehensive answers to custodial challenges that may arise from complex integrated clinical systems.

In re Vee Vinhnee noted (The Sedona Conference 2008):

- The trial judge declined to admit the plaintiff's computerized business records.
- The records were not adequately authenticated at trial:
  - The witness was not qualified sufficiently.
  - The witness did not have the requisite degree of expertise in a range of areas relating to the nature of the computer equipment and software.
  - There was no evidence that the business conducted its operations relying upon the accuracy of the computer to retain and retrieve the information in question.

The plaintiff failed, when offered the opportunity, to rectify the lack of evidentiary foundation.

Defining a qualified custodian for various components of a health service organization's electronic health record needs to take into consideration the court's expectation of that custodian and the requisite knowledge necessary to fulfill that obligation. Adequate familiarity with the software complexities may require a cross-disciplinary approach and more than one person to satisfy the custodian role.

3.9.1.10 Data Integrity

Describing all the potential areas of risk to data integrity for EHRs is beyond the scope of this publication and varies from application to application. Despite the usual strict policies, it is all too commonplace to find login ID and passwords taped to workstations that allow access to PHI. Less blatant penetration or inappropriate access channels into clinical applications are clearly possible and require the minimum threshold of the HIPAA-defined administrative, physical, and technical security safeguards.

While computerized data raise unique issues concerning accuracy and authenticity, problems may be exacerbated when it comes to the healthcare industry because of the history of decentralized recordkeeping, lack of clear definition of a legal health record, and the more elusive definition of a legal EHR (Brady et al. 2008). Accuracy of health information may be impaired by incomplete data entry, mistakes in output or reporting instructions, programming errors, illogic in decision support tools, damage and contamination of storage media, power outages, and equipment malfunctions. These errors may be a result of human and system software failures. The integrity of data may also be compromised in the course of litigation by improper search and retrieval techniques, data conversion, or mishandling.

The proponent of computerized evidence has the burden of laying a proper foundation by establishing its accuracy, and the judge has to consider the accuracy and reliability of computerized electronic information systems.

3.9.1.11 System Safety

Only recently has the medical literature begun to address some of the unintended consequences HIT may have, which impact discussions of the integrity of ESI in EHRs. Evaluation researchers consistently identify the consequences of HIT safety and the sociotechnical interactions. Many urge the need to carefully track ongoing usage patterns to provide assistance to managers and IT designers in addressing emerging consequences before they harm patients or compromise quality (Harrison et al. 2007; Koppel et al. 2008a; Campbell et al. 2007). Ethnographic informatics researchers have identified 22 widely used CPOE system–facilitated types of medication error risks (Koppel et al. 2005). In one qualitative study of barcode medication administration systems, authors identified threats to patient safety including description of 15 types of clinical workarounds and 31 types of causes of workarounds (Koppel et al.

2008b). Scholarly investigators have coined the term "e-iatrogenesis" as the most critical unintended consequence of CPOE and other health information technologies (Weiner et al. 2007).

In February 2010, the ONC HIT Policy Committee Certification and Adoption Working Group devoted comprehensive hearings related to HIT system safety and reliability. Policy makers strongly suggest that Stage 2, meaningful use criteria include requirements for auditable training programs and training for processes for reporting patient safety incidents and unsafe HIT conditions such as focus on hazards and near misses (ONC 2010). Policy makers expect reporting of potential HIT hazards and incidents to national patient safety organizations (PSOs). It is expected that this reporting shall be encouraged by health service organizations and not laden with undue prejudice by being branded a disruptive force or non-team player for reporting incidents. Additionally, PSOs would be provided with the cloak of federal protections under the Patient Safety and Quality Improvement Act of 2005 (Public Law 109-41).

> . . . the Patient Safety Act includes "reporter protections" that give an employee a "right of action" if the employer takes an adverse personnel action for filing a report with a PSO. ONC staff can find the provision at 42 U.S.C. 2699b-22e (Section 922(e) of the Public Health Service Act. While the identifiable information held by the PSO is confidential and privileged, ONC can benefit from the knowledge developed by the PSO. The PSO can aggregate, analyze, and publicly release information and "lessons learned" as long as the information is made contextually non-identifiable. Information that is confidential and privileged can only be disclosed if there is a specific permission in the patient safety rule and, in some cases, there are requirements for how they can take place (for example, to make disclosures of protected information to vendors as your statement suggests requires specific procedures to be followed). The goal of transparent, non-punitive anonymous reporting allows for hazard analysis of risk associated with facility (or system) specific configurations and vendor related implementations errors.

Knowledge of e-discovery best practices must be a core competency for the healthcare legal professional that mandates further development and innovative models, especially with implications of environmental and policy directives.

More recently, the professors of law and ethics have contributed to the discussions of concern surrounding technologies and provider liabilities. George Annas (2006) writes that "physicians do not control all possible risks of injury in the hospital setting. Therefore, it is more appropriate to focus on the hospital and to define the scope of the right to safety as a reflection of corporate responsibility: the obligation of a hospital to maintain a safe environment for patients and for their healthcare providers."

Hoffman and Podgurski (2009) provide a comprehensive analysis of liability risks associated with use of complex HIT, and describe significant concerns for providers and considerations for federal regulations designed to ensure the quality and safety of EHR systems.

Special attention must be noted with ESI in an EHR's included metadata. Acts such as just opening a record for review will modify metadata and make it less meaningful or misleading for authenticity purposes. Accordingly, careful attention should be paid to the methods used to preserve and authenticate metadata.

Independent obligations of data integrity are found under compliance regulations, such as HIPAA's requirement that the record cannot be altered or destroyed in an unauthorized manner:

- 45 CFR 164.312(c)—Protect e-PHI from alteration or destruction in an unauthorized manner (at rest)
- 45 CFR 164.312(e)(2)—Implement security measures to ensure that electronically transmitted e-PHI is not improperly modified without detection until disposed of (in motion)

It is only recently that Certification Commission for Health Information Technology (CCHIT) certification standards for the ambulatory clinical software products require maintaining original documents and modified notes (CCHIT 2009). The certification criterion AM 08.08 (Category: Manage clinical documents and notes) reads:

> The system shall provide the ability to identify the full content of a modified note, both the original content and the content resulting after any changes, corrections, clarifications, addenda, etc. to a finalized note.

The necessity for electronic health data quality and integrity has been tackled from angles of compliance, evidence-based metric reporting, clinical communications, revenue cycle management, risk mitigation concerning fraud (RTI International 2007), and medical malpractice (Vigoda and Lubarsky 2006, 2006; Vigoda et al. 2008; Korin and Quattrone 2007). Focus on data integrity for the primary uses of e-PHI and patient care delivery is an obvious priority for healthcare organizations. Counsel should expect that the secondary uses of the data, including litigation, will be more easily satisfied with such principled expectations of clinical applications.

3.9.1.12 Doctrine of Hearsay of Computer-Generated Records and System Reliability

Modern EHR systems routinely generate their own information from embedded system logic, interfaces with other clinical or administrative systems, and reports and outputs, independent of any declarant or other witness. The reliability and integrity of EHR system–generated information is not subject to testing by cross-examination.

The courts have acknowledged the distinction between computer-generated and computer-stored information. "If the system made the statement it is 'computer generated.' If a person inputs a statement into the system that then preserves a record of it, it is 'computer stored' evidence" (Paul 2008). Underlying the distinction is the idea that computer-*stored* evidence is a repetition of the data originally entered by a human language writer, while computer-*generated* evidence is the product of electronic processes, or the statements an information system makes in its reading and writing protocols.

Paul points out that when human judgments are incorporated into computer-generated statements, they may have implications for the eventual outputs, or record: "The decision of human programmers might severely affect what an information system generates as information, many steps later when it inserts information into a record" (Paul 2008).

Paul elegantly describes a culture in the courts to bypass the authentication and trustworthiness requirements explicit in FRE 803(6) that allows admission of information into evidence: "Unless the source of the information or the method or circumstances of the preparation indicate lack of trustworthiness." He adds that:

> the law now routinely lets such statements into evidence, after defining them outside the hearsay rule simply because the assertions are 'not made by people,' or after utilizing a business-records exception that was never intended to apply to such statements in the first place. In fact, the nature of these assertions has yet to be fully explored by the law. New rules about the admissibility of such out-of-court statements are necessary. There is a need for a new doctrine, a twenty-first-century manifestation of the hearsay rule if you will, here called 'systems reliability.'

Future courts may consider the primary authenticity issue in business records from the EHR what has or may have happened in the record in the interval between when it was entered in the system and the time of disclosure, discovery, or trial. "[The health] record being proffered must be shown to continue to be an accurate representation of the record that was originally created" by the clinical team members and HIT system reliability (Brady 2007). The focus should be on the circumstances of the preservation of the record during the time the evidentiary health record is initially archived, to provide assurance that the document being proffered at discovery is the same as the document that was originally created.

In order to provide more clarity in the matter of EHR system reliability, examples are provided of recent cases, qualitative research expert findings, and pending regulatory safety oversight. These discussions and exemplars are not meant to be a representative sample of *all* EHR applications but rather a reflection of possible issues related to system reliability when determining issues of evidence for the courts. They may provide a better understanding of how our authenticity rules may impact the management of the integrity of electronic health information systems. Paul (2008) demonstrates that under our current rules of evidence, very little is required to establish the authenticity of a computer file. In fact, the paper-based rules inadvertently allow almost all ESI to be admitted into evidence with few if any safeguards as to authenticity. He appropriately asserts that these ambiguities leave our legal system open to abuse and uncertainty that the rules of evidence are supposed to prevent. Additionally, the fact finder will be obligated to identify relevant issues related to clinical system software reliability.

Adapted from Brady et al. (2008):

> In *Rush University Medical Center. v. Minnesota Mining and Manufacturing Co. (3M)*, No. 04-c-6878 (N.D. Ill. Nov. 21, 2007), an Illinois District Court held that the Rush University's Consumer Fraud Act claim against Minnesota Mining and Manufacturing (3M) was time barred by the Act's three-year statute of limitation period. On December 24, 1998, after nearly three years of negotiations with 3M, Rush signed a contract with the EHR vendor to license 3M's Care Innovation system, an integrated clinical information system designed to give medical providers improved medical electronic access to patient records. During the negotiations leading up to the parties' agreement, 3M made certain representations to Rush that caused Rush to believe that 3M had the capabilities to provide for all of Rush's requested functions. The Care Innovation system went "live" at Rush by the fall of 1999. The parties' contract required the 3M Care Innovation System to link Rush's different clinical and administrative systems into a single integrated patient information system. On

October 26, 2004, Rush filed a complaint alleging that the Care Innovation system that 3M provided lacked some or most of the functionalities that 3M had contractually agreed to provide.

The following is a review of memorandum in opposition to defendant's motion for partial summary judgment (*Rush* 2007):

> In the mid-1990s, Rush University Medical Center had to decide to whom to turn in order to realize the potential that the computer age offers hospitals. Like many other hospitals, Rush had already computerized certain functions by buying a number of clinical and administrative systems from different companies. Nevertheless, these systems were not linked into an integrated patient data system, and Rush had no single "clinical data repository" ("CDR") from which physicians, nurses, and others could obtain most of the information on patients' medical history and treatment. Mover, once it linked its existing systems to a CDR, Rush would still need to obtain the "functionalities" that would enable doctors, nurses, researchers, and administrators to interact with the clinical information in the CDR and would need "workflow" solutions to accommodate the way in which patient care is delivered at Rush. Only with such "functionalities" and with such "workflow" solutions could a system help Rush clinicians make better treatment decisions, avert medical errors, avoid unnecessary treatment, access patient information from the Internet, analyze data for research and quality studies, reduce costs, and otherwise carry out the hospital's mission.

Brady et al. (2008) further summarize:

> Rush brought claims for breach of contract, breach of warranty, and statutory fraud. 3M denied all allegations and moved for summary judgment. The court found that there was a genuine controversy that existed as to whether 3M acted with gross negligence or willful misconduct and so it granted the 3M's motion in part and denied it in part. This case provides an excellent example of the impact poorly procured EHRs have on healthcare operations. The court's decision demonstrated that the functional requirements for an EHR should be clearly delineated and set forth in the contract that the healthcare provider signs with the vendor. There should also be timelines for the review of the status of implementation. In addition, system performance should be closely monitored.

Another example of clinical system reliability was evident when, in August 2009, shareholders filed suit against EHR vendor Allscripts-Misys (*Compl., Plumbers & Pipefitters Local Union No. 630 Pension-Annuity Trust Fund v.*

Allscripts-Misys Healthcare Solutions, Inc., No. 09-4726 (N.D. Ill. Aug. 4, 2009)). The shareholders of Allscripts-Misys Healthcare Solutions alleged that the company violated federal securities laws when it released the newest version of its Touchworks software. In the class action complaint, the shareholders argued that Allscripts' executive leadership provided an erroneous impression of the company's financial position because they failed to disclose that Allscripts encountered continued delays in installation due to system reliability issues for end-user clinicians (Monegain 2009).

> At a user conference in Orlando, Fla., July 30–31, 2009 Allscripts CEO Glen Tullman told some of the attendees that Allscripts might have rushed version 11 of Touchworks to market too quickly. He said the company was caught off guard by providers who found new uses for the product. Tullman and Faisal Mushtaq, the company's senior vice president of product development, said Allscripts has invested roughly $14 million to improve stability and performance, and they expect the next version, to be rolled out soon, to work more smoothly.

Although the *Rush* case may be construed as just another contract dispute case and the *Allscripts* case considered an example of disgruntled shareholders due to development and implementation delays, both are indirect examples of system failures that affect organizations and other stakeholders. The claim that a vendor was taken "off guard by providers who found new uses for the product" suggests little regard to usability validation and testing prior to in situ use in clinical environments of software updates that directly affect patient safety (Monegain 2009). The rational expectation of an organization that system fidelity is necessary for safe clinical workflow and thoughtflow (Ball and Bierstock 2007) solutions demands that EHRs help clinicians make better treatment decisions and mitigate, *not* cause medical errors. Ball and Bierstock (2007), world-renowned informatics scholars, describe, "What is still missing is not just the knowledge of how physicians work. For these systems to work well, developers must understand how physicians think and then work."

Ball and Bierstock add:

> That knowledge is 'thoughtflow,' the process by which physicians obtain, assess, prioritize and act on information. Thoughtflow is at the center of all patient care considerations and actions. After decisions are made, individual clinician workflow preferences evolve based on an individual's specialty, training and established practices. In effect, because thoughtflow is the source of workflow, thoughtflow is a key underlying factor in clinician adoption of technology.

. . . [A]s long as vendors and clinical champions impose workflow without considering thoughtflow, clinicians will resist using these systems. What's worse, the system may give rise to errors, such as order sets signed without being carefully read, data entered inaccurately or orders entered on the wrong patient.

. . . [S]ystems designers need to collaborate with clinicians to create systems that clinicians will use, and that reflect and reinforce their experiential expertise. Acknowledging human factors and understanding thoughtflow are key to meeting this challenge, with information technology as the enabler.

Scholarly research in the area has only begun to identify system errors that affect patient safety (Walker et al. 2008), however, many of the complexities of the sociotechnical issues have been identified (Harrison et al. 2007). More recently, legal scholars are providing independent insight into the potential liabilities and hazards of EHR systems (Hoffman and Podgarski 2009). Regulatory oversight agencies—for example, the Joint Commission in the form of a sentinel event report (Joint Commission 2008) and the ONC HIT Policy Committee recommendations to the HHS Secretary—are providing early guidance to mitigating risk related to HIT systems.

In April 2010, the ONC HIT Policy Committee's Certification/Adoption Working Group presented draft recommendations for future "meaningful use" regulatory requirements related to HIT safety reporting. The working group members, through public hearings, acknowledged that healthcare organizations and clinicians represent the primary source of information about unsafe conditions related to HIT software.

> Recommendation 1.0—A national, transparent oversight process and information system is proposed, similar to a Patient Safety Organization (PSO), with the following components (ONC HIT Policy Committee 2010):
> - Confidential reporting with liability protection (e.g., whistle-blower protection)
> - Ability to investigate serious incidents
> - Provision of standardized data reporting formats that facilitate analysis and evaluation
> - Receive reports from patients, clinicians, vendors, and healthcare organizations

- A reporting process to cover multiple factors including usability, processes, and training
- Receive reports about all health information technology (HIT) systems
- Receive reports from all Software Sources (vendors, self-developed, and open source)
- Ability to disseminate information about reported hazards

Recommendation 2.0—Stage 2 of meaningful use should include a requirement that EPs and hospitals report HIT-related patient safety issues to an ONC authorized testing and certification body (ONC-ATCB).

Recommendation 2.1—Certification criteria for EHRs should include functionality that makes it easier for clinician-users to immediately report any problems/concerns (a "feedback button").

Recommendation 2.2—The Regional Extension Centers should provide HIT-related patient safety reporting training.

Recommendation 3.0—Stage 2 EHR certification criteria should include requirements that vendors maintain records on all patient safety concerns reported by their customers, and that vendors have established processes to promptly provide all impacted customers with safety alerts.

Recommendation 4.0—The HIT Standards Committee should consider the concept of "traceability" of interface transactions.

Recommendation 5.0—ONC work with the Regional Extension Centers and with organizations such as the American Medical Informatics Association (AMIA) to create a set of best safety practices for selecting, installing, using, and maintaining HIT, and disseminate those best practices to providers.

Recommendation 6.0—ONC should discuss HIT patient safety concepts with these organizations to determine if they are examining whether large institutions have a patient safety review committee, and whether processes are in place that encourage reporting of problems.

Recommendation 7.0—For each stage, certification criteria should be finalized at least 18 months prior to the beginning of the eligibility period.

Recommendation 8.0—ONC work with the FDA and representatives of patient, clinician, vendor, and healthcare organizations to determine the role that the FDA should play to improve the safe use of Certified EHR Technology.

Recommendation 9.0—ONC continue its efforts to encourage implementation of EHR systems.

Many of the ONC HIT Certification and Adoption Committee suggested that the HHS HIT Policy Committee aim to impact determination, validation, and monitoring of clinical system reliability and future litigation with respect to patient safety.

3.9.1.13 Inputs versus Outputs

Consideration of subtle but significant changes in data entry and retrieval processes are discussed as the healthcare industry migrates to electronic platforms. The data input and retrieval locations have traditionally been one and the same in the paper medical record environment. The provider, nurse, and pharmacist all interpret the same paper record for clinical needs, as do risk management and counsel for potential litigation purposes. In an electronic environment; however, the input and retrieval screens vary significantly across HIT applications. Rarely does the data entry screen look and behave to the same for all users across organizations. Risks of differently filtered data and customized data arise from EHRs when the data entry and data retrieval screens diverge.

A typical CPOE allows a provider to place an order for medication with systems expectation of the attestation of accuracy. The pharmacist may view the order and its attributes in a different formation from the physician's. The pharmacist may review the original physician's order and amend the order based on the organization's use of the system (for example, change a brand name to a generic drug). Finally, the nurse delivering the medication to the patient may see a third version of the order with comments and order that were not explicitly attested to by the primary ordering physician. An example of different information that may be provided for the nurse may be product concentration calculated in milliliters. Every time the attributes of the orders are interfaced, pulled from different tables based on provider type, causing changes to the original order, there is an increased risk to the data integrity from the clinician's original intent.

The array of forms of data input and output introduce risk to data integrity for care delivery and e-evidence purposes. Determining who saw what and when, and what action was intended versus what action was performed may only be possible from a patient encounter when all the screen views are provided for interpretation by the fact finder.

Considerable professional expertise and training is required to interpret the variations in formats of the human-computer interfaces from clinical software systems. Using and understanding the data from various formats is not always explicit or intuitive for the end user, let alone counsel. In addition to aggregate views based on clinical roles, many EHR systems allow data to be filtered and sorted at an individual level. Most systems do not capture or retain metadata for filters at the provider level. Disagreement may arise in determining what is considered the evidentiary record. An accurate reconstruction of the record may not be possible from many EHRs.

3.9.1.14 Original Writing Rule and FRE 1001(3)

An original writing or recording and its versions are intended to have the same effect by a person executing and issuing it. An original photograph includes the negative or any print therefrom. If data are stored in a computer or similar device, any printout or other output readable by sight, shown to reflect the data accurately, is an original. The FRE have explicit criteria with respect to the nature of printed or other outputs to satisfy the best evidence rules.

3.9.1.15 Computer Records as Evidence, FRE 1001(3)

If data are stored in a computer or similar device, any printout or other output readable by sight, shown to reflect the data accurately, is an original (Kerr 2001). Thus, an accurate printout of computer data always satisfies the best evidence rule. Significant controversy may arise as to whether outputs from present-day clinical documentation and printouts are accurate for evidentiary purposes.

A duplicate is a counterpart produced by:

1. The same impression as the original
2. The same matrix
3. Photography, including enlargements and miniatures, or by mechanical or electronic re-recording
4. Chemical reproduction
5. By other equivalent techniques

3.9.2.16 Rule 1003, Admissibility of Duplicates

A duplicate is admissible to the same extent as an original unless a genuine question is raised as to the authenticity of the original, or under circumstances that would be unfair to admit the duplicate in lieu of the original.

Significant discussions arise from the concept of duplicates from EHR systems. Is a print report an admissible duplicate? How should HIM handle copies of records from outside sources, in electronic or paper form, that have the potential to be relied upon for clinical decision making? Should outside sources be treated differently if provided in a paper versus an electronic medium? What are the implications of such reliance on the NHIN, HIEs, and use of such data in disease and clinical disease repositories as mandated under the ARRA and anticipated regulations?

Controversy may arise in determining what is a duplicate of an EHR. Many clinicians would claim that navigating the ESI in native and live format constitutes an original because it most closely reflects what the clinician observed at the time the record was created. Some HIT systems allow for a filter or sort view of input data entry elements ordered chronologically. Does a printout of data in this format satisfy evidence rules for originals?

Healthcare legal experts recommend that organizations define what information from outside sources is included in its official business record (Herrin 2008a). Healthcare legal experts recommend that the HIM department, in collaboration with legal counsel, clearly define and establish policies as to which records, if any, shall be incorporated into the organization's electronic record to support professional practice and decision making. Healthcare legal experts recommend that records from outside sources (such as personal health records, CDs, and external drives) that will be used by a provider for care delivery decision making be officially designated as part of the organization's legal EHR and disclosed in accordance with organization policy and procedure (Herrin 2008c):

> If a health care provider accepts medical records from outside sources, it must have a protocol to help determine whether each record was actually used by a clinician in developing the plan of care or in treating the patient. In the paper environment, it is (relatively) easy for a clinician to indicate whether he or she reviewed an external record of care. In the electronic environment, however, it is almost impossible to do so, particularly when the external information comes preloaded on a flash drive or compact disc that has its own loading and viewing software—both of which formats are increasing in popularity with PHR users. Whether

a health care provider has accessed records of a patient's previous care via the Internet is also virtually impossible to determine, but we think this question is qualitatively different as such information never really becomes resident on the viewing clinician's computer, but instead resides in cyberspace when being viewed. We recommend that the clinician be required, pursuant to policy, to make an entry in the medical record noting the investigation of remote PHRs and identify any useful data derived therefrom.

Additional discussion (Herrin 2008b; Dougherty and Washington 2008) arises from interpretation of Rule 803(6)'s text: "information transmitted by a person with knowledge, if kept in the course of a regularly conducted business activity, and if it was the regular practice of that business activity to make the memorandum, report, record, or data compilation, all as shown by the testimony of the custodian or other qualified witness."

Herrin (2008b) simplifies the admissibility of outside records perceived reliability of the resource. "Exceptions to hearsay (of which Rule 803(6) is one) are based on the intrinsic reliability of the information." If a health service organization "relied on it to provide care as if it were made by a person with knowledge," the provider assumed an implicit level of reliability of the outside information source. Herrin's caveat to this exemption to the hearsay rule is, "it does not mean that the information is true, just that it is admissible."

3.9.1.17 Challenges: Limits of Technology

Many evidentiary challenges arise from the limitations of health information technologies. Unique identifiers are difficult to control with data production from EHRs, for example, identifying subtle but potentially relevant changes in outputs because of version control. Synchronized timestamps may not be standard. No creator or time stamp assurances exist for clinicians who upload outside e-PHI into HIEs. Other technology limitations may arise from system metadata, digital signatures, or storage media. Fortunately, for computer forensics experts, these limitations allow a sense of job security. Craig Ball, articulates the evidentiary value of metadata (2006):

Metadata is discoverable evidence that we are obliged to preserve and produce. Metadata sheds light on the origins, context, authenticity, reliability and distribution of electronic evidence, as well as providing clues to human behavior. It's the electronic equivalent of DNA, ballistics and fingerprint evidence, with a comparable power to exonerate and incriminate.

Discussions of the limitations of metadata derived from clinical software systems have ranged from concerns of reliability and accuracy for tracking provider behaviors such as review of radiographs (McLean et al. 2008) to other audit trails that may not accurately reflect clinical behavior (McLean 2008), to how HIT systems metadata intersect with the law (Gelzer 2008). For example, despite describing evidentiary elements in the EHR metadata, only a quarter of the experts in one investigation reported that the functionality existed to print metadata from the components of the legal EHR (Ball 2008). George Paul (2008) weighs in on the limits of technology in authentication:

> First, judges may well begin demanding authentication foundations that do more than constitute trivial showings. They may start ruling that, although it is rational, it is not allowable for juries to in effect guess that a record of information is authentic if an authenticating witness cannot testify with any personal knowledge about integrity of information, dates and times, or the identity of authors, signers, or transmitters. This higher standard has already appeared in at least one case, and may increase in the future, and is exemplified by *In re Vee Vinhnee* (2005). . . . Unless you know how to oppose the authentication foundation of your opponent, you will miss out on this opportunity to exclude evidence from being admitted. But remember that the main fight in any battle over truth is not the concept of admissibility, but rather the weight of evidence.

3.9.1.18 Summary

The process of litigation preparedness happens long before the triggers for litigation. It requires organizations to have an understanding of responsibilities and to define policies with respect to their regulatory and business environment. Litigation readiness and stringency of the evidentiary support of an organization's electronic records is a direct function of litigation risk. Few would argue against requirements that health records have the highest level of data integrity, security, and retention and litigation hold capabilities. Best practices for addressing EHR evidentiary issues include:

1. Identify evidentiary hurdles of ESI in electronic health record early.
2. Conduct e-discovery with a focus on authentication and admissibility.
3. Seek legal counsel far in advance of litigation for health information management issues.
4. Revise electronic health record management policies that are vague or poorly implemented.
5. Consider the methods of authentication of electronic health records that might be used by the proponent of the ESI.

6. Identify the potential ways litigators will discount ESI and might draw adverse presumptions.
7. Train and hire teams of qualified custodians and information professionals that include HIT, HIM, health informatics, compliance, and privacy officers.
8. Maintain and audit secure HIT systems for retention and preservation.
9. Be prepared for authentication and admissibility challenges of EHRs at the summary judgment stage.
10. Design e-health business practices that generate authentic and admissible evidence.
11. Address evidentiary concerns before, during, and after migration from paper to electronic files.
12. Create enterprise databases and data maps for operational and litigation needs.
13. Prepare to have full disclosure and advocate the system (un)reliability as a trustworthiness or competency determination.

References

42 CFR 482.24: Medical record services. 2006.

42 CFR 482.24(c)(1): Medical record services. 2008.

45 CFR 170: Initial set of standards, implementation specifications, and certification criteria for electronic health record technology. 2010.

71 FR 68687. 2006.

Advisory Committee Note to 1983 Amendment to Rule 26(b).

Advisory Committee Note to 1993 Amendment to Rule 26(b).

Advisory Committee Note to 2000 Amendment to Rule 26(b)(1).

Advisory Committee Note to 2006 Amendment to Rule 26(b)(2)(B).

Advisory Committee Note to 2006 Amendment to Rule 26(b)(2)(C).

Advisory Committee Note to 2006 Amendment to Rule 26(b)(5).

Advisory Committee Note to 2006 Amendment of Rule 34(a).

Advisory Committee Note to 2006 Amendment to Rule 34(b).

Advisory Committee Note to 2006 Amendment to Rule 37.

Advisory Committee Note to 2006 Amendment to Rule 45.

Aguilar v. ICE Div., 2008 WL 5062700 (S.D.N.Y. 2008).

AHIMA e-HIM Workgroup on Assessing and Improving Healthcare Data in the EHR. 2007. Practice brief: Assessing and improving EHR data quality. Journal of AHIMA 78(3):69–72.

Ak-Chin Indian Community v. United States, 85 Fed. Cl. 397 (Ct. Ct. 2009).

Amarasingham, R., M. Diener-West, M. Weiner, H. Lehmann, J.E. Herbers, and N.R. Powe. 2006. Clinical information technology capabilities in four U.S. hospitals: Testing a new structural performance measure. Medical Care 44(3):216–224.

American Society for the Prevention of Cruelty to Animals v. Ringling Bros. and Barnum & Bailey Circus, civil action no. 03-2006 (D.D.C. 2008).

Annas, G.J. 2006. The patient's right to safety: Improving the quality of care through litigation against hospitals. The New England Journal of Medicine 354(19):2063–2066.

Arista Records, LLC v. Usenet.com Inc., 2009 WL 185992 (S.D.N.Y. 2009).

Ball, C. 2006. Understanding metadata: Knowing metadata's different forms and evidentiary significance is now an essential skill for litigators. Law Technology News 36(36).

Ball, K. Organizational Approaches to Early Litigation Readiness for Electronic Discovery of Electronic Health Records: A Modified Delphi Study. Baltimore, MD: Johns Hopkins University; 2008.

Ball, M.J., and S. Bierstock. 2007. Clinical use of enabling technology: Creating a new healthcare system though the use of enabling technologies requires changes in a profound scale. JHIM 21(3):68–71.

Ball, K., G.E. DeLoss, E.F. Shay, and E. Zych. 2008 (May 8). The American Health Lawyers Association's Health Information Technology Practice Group Webinar: EHRs and e-discovery: The readiness is all.

Bierman, E., and M. Buenafe. 2009. FDA and health IT: As role of health IT gains new significance, regulators will be keeping watch. Health Lawyers News 13(5):30–32.

Board of Regents v. BASF Corp., 2007 WL 3342423 (D. Neb. 2007).

Brady, K. 2007. Admissibility problems with ESI? The answer just might be in a "Grimm" fairy tale. Digital Discovery and E-Evidence: BNA 7(6):96.

Brady, K., K. Ball, R.J. Hedges, and A. Estaban. 2008. E-discovery in healthcare litigation: What is ahead for ESI, PHI and EHR? The Sedona Conference Journal.

Brady, K., and P. Grimm. 2007. Admissibility of electronic evidence. Paper presented at CGOC. http://www.cgoc.com/resources/admissibility-electronic-evidence.

Bray & Gillespie Management LLC v. Lexington Ins. Co., civil action no. 07-222-Orl-35KRS (M.D. Fl. 2009).

Cache La Poudre Feed, LLC v. Land O' Lakes Inc., 244 F.R.D. 614 (D. Colo. 2007).

Campbell, E.M., D.F. Sittig, J.S. Ash, K.P. Guappone, and R.H. Dykstra. 2006. Types of unintended consequences related to computerized provider order entry. Journal of the American Medical Informatics Association 13(5):547–556.

Campbell, E.M., D.F. Sittig, J.S. Ash, K.P. Guappone, and R.H. Dykstra. 2007. In reply to: "e-iatrogenesis: The most critical consequence of CPOE and other HIT." Journal of the American Medical Informatics Association 14(3):389.

Cason-Merenda v. Detroit Med. Ctr., 2008 WL 2714239 (E.D. Mich. 2008).

Centers for Medicare and Medicaid Services. 2010. Clinical Laboratory Improvement Amendments of 1988 (CLIA)—Issuance of Revised Survey Procedures and Interpretive Guidelines for Laboratories and Laboratory Services in Appendix C of the State Operations Manual to Facilitate the Electronic Exchange of Laboratory Information. https://www.cms.gov/SurveyCertificationGenInfo/downloads/SCLetter10-12.pdf.

Certification Commission for Health Information Technology. 2009. CCHIT criteria proposed final: Ambulatory 2009. http://www.cchit.org.

Chaudhry, B., J. Wang, S. Wu, M. Maglione, W. Mojica, E. Roth, S.C. Morton, and P.G. Shekelle. 2006. Systematic review: Impact of health information technology on quality, efficiency, and costs of medical care. Annals of Internal Medicine 144(10):742–752.

In re Classicstar Mare Lease Litigation, 2009 WL 250954 (E.D. Kan. 2009).

Clinical Laboratory Improvement Amendments, Subpart K. http://wwwn.cdc.gov/clia/regs/subpart_k.aspx#493.1291.

Columbia Pictures, Inc. v. Bunnell, 245 F.R.D. 443 (C.D. Cal. 2007).

Columbia Pictures, Indus. v. Bunnell, 2007 U.S. Dist. LEXIS 63620 (C.D. Cal. Aug. 24, 2007).

Compl., Plumbers & Pipefitters Local Union No. 630 Pension-Annuity Trust Fund v. Allscripts-Misys Healthcare Solutions, Inc., No. 09-4726 (N.D. Ill. 2009).

Convolve, Inc. v. Compaq Computer Corp., 223 F.R.D. 162 (S.D.N.Y. 2004).

Crawford-El v. Britton, 523 U.S. 574, 598 (1996).

Crowley, C. 2010 (March 25–26). Mapping your client's data. Fourth Annual The Sedona Conference Institute Program on Getting Ahead of the e-Discovery Curve.

Cumberland Truck Equip. v. Detroit Diesel Corp., 2008 WL 511194 (E.D. Mich. 2008).

D.N.J. L. Civ. R. 26.1(d)(3)(a).

Dougherty, M. 2007 (Oct. 6). Opening remarks. AHIMA Legal EHR Conference.

Dougherty, M., and L. Washington. 2008. Defining and disclosing the designated record set and the legal health record. Journal of AHIMA 79(4):65–68.

Dougherty, M., H. Rhodes, and M. O'Neill. 2007. Portrait of a legal EHR: Developing a legal EHR conformance profile. Journal of AHIMA 78(6):66–67.

In re Ebay Seller Antitrust Litigation, 2007 WL 2852364 (N.D. Ca. 2007).

Equity Analytics, LLC v. Lundin, 248 F.R.D. 331 (D.D.C. 2008).

ex rel. Edmondson v. Tyson Foods, Inc., 2007 WL 1498973 (N.D. Okla. 2007).

Facciola, J.M. 2010 (March). Ethical considerations pertaining to counsel's entering into agreements that particular procedures: Do not waive attorney-client or work product privileges. Paper presented at the Fourth Annual The Sedona Conference Institute Program on Getting Ahead of the e-Discovery Curve.

In re Fannie May Securities Litigation, 2009 WL 21528 (D.C. Cir. 2009).

Federal Rule of Civil Procedure 1. 1938.

Fox Cable Networks, Inc. v. Goen Technologies Corp., 2008 WL 2165179 (D.N.J. 2008).

Gelzer, R.D. 2008. Metadata, law, and the real world. Journal of AHIMA 79(2):56–57, 64; quiz 65–66.

Grossman, J.M. 2007. Physicians' use of electronic medical records for quality reporting. Paper presented at the Division of Health Sciences Informatics Grand Rounds, Johns Hopkins University, School of Medicine.

Haka v. Lincoln County, 246 F.R.D. 577 (W.D. Wisc. 2007).

Hall, M.A., and K.A. Schulman. 2009. Ownership of medical information. Journal of the American Medical Association 301(12):1282–1284.

Harrison, M.I., R. Koppel, and S. Bar-Lev. 2007. Unintended consequences of information technologies in health care: An interactive sociotechnical analysis. Journal of the American Medical Informatics Association 14(5):542–549.

Hawaiian Airlines, Inc. v. Mesa Air Group, Inc., 2007 WL 3172642 (Bankr.D. Haw. 2007).

Hedges, R.J. 2007. Discovery of Electronically Stored Information: Surveying the Legal Landscape. Washington, D.C.: BNA Books.

Herrin, B.S. 2008a. Professional practice solutions: Releasing records from other providers. Journal of AHIMA 79(11):55.

Herrin, B.S. 2008b (Aug. 18). The legal EHR: Beyond definition. The American Health Information Management Association Legal EHR Conference.

Herrin, B.S. 2008c. Unsolicited medical information: Use it or lose it? Legal HIM-formation 4(5):1–2.

HHS-CMS Pub 100-07. State Operations Provider Certification. 2009 (June 5).

HHS-ONC Policy, Adoption and Certification Working Group. 2010 (March 25).

HL7 RM-ES. 2010. HL7 EHR Records Management and Evidentiary Support Functional Profile Release 1. https://www.hl7.org/store/index.cfm?ref=nav.

Hoffman, S., and A. Podgurski. 2008. Finding a cure: The case for regulation and oversight of electronic health record systems. Harvard Journal Law and Technolology 22(1):1–63.

Hoffman, S., and A. Podgurski. 2009. E-Health hazards: Provider liability and electronic health record systems. Berkeley Technology Law Journal 24:1523–1581. http://ssrn.com/abstract=1463671.

In re Honeywell Int'l Inc., 2003 U.S. Dist. LEXIS 20602 (S.D.N.Y. 2003).

Hopson v. City of Baltimore, 232 F.R.D. 228 (D. Md. 2005).

Jenders, R.A., J.A. Osheroff, D.F. Sittig, E.A. Pifer, and J.M. Teich. 2007. Recommendations for clinical decision support deployment: Synthesis of a roundtable of medical directors of information systems. Proceedings of the American Medical Informatics Association Annual Symposium, pp. 359–363.

John B. v. Goetz, 531 F.3d 448 (6th Cir. 2008).

The Joint Commission. 2008 (Dec. 11). Issue 42: Safely implementing health information and converging technologies. http://www.jointcommission.org/sentinel_event_alert_issue_42_safely_implementing_health_information_and_converging_technologies.

K&L Gates. 2004 (Dec. 15). Court directs production in native electronic form notwithstanding prior hard copy production: Electronic discovery law. http://www.ediscoverylaw.com/2004/12/articles/case-summaries/court-directs-production-in-native-electronic-form-notwithstanding-prior-hard-copy-production.

Kerr, O.S. 2001. Computer Records and Federal Rules of Evidence. http://www.usdoj.gov/criminal/cybercrime/usamarch2001_4.htm.

King, P., and T. Bunsen. 2009 (Aug. 17). E-discovery. Adaptation from case presentation, Risk Management and Legal Affairs, NorthShore University Health System. AHIMA Legal EHR Conference, Chicago.

Knifesource LLC v. Wachovia Bank, N.A., 2007 U.S. Dist. LEXIS 58829 (D.S.C. 2007).

Koppel, R., and D. Kreda. 2009. Health care information technology vendors' "hold harmless" clause: Implications for patients and clinicians. The Journal of the American Medical Association 301(12):1276–1278.

Koppel, R., C.E. Leonard, A.R. Localio, A. Cohen, R. Auten, and B.L. Strom. 2008a. Identifying and quantifying medication errors: Evaluation of rapidly discontinued medication orders submitted to a computerized physician order entry system. JAMIA 15(4):461–465.

Koppel, R., J.P. Metlay, A. Cohen, B. Abaluck, A.R. Localio, S.E. Kimmel, and B.L. Strom. 2005. Role of computerized physician order entry systems in facilitating medication errors. The Journal of the American Medical Association 293(10):1197–1203.

Koppel, R., T. Wetterneck, J.L. Telles, and B.T. Karsh. 2008b. Workarounds to barcode medication administration systems: Their occurrences, causes, and threats to patient safety. JAMIA 15(4):408–423.

Korin, J.B., and M.S. Quattrone. 2007. Litigation in the decade of electronic health records. New Jersey Law Journal 188(11):183.

Lender, D. 2006 (May). Duty to preserve: Should your client clam up when you make a mistake and hope it all goes away? The Federal Lawyer. http://www.weil.com/news/pubdetail.aspx?pub=3327.

Lorraine v. Markel Am. Ins. Co., 241 F.R.D. 534 (D. Md. 2007).

Mancia v. Mayflower Textile Services Co., 253 F.R.D. 354 (D. Md. 2008).

McLean, T.R. 2008 (Sept. 16). Metadata: An Orwellian big brother within electronic medical records. MDNG Primary Care. http://www.hcplive.com/publications/mdng-primarycare/2008/Sep2008/PC_Metadata_within_EMRs.

McLean, T.R., L. Burton, C.C. Haller, and P.B. McLean. 2008. Electronic medical record metadata: Uses and liability. Journal of the American College of Surgeons 206(3):405–411.

McPeek v. Ashcroft, 202 F.R.D. 31 (D.D.C. 2001).

Medical Products Agency Working Group on Medical Information Systems. 2009. Proposal for Guidelines Regarding Classification of Software Based Information Systems Used in Health Care. http://www.lakemedelsverket.se/upload/foretag/medicinteknik/en/Medical-Information-Systems-Report_2009-06-18.pdf.

Mitchell, J. 2007. Data source mapping workshop. CGOC Conference: Data Source Synchronization for Preservation, Discovery & Retention.

Monegain, B. 2009 (Aug. 5). Allscripts shareholders file class action suit. Healthcare IT News. http://www.healthcareitnews.com/news/allscripts-shareholders-file-class-action-suit.

Muro v. Target Corp., 2007 WL 3254463 (N.D. Ill. 2007).

In re Napster Inc. Copyright Litigation, 2006 WL 3050864, *9 (N.D. Ca. 2006).

Office of the National Coordinator for Health Information Technology Policy Committee. 2009 (July 16). Meeting. http://healthit.hhs.gov/portal/server.pt/community/healthit_hhs_gov__home/1204.

Office of the National Coordinator for Health Information Technology Policy Committee. 2010 (April 21). Meeting. http://healthit.hhs.gov/portal/server.pt/community/healthit_hhs_gov__home/1204.

Palgut v. City of Colorado Springs, 2007 WL 4277564 (D. Colo. 2007).

Paterno, M.D., S.M. Maviglia, P.N. Gorman, D.L. Seger, E. Yoshida, A.C. Seger, D.W. Bates, and T.K. Gandhi. 2009. Tiering drug-drug interaction alerts by severity increases compliance rates. Journal of the American Medical Informatics Association 16(1):40–46.

Patient Safety and Quality Improvement Act of 2005. Public Law 109-41.

Paul, G.L. 2008. Foundations of Digital Evidence. Chicago: ABA Publishing.

Peskoff v. Faber, 240 F.R.D. 26 (D.D.C. 2007).

Peskoff v. Faber, 244 F.R.D. 54 (D.D.C. 2007).

Regan-Touhy v. Walgreen Co., 526 F.3d 641 (10th Cir. *2008).*

Rhoads Industries, Inc. v. Building Materials Corp., 2008 WL 96404 (E.D. Pa. 2008).

Rhoads Industries, Inc. v. Building Materials Corp., 2008 WL 4916026 (E.D. Pa. 2008).

RLI Ins. Co. v. Indian River School Dist., 2007 WL 3112417 (D. Del. 2007).

Roach, W.H., and AHIMA. 2006. Medical Records and the Law. Sudbury, Mass.: Jones and Bartlett Publishers.

Rollins, G. 2007. Printing electronic records: Managing the hassle and the risk. Journal of AHIMA 78(5):36, 38, 40.

RTI International. 2007. Recommended Requirements for Enhancing Data Quality in Electronic Health Records. Report for the Office of the National Coordinator for Health Information Technology.

Rush University Medical Center v. Minnesota Mining and Manufacturing Co. (3M), No. 04-c-6878, 2007 WL 4198233 (N.D. Ill. 2007).

SEC v. Collins & Aikman Corp., 2009 U.S. Dist. LEXIS 3367 (S.D.N.Y. 2009).

The Sedona Conference. 2007a. The Sedona Principles Second Edition: Best Practices Recommendations & Principles for Addressing Electronic Document Production. http://www.thesedonaconference.org/content/miscFiles/TSC_PRINCP_2nd_ed_607.pdf.

The Sedona Conference. 2007b. The Sedona Conference Commentary on Legal Holds: The Trigger and the Process. http://www.thesedonaconference.org/content/miscFiles/Legal_holds.pdf.

The Sedona Conference. 2008a. The Sedona Conference Cooperation Proclamation. http://www.thesedonaconference.org/content/tsc_cooperation_proclamation/proclamation.pdf.

The Sedona Conference. 2008b. The Sedona Conference Commentary on Non-Party Production & Rule 45 Subpoenas.

The Sedona Conference. 2008c. The Sedona Conference Commentary on ESI Evidence & Admissibility.

Shay, E.F. 2007. Ensuring health record integrity. Paper presented at AHIMA Annual Convention.

Shortliffe, E.H., and J.J. Cimino, eds. 2006. Biomedical Informatics: Computer Applications in Health Care and Biomedicine, 3rd ed. New York: Springer.

Shuren, J. 2010. Testimony during a hearing on health information technology safety. Office of the National Coordinator HIT Policy Committee and Adoption and Certification Working Group.

Silverstein, S. 2009. The syndrome of inappropriate overconfidence in computing: An invasion of medicine by the information technology industry? The Journal of American Physicians and Surgeons 14(2).

Spieker v. Quest Cherokee, LLC, 2008 WL 4758604 (D. Kan. 2008).

State of Texas v. City of Frisco, 2008 WL 828055 (E.D. Tex. 2008).

SubAir Systems, LLC v. PrecisionAire Systems, Inc., civil action no. 06-2620 (D.S.C. 2009).

Thomas, J., and R. Hedges. 2010. Victor Stanley revisited: Judge Grimm's analysis of the law governing spoliation sanctions. Digital Discovery & e-Evidence 10(17):4. http://www.crowell.com/documents/Victor-Stanley-Revisited-Judge-Grimms-Analysis-of-%20the-Law-Governing-Spoliation-Sanctions.pdf.

Tomlinson v. El Paso Corp., 254 F.R.D. 474 (D. Colo. 2007).

United States v. O'Keefe, 2008 WL 44972 (D.D.C. 2008).

In re Vee Vinhnee, Debtor American Express Travel Related Services Company Inc. v. Vee Vinhnee, 336 B.R. 437 (9th Cir. BAP 2005).

Victor Stanley, Inc. v. CreativePipe, Inc., 250 F.R.D. 251 (D. Md. 2008).

Vigoda, M.M., and D.A. Lubarsky. 2006. Failure to recognize loss of incoming data in an anesthesia record-keeping system may have increased medical liability. Anesthesia and Analgesia 102(6):1798–1802.

Vigoda, M., J.C. Dennis, and M. Dougherty. 2008. E-record, e-liability: Addressing medico-legal issues in electronic records. Journal of AHIMA 79(10):48, 52; quiz 55–56.

Wachtel v. Health Net, Inc., 239 F.R.D. 81 (D.N.J. 2006).

Wagner, L. and C. Kenreigh. 2005. CPOE: Fallible, not foolproof: Clinical decision support for e-prescribing. Medscape Pharmacists 6(2). http://www.medscape.com/viewarticle/516367_2.

Walker, J.M., P. Carayon, N. Leveson, R.A. Paulus, J. Tooker, H. Chin, A. Bothe Jr., and W.F. Stewart. 2008. EHR safety: The way forward to safe and effective systems. Journal of the American Medical Informatics Association 15(3): 272–277.

Weiner, J.P., T. Kfuri, K. Chan, and J.B. Fowles. 2007. "E-iatrogenesis": The most critical unintended consequence of CPOE and other HIT. Journal of the American Medical Informatics Association 14(3):387–388; discussion 389.

Withers, K.J. 2006. Electronically stored information: The December 2006 amendments to the federal rules of civil procedure. Northwestern Journal of Technology and Intellectual Property 4(2):171–211.

Youle v. Ryan, 349 Ill. App. 3d 377, 380, 811 N.E.2d 1281, 1283 (2004).

Zubulake v. UBS Warburg LLC, 220 F.R.D. 212 (S.D.N.Y. 2003).

Litigation Response Planning

Chapter Objectives

The purpose of this chapter is to describe the state of healthcare IT adoption within the United States as well to assist organizations in planning for e-discovery and regulatory investigations. This chapter provides a framework for developing a litigation response plan (LRP) and identifying members who may serve on the organization's litigation response team (LRT).

The objectives of this chapter are to:

- Provide an understanding of the scope and framework of healthcare IT adoption
- Introduce the concept of the nationwide health information network (NHIN) and the future structure for the exchange of health information
- Establish the business case for litigation response planning in healthcare
- Define a litigation response plan
- Outline practical steps in development of a litigation response plan
- Describe a litigation response team and its suggested composition
- Discuss the relationship between health informatics and litigation and provide various definitions of informatics
- Outline the flow of litigation and related federal rules and application of case law

A series of questions are put forth for discussion by the LRT along with recommendations for review of reference materials that contain a mock pretrial conference to highlight the unique recordkeeping issues and challenges of electronically stored records.

4.1 Overview

Concomitant with enactment of federal amendments and the increasing adoption of e-discovery rules at the state and local levels, the use and discovery of electronically stored information (ESI) in litigation is growing at a rapid pace. Meanwhile, the healthcare industry faces new and greater challenges with regard to the discovery and management of ESI. Given a legislative mandate for implementation of a certified electronic health record (EHR) by 2015, today's EHR systems are now undergoing a period of transformation and rapid development. ARRA, HIPAA, and the HITECH Act will pose privacy, security, and regulatory challenges, while increasing adoption of Web 2.0 and Cloud computing will add increased litigation complexities and implications.

Billions will be spent on healthcare IT during the next several years with an eye toward a patient-centered healthcare system that integrates **personal health records (PHRs)** into an organization's EHR. The healthcare delivery system of tomorrow will look and feel very different than it does today. As described in the 2009 National Committee on Vital and Health Statistics (NCVHS) report of hearing on meaningful use of HIT, the healthcare system of tomorrow will be comprised of registries and hubs for the exchange of health information, **electronic prescribing (e-prescribing)** will be commonplace, and quality will be measured and reported electronically in real time with feedback to the provider and the individual to influence real-time quality and safety improvements (NCVHS 2009). Ultimately, the establishment of health information exchanges (HIEs), regional health information organizations (RHIOs), and beacon communities coupled with technological improvements to support public health reporting, the NHIN will become a reality within the United States, providing a means by which all health information can be captured and exchanged securely. See figure 4.1. The model is still evolving, depicts the operational structure of the NHIN of tomorrow, and provides a contextual overview of how health information will be exchanged in the future (Abbott 2010).

One important aspect of the NHIN is that, contrary to popular belief, it will not be a giant repository of individually identifiable personal health information (PHI). Rather, the NHIN will be an integrated standardized network for the flow of PHI from one place to another in a secure and protected manner. The NHIN will operate much in the same manner as automated teller machines (ATMs) exchange information between banks and distribute cash to an individual (Abbott 2010).

The NCVHS vision of the transformation of health and healthcare, coupled with the increasing adoption of and reliance by physicians and other providers upon new technologies, e-mail, digital voice, instant messaging, mobile devices, and **telehealth** applications for the management of patient information and making decisions about the patient's care, are continuingly reshaping and redesigning the healthcare delivery landscape. As a result, the healthcare organization can no longer afford to put off plans for developing e-discovery and litigation management plans. Soon the use of electronically stored information in litigation will be routine.

Figure 4.1. The NHIN

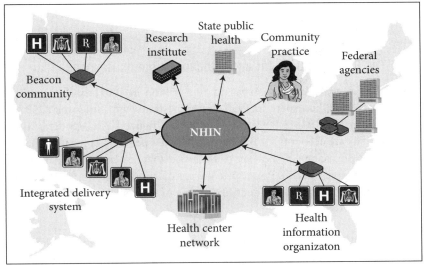

Source: Charles Friedman, MD, American College of Medical Informatics Annual Meeting, February 2009.

The 2010 federal report entitled "Designing a Digital Future: Federally Funded Research and Development in Networking and Information Technology" assesses the status and direction of the federal Networking and Information Technology Research and Development (NITRD) program (White House Office of Science and Technology Policy n.d.). This report summarizes conclusions about the status of healthcare IT adoption including (PCAST 2010):

- Department of Health and Human Services (HHS) efforts for meaningful use and HITECH response have established a strong foundation for future success.
- Existing efforts at developing standards-based data exchange is not robust enough to achieve a "network effect" of health IT. Future success will depend on vigorous adherence to the development and dissemination of a "universal exchange language."
- Federal leadership is needed for developing infrastructure and the necessary universal exchange language for data exchange.
- HHS should leverage lessons learned from other sectors of society, including the use of tagged metadata, to expand the successes of data exchange.
- The Office of the National Coordinator (ONC) should act to develop a process to achieve a universal exchange language that ensures it is available and included in Meaningful Use Stage 2 and Stage 3.

- The US government should start leveraging the requirements identified for the Centers for Medicare and Medicaid Services (CMS). (HIMSS 2010)

4.1.1 The Business Case for a Healthcare Litigation Response Plan

US healthcare expenditures surpassed $2.2 trillion in 2007, more than three times the $714 billion spent in 1990, and more than eight times the $253 billion spent in 1980 (CMS 2009). As depicted in figure 4.2, CMS determined that hospital care accounts for the largest share (31 percent) of health expenditures, while physician services comprise the next largest component at 21 percent of the national health. Prescription drugs currently account for 10 percent of total expenditures and are identified as one of the fastest-growing segments of healthcare costs.

As the government, employers, and consumers struggle to find ways to reduce healthcare costs while increasing the expectations for improved safety and quality, US healthcare reform is becoming a major policy priority. While the 2010 PACA focuses on many issues such as healthcare coverage, it also further mandates the development and implementation of electronic systems in healthcare (111th Congress of the United States 2010).

Figure 4.2.   National health expenditures

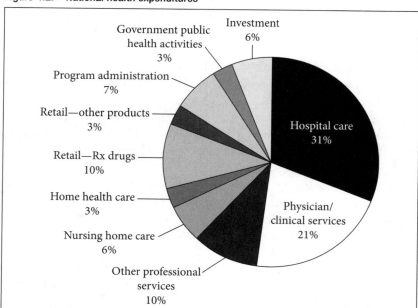

Source: CMS 2009.

The efforts of trial lawyers to target providers for profit is a contributing factor to the rising costs of US healthcare (Konig 2005). The Heartland Institute conducted a project with the Manhattan Institute's Center for Legal Policy and concluded that, "while the excesses of the litigation industry alone cannot explain America's mounting medical costs . . . healthcare litigation is a large, and growing, contributor to our health-care bill" (Trial Lawyers, Inc. 2005).

Several areas of high cost associated with litigation were identified in the Trial Lawyers, Inc. 2005 healthcare report including:

- Medical malpractice liability—The **"tort tax"** on doctors and hospitals over time has grown much faster than overall healthcare inflation. For example, in 2003, the cost to the average American family of four was more than $3,300 a year.
- **Defensive medicine**—This practice inflates overall healthcare costs by encouraging unnecessary procedures and referrals by doctors and hospitals in an attempt to limit their exposure to future litigation.
- Ineffective litigation process—The litigation industry does a poor job compensating the victims it is supposed to be protecting. It was noted that most medical malpractice claimants are not harmed by avoidable doctor error, and that most medical malpractice victims never sue. For those claimants who are harmed and do sue, however, typically a plaintiff will wait years to recover damages and then will receive less than 50 cents on the dollar, with lawyers' and administrative fees accounting for the majority of settlements and verdicts.
- Vaccination litigation—Liability over the use of vaccines is particularly susceptible to litigation, despite the fact that Congress has shielded some existing vaccines from liability. With the emphasis today on improving safety and quality, however, the investment in the development of new vaccines and other drugs vital to public health threats is vulnerable

Trial Lawyers, Inc. (2005) ultimately concluded that the litigation process operates in such a way that it punishes indiscriminately and, in the end, it does not deter bad conduct but rather contributes to increasing healthcare costs and creates barriers to access by reducing the supply of doctors. Additionally, consumers are not made safer through product liability litigation over drugs and medical devices. Instead, "such suits inevitably drive innovation from the marketplace that would lead to net health improvements—not only for US society but for the entire world" (Trial Lawyers, Inc. 2005).

As evidenced by the findings of the Trial Lawyers report, measures must be undertaken to improve the litigation process. Not only will improving the litigation process result in the more timely and just resolution of disputes, but also the litigation industry will do a better job of protecting and defending the plaintiff and, at the same time, contribute to overall improvement in the safety and quality of US healthcare delivery systems.

4.2 What Is a Litigation Response Plan?

Even under the best of circumstances, e-discovery is a costly and daunting endeavor. And while the litigation process can be expensive, it is also important to remember that the courts can impose penalties and sanctions for Federal Rules of Civil Procedure (FRCP) violations. In recent years, landmark discovery decisions such as *Zubulake v. UBS Warburg*, 229 F.R.D. 422 (S.D.N.Y 2003), *Coleman (Parent) Holdings, Inc. v. Morgan Stanley & Co., Inc.*, 2005 WL 674885 (Fla. Cir. Ct. 2005), and *Qualcomm Inc. v. Broadcom Corp.*, 2008 WL 66932 (S.D. Cal. Jan. 7, 2008) have demonstrated how a court can become weary and impatient, according to e-discovery author and national practice leader, Ralph Losey:

> The courts tire of mistakes and delay, and are increasing the pressure upon litigants to get their ESI house in order. Strict compliance is starting to be enforced by judges across the country who no longer tolerate the 'pure heart, empty head' defense in the area of e-discovery. (Losey 2008 at 34) The *Zubulake, Coleman,* and *Qualcomm* cases demonstrate how important it is for an organization to prepare for litigation in advance and to ensure that a process is in place for the accurate identification, collection, preservation, and production of responsive ESI. The costly verdicts and decisions rendered in *Zubulake, Coleman,* and *Qualcomm,* along with the growing number of other e-discovery decisions, are capturing the attention of legal counsel and senior management throughout the country.

The litigation response plan (LRP) is a key component of the organization's risk management and records-management programs. The LRP is the primary source document and roadmap for the organization's litigation response team and ensures that a company meets its legal obligations while minimizing the expense and burden of electronic discovery and litigation. The purpose of the LRP is to:

- Establish a written policy to follow upon receipt of a discovery request, preservation order, or other legal notice
- Provide a common understanding and a framework for inside counsel, outside counsel, and information technology, including accounting for electronic documents for both current and anticipated litigation, and document methodologies for producing and gathering electronic evidence

- Collect, assimilate, and document all legal strategies and corporate infrastructures, including computer infrastructures
- Map the current network landscape for obtaining the information within the organization, including site information, backup protocols, and archiving systems
- Identify the specific steps and assignments for preserving backup tapes, archiving e-mails, and suspending the company's records management program
- Ensure that any third-party consultants or other individuals within the organization can provide expert witness testimony in the event that the discovery strategy implementations come into question
- Create a procedure for lifting the litigation hold and restoring the records management program

When carefully constructed, the LRP will provide the organization with a focused and clear understanding of its legal obligations while minimizing time, litigation expenses, and business disruption.

4.2.1 Planning for e-Discovery and Litigation

It is unrealistic to believe that an organization will not, at some point in the future, be subject to litigation or the target of regulatory investigation. Therefore, planning is one of the most important components of e-discovery and litigation.

The lack of planning for e-discovery, litigation, and/or a regulatory investigation is not only unwise, but it could actually have a negative effect upon the organization by adding time, expense, and possible exposure and liability to the organization. Lack of a mechanism to preserve evidence relevant to current or reasonably anticipated litigation could result in sanctions, spoliation claims, and an adverse inference instruction to a jury.

Today's digital world is making it much more challenging for HIM and IT professionals to meet their responsibilities to preserve and produce information for litigation than it was in the paper era. As discussed in chapter 1, a host of factors make e-discovery different from the traditional paper-based process:

- Dynamic vs. static nature of data—Electronic data are fleeting and dynamic and can change automatically based upon changes made to other data or systems.
- Volume of data—The volume of information that can be compressed and saved onto a single computer thumb drive dwarfs what is maintained in the traditional paper-based medical record department and warehouse.

- **Metadata**—The computer is today's expert witness. Computer and system files contain metadata. Metadata is invisible to the user and contains information about the data or computer system, will vary by file type, and can represent information about system function and user input.
- Replication of computer files—It is very easy to replicate a computer file, allowing for the widespread dispersal of exact or near-exact duplicates to innumerable locations and various media.
- Lack of true deletion capability—An electronic file can persist long after the user believes the file was erased. Additionally, the file can be recreated without any knowledge of said user.
- **Legacy systems** and technological obsolescence—Electronic information relies on hardware devices to translate the stored binary and coded data into a readable format. As a result, the organization must continually plan and evaluate what and how much information can be stored and maintained on a legacy system or migrated to a new system. This is especially challenging because, in today's healthcare environment, many EHR systems are designated obsolete even before the product is fully implemented and functional within the organization.

The changing care delivery landscape, combined with the 2015 EHR mandate, dictates that the time for the healthcare organization to plan and prepare for e-discovery is now. Does the evolution and adoption of EHR systems, coupled with the unique properties of electronic data versus paper, mean that the management of today's digital information in the context of future litigation is impossible? No. On the contrary, doing so today will enhance the development and adoption of the EHR systems of tomorrow. The lessons and experiences an organization will learn in response to litigation will position it for the future and better enable the organization to negotiate with an EHR vendor as to its requirements for EHR system functionality.

Legal counsel should play a crucial role in establishing organizational LRPs and must be supported by the risk management, IT, HIM, and compliance departments. Any organization is likely to be the subject of litigation. Therefore, it is vital for an organization to plan for litigation. The best way to do this is:

1. Begin with a positive attitude—Planning for future litigation today will greatly reduce risk and exposure in the future.
2. Conduct a risk assessment—Ask legal counsel to prepare and summarize on a matrix all applicable federal, state, and local rules governing e-discovery and regulatory compliance and then educate senior management about the findings.

3. Review and evaluate prior cases or claims—Along with legal counsel and risk management, conduct an audit of past claims and settlement amounts. Identify and determine the nature and types of cases that were brought against the organization. Examine how and why these cases were brought and what could or should have been done differently. Evaluate the type, format, and form of information that was produced for litigation. If the information produced was in paper form, determine if this information is being maintained electronically and who is responsible for maintaining such data.

4. Develop an implementation strategy—Once legal counsel and risk management complete their review and assessment of the litigation process, consider appointing a multidisciplinary team that will work to ensure the efficient and effective management of the e-discovery process within the organization.

Soon after legal counsel conducts its initial assessment, the governing board, senior and middle management, and impacted departments should be interviewed to gain their perspective about how information is managed within the organization and how effective the organization is in reviewing and responding to potential risk and quality matters. Senior management should advise legal counsel as to how they want the organization to proceed with implementing an LRP, including having legal counsel lead the project, enlisting an outside consultant, or a combination of the two. Whatever implementation strategy is ultimately undertaken, legal counsel or an outside consultant should also solicit input and feedback from senior management, risk management, HIM, IT, quality, and compliance as to what can be done to improve processes within the organization in preparation for e-discovery.

The implementation strategy should begin with series of interviews with risk management, IT, HIM, and compliance. In their interviews with legal counsel (or a designee), staff within the organization should be knowledgeable about how information is managed and should be able to discuss or provide the information listed in figure 4.3.

Ultimately, the process by which the organization will respond to an e-discovery request will be dependent on the type, nature, and complexity of the case as well as the jurisdiction of the court. Because the vast majority of healthcare litigation is heard at the state and local levels, the existence of any state and local rules governing the discovery of ESI should also be a factor to consider in how the organization will respond to litigation.

Figure 4.3.   Planning for e-discovery

List of Information to be Discussed and/or Provided to Legal Counsel

1. Description of the organization's technological infrastructure, including a synopsis of all current hardware and software applications by department.

2. Summary of the type, nature, and location of all information systems that include voice, backup, legacy, and orphan systems.

3. Summary of the location(s) and/or name(s) of all records custodians in the organization.

    i. Describe how well information systems meet user needs.

    ii. Describe the mechanisms the information system user has to store, maintain, and retrieve data, such as desktop, flash drives, shared folders on a disk drive, mobile devices, etc.

4. All organizational policies and procedures related to records retention storage, management, and destruction.

    i. Provide legal counsel with current copy of the organization's Information Management Plan.

5. Summarize and provide legal counsel current copies of the IT and HIM departments' policy and procedure manuals.

6. Undergo and provide legal counsel with an internal study that determines the burdens and actual operational costs to search and produce potentially responsive information.

    i. Provide a breakdown of the actual costs and fees associated with the production of paper-based records.

    ii. Ask the cost accounting and IT departments to do a study to determine the actual costs and burdens of production of electronic information from current systems vs. legacy systems.

4.2.2 Developing the Litigation Response Plan

Many outside e-discovery vendors, consultants, and legal firms provide consulting services for creating and defining e-discovery projects, including drafting LRPs. Whatever approach is taken, the LRP must include input from key company individuals such as senior management, internal and outside counsel, risk management, IT, and HIM, and it must document their individual credentials and experience. If desired, the organization may also solicit input from other key functions and departments such as corporate compliance, nursing, laboratory, radiology, pathology, human resources, other outside consultants, business associates, and the medical staff. These individuals, depending on their role and function, may also provide insight and information about the location of potentially relevant electronic information.

The decision as to whether or not to involve the medical staff in developing the LRP can be ambiguous, as many physicians harbor negative feelings about litigation and the discovery process. However, when the medical staff is involved in litigation planning, many physicians will become less apprehensive of the litigation process. Once they are educated about e-discovery and the process the organization undergoes to respond to an e-discovery request, some physicians begin to view the EHR system not only as a necessary care delivery mechanism but also as a tool to assist in litigation. In some organizations, after a physician has worked collaboratively with legal counsel and risk management in the development of the LRP, the medical staff not only takes ownership in the development of the LRP, but some physicians also begin to view legal counsel and the risk management department as allies.

4.3 The Litigation Response Team

Once the strategy for implementation is established and preliminary interviews with key personnel within the organization have been completed, the next step is the appointment of a team of interdisciplinary professionals to serve as the organization's litigation response team.

The role of the LRT will be to establish and execute the LRP. The LRT should be **transdisciplinary** in nature and should also work collaboratively with legal counsel and risk management in the identification, preservation, search, retrieval, and production of responsive electronic and other potentially relevant information. The LRT should, on an ongoing basis, provide input to legal counsel and the organization's records management committee about the forms, formats, methods, status, costs, location, and burden of production of potentially responsive information.

4.3.1 Core Composition of the LRT

Depending on the nature, scope, and complexity of the organization, the composition of the LRT will vary. At a minimum, the healthcare organization's LRT should be integrated in nature and comprised of individuals from the following departments:

1. Legal counsel/risk management
2. Health information management
3. Information technology

This team of professionals will be responsible not only for implementing e-discovery within the organization, but also for the ongoing review, auditing, and monitoring of the process. Depending on the type, structure, and

Figure 4.4. Core departments on e-discovery litigation response team

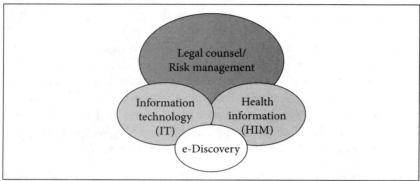

complexity of the healthcare organization, the organization may appoint other members to the LRT such as:

1. **Chief medical information officer (CMIO)**
2. **Compliance officer**
3. Executive management (chief operating officer, chief information officer)
4. Executive nursing management
5. Financial officer
6. Other designated department heads (business office, radiology, laboratory/pathology, emergency services)
7. Medical staff
8. HR representative
9. Analysts and specialists from other departments such as legal, risk management, and/or compliance

4.3.2 The Integrated LRT

To ensure success, the LRT leader must be able to work effectively with legal counsel and executive management. The roles and responsibilities of the LRT members must be well defined. In addition, the organization must ensure that the information management plan is current and reviewed at least annually along with any related information management policies and procedures. Figure 4.5 is a depiction and description of the structure, roles, and responsibilities of a transdisciplinary LRT.

A. Governing board—The ultimate responsibility for management of the organization's LRP should rest with the governing board. If the litigation process is managed effectively, there will be very little need, if any, for the governing board to become involved with or apprised

Figure 4.5. Roles and responsibilities of an integrated litigation response team

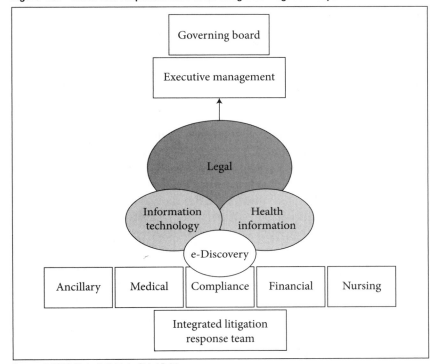

about litigation matters. If or when a matter becomes very large (millions of dollars) or of concern to the organization (loss of image/negative publicity), however, then the board should be apprised. The governing board should have final approval of the organization's LRP.

B. Executive management—The CEO or a designee should work closely with legal counsel and risk management in the ongoing review of e-discovery litigation. The status of e-discovery litigation should be reported to the governing board on a regular basis.

C. Legal counsel/risk management—The e-discovery of information can be a complex, time-consuming, and costly endeavor with varying legal rules. Legal counsel may be involved in a single or a number of meet and confer conferences with opposing counsel and the court and because of this, legal counsel must play an integral role in the process. Depending on the size and structure of organization, legal counsel and risk management may operate as a single department or separately. The e-discovery operating structure should be tailored to the needs of the organization. It is advisable to appoint a member of legal counsel to the organization's e-discovery team. Legal counsel can provide

the necessary legal oversight while working collectively and collaboratively with IT and HIM to ensure relevant information is identified,
preserved, and produced in the face of pending litigation.

D. Information technology—The IT department can assist legal counsel
in describing to a court how the organization's technical systems are
structured, maintained, and operated. IT should also be able to detail
how data are accessed, stored, retrieved, and destroyed. The IT department can play an integral role in developing and maintaining the organization's information management plan and should work closely with
the HIM department to understand and articulate the records management requirements for the organization.

E. Health information management—The HIM department will provide
authoritative and technical knowledge about how both paper and electronic health information are managed. Traditionally, the HIM department has been recognized as the official custodian of the patient's
medical records. In most organizations, the HIM department accepts
and processes subpoenas for the patient medical records. In this role,
the HIM department generally will work closely with risk management.
The HIM department must play an integral role in the discovery process. HIM should work closely with legal counsel on the identification,
preservation, and production of all information (electronic and paper)
relevant to litigation. The HIM director should maintain ongoing
knowledge about the flow, forms, formats, and locations of information and records maintained by the organization. The HIM department
should work closely with IT and be involved in developing the organization's information management plan and its ongoing maintenance.

F. Ancillary departments—Depending on the structure of the organization, management from ancillary departments may support the IT and
HIM departments in ensuring that relevant information is identified,
preserved, and retained in the face of pending litigation. The role of
ancillary department management in an e-discovery team and an organizational response to e-discovery requests for information should
be established by the organization. Each ancillary department should
develop its own policies to describe the methods (automated, handwritten) by which entries are made into the medical record, and the
organizational process for ensuring the quality and integrity of the data.

G. Medical staff—The organization should establish the role of the medical staff in an e-discovery team and how it will respond to e-discovery
requests. Many healthcare organizations designate a member of its
medical staff or an individual with extensive clinical background to
function as the CMIO for the organization. The role of the CMIO is to
provide a concentrated focus on issues of quality, safety, usability, and

process improvement to ensure the medical staff and other clinicians within the organization are fully engaged in the usage and applications of the organization's information management systems. The CMIO can be a valuable resource to legal counsel in understanding the applications and functionality of the organization's information systems and the impact they have in the delivery of a patient's care. Whenever members of the organization's medical staff are named in a legal notice received by the organization, the organization's risk management department and/or legal counsel should notify the physician(s) of the impending litigation and instruct them to preserve all information that may be relevant to the case. The medical staff should also describe its practice for documentation of entries into the medical record (automated, handwritten) and the process with which the medical staff reviews documentation to ensure the quality, timeliness, and appropriateness of the information.

H. **Compliance**—Depending on the structure and complexity of the organization, the compliance officer may or may not be designated to be an active member of the organization's e-discovery team. Regardless of that structure, the potential involvement of compliance in e-discovery cannot be overlooked. The compliance office should work closely with IT and HIM to understand the coding and billing systems utilized by the organization as well as ensure ongoing compliance with HIPAA and other applicable laws such as Anti-Kickback, Stark, Medicare Recovery Audit Contractor (RAC) Program, and Medicare and Medicaid program compliance. Additionally, IT and HIM should work closely with the compliance office to ensure the organization is aware of any/all potential compliance issues. For example, whenever the HIM department is in receipt of notice of a governmental investigation (HHS subpoena for patient medical records), the compliance office should be immediately notified. The compliance office and/or legal counsel will work closely with the IT and HIM departments to ensure an appropriate response for any governmental requests for information.

I. Financial management—Depending on the structure, complexity, and profit structure (nonprofit versus for-profit) of the organization, the financial office may or may not be designated to be an active member of the organization's e-discovery team. The impact of the **Sarbanes-Oxley Act (SOX)** on a for-profit healthcare organization is significant. The finance office of a for-profit healthcare organization should take an active role in the organization's e-discovery, litigation hold, and document retention practices. Enactment of SOX has established a new era of increased regulatory scrutiny for for-profit healthcare organizations. Criminal penalties may result from SOX noncompliance. A publicly traded company is now required to closely monitor electronic and paper document retention, and any for-profit healthcare organizations that blindly destroy documents, e-mails, voicemails, backup tapes, and such are at risk for sanctions and possible criminal prosecution.

J. Nursing—Depending on the structure of the organization, the nursing office may support the IT and HIM departments to ensure that relevant information is identified, preserved, and retained. The role of the nursing office on the e-discovery team and organizational response to an e-discovery request for information should be established by the organization. The nursing office should also develop its own policies that describe the methods (automated, handwritten) by which nursing personnel make entry into the medical record, and the organizational process for ensuring the quality and integrity of the data.

4.4 The Litigation Process and Health Informatics

Chapter 3 discusses some of the rules that surround the pretrial litigation process. As the US healthcare system transitions toward adoption of EHRs and ultimately the establishment of the NHIN, it is critical that all healthcare organizations, providers, and HIM and IT professionals possess a perfunctory understanding of both the litigation process and health informatics. In the very near future, healthcare organizations and practitioners alike will be expected to possess a basic understanding about how electronic data are structured, used, captured, and exchanged in order to articulate a position in a court of law.

What is health informatics and why is it important to e-discovery? While no universally accepted definition for health informatics currently exists, a few of the most commonly recognized and accepted definitions are outlined below:

- "A scientific discipline that deals with the collection, storage, retrieval, communication and optimal use of health related data, information and knowledge. The discipline utilizes the methods and technologies of the information sciences for the purpose of problem solving, decision making and assuring highest quality health care in all basic and applied areas of the biomedical sciences." (Shortliffe and Cimino 2006)
- "A discipline concerned with the systematic processing of data, information and knowledge in medicine and health care. The domain of medical informatics covers computational and information aspects of process and structures in medicine and healthcare." (Hausman, Haux, and Albert 1996)

- "Health Informatics (HI) is a science that defines how health information is technically captured, transmitted and utilized. Health informatics can be considered 'transdisciplinary' and focuses on information systems, informatics principles, and information technology as it is applied to the continuum of healthcare delivery. It is an integrated discipline with specialty domains that include management science, management engineering principles, healthcare delivery and public health, patient safety, information science and computer technology." (CAHIIM 2010)
- "Biomedical informatics is the interdisciplinary science of acquiring, structuring, analyzing and providing access to biomedical data, information and knowledge. As an academic discipline, biomedical informatics is grounded in the principles of computer science, information science, cognitive science, social science, and engineering, as well as the clinical and basic biological sciences." (Vanderbilt University Department of Biomedical Informatics 2002)

Figure 4.6 illustrates health informatics as both a science and a discipline.

Figure 4.6.   Informatics applications and research areas

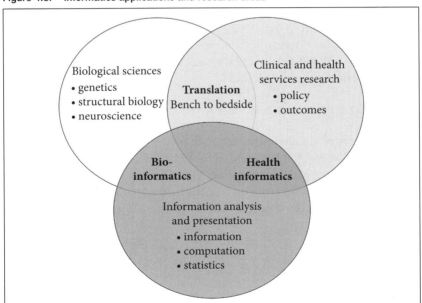

Source: Vanderbilt University Department of Biomedical Informatics, 2002.

Health informatics is important to e-discovery because there are vast differences between paper documents and ESI, and in the future, a provider must be able to describe and articulate to a court of law the process by which a patient's health information was used or relied upon in decision making.

Organizational processes must provide for timely notice to data owners (or records custodians) of their preservation obligations, and individuals must be prepared to speak on behalf of the organization as to how systems operate and how data are used. Persons possessing requisite knowledge of health informatics principals will be an invaluable asset to the organization and legal counsel.

4.4.1 The Flow of Litigation

As depicted in figure 4.7, litigation is a three-phase process: pre-litigation, litigation, and post-litigation. Within each phase are sets of tasks and responsibilities that, without careful consideration, can become time-consuming and costly endeavors.

As discussed in chapter 3, the process by which information will be placed on legal hold will be anything but simple in the electronic era of tomorrow. Therefore, in the next section we will examine phases 2 and 3 from the flow of litigation flowchart in figure 4.7 and discuss three important federal rules: the 26(f) conference, the 16(b) conference, and the 30(b)(6)rule. Finally, we will conclude with a discussion of the roles and responsibilities of the LRT in establishing and lifting the legal hold.

The purpose of this section is twofold:

1. To review and discuss the litigation process
2. To utilize FRCP rules 26(f), 16(b), and 30(b)(6) as an anchor for review discussion within the organization with regard to the development of the organizational content of the litigation response plan and actions the organization may choose to take in response to threatened or impending litigation

4.4.1.1 The Pretrial Litigation Process

The FRCP provide a good foundation for understanding the pretrial litigation process by which electronic discovery is conducted within the federal court system. However, each state or local court system may (or will) establish its own procedures for electronic discovery and admission of electronic records into a court of law. Therefore, healthcare organizations and providers must begin establishing transdisciplinary teams and policies, procedures, and processes that support the retention, destruction, preservation, and discovery process now.

4.4.1.2 The Meet and Confer or Rule 26(f) Conference

Prior to trial and very early on in the litigation process, the parties' legal counsel will meet to discuss discovery. A judge, magistrate, or special master will oversee e-discovery litigation between parties at a session known as the **meet and confer** (or Rule 26(f)) session. The purpose of this session is to provide an opportunity for the parties to meet, discuss, and agree upon matters and the approach to be taken with regard to the discovery of ESI. The end result of the meet and confer session should be the development of the legal plan for discovery, also known as the Form 35. "The Rule 26(f) discovery conference is not merely a perfunctory exercise. Rather, it is an opportunity for the parties to educate themselves and their adversaries, anticipate and resolve electronic discovery disputes before they escalate, expedite the progress of their case, and assess and manage litigation costs" (Scheindlin et al. 2009).

The meet and confer session may be conducted in as little as a one session or can be ongoing. The actual number of meet and confer sessions will be dependent on a multitude of factors impacting the case, including, but not limited to, the size, scope, and complexity of case as well as the knowledge, education, and experience of the judge, magistrate, special master, and attorneys involved in the e-discovery litigation. Although the court can oversee the process, "[t]he obligation to address electronic discovery at the Rule 26(f) meet and confer rests with the litigants" (Scheindlin et al. 2009).

Therefore, before an e-discovery meet and confer conference takes place, it is important that legal counsel are educated and knowledgeable about the organization's information systems and records management policies even though in today's current legal environment, and despite the ubiquity of electronic discovery disputes, courts focus on e-discovery to varying degrees. Some jurisdictions have set forth local rules with exhaustive lists of topics for parties to address at the Rule 26(f) meet and confer, while others merely recite Rule 26(f) without further comment.

See table 4.1 for additional items for consideration and discussion by the LRT.

Figure 4.7   Flow of litigation

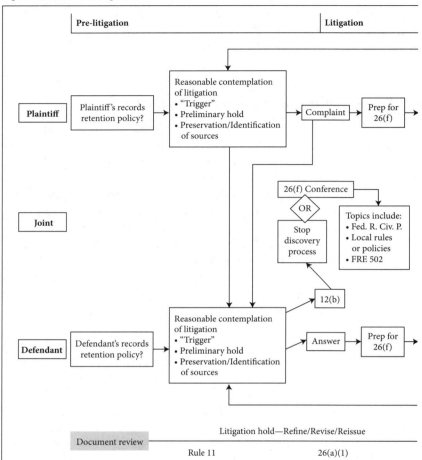

4.4.1.2.1 Discussion and Actions of the LRT

1. Determine whether the content of the organization's litigation response plan shall include policies and the conditions as to how, when, and if a meet and confer session should be held between the parties.

2. Identify and outline all state and local rules governing the process for the discovery of electronically stored information and include a description of all state and local rules in the content of the litigation response plan.

Figure 4.7 Flow of litigation (continued)

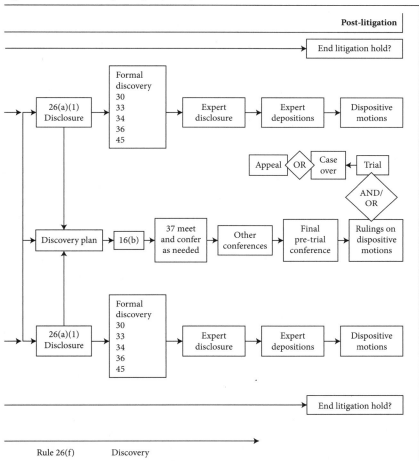

a. Ask legal counsel and risk management to identify how, when, and if measures should be taken to facilitate earlier discussion between parties of the discovery of electronically stored information.

b. Conduct a transdisciplinary team review of the organization's current policies and procedures with regard to processing of subpoenas and the preservation of records. Ask the HIM department to review and outline the current process by which the organization responds to subpoenas and/or identifies cases in which the organization may be named as a party to litigation.

Table 4.1.   Additional items for consideration and discussion by the LRT

Topic	Litigation Response Planning Issues for Consideration and Discussion by the LRT
Characteristics of ESI	ESI is vastly different than paper media. It is much more easily manipulated, communicated, stored and best utilized in digital form and requiring the use of computer hardware and software.
	ESI must be distinguished from information derived from conventional media such as paper documents, photographs, microfilm, and analog recordings. The volume of ESI is significantly greater than that of paper documents.
	(Q) What will be the standard procedures and method(s) by which the organization will disclose versus discover information?
Definition of Official Custodian of the Record	In the traditional, paper-based realm of healthcare discovery, designation of the official custodian of the medical record was clear. In virtually all healthcare organizations, the HIM department served in this capacity. The mechanics of the traditional paper-based discovery process have been tied closely with the identification of the official custodian of the medical record.
	In today's ESI realm, the role of official custodian of the medical record is not nearly as clear. The loss of a clear designation of the official custodian of the medical record will generate problems with the retention, preservation, and production of ESI.
	With ESI there are three basic levels of custodianship:
	1. Level 1—Primary/Direct Custodianship: Those person(s) who work with the data directly or have direct involvement/knowledge of the events the case. For example, a staff nurse who has made an entry into the medical record and is knowledgeable about the events of a case in litigation.
	2. Level 2—HIM and Information Technology Department Functions
	a. HIM Department: The HIM department historically has been the designated official custodian of the medical record. The HIM department has played an important role in the processing of subpoenas for the organization, whether or not the organization was named in litigation. In today's new realm of electronic discovery, the HIM department should be designated to maintain the administrative and technical knowledge about how the ESI is managed and used within the organization. The HIM department should be responsible for content and compliance responsibilities associated with the management of ESI. The HIM department should be knowledgeable about the forms, format, and locations of potentially responsive ESI.
	b. Systems Analysts: Those staff within the IT department who are knowledgeable of the organization's overall information systems. They understand the overall relationships between the different files, structure, and storage mechanisms of the organization's information management systems. An IT systems analyst may know very little about the specific content of the information, or how it is managed, but understands how the organization's systems operate on a global level.

Topic	Litigation Response Planning Issues for Consideration and Discussion by the LRT
Definition of Official Custodian of the Record (continued)	c. IT Staff: Those staff within the IT department who serve as the official custodians of the active, physical ESI. Examples of this are the computers, servers, back-up/legacy systems, communications and voice-systems, near-line media, etc. The IT staff who serve in this capacity will play an essential role in the discovery of ESI. These personnel actually run the organization's information management systems on a day-to-day basis, and make sure that the hardware and software are operating correctly, but may know very little about how the specific content of the information, or how it is managed, but they understand how the organization's systems operate on a technical level. 3. Level 3—Business Associates/Third Parties: Those outsource contractors and others who serve a variety of functions associated with a party's information, but who themselves are not parties to the litigation. Examples include Internet service providers (ISPs), application service providers (ASPs) such as a claims clearinghouse, and other providers who provide services ranging from offsite data storage to complete outsourcing of the IT department. (Q) How will the organization define and delineate official custodianship of its health and business records? (Q) How will the organization communicate to its business associates of a potential need to identify, preserve, and produce potentially responsive for e-discovery litigation?
Preservation and Legal Holds	The organization has a legal duty to preserve all potentially responsive information in the face of threatened or impending litigation. The scope of that duty encompasses all potential evidence related to those identifiable facts, and may shift as litigation develops. (Q) What potential triggers will initiate a potential litigation investigation and possible legal hold? (Q) Who within in the organization will be responsible for establishing a litigation hold? (Q) How will all potential evidence be assimilated, indexed, and produced? (Q) Who will monitor the legal hold and reissue or lift it as pertinent facts change over time? (Q) At what point in the process should the legal counsel of the parties negotiate a stipulated plan for the preservation of data to make sure the opposing side understands its obligations, and to limit is own potential liability?
Form(s) of Production	In the traditional paper-based world of discovery, the physical form of production occurred generally only through paper. Documents were entered into evidence by one of the following ways: 1. Admission under the Business Records Rule, Fed. R. Evid. 803(6) (Medical Records) 2. Authenticated and admitted under the Best Evidence Rules, Fed. R. Evid. 1001 and 1001(3)

(continued)

Table 4.1.   Additional items for consideration and discussion by the LRT (continued)

Topic	Litigation Response Planning Issues for Consideration and Discussion by the LRT
Form(s) of Production (continued)	3. Authenticated, Bates-stamped, indexed, and labeled to correspond to the categories of a document request
	The FRCP and Uniform Rules provide that legal counsel meet and confer early in litigation and agree upon the form(s) and manner of production of ESI.
	(Q) At what point in litigation involving production of ESI will legal counsel meet with HIM and IT to discuss the forms, format, and location of all potentially responsive information?
	(Q) How will legal counsel, HIM, and IT work together to identify the most cost-efficient and effective means to produce potentially responsive information?
Reasonably Accessible Information vs. Not Reasonably Accessible Information	The FRCP and Uniform Rules both contain provisions for two-tiered discovery. The management of ESI provides for some unique challenges not presented by paper-based and other traditional media (microfilm, pictures, etc.). All ESI must be rendered usable through technology, that being computer, operating system or application software.
	If ESI is readily available through appropriate technology and able to be used and read, it is considered accessible.
	Much of the ESI subject to discovery is not easily rendered usable unless appropriate technologies are employed to render the data into usable form. There is usually a significant cost and burden to render the ESI usable. This type of ESI is considered not reasonably accessible.
	(Q) How will the organization account for and determine its true costs to search, cull, and produce data that are reasonably accessible versus data that are not reasonably accessible?
Form(s) of Production	In the traditional paper-based world of discovery, the physical form of production occurred generally only through paper. Documents were entered into evidence by one of the follows ways:
	1. Admission under the Business Records Rule – Fed. R. Evid. 803(6) (Medical Records)
	2. Authenticated and admitted under the Best Evidence Rules – Fed. R. Evid. 1001 and 1001(3)
	3. Authenticated, Bates-stamped, indexed, and labeled to correspond to the categories of a document request.
	The FRCP and Uniform Rules provide that legal counsel meet and confer early in litigation and agree upon the form(s) and manner of production of ESI.
	(Q) At what point in litigation involving production of EST will legal counsel meet with HIM and IT to discuss the forms format and location of all potentially responsive information?
	(Q) How will legal counsel, HIM and IT work together to identify the most cost-efficient and effective means to produce potentially responsive information?

Topic	Litigation Response Planning Issues for Consideration and Discussion by the LRT
Cost Shifting	In traditional paper-based document discovery, the FRCP interpreted the common law rule that "each party bear its own costs." For the healthcare organization, the costs were in the locating of responsive documents, assembling them into proper order, Bates stamping, and presenting to the requesting party for inspection and copying. The requesting party bore the cost of analyzing the documents and the cost of photocopying and delivering the documents.
	With the advent of e-discovery, it should be recognized that the traditional cost paradigm associated with the production of paper documents has shifted and the traditional cost paradigms associated with paper-based discovery do not apply to e-discovery.
	The FRCP and Uniform Rules contain provisions to balance ESI discovery costs between the parties. If a party shows good cause, the court can order the search, retrieval, and/or testing and sampling of inaccessible information.
	The true costs to cull, search, retrieve, and produce ESI can be very expensive and will depend greatly on the location, form, accessibility, and format of the information.
	An organization without appropriate technologies or methods to index, classify, store, cull, search, retrieve, and produce potentially responsive information could face enormous costs and burdens, and even risk imposition of sanctions and penalties.
	(Q) In response to a request of ESI, how will the organization locate, index, cull, search, classify, and produce all potentially responsive information?
	(Q) What benefit (if any) would there be to the organization through installation of an enterprise content management (ECM) system?
	(Q) How will the organization determine its true costs to index, classify, store, cull, search, retrieve, and produce ESI?
	(Q) If asked, how would the organization describe the good faith operation of its information management systems?
E-mail	On September 27, 2007, the Financial Industry Regulatory Authority (FINRA) issued a $12.5 million fine to Morgan Stanley for the mishandling of e-mail dated before the September 11, 2001, terrorist attacks. This settlement provides for a $9.5 million allocation to two groups of customers that made arbitration claims against the company and a $3 million fine for failing to provide e-mail and supervisory materials.
	The effects resulting from the mismanagement of company e-mail can be devastating to an organization. E-mails have become a proverbial "cache to the cash" for a savvy litigant.
	(Q) What systems and processes are in place for the management, storage, and retention of company e-mail?
	(Q) What is the organization's policy with regard to the use and transmission of PHI in company e-mail?
	(Q) What are the organization's current policies and practices with regard to the screening and monitoring of company e-mail?

(continued)

Table 4.1.   Additional items for consideration and discussion by the LRT (continued)

Topic	Litigation Response Planning Issues for Consideration and Discussion by the LRT
Nonapparent and Ancillary ESI The Role, Usage and Retention of Metadata	Not only is the volume of ESI greater than that of paper, management of ESI brings about a need for ancillary electronic information systems and procedures in which to manage the primary information. Operating system and application software require that electronic files be labeled so that the information can be stored, retrieved, viewed, and communicated. This process creates bits of information about the data known as metadata. Metadata can be a useful way to authenticate the integrity of data. (Q) How will the organization store, retain, and manage its metadata? (Q) What will the role of metadata (if any) be in a HIPAA accounting for disclosures? (Q) Should the organization establish a metadata repository?
Nonapparent and Ancillary ESI The Role, Usage and Retention of Ephemeral Data	Recent court opinion suggests that short-lived data (such as RAM) are potentially discoverable and should be preserved if the information does not exist in any other form or cannot be obtained through any other means or source. The potential for the discovery of ephemeral data could pose a significant burden upon the organization. (Q) Under what possible circumstances (if any) could the organization be ordered to preserve and produce ephemeral data for a legal proceeding? (Q) What are the locations, sources, and types of ephemeral data that exist within the organization?
Legacy Data/ Systems	In certain cases, the retrieval and/or restoration of ESI, which is contained on a legacy system or backup tape, may be warranted. Access to ESI contained on a legacy system could solely depend on the availability of the retired operating system and application software. Large volumes of ESI virtually become inaccessible and place significant burden on the organization when that ESI, which is needed for business/legal purposes, is not migrated appropriately. (Q) What provisions will the organization establish to provide for the efficient and effective migration of legacy data? (Q) How long will legacy data not needed for business/legal purposes be retained? (Q) What will be the mechanism for destruction of legacy data?
Backup Media	As evidenced in the *Zubulake* decision, one of the biggest problems facing organizations today is the common practice of replicating ESI in wholesale, as a mirror image in the event of a disaster. While creating mirror image backup tapes may be a good procedure for the short term, the long-term implications of retaining them may be disastrous. In essence, the organization's backup tape may not "back" the organization at all. It is important to remember that routine maintenance of backup tapes makes backup tape information potentially discoverable and the organization could be ordered to search and restore its backup tapes for a legal proceeding. (Q) What is and should be organizational practice with regard to the disposition and processing of its backup tapes and other media?

Topic	Litigation Response Planning Issues for Consideration and Discussion by the LRT
Screening ESI for Privilege	One of the greatest costs associated with the discovery of ESI is the potential waiver of privilege that could result from the inadvertent production of privileged material.
	Shifting costs to the requesting party or through the use of technology can mitigate some e-discovery costs. But, currently there is no technology to screen for privilege. The costs to screen for privilege must be borne by the organization. There is tremendous cost associated with screening ESI for privilege. For example, the review and parsing out of a person's e-mail account to separate the nonprivileged messages from the privileged ones. In a healthcare organization, counsel will need to take added measures to ensure that no unauthorized PHI is inadvertently produced to a requesting party.
	(Q) What will organizational policy and procedure be with regard to the screening for privilege?
Voicemail	Voicemail messages are admissible into a court of law and they are utilized routinely within the healthcare setting. It is not possible to predict whether a court will impose broad or narrow obligations to preserve and produce electronic information.
	(Q) Does the organization have a policy in place that delineates the use and retention of voicemail?
	(Q) Does the organization have a policy that describes how long original dictated voice files are maintained after they have been dictated and the report has been typed?
	(Q) What (if any) recordings of conversations are maintained by the organization, such as utilization review and case management calls and/or calls from members of a health plan?
EHR Implementation	When planning for an EHR implementation, the terms and conditions of the contract should be clearly stipulated and agreed upon in advance. Many organizations maintain clauses that provide for penalties for noncompliance with the terms and conditions of the EHR contract. The organization should establish a process by which to monitor the progress of the EHR implementation and communicate with the vendor and legal counsel when/if problems arise.
	(Q) Who are the person(s) responsible for the implementation of the EHR?
	(Q) Are all parties involved with the implementation of the EHR knowledgeable about the EHR implementation plan?
	(Q) Who from within the organization, will be responsible for monitoring EHR contract compliance?
	(Q) What is the statute of limitations for filing an action against the EHR vendor for nonperformance?
Third-Party ESI—Burden and Costs for Production	The rulings in *Guy Chemical* and *In re Honeywell Int'l Inc.* evidence that non-party production of ESI will become a cost of doing business for all organizations.
	(Q) How will the organization respond to third-party subpoenas for ESI?
	(Q) What measures will the organization take to determine the burden and cost of production of third-party ESI?

3. Identify the barriers that preclude legal counsel from meeting earlier in the litigation process to discuss the discovery of electronically stored information.
   a. Ask legal counsel and risk management what steps can and should be taken to facilitate cooperation between the parties in discovery.
4. Appoint those individuals who will be designated to participate in a meet and confer session. Ensure all appointed individuals have been educated and trained by legal counsel about the activities and questions that may take place at a meet and confer session. Ensure that all individuals who have been designated to participate in a meet and confer session are knowledgeable about the organization's information systems and the locations and uses of information within the organization.

4.4.1.3 The Pretrial Conference or Rule 16(b) Session

The pretrial conference (Rule 16(b) session) is presided over by a judge, magistrate, or special master and occurs after the parties have met (meet and confer or Rule 26(f) session) and agreed upon a plan for discovery (Form 35). "Specifically, Rule 26(f)(1) requires the parties to meet and confer to develop a proposed discovery plan prior to the Rule 16 pretrial conference, which is typically scheduled by the court at the outset of litigation for the purpose of creating a scheduling order for discovery and other pretrial matters" (Scheindlin et al. 2009).

The purpose of a pretrial conference is to:

- Present to the court the parties' plan for discovery (Form 35)
- Clarify the scope and complexity of the document requests
- Better understand the opposing party's technical landscape
- Review, discuss, and resolve any production format disagreements, which may reduce liability and discovery costs later
- Reduce unnecessary waste and reproduction of documents
- Preempt the negative impact and consequences of inadvertent production of confidential or privileged documents

As EHR adoption evolves, both the meet and confer (Rule 26(f)) and the pretrial conference (Rule 16(b)), or some state or local form thereof, will become routine. The parties must understand and discuss relevant issues related to EHR system reliability as well as the nature and degree of whether an EHR system or technological application is relevant in the harm or death of a patient (Paul 2008). Until then, the pretrial conference should be held any time either party anticipates that ESI may be relevant to a lawsuit.

4.4.1.3.1 Discussion and Actions of the LRT

1. Determining whether or not the content of the organization's LRP shall include discussion and a description of what a pretrial conference is, and the roles and responsibilities of legal counsel and the LRT in preparation for a pretrial conference.

2. Ensuring state and local rules governing the process for the discovery of ESI have been adequately described and referenced in the LRP.

   a. Ask legal counsel and risk management to determine whether the judges presiding over the case have established any specific forms or procedures they require.

   b. Determine to what extent legal counsel and risk management can and will educate the judges on the process of e-discovery.

3. Identifying the barriers that will preclude legal counsel from developing a discovery plan (Form 35) early on in the process.

   a. Ask legal counsel and risk management what steps should be taken to facilitate cooperation between the parties in discovery.

4. Designating individuals to participate in the pretrial conference. Ensuring all appointed individuals have been educated and trained by legal counsel about the purpose of a pretrial conference, and the types of activities and questions that may take place at the pretrial conference. Ensuring that all individuals who have been designated to participate in a pretrial conference are knowledgeable about the status of the case and possess a good understanding of the process and agreed upon by the parties.

4.4.1.4 Questions for Consideration by the LRT

Summarized below is a list of questions and considerations for discussion between the court and the parties to assist the LRT in preparing for a pretrial conference.

I. Data Preservation

   - Do the parties maintain a standardized protocol or plan for the discovery of ESI?
   - In what form(s) does the relevant information currently exist, such as paper or hybrid? Does the organization maintain a plan for information management?
   - At what point could the parties reasonably have anticipated litigation?
   - What steps have the parties undertaken to preserve relevant ESI? Was a litigation hold established? If so, on what date?

- What protocols for data retention and deletion are in place? Is information from deleted records archived on backup tapes?
- Are the parties aware of the location and format of all potentially relevant electronic evidence? What legacy systems are in place?
- Who are the directors of IT and HIM? If a deposition regarding the organization's information management and records retention policies is necessary, who will participate?

II. Scope of Discovery

- Should the parties agree upon a neutral third party or ask the court to appoint a special master to oversee the discovery process?
- What are the roles and responsibilities of the IT and HIM in the culling, searching, and retrieval of relevant ESI?
- How far back in time should the party search, cull, preserve, and produce ESI?
- Who are the most likely custodians of relevant electronic evidence?
- What type of computer systems capable of electronic data storage does each party have? Are these systems summarized in the organization's information management plan?
- Should the search and production of potentially relevant information be extended into backup tapes or archived records of all computer activity?
- Should the scope of the discovery be limited by the type of computer device and to a class of users?
  — For example, should hard drives, laptops, or other mobile devices be produced for examination?
- What search terms should be employed to limit responsive documents?
- Should a party produce the physical electronic evidence even though data may have been deleted? Will the situation require that a computer forensic specialist recover the deleted data?
- Should SPAM or virus filters be applied to e-mails and attachments?

III. Screening for Privileged or Confidential Documents

- Have the parties entered into an agreement for the screening and production of ESI that may contain privileged or confidential information, including that protected by HIPAA?
  — Examples include peer review protections, attorney-client communications, licenses, copyrights, and trade secrets.
- Do the parties want to waive any privileges?
- Do the parties want to allow for a quick peek of potentially confidential documents?
- Do the parties want to enter into a clawback agreement for the inadvertent production of confidential documents?

- What protective orders or confidentiality agreements are necessary?
- What should happen if trial preparation materials are inadvertently disclosed?

IV. Chain of Custody Issues
- How does the EHR record and trace the individuals who have accessed information and when?
- Will either party hire an outside e-discovery service provider? If so, how will the service provider handle chain of custody?
- If the documents will be handled internally, how will the chain of custody be handled?

V. Costs
- Does the organization have a mechanism in place to identify the true costs and burdens of production?
- Who should bear the costs of production?

VI. Timeliness
- What is a reasonable time to search a party's entire electronic database, and to review and organize the relevant documents?
- Should the normal limits as provided under FRCP Rule 26 be expanded upon when data with limited accessibility are involved?

VII. Production
- How will the documents be produced? Native file format, PDF, or TIFF images, or by some other mechanism?
- Should the parties produce data with the metadata attached or hidden? Which metadata fields or messages should be produced?
- Should production be on a read-only medium such as a CD-ROM, or by some other means?
- Will a litigation support load file be required?

4.4.1.5 The Role of the 30(b)(6) Witness

The storage and maintenance of EHRs will add new set of roles and responsibilities for the LRT and HIM and IT professionals. As EHRs and HIEs become commonplace, it is critically important for the court to understand the steps the defendant or a plaintiff takes to identify, preserve, collect, and produce documents. One way the court can determine whether the discovery process was completed in good faith is to conduct a detailed inquiry into a corporation's information management and retrieval systems. The 30(b)(6) witness is the target of this inquiry.

The 30(b)(6) witness' role is to testify not on the facts of the case, but on a company's operations, such as IT infrastructure or how information is stored, maintained, and used within the organization and processed through the HIE. A 30(b)(6) witness' testimony represents the knowledge of the entity, not of the person being deposed. In the context of e-discovery, the 30(b)(6) witness is often called to testify on the steps the corporation took to find and produce responsive documents to ensure good-faith discovery.

The HIM and IT manager may be called to be a 30 (b)(6) witness for the organization. The 30(b)(6) deposition differs from other depositions in that HIM managers are familiar with and may be or have been the "official custodian or keeper of the record."

It is vitally important that legal counsel educate the both the HIM and IT managers on the discovery process and the procedures that the court will follow to preserve and submit EHRs and other relevant ESI. In order to prepare HIM and IT managers to become potential 30(b)(6) witnesses, the discussion and actions of the LRT are summarized below.

4.4.1.5.1 Discussion and Actions of the LRT

1. Ensure the content of the litigation response adequately describes what a 30(b)(6) witness is and the role of a 30(b)(6) witness to speak on behalf of the organization.
   a. Identify which individuals will be potential 30(b)(6) witnesses.
   b. Instruct legal counsel to educate and train individuals on how to be a 30(b)(6) witness.
   c. Develop sample questions that may be asked of a 30(b)(6) witness and have legal counsel conduct mock trial sessions with potential witnesses.
2. Outline any state and local rules governing the process for the discovery of ESI and ensure the 30(b)(6) witness is knowledgeable in this area. Include a description of all state and local rules in the content of the litigation response plan.
3. Identify any obstacles or barriers to the education and training of potential 30(b)(6) witnesses.
4. Establish a policy and procedure that ensure that when a potential 30(b)(6) witness leaves the organization, competent individuals have been identified and are ready to fulfill the role of a 30(b)(6) witness if necessary.
   a. Ensure appropriate policies are in place to ensure the confidentially and nondisclosure of organizational information are maintained by a potential 30(b)(6) witness when he/she leaves the organization.

4.4.1.6 Managing the Legal Hold

As stated in chapter 3, the organization is responsible for formulating policies and establishing the processes necessary for identifying the triggers of and communicating and auditing an effective legal hold. The process by which data are placed on legal hold will be anything but simple and straightforward in the initial stages of EHR and HIE adoption and until vendors can establish mechanisms within their systems to identify and manage cases in which a legal hold is in place.

According to The Sedona Conference, "The duty to preserve typically arises from the common law duty to avoid spoliation of relevant evidence for use at trial; the inherent power of courts; and court rules governing the imposition of sanctions" (The Sedona Conference 2007a, 1).

When does the organization's duty to preserve relevant information from an EHR or HIE begin? According to The Sedona Conference (2007a, 5):

> The duty to preserve relevant information arises when litigation is "reasonably anticipated." The duty to preserve relevant information is certainly triggered when a complaint is served or a governmental proceeding is initiated or a subpoena is received. However, the duty to preserve could well arise before a complaint is served or a subpoena is received and regardless of whether the organization is bringing the action, is the target of the action or is a third party possessing relevant evidence. The touchstone is "reasonable anticipation."

> Determining when a duty to preserve is triggered is fact intensive and is not amenable to a one-size-fits-all or a checklist approach. A particular organization will likely not be able to resolve the question the same way each time it arises. In general, determining when the duty to preserve arises will require an approach that considers a number of factors, including (but not necessarily limited to) the level of knowledge within the organization about the claim, the risk to the organization of the claim, the risk of losing information if a litigation hold is not implemented, and the number and complexity of sources where information is reasonably likely to be found. Weighing these factors will enable an organization to make a determination regarding when litigation is reasonably anticipated and when a duty to take affirmative steps to preserve relevant information has arisen.

The identification and preservation of all relevant ESI are absolutely necessary in order for the court to carry out its truth-seeking function. Until such time that the admission of EHR and HIE data into a court of law is ubiquitous, it will be up to the parties and the courts to work together to establish systems and processes that can strike a balance between obligations not to obstruct justice and to avoid spoliation claims.

The LRT plays a crucial role in assisting legal counsel and risk management in the ongoing review of the legal hold process in evaluating where data reside and identifying the data owners responsible for the preservation of relevant ESI. Outlined below is a summary of the discussion and actions to be taken by the LRT in management of the legal hold.

4.4.1.6.1 Discussion and Actions of the LRT

1. Ensure the content of the litigation response adequately describes under which conditions and circumstances a legal hold will be placed on EHR, HIE, and other relevant information.
   a. Identify those individual(s) or departments (legal counsel and/or risk management) who will be responsible for making the determination when a legal hold will be placed upon a patient's record and/or other data relevant to litigation.
   b. Develop organizational policies and procedures regarding the establishment of legal holds.
      i. Identify to what extent (if any) the organization will be required to notify the HIE of EHR data that have been placed under legal hold.
   c. Develop standardized letters and methods of communication to inform the data owners, records custodians, or potential witnesses of the establishment of the legal hold and the individual's preservation obligations. The type of standardized legal hold notification letters to be developed should include the following:
      i. Internal notification of legal hold—A letter issued by legal counsel or another individual appointed that is sent to data owners, key custodians, or other potential witnesses. A copy of this letter should also be sent to HIM and IT personnel who may be responsible for retaining electronic and other hard-copy data. The following information should be outlined in the internal notification letter:
         1. High-level description of the matter and allegations
         2. Description of the nature, scope, and complexity of the case along with what data and records are subject to the legal hold and for what period of time

3. Description of the organizational process and policy by which the data owners, custodians, or potential witnesses should retain the data

4. Outline of organizational policy for notification to legal counsel and/or risk management of the form and location of any/all potentially relevant information

   a. Request individuals receiving legal hold notification also identify all other personnel or providers who may have knowledge or relevant data.

   b. Ask for a detailed listing of all potential locations where data might exist with a description of the type of data, form, and format.

   c. Identify data sources that are easily accessible versus not reasonably accessible.

5. Statement that outlines the organization's preservation obligations and that legal hold supersedes any current records retention and destruction policies

6. Contact information for LRT and/or individual who will be responsible for the ongoing review of the legal hold

The internal notification letter should also include some sort of written or electronic verification acknowledging that the individual has received, read, reviewed, and fully intends to comply with the legal hold obligations.

ii. Notification of revised legal hold—A followup letter issued by legal counsel or another appointed individual within the organization that is sent to designated individuals within the organization for the purpose of broadening or narrowing the legal hold in response to conditions or circumstances that may have changed or become known in the case. A copy of this letter should also be sent to HIM and IT personnel who may be responsible for retaining electronic and hard-copy data. The following information should be outlined in the revised legal hold letter:

1. Description of the matter and allegations

2. Identification of any/all new responsibilities of the individuals with regard to their preservation obligations

3. Description of the organizational process and policy by which the data owners, custodians, or potential witnesses should retain the data

4. Delineation of the expected time period for which the legal hold will remain in effect

The revised legal letter should also include some sort of written or electronic verification acknowledging that the individual(s) have received, read, reviewed, and fully intends to comply with the revised legal hold obligations.

iii. Legal hold reminder notice—Once a legal hold has been established, it should be reviewed by the LRT and/or another designated individual within the organization until such time that it has been officially lifted. In addition, the organization's LRP should also clearly outline the organizational process by which legal holds are reviewed and communicated within the organization. Legal hold reminder notices can be communicated on a monthly, quarterly, or semiannual basis and should be consistently administered, managed, and communicated. The legal hold reminder notice should be sent to all data owners, records custodians, and/or potential witnesses to remind them of their legal hold obligations and include the following information:

1. Description of the matter and allegations
2. Brief description of the status of the case
3. Reminder of the organizational process and policy by which the data owners, custodians, or potential witnesses should retain the data
4. Reminder of the expected time period the legal hold is expected to remain in effect

Documentation of the date(s) and persons to whom the legal hold reminder notice was sent should be maintained by the LRT and/or the individual designated to review and manage the status of all legal holds.

iv. External notification of legal hold letter—A letter issued by legal counsel or another appointed individual within the organization that is sent to HIPAA business associates and/or other third parties that the organization believes may possess data relevant to litigation. A copy of this letter should also be sent to legal counsel, risk management, or a designated member of the LRT personnel who may be responsible for the ongoing review of all legal hold notices. The following information should be outlined in the external notification letter:

1. High level description of the matter and allegations
2. Description of the nature, scope, and complexity of the case along with what data and records are subject to the legal hold and for what period of time

3. Description of the organizational process and policy by which the third party should retain the data

4. Outline of organizational policy for notification to legal counsel and risk management of the form and location of all potentially relevant information

5. Statement that outlines the third party organization's preservation obligations and states that legal hold supersedes any/all current records retention and destruction policies

6. Contact information for LRT and individuals who will be responsible for the ongoing review of the legal hold

The external notification letter should also include some sort of written or electronic verification acknowledging that the organization has received it, read, reviewed, and fully intends to comply with the legal hold obligations.

In preparation for the evolving role of HIM and IT in litigation, in 2008, the AHIMA e-Discovery Task Force established a model policy to assist healthcare organizations and legal counsel to prepare for the pretrial conference. This tool was designed for HIM and IT professionals and other members of the LRT with a standard protocol in which they can better assist legal counsel and help to assure compliance with the FRCP.

4.4.2 Application of Case Law

The judicial decision in the multidistrict pharmaceutical products liability litigation, *In re Seroquel, Products Liability Litigation,* 224 F.R.D. 650 (M.D. Fla. 2007) provides an excellent example of what can happen when parties fail to cooperate in discovery and when a defendant engages in pretrial tactics such as "purposeful sluggishness." Based on a perceived "failure to timely comply with numerous discovery obligations since the inception of this litigation," (*In re Seroquel* M.D. Fla. 2007) the plaintiffs moved for sanctions. Although neither party was sanctioned under Rule 16(f)(1)(B), the court lost confidence in the parties after it became frustrated over their lack of cooperation and the conduct they exhibited at the meet and confer and pretrial conferences. The parties' conduct weighed heavily against them in later stages of litigation.

In making its sanction determinations, the court evaluated the discovery process leading up to the parties' dispute (*In re Seroquel* M.D. Fla. 2007). US Magistrate Judge David A. Baker admonished the parties for their failure to resolve their discovery and scheduling issues through the meet and confer process. In rendering his decision, Judge Baker relied heavily on the second edition of *The*

Sedona Principles (The Sedona Conference 2007a) and the *Manual for Complex Litigation* (4th Edition) and specifically cited §11.446 Discovery of Computerized Data, which is summarized as follows:

- Computerized data have become commonplace in litigation. The sheer volume of such data, when compared with conventional paper documentation, can be staggering. . . . One gigabyte is the equivalent of 500,000 typewritten pages. Large corporate computer networks create backup data measured in terabytes, or 1,000,000 megabytes; each terabyte represents the equivalent of 500 billion [sic] typewritten pages of plain text.
- Digital or electronic information can be stored in any of the following: mainframe computers, network servers, personal computers, hand-held devices, automobiles, or household appliances; or it can be accessible via the Internet, from private networks, or from third parties. Any discovery plan must address issues relating to such information, including the search for it and its location, retrieval, form of production, inspection, preservation, and use at trial.

For the most part, such data will reflect information generated and maintained in the ordinary course of business. As such, discovery of relevant and non-privileged data is routine and within the commonly understood scope of Rules 26 and 34. Other data are generated and stored as a byproduct of the various information technologies commonly employed by parties in the ordinary course of business, but not routinely retrieved and used for business purposes. Such data include:

> *Metadata, or information about information.* This includes the information embedded in a routine computer file reflecting the file creation date, when it was last accessed or edited, by whom, and sometimes previous versions or editorial changes. This information is not apparent on a screen or in a normal printout of the file, and it is often generated and maintained without the knowledge of the file user . . . (Marcus, et al. 2004, Sec. 11,446)

4.4.2.1 The 16(b) Pretrial Conference—The Role of the Judge in Electronic Discovery

The *In re Seroquel* litigation provides an excellent example of the important role a judge has in facilitation of the timely and just resolution of a matter by encouraging the parties to discuss the scope of proposed computer-based discovery early in the case, particularly any discovery of data beyond those available to the responding parties in the ordinary course of business.

As stated in *In re Seroquel:*

> The requesting parties should identify the information they require as narrowly and precisely as possible, and the responding parties should be forthcoming and explicit in identifying what data are available from what sources, to allow formulation of a realistic computer-based discovery plan. Rule 26(b)(2)(iii) allows the court to limit or modify the extent of otherwise allowable discovery if the burdens outweigh the likely benefit-the rule should be used to discourage costly, speculative, duplicative, or unduly burdensome discovery of computer data and systems . . .

> There are several reasons to encourage parties to produce and exchange data in electronic form: Production of computer data on disks, CD-ROMS, or by file transfers significantly reduces the costs of copying, transport, storage, and management-protocols may be established by the parties to facilitate the handling of documents from initial production to use in depositions and pretrial procedures to presentation at trial
> - Computerized data are far more easily searched, located, and organized than paper data
> - Computerized data may form the contents for a common document depository

> The goal is to maximize these potential advantages while *minimizing the potential problems of incompatibility among various computer systems, programs, and data, and minimizing problems with intrusiveness, data integrity, and information overload . . .*

> The relatively inexpensive production of computer-readable images may suffice for the vast majority of requested data. Dynamic data may need to be produced in native format, or in a modified format in which the integrity of the data can be maintained and the data can be manipulated for analysis. If raw data are produced, appropriate applications, file structures, manuals, and other tools necessary for the proper translation and use of the data must be provided. *Files (such as e-mail) for which metadata is essential to the understanding of the primary data, should be identified and produced in an appropriate format.*

Judge Baker determined that "[the defendant] and its counsel had a responsibility at the outset of litigation to 'take affirmative steps to monitor compliance so that all sources of discoverable information are identified and searched' and also commented 'the failure of the defendant to investigate and understand its own records and documents and to prepare them for production did not meet the expectations of the Court as discussed at the September 2006 Conference'" (*In re Seroquel* M.D. Fla. 2007).

Judge Baker further held that sanctionable conduct exhibited by the defendant included:

- Producing ESI without its corresponding metadata
- Producing multipage TIFF images, some of which consisted of more than 20,000 pages
- Producing electronic documents without apparent sequential numbering
- Producing 8 percent of the entire production as one lengthy document that could be only opened with a very powerful workstation
- Producing electronic files with no load files, rendering production inaccessible and unusable (*In re Seroquel* M.D. Fla. 2007)

With regard to Judge Baker's assertions, the defendant responded that the plaintiffs were not cooperating in good faith and, therefore, did not meet the standard for imposing sanctions (*In re Seroquel* M.D. Fla. 2007).

With regard to the defendant's assertions, Judge Baker determined:

- The key word search employed by the plaintiff was "plainly inadequate."
- Despite an offer from the defendant to run additional search terms for the plaintiff, the plaintiff limited its search terms to 60, being described to be "stubbornly unresponsive."

The court noted that these and many of the other technical problems "likely could have been resolved far sooner and less expensively had [the defendant] cooperated by fostering consultation between the technical staffs responsible for production. Instead [the defendant] shielded its third party technical contractor from all contact with the Plaintiffs. This approach is antithetical to the Sedona Principles and is not an indicium of good faith" (*In re Seroquel* M.D. Fla. 2007).

Although the FRCP do not require judges to address e-discovery in the Rule 16 scheduling order, the importance of the pretrial conference must not be overlooked. Under Rule 16(f)(1)(B), the court can impose broad sanctions upon a party or its attorney if either is "substantially unprepared to participate—or does not participate in good faith—in the [Rule 16 pretrial] conference" as *In re Seroquel* demonstrates.

Furthermore, under Rule 37, the court also may impose broad sanctions for discovery-related abuses. The conduct of the parties at the pretrial conference will set the stage for the trial and will provide the court with a glimpse as to how prepared the parties are and to what extent, if any, the discovery disputes involve electronically stored information.

In re Seroquel is an important case to evaluate from a litigation response planning perspective. It provides an example of how the failure to plan for discovery, and "purposeful sluggishness" will result in delays, added expense, and possibly lead to court-imposed sanctions.

The *In re Seroquel* case demonstrates the importance of cooperation and communication in discovery. Prior to a pretrial conference, the parties must be prepared to present to the Court the nature of the case, the possibility of settlement, and discuss the nature and length of discovery necessary to prepare the case for trial. The pretrial conference will set the stage for the litigation process and, as in *In re Seroquel*, the judge may evaluate the parties' pretrial conference behavior and the consequences for failing to cooperate can be severe including, but not limited to, the imposition of sanctions and penalties.

4.5 e-Mail

As evidenced by the $28 million dollar jury verdict in *Zubulake* (S.D.N.Y. 2003), the e-mail system has become a veritable "cache to the cash." Given the ubiquitous nature of e-mail, there appears to be no end in sight to the digital information explosion and there is a need to develop and improve the methodologies by which information contained within e-mail can be searched and retrieved.

From 2004 to 2007, the average amount of data contained within a Fortune 1000 corporation grew by 526 percent, going from 190 terabytes to 1 **petabyte** (1,000 terabytes). During this same time period, the amount of digital information in midsize American companies grew by a whopping 5,000 percent, going from 2 terabytes to 100 terabytes. Globally, the data set grew by 3,200 percent, going from 5 exabytes (5 billion gigabytes) to 161 exabytes (Scheindlin et al. 2009). Today, the consumer can purchase a one terabyte hard drive for under $100. The National Archives and Records Administration (NARA) reported that as of January 20, 2009, it "expected to receive substantially over a hundred million e-mails from the [former] incumbent White House. At the present rate of e-mail creation, it expects to receive over *one billion* e-mails over the course of the next decade as permanently accessioned records of the government" (Paul and Baron 2007).

The costs to search, retrieve, and review e-mail are staggering (Paul and Baron 2007).

To illustrate:

e-Mail Search

Take then, for example, litigation in which the universe subject to search stands at 1 billion e-mail records, at least 25% of which have one or more attachments of varying length (1–300 pages). . . .

At an assumed billing rate of $100/hour, the costs to review 1 billion e-mails at a rate of 50 e-mails/per person/hour would take 100 people, working 10 hours a day, 7 days a week, 50 weeks a year over 54.95 years to complete. The cost of the review would be $2 billion. If the cost of the labor is lowered to $10/hour by going "offshore," the cost would still be over $200 million.

The thought of searching through a billion e-mails today is unfathomable, yet, just 10 years ago, some parties had *already* crossed the billion electronic document threshold. In 2000, John H. Jessen, Founder and Chairman of the Board of Daticon EED, reported (Jessen 2000):

One Billion e-Mails

We have had about half a dozen cases now where the total number of electronic things brought into play—not that were available in a global set—but which were available after a reasonable review of the set—went over one billion. A billion pieces of discovery material. . . .

Those kind of numbers introduce a whole host of issues about scope and management. How do you manage a billion things? . . .

In the movement toward the EHR, it is conceivable to think that a search through a patient record could exceed the one-billion-electronic-document threshold. It is realistic to expect that an EHR vendor will develop and deploy mechanisms by which EHRs can easily and efficiently be searched, and possibility integrate EHR search capabilities with the organization's e-mail system.

Policies and procedures regarding the deletion and retention of e-mail, including how and by which mechanisms e-mail is searched, must be instituted. And, as Paul and Baron (2007) conclude in *Information Inflation*, "The numbers add up to more of a burden than any party should assume, no matter how rich in resources, without changes being made to the way cases are litigated and to techniques used in discovery."

The time, burdens, and costs involved in the searching and discovery of e-mail beckon the need for a rethinking in how searches are performed on the EHR as well as e-mail.

4.6 Voicemail

Since 1970, when the FRCP were amended, the courts have routinely allowed voicemails to be admitted into evidence (see *Anti-Monopoly, Inc. v. Hasbro, Inc.* No. 94 Civ. 2120, 1995 WL 649934, 2 ([S.D.N.Y. Nov. 3, 1995]; Bennett 2003). A voicemail maintains equal footing to other forms of ESI in the eyes of the court.

According to Bennett (2003), "The preservation, review and production of voicemail records may be even harder to handle than other electronic records." Voicemail records have long moved from simple tape recordings to digitized, manipulable records . . . and the preservation, review and production of voicemail records may be even harder to handle than other electronic records" (Jessen 2000).

The LRT should discuss the use and storage capacity of its voicemail and EHR transcription systems. If it has not done so already, the organization should establish a retention policy, describing how long voice files are maintained on the organization's voicemail and EHR transcription systems.

4.7 EHR Planning and Implementation

The HITECH stimulus funding incentives provide motivation for clinicians and other providers to invest in EHRs. As *Rush University Medical Center. v. Minnesota Mining and Manufacturing Co. (3M)*, No. 04 C 6878 (N.D. Ill. Nov. 21, 2007) demonstrates, let the buyer beware when it comes to negotiating with EHR vendors, because purchasing contracts are built by vendors. The buyer should seek legal review before entering into and implementing a new EHR system.

Rush University Medical Center (N.D. Ill. Nov. 21, 2007) involved a Consumer Fraud Act claim against integrated EHR system vendor 3M. After nearly three years of negotiations with the defendant, on December 24, 1998, the plaintiff signed a contract with the defendant to license its Care Innovation system. The plaintiff required the vendor to link the plaintiff's different clinical and administrative systems into a single integrated patient information system. Within one year after signing the contract with the defendant, the Care Innovation system went live in the fall of 1999.

On October 26, 2004, the plaintiff filed suit alleging that the defendant's Care Innovation system lacked some or most of the functionalities it promised to provide. The plaintiff asserted claims for breach of contract, breach of warranty, and statutory fraud. The defendant denied all allegations and moved for summary judgment.

The Northern District of Illinois granted the defendant's motion in part and denied it in part. The court turned first to the defendant's argument that the plaintiff's claims were barred by the three-year statute of limitations period. The court held that, "By September, 2001, after [the plaintiff] had used the Care Innovation system for nearly two years, it had all the information it needed to draw the conclusion that defendant had misrepresented its capabilities with regards to Care Innovation's functionalities."

The court addressed the defendant's argument that the plaintiff was not entitled to seek damages outside of the contract signed by the parties. The court held that, "Because we find a genuine controversy exists as to whether [the defendant] acted with gross negligence or willful misconduct, we refuse to limit [plaintiff's] potential damages at this time."

The court said, "We are unwilling at the summary judgment stage, to conclude as a matter of law, that 3M did not act with gross negligence or willful misconduct when it made representations to Rush about either Care Innovation's capabilities or 3M's commitment to Care Innovation."

Rush University Medical Center provides a notice to all potential purchasers of an EHR system—that the functional requirements, timelines for implementation, and scope of damages must be clearly delineated in the EHR purchase contract. Once the EHR system is in operation, the performance of the product and the status of implementation should be closely monitored.

4.8 Issues for Discussion by the Litigation Response Team

The foundational principles listed in table 4.1 are further explored in the AHIMA LRP practice briefs found in appendices A–C of this book.

References

42 CFR 482.24: Medical record services. 2006.

42 CFR 482.24(c)(1): Medical record services. 2008.

45 CFR 170: Initial set of standards, implementation specifications, and certification criteria for electronic health record technology. 2010.

71 FR 68687. 2006.

Advisory Committee Note to 1983 Amendment to Rule 26(b).

Advisory Committee Note to 1993 Amendment to Rule 26(b).

Advisory Committee Note to 2000 Amendment to Rule 26(b)(1).

Advisory Committee Note to 2006 Amendment to Rule 26(b)(2)(B).

Advisory Committee Note to 2006 Amendment to Rule 26(b)(2)(C).

Advisory Committee Note to 2006 Amendment to Rule 26(b)(5).

Advisory Committee Note to 2006 Amendment of Rule 34(a).

Advisory Committee Note to 2006 Amendment to Rule 34(b).

Advisory Committee Note to 2006 Amendment to Rule 37.

Advisory Committee Note to 2006 Amendment to Rule 45.

Aguilar v. ICE Div., 2008 WL 5062700 (S.D.N.Y. 2008).

AHIMA e-HIM Workgroup on Assessing and Improving Healthcare Data in the EHR. 2007. Practice brief: Assessing and improving EHR data quality. Journal of AHIMA 78(3):69–72.

Ak-Chin Indian Community v. United States, 85 Fed. Cl. 397 (Ct. Ct. 2009).

Amarasingham, R., M. Diener-West, M. Weiner, H. Lehmann, J.E. Herbers, and N.R. Powe. 2006. Clinical information technology capabilities in four U.S. hospitals: Testing a new structural performance measure. Medical Care 44(3):216–224.

American Society for the Prevention of Cruelty to Animals v. Ringling Bros. and Barnum & Bailey Circus, civil action no. 03-2006 (D.D.C. 2008).

Annas, G.J. 2006. The patient's right to safety: Improving the quality of care through litigation against hospitals. The New England Journal of Medicine 354(19):2063–2066.

Anti-Monopoly, Inc. v. Hasbro, Inc., No. 94 Civ. 2120, 1995 WL 649934 (S.D.N.Y. Nov. 3, 1995).

Arista Records, LLC v. Usenet.com Inc., 2009 WL 185992 (S.D.N.Y. 2009).

Ball, C. 2006. Understanding metadata: Knowing metadata's different forms and evidentiary significance is now an essential skill for litigators. Law Technology News 36(36).

Ball, K. Organizational Approaches to Early Litigation Readiness for Electronic Discovery of Electronic Health Records: A Modified Delphi Study. Baltimore, MD: Johns Hopkins University; 2008.

Ball, M.J., and S. Bierstock. 2007. Clinical use of enabling technology: Creating a new healthcare system though the use of enabling technologies requires changes in a profound scale. JHIM 21(3):68–71.

Ball, K., G.E. DeLoss, E.F. Shay, and E. Zych. 2008 (May 8). The American Health Lawyers Association's Health Information Technology Practice Group Webinar: EHRs and e-discovery: The readiness is all.

Bierman, E., and M. Buenafe. 2009. FDA and health IT: As role of health IT gains new significance, regulators will be keeping watch. Health Lawyers News 13(5):30–32.

Board of Regents v. BASF Corp., 2007 WL 3342423 (D. Neb. 2007).

Brady, K. 2007. Admissibility problems with ESI? The answer just might be in a "Grimm" fairy tale. Digital Discovery and E-Evidence: BNA 7(6):96.

Brady, K., K. Ball, R.J. Hedges, and A. Estaban. 2008. E-discovery in healthcare litigation: What is ahead for ESI, PHI and EHR? The Sedona Conference Journal.

Brady, K., and P. Grimm. 2007. Admissibility of electronic evidence. Paper presented at CGOC. http://www.cgoc.com/resources/admissibility-electronic-evidence.

Bray & Gillespie Management LLC v. Lexington Ins. Co., civil action no. 07-222-Orl-35KRS (M.D. Fl. 2009).

Cache La Poudre Feed, LLC v. Land O' Lakes Inc., 244 F.R.D. 614 (D. Colo. 2007).

Campbell, E.M., D.F. Sittig, J.S. Ash, K.P. Guappone, and R.H. Dykstra. 2006. Types of unintended consequences related to computerized provider order entry. Journal of the American Medical Informatics Association 13(5):547–556.

Campbell, E.M., D.F. Sittig, J.S. Ash, K.P. Guappone, and R.H. Dykstra. 2007. In reply to: "e-iatrogenesis: The most critical consequence of CPOE and other HIT." Journal of the American Medical Informatics Association 14(3):389.

Cason-Merenda v. Detroit Med. Ctr., 2008 WL 2714239 (E.D. Mich. 2008).

Centers for Medicare and Medicaid Services. 2010. Clinical Laboratory Improvement Amendments of 1988 (CLIA)—Issuance of Revised Survey Procedures and Interpretive Guidelines for Laboratories and Laboratory Services in Appendix C of the State Operations Manual to Facilitate the Electronic Exchange of Laboratory Information. https://www.cms.gov/SurveyCertificationGenInfo/downloads/SCLetter10-12.pdf.

Certification Commission for Health Information Technology. 2009. CCHIT criteria proposed final: Ambulatory 2009. http://www.cchit.org.

Chaudhry, B., J. Wang, S. Wu, M. Maglione, W. Mojica, E. Roth, S.C. Morton, and P.G. Shekelle. 2006. Systematic review: Impact of health information technology on quality, efficiency, and costs of medical care. Annals of Internal Medicine 144(10):742–752.

In re Classicstar Mare Lease Litigation, 2009 WL 250954 (E.D. Kan. 2009).

Clinical Laboratory Improvement Amendments, Subpart K. http://wwwn.cdc.gov/clia/regs/subpart_k.aspx#493.1291.

Columbia Pictures, Inc. v. Bunnell, 245 F.R.D. 443 (C.D. Cal. 2007).

Columbia Pictures, Indus. v. Bunnell, 2007 U.S. Dist. LEXIS 63620 (C.D. Cal. Aug. 24, 2007).

Compl., Plumbers & Pipefitters Local Union No. 630 Pension-Annuity Trust Fund v. Allscripts-Misys Healthcare Solutions, Inc., No. 09-4726 (N.D. Ill. 2009).

Convolve, Inc. v. Compaq Computer Corp., 223 F.R.D. 162 (S.D.N.Y. 2004).

Crawford-El v. Britton, 523 U.S. 574, 598 (1996).

Crowley, C. 2010 (March 25–26). Mapping your client's data. Fourth Annual The Sedona Conference Institute Program on Getting Ahead of the e-Discovery Curve.

Cumberland Truck Equip. v. Detroit Diesel Corp., 2008 WL 511194 (E.D. Mich. 2008).

D.N.J. L. Civ. R. 26.1(d)(3)(a).

Dougherty, M. 2007 (Oct. 6). Opening remarks. AHIMA Legal EHR Conference.

Dougherty, M., and L. Washington. 2008. Defining and disclosing the designated record set and the legal health record. Journal of AHIMA 79(4):65–68.

Dougherty, M., H. Rhodes, and M. O'Neill. 2007. Portrait of a legal EHR: Developing a legal EHR conformance profile. Journal of AHIMA 78(6):66–67.

In re Ebay Seller Antitrust Litigation, 2007 WL 2852364 (N.D. Ca. 2007).

Equity Analytics, LLC v. Lundin, 248 F.R.D. 331 (D.D.C. 2008).

ex rel. Edmondson v. Tyson Foods, Inc., 2007 WL 1498973 (N.D. Okla. 2007).

Facciola, J.M. 2010 (March). Ethical considerations pertaining to counsel's entering into agreements that particular procedures: Do not waive attorney-client or work product privileges. Paper presented at the Fourth Annual The Sedona Conference Institute Program on Getting Ahead of the e-Discovery Curve.

In re Fannie May Securities Litigation, 2009 WL 21528 (D.C. Cir. 2009).

Federal Rule of Civil Procedure 1. 1938.

Fox Cable Networks, Inc. v. Goen Technologies Corp., 2008 WL 2165179 (D.N.J. 2008).

Gelzer, R.D. 2008. Metadata, law, and the real world. Journal of AHIMA 79(2):56–57, 64; quiz 65–66.

Grossman, J.M. 2007. Physicians' use of electronic medical records for quality reporting. Paper presented at the Division of Health Sciences Informatics Grand Rounds, Johns Hopkins University, School of Medicine.

Haka v. Lincoln County, 246 F.R.D. 577 (W.D. Wisc. 2007).

Hall, M.A., and K.A. Schulman. 2009. Ownership of medical information. Journal of the American Medical Association 301(12):1282–1284.

Harrison, M.I., R. Koppel, and S. Bar-Lev. 2007. Unintended consequences of information technologies in health care: An interactive sociotechnical analysis. Journal of the American Medical Informatics Association 14(5):542–549.

Hawaiian Airlines, Inc. v. Mesa Air Group, Inc., 2007 WL 3172642 (Bankr.D. Haw. 2007).

Hedges, R.J. 2007. Discovery of Electronically Stored Information: Surveying the Legal Landscape. Washington, D.C.: BNA Books.

Herrin, B.S. 2008a. Professional practice solutions: Releasing records from other providers. Journal of AHIMA 79(11):55.

Herrin, B.S. 2008b (Aug. 18). The legal EHR: Beyond definition. The American Health Information Management Association Legal EHR Conference.

Herrin, B.S. 2008c. Unsolicited medical information: Use it or lose it? Legal HIM-formation 4(5):1–2.

HHS-ONC Policy, Adoption and Certification Working Group. 2010 (March 25).

HL7 RM-ES. 2010. HL7 EHR Records Management and Evidentiary Support Functional Profile Release 1. https://www.hl7.org/store/index.cfm?ref=nav.

Hoffman, S., and A. Podgurski. 2008. Finding a cure: The case for regulation and oversight of electronic health record systems. Harvard Journal Law and Technolology 22(1):1–63.

Hoffman, S., and A. Podgurski. 2009. E-Health hazards: Provider liability and electronic health record systems. Berkeley Technology Law Journal 24:1523–1581. http://ssrn.com/abstract=1463671.

In re Honeywell Int'l Inc., 2003 U.S. Dist. LEXIS 20602 (S.D.N.Y. 2003).

Hopson v. City of Baltimore, 232 F.R.D. 228 (D. Md. 2005).

Jenders, R.A., J.A. Osheroff, D.F. Sittig, E.A. Pifer, and J.M. Teich. 2007. Recommendations for clinical decision support deployment: Synthesis of a roundtable of medical directors of information systems. Proceedings of the American Medical Informatics Association Annual Symposium, pp. 359–363.

John B. v. Goetz, 531 F.3d 448 (6th Cir. 2008).

The Joint Commission. 2008 (Dec. 11). Issue 42: Safely implementing health information and converging technologies. http://www.jointcommission.org/sentinel_event_alert_issue_42_safely_implementing_health_information_and_converging_technologies.

K&L Gates. 2004 (Dec. 15). Court directs production in native electronic form notwithstanding prior hard copy production: Electronic discovery law. http://www.ediscoverylaw.com/2004/12/articles/case-summaries/court-directs-production-in-native-electronic-form-notwithstanding-prior-hard-copy-production.

Kerr, O.S. 2001. Computer Records and Federal Rules of Evidence. http://www.usdoj.gov/criminal/cybercrime/usamarch2001_4.htm.

King, P., and T. Bunsen. 2009 (Aug. 17). E-discovery. Adaptation from case presentation, Risk Management and Legal Affairs, NorthShore University Health System. AHIMA Legal EHR Conference, Chicago.

Knifesource LLC v. Wachovia Bank, N.A., 2007 U.S. Dist. LEXIS 58829 (D.S.C. 2007).

Koppel, R., and D. Kreda. 2009. Health care information technology vendors' "hold harmless" clause: Implications for patients and clinicians. The Journal of the American Medical Association 301(12):1276–1278.

Koppel, R., C.E. Leonard, A.R. Localio, A. Cohen, R. Auten, and B.L. Strom. 2008a. Identifying and quantifying medication errors: Evaluation of rapidly discontinued medication orders submitted to a computerized physician order entry system. JAMIA 15(4):461–465.

Koppel, R., J.P. Metlay, A. Cohen, B. Abaluck, A.R. Localio, S.E. Kimmel, and B.L. Strom. 2005. Role of computerized physician order entry systems in facilitating medication errors. The Journal of the American Medical Association 293(10):1197–1203.

Koppel, R., T. Wetterneck, J.L. Telles, and B.T. Karsh. 2008b. Workarounds to barcode medication administration systems: Their occurrences, causes, and threats to patient safety. JAMIA 15(4):408–423.

Korin, J.B., and M.S. Quattrone. 2007. Litigation in the decade of electronic health records. New Jersey Law Journal 188(11):183.

Lender, D. 2006 (May). Duty to preserve: Should your client clam up when you make a mistake and hope it all goes away? The Federal Lawyer. http://www.weil.com/news/pubdetail.aspx?pub=3327.

Lorraine v. Markel Am. Ins. Co., 241 F.R.D. 534 (D. Md. 2007).

Mancia v. Mayflower Textile Services Co., 253 F.R.D. 354 (D. Md. 2008).

McLean, T.R. 2008 (Sept. 16). Metadata: An Orwellian big brother within electronic medical records. MDNG Primary Care. http://www.hcplive.com/publications/mdng-primarycare/2008/Sep2008/PC_Metadata_within_EMRs.

McLean, T.R., L. Burton, C.C. Haller, and P.B. McLean. 2008. Electronic medical record metadata: Uses and liability. Journal of the American College of Surgeons 206(3):405–411.

McPeek v. Ashcroft, 202 F.R.D. 31 (D.D.C. 2001).

Medical Products Agency Working Group on Medical Information Systems. 2009. Proposal for Guidelines Regarding Classification of Software Based Information Systems Used in Health Care. http://www.lakemedelsverket.se/upload/foretag/medicinteknik/en/Medical-Information-Systems-Report_2009-06-18.pdf.

Mitchell, J. 2007. Data source mapping workshop. CGOC Conference: Data Source Synchronization for Preservation, Discovery & Retention.

Monegain, B. 2009 (Aug. 5). Allscripts shareholders file class action suit. Healthcare IT News. http://www.healthcareitnews.com/news/allscripts-shareholders-file-class-action-suit.

Muro v. Target Corp., 2007 WL 3254463 (N.D. Ill. 2007).

In re Napster Inc. Copyright Litigation, 2006 WL 3050864, *9 (N.D. Ca. 2006).

Office of the National Coordinator for Health Information Technology Policy Committee. 2009 (July 16). Meeting. http://healthit.hhs.gov/portal/server.pt/community/healthit_hhs_gov__home/1204.

Office of the National Coordinator for Health Information Technology Policy Committee. 2010 (April 21). Meeting. http://healthit.hhs.gov/portal/server.pt/community/healthit_hhs_gov__home/1204.

Palgut v. City of Colorado Springs, 2007 WL 4277564 (D. Colo. 2007).

Paterno, M.D., S.M. Maviglia, P.N. Gorman, D.L. Seger, E. Yoshida, A.C. Seger, D.W. Bates, and T.K. Gandhi. 2009. Tiering drug-drug interaction alerts by severity increases compliance rates. Journal of the American Medical Informatics Association 16(1):40–46.

Patient Safety and Quality Improvement Act of 2005. Public Law 109-41.

Paul, G.L. 2008. Foundations of Digital Evidence. Chicago: ABA Publishing.

Peskoff v. Faber, 240 F.R.D. 26 (D.D.C. 2007).

Peskoff v. Faber, 244 F.R.D. 54 (D.D.C. 2007).

Regan-Touhy v. Walgreen Co., 526 F.3d 641 (10th Cir. *2008).*

Rhoads Industries, Inc. v. Building Materials Corp., 2008 WL 96404 (E.D. Pa. 2008).

Rhoads Industries, Inc. v. Building Materials Corp., 2008 WL 4916026 (E.D. Pa. 2008).

RLI Ins. Co. v. Indian River School Dist., 2007 WL 3112417 (D. Del. 2007).

Roach, W.H., and AHIMA. 2006. Medical Records and the Law. Sudbury, Mass.: Jones and Bartlett Publishers.

Rollins, G. 2007. Printing electronic records: Managing the hassle and the risk. Journal of AHIMA 78(5):36, 38, 40.

RTI International. 2007. Recommended Requirements for Enhancing Data Quality in Electronic Health Records. Report for the Office of the National Coordinator for Health Information Technology.

Rush University Medical Center v. Minnesota Mining and Manufacturing Co. (3M), No. 04-c-6878, 2007 WL 4198233 (N.D. Ill. 2007).

SEC v. Collins & Aikman Corp., 2009 U.S. Dist. LEXIS 3367 (S.D.N.Y. 2009).

The Sedona Conference. 2007a. The Sedona Principles Second Edition: Best Practices Recommendations & Principles for Addressing Electronic Document Production. http://www.thesedonaconference.org/content/miscFiles/TSC_PRINCP_2nd_ed_607.pdf.

The Sedona Conference. 2007b. The Sedona Conference Commentary on Legal Holds: The Trigger and the Process. http://www.thesedonaconference.org/content/miscFiles/Legal_holds.pdf.

The Sedona Conference. 2008a. The Sedona Conference Cooperation Proclamation. http://www.thesedonaconference.org/content/tsc_cooperation_proclamation/proclamation.pdf.

The Sedona Conference. 2008b. The Sedona Conference Commentary on Non-Party Production & Rule 45 Subpoenas.

The Sedona Conference. 2008c. The Sedona Conference Commentary on ESI Evidence & Admissibility.

In re Seroquel Products Liability Litigation, 224 F.R.D. 650 (M.D. Fla. 2007).

Shay, E.F. 2007. Ensuring health record integrity. Paper presented at AHIMA Annual Convention.

Shortliffe, E.H., and J.J. Cimino, eds. 2006. Biomedical Informatics: Computer Applications in Health Care and Biomedicine, 3rd ed. New York: Springer.

Shuren, J. 2010. Testimony during a hearing on health information technology safety. Office of the National Coordinator HIT Policy Committee and Adoption and Certification Working Group.

Silverstein, S. 2009. The syndrome of inappropriate overconfidence in computing: An invasion of medicine by the information technology industry? The Journal of American Physicians and Surgeons 14(2).

Spieker v. Quest Cherokee, LLC, 2008 WL 4758604 (D. Kan. 2008).

State of Texas v. City of Frisco, 2008 WL 828055 (E.D. Tex. 2008).

SubAir Systems, LLC v. PrecisionAire Systems, Inc., civil action no. 06-2620 (D.S.C. 2009).

Thomas, J., and R. Hedges. 2010. Victor Stanley revisited: Judge Grimm's analysis of the law governing spoliation sanctions. Digital Discovery & e-Evidence 10(17):4. http://www.crowell.com/documents/Victor-Stanley-Revisited-Judge-Grimms-Analysis-of-%20the-Law-Governing-Spoliation-Sanctions.pdf.

Tomlinson v. El Paso Corp., 254 F.R.D. 474 (D. Colo. 2007).

United States v. O'Keefe, 2008 WL 44972 (D.D.C. 2008).

In re Vee Vinhnee, Debtor American Express Travel Related Services Company Inc. v. Vee Vinhnee, 336 B.R. 437 (9th Cir. BAP 2005).

Victor Stanley, Inc. v. CreativePipe, Inc., 250 F.R.D. 251 (D. Md. 2008).

Vigoda, M.M., and D.A. Lubarsky. 2006. Failure to recognize loss of incoming data in an anesthesia record-keeping system may have increased medical liability. Anesthesia and Analgesia 102(6):1798–1802.

Vigoda, M., J.C. Dennis, and M. Dougherty. 2008. E-record, e-liability: Addressing medico-legal issues in electronic records. Journal of AHIMA 79(10):48, 52; quiz 55–56.

Wachtel v. Health Net, Inc., 239 F.R.D. 81 (D.N.J. 2006).

Wagner, L. and C. Kenreigh. 2005. CPOE: Fallible, not foolproof: Clinical decision support for e-prescribing. Medscape Pharmacists 6(2). http://www.medscape.com/viewarticle/516367_2.

Walker, J.M., P. Carayon, N. Leveson, R.A. Paulus, J. Tooker, H. Chin, A. Bothe Jr., and W.F. Stewart. 2008. EHR safety: The way forward to safe and effective systems. Journal of the American Medical Informatics Association 15(3): 272–277.

Weiner, J.P., T. Kfuri, K. Chan, and J.B. Fowles. 2007. "E-iatrogenesis": The most critical unintended consequence of CPOE and other HIT. Journal of the American Medical Informatics Association 14(3):387–388; discussion 389.

Withers, K.J. 2006. Electronically stored information: The December 2006 amendments to the federal rules of civil procedure. Northwestern Journal of Technology and Intellectual Property 4(2):171–211.

Youle v. Ryan, 349 Ill. App. 3d 377, 380, 811 N.E.2d 1281, 1283 (2004).

Zubulake v. UBS Warburg LLC, 220 F.R.D. 212 (S.D.N.Y. 2003).

Content and Records Management and Electronic Discovery

Chapter Objectives

Adherence to sound content and record management principles is an important strategy for managing e-discovery requests. This chapter provides the foundational principles for content and record management in healthcare and related compliance issues.

⇒ Define content and records management
⇒ Describe the impact of content and records management on e-discovery
⇒ Identify major regulatory or legislative programs for healthcare that are impacted by content and record management practices
⇒ Understand the stages of the information lifecycle
⇒ Understand the importance of a record management program and the major record categories in healthcare
⇒ Describe the roles of a records manager, custodian, and steward
⇒ Recognize the importance of education, training, and documentation to support a content and records management program

5.1 Overview

The demands of e-discovery and compliance have highlighted the importance of having an overarching strategy to aggressively manage information and records throughout their lifecycle. The strategy, called content and record management, is a way to capture, structure, store, retrieve, archive, and destroy content across the organization. The ability to manage information holistically across the healthcare enterprise increases information's value, reduces risk, and improves operational efficiency (Dimick 2009). Ultimately, healthcare organizations must begin to see their information as a valuable asset to be managed and protected.

It is estimated that more than 90 percent of all information created and used in organizations today is electronic (The Sedona Conference 2007). To avoid fragmented, chaotic information processes, healthcare organizations must adopt an integrated set of strategies, standards, best practices, and technologies for managing patient-centric and organizational information (AHIMA 2008).

5.1.1 What Is Content and Records Management?

Healthcare organizations can take a cue from other industries in the resurgence of the importance of record management. This following section provides an overview of content and records management from a general business perspective.

Content and records management combines two concepts; electronic records management and enterprise content management. At the foundational level, the two main components are defined as follows:

- **Electronic records management (ERM)** is the electronic management of digital and analog records contained in information technology (IT) systems using computer equipment and software according to accepted principles and practices of records management. **Records management** is the field of management "responsible for the efficient and systematic control of the creation, receipt, maintenance, use, and disposition of analog and digital records, including processes for capturing and maintaining evidence of and information about business activities and transactions in the form of records" (Sprehe 2002).
- **Enterprise content management (ECM)** includes the technologies, tools, and methods used to capture, manage, store, preserve, and deliver content across an enterprise (AIIM International and ARMA International 2006). Content is generally considered the intellectual substance of a document. A record is defined as information created or received in the transaction of business and maintained as evidence in pursuance of legal obligations (AHIMA 2008).

In the days before typewriters and word processors, most records were handwritten and the volume was manageable. With the proliferation of photocopiers, record volume increased, largely due to ease of duplication, presenting records management issues not previously faced by businesses. Then, along came technology—mainframes, personal computers, networks, e-mail—and records management issues increased substantially. Many businesses, however, did not immediately focus on records management issues; after all, they were not in business to manage records. Proper records management comes at a cost, and most businesses fail to allocate sufficient funds in budgets to appropriately manage business records. Despite increased pressure from regulators and the courts, almost half of US organizations today have not adopted and implemented policies that minimize risk and increase productivity.

Most businesses, however, eventually came to realize that records are one of their most important assets—a critical ingredient to their livelihood and essential to every aspect of operation, and that without proper management of records, they would face many risks. Risks include inability to properly defend or prosecute legal claims. This realization has moved to the front burner in the last few years with the 2006 amendments of the Federal Rules of Civil Procedure (FRCP) that specifically address electronically stored information (ESI). There have been similar rule amendments by numerous governmental agencies (state and federal) arising from investigations, international privacy and cross-border data issues, and developing case law.

Businesses generate more records today than ever. Most of those records are in the form of ESI and are never printed to paper. Many of the records, such as databases and complex spreadsheets, are not even conducive to printing on paper. Further complicating efficient management of business records are outsourcing of IT functions, computing, Software-as-a-Service, and other technology advancements, which mean much of a business' data may be in their control, but not in their possession or custody.

Throughout an enterprise, businesses need to capture, manage, process, store, locate, produce, and ultimately dispose of numerous types of content existing in a large number of locations on disparate types of media in many formats for a variety of uses. This information may be in the possession of numerous third-party entities through contractual relationships. Implementation of ECM can be complicated and costly. Proper implementation must take place over time in a well-planned process, ensuring management buy-in and involvement of all stakeholders. Stakeholders should include IT, compliance, legal, records and information management (including HIM), representatives of impacted business units, and possibly human resources and other departments.

ECM technologies have developed as a result of the growing need and rapidly increasing complexity of IT infrastructures. The goal in implementing any ECM solution is to leverage existing investments in infrastructure, such as e-mail configurations, enterprise business process operations, and storage and server architecture, while also aligning the solution with ongoing business and legal requirements and needs. Ideally, in developing an ECM solution, paramount to the planning process will be an analysis of how business people and processes use the content and an understanding of business context. Early stages should include figuring out what information exists, how it is created, where it is located, how it is stored, its business use and purpose, and how it is ordinarily retrieved. Developing a system that addresses these details will go a long way in achieving widespread adoption of the solution, which is critical to its success.

5.2 Content and Record Practices Impacting e-Discovery

The domain of content and records management is complex. This section will focus on the critical issues that have the most impact on e-discovery rather than comprehensively addressing all aspects of content and record management. The importance of many of these issues has increased as case law has highlighted weaknesses in organizational programs that resulted in negative rulings or outcomes.

5.2.1 Data Governance

The building blocks for any effective e-discovery program is data governance, which supports compliance and legal efforts by establishing authority and decision making, and organizing data for retrieval and retention (Nunn 2009). From an e-discovery perspective, the ability to accurately and comprehensively locate information that may be relevant to litigation will reduce e-discovery costs and reduce the risks such as spoliation challenges.

The electronic discovery reference model shown in figure 5.1 illustrates the importance of information management on the front end. With litigation there is often a large volume of information to identify, preserve, and collect. The goal is to know where information is located and then filter out information so only relevant pieces are available for analysis by legal counsel. By reducing the unnecessary information analyzed by legal resources, litigation expenses are reduced. This typically is considered a significant area for return on investment for a content and records management program and officer.

Healthcare organizations increasingly struggle to manage huge volumes of e-mails, thousands of documents on shared drives, hundreds of source and feeder systems that pour data into the EHR systems, data warehouses, and

Figure 5.1. Electronic discovery reference model

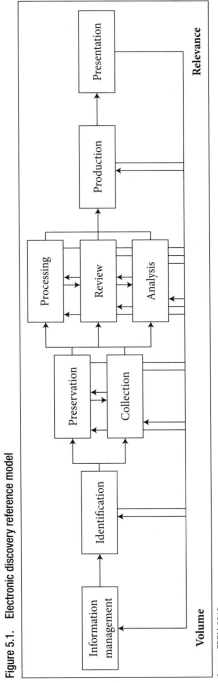

Source: EDRM 2010.

decision-support systems (Nunn 2009). A data governance program provides the necessary infrastructure to manage information assets and establish a long-term vision for aligning governance of data with the strategic direction of the organization.

Data governance can be defined as the authority and decision-making structure within an organization for information-related matters and outlines the following 10 universal components of a data governance program (Data Governance Institute n.d.):

Rules and Rules of Engagement
Mission and Vision
Goals, Governance Metrics and Success Measures and Funding Strategies
Data Rules and Definitions (data-related policies, standards, compliance requirements, business rules, and data definitions)
Decision Rights (who gets to make the decision and when using what process)
Accountabilities
Controls (preventive, detective, or corrective controls built into the process)
People and Organizational Bodies
Data Stakeholders (groups that create data, use data, and set rules and requirements for data)
A Data Governance Office (facilitates and supports data governance activities)
Data Stewards (a set of data stakeholders who come together to make data related decisions)
Processes of Governing Data
Proactive, Reactive, and Ongoing Data Governance (formal documented repeatable procedures)
 • Aligning policies, requirements, and controls
 • Establishing decision rights
 • Establishing accountability
 • Performing stewardship
 • Managing change
 • Defining data
 • Resolving issues
 • Specifying data quality requirements
 • Building governance into technology
 • Stakeholder care

- Communications
- Measuring and reporting value

5.2.2 Corporate Compliance and Electronic Regulatory Scrutiny

Compliance has become a priority for many healthcare corporations in relation to tax reports, privacy regulations, data security obligation, scrutiny of corporate conduct, and responsibilities of records management. The subsequent discussions provide a few pertinent areas where health service organizations can mitigate risk related to regulatory investigations, audits, and litigation and related issues of e-discovery by instituting best records management practices.

Sarbanes-Oxley (SOX) and other regulatory and legal mandates (Health Insurance Portability and Accountability Act [HIPAA], Gramm-Leach-Bliley Act, state laws) are strongly influencing governance in both for-profit and nonprofit healthcare organizations. The governance personnel and bodies of healthcare organizations are finally noticing and formalizing recordkeeping requirements and are shifting to compliance in fear of civil and criminal penalties.

Figure 5.2 depicts a basic environmental scan and framework for understanding the complexities and profound influences that various external regulatory and legal decisions have on healthcare records management and the ESI contained in the legal EHR. The organization's capacity to manage information is a direct function of its internal records management and compliance processes. Capacity to manage potential, expected, or unexpected events has many circuitous and direct relationships with the outcomes of various healthcare investigations and dealings with regulators. These events may be a consequence of accreditation processes, audits, and reform laws and thus are not limited to patient complaints.

SOX emphasizes many of the issues critical to good corporate governance. Whether it is a private, public, or nonprofit entity, every healthcare organization has business, ethical, and fiduciary duties requiring it to make sure that solid corporate governance policies are in place. Even many charitable foundations are expected to implement some of the corporate governance and accounting policies established by SOX. Similarly, many states either have proposed or are considering enacting similar legislation. SOX protects the rights of a whistleblower to report wrongdoing to federal investigators without the risk of retaliation (Sarbanes-Oxley Act of 2002).

Figure 5.2.   Process, outcome, and capacity for compliance

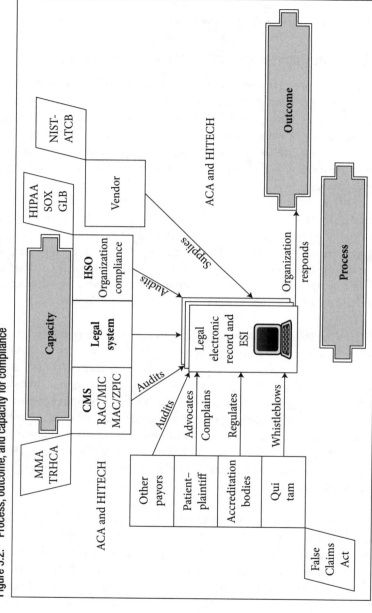

Source: © 2011 Katherine L. Ball.

5.2.2.1 Sarbanes-Oxley Act

The three rules of SOX affect the management of electronic records. The first rule deals with destruction, alteration, or falsification of records.

> Sec. 802(a):

> Whoever knowingly alters, destroys, mutilates, conceals, covers up, falsifies, or makes a false entry in any record, document, or tangible object with the intent to impede, obstruct, or influence the investigation or proper administration of any matter within the jurisdiction of *any department or agency of the United States* or any case filed under title 11, or in relation to or contemplation of any such matter or case, shall be fined under this title, imprisoned not more than 20 years, or both.

The second rule defines the retention period for records storage. Best practices indicate that corporations should securely store all business records using the same guidelines set for public accountants.

> Sec. 802(a)(1):

> Any accountant who conducts an audit of an issuer of securities to which section 10A(a) of the Securities Exchange Act of 1934 (15 USC 78j-1(a)) applies, shall maintain all audit or review workpapers for a period of 5 years from the end of the fiscal period in which the audit or review was concluded.

The third rule refers to the type of business records that need to be stored, meaning all business records and communications, including electronic communications.

> Sec. 802(a)(2):

> The Securities and Exchange Commission shall promulgate, within 180 days, such rules and regulations, as are reasonably necessary, relating to the retention of relevant records such as workpapers, documents that form the basis of an audit or review, memoranda, correspondence, communications, other documents, and records (including electronic records) which are created, sent, or received in connection with an audit or review and contain conclusions, opinions, analyses, or financial data relating to such an audit or review.

5.2.2.2 Gramm-Leach-Bliley Act

The Gramm-Leach-Bliley Act (GLBA), also known as the Financial Services Modernization Act of 1999, provides privacy protections against the disclosure of private client (patient) information to third parties. It also requires institutions to have administrative, physical, and technical safeguards to protect the confidentiality and integrity of personal client (patient) information. The GLBA codifies protections against obtaining personal information through false pretenses. Health service organizations must comply with the safeguards defined under GLBA.

The Federal Trade Commission (FTC) may bring an administrative enforcement action against any financial or insurance institution for noncompliance with the safeguards rules. Penalties for violating safeguards rules may include harm caused by the loss of privacy, for example, a breach of security resulting in an identity theft, an area of increasing concern to healthcare governance (GLBA 1999b).

5.2.2.3 CMS Program Integrity Initiatives: RAC MIC, MAC, and ZPIC

Healthcare institutions and their legal EHR are not only subject to compliance with laws and regulatory mandates for retention, destruction, and alteration; additionally, the legal EHR is subject to the routine audit. The audits may result from complaint-based investigations (for example, Centers for Medicare and Medicaid Services [CMS] evaluation of HIPAA security and Office of Civil Rights for HIPAA Privacy Rules complaints), or fraud allegations under the False Claims Act, CMS recovery audits, or qui tam whistleblower investigations. Academic medical centers face even further scrutiny of the legal EHR from investigations into clinical trial billing and research clinical databases derived from legal EHR data.

With the Tax Relief and Health Care Act of 2006 and Section 306 of the Medicare Prescription Drug, Improvement, and Modernization Act of 2003 (MMA), Congress mandated the **recovery audit contractor (RAC)** program to detect and correct improper payments in the Medicare program. This is summarized as below:

I. SEC. 302. EXTENSION AND EXPANSION OF RECOVERY AUDIT CONTRACTOR PROGRAM UNDER THE MEDICARE INTEGRITY PROGRAM.

(b) [42 U.S.C. 1395 ddd note] Access to Coordination of Benefits Contractor Database.—The Secretary of Health and Human Services shall provide for access by recovery audit contractors conducting audit and recovery activities under section 1893(h) of the Social Security Act, as added by subsection (a), to the database of the Coordination of Benefits Contractor of the Centers for Medicare & Medicaid Services with respect to the audit and recovery periods described in paragraph (4) of such section 1893(h) (Tax Relief and Health Care Act 2006).

Section 306 directed the Department of Health and Human Services (HHS) to conduct a 3-year demonstration program using RACs to determine whether their use was cost-effective in ensuring correct payments to providers and suppliers. The RACs detect and correct improper payments in the Medicare FFS program. The demonstration was operated in New York, Massachusetts, Florida, South Carolina, and California, ending on March 27, 2008 (HHS 2008). CMS has implemented the permanent RAC program. The RACs identify claims that clearly contain improper payments and those that likely contain improper payments. "In the case of clear improper payments, the RAC contacts the provider and requests a refund of any overpayment amounts and pays the provider any underpayment amounts. In the case of claims that contain likely improper payments, the RAC requests the medical record from the provider, reviews the claim and medical record, and then makes a determination as to whether the claim contains an overpayment, an underpayment, or a correct payment" (HHS 2008).

The alphabet soup of compliance includes other CMS Program Integrity Initiatives. In February 2006, the Deficit Reduction Act (DRA) of 2005 was signed into law and created the Medicaid Integrity Program (MIP) under Section 1936 of the Social Security Act. The MIP directs the CMS to enter into contracts to review Medicaid provider documentation and billing behaviors, audit claims, identify overpayments, and educate providers on Medicaid program integrity issues (HHS 2008). Audit Medicaid Integrity Contractors (Audit MICs) are entities with which CMS contracts to perform audits of Medicaid providers. The overall goal of the provider audits is to identify overpayments and to ultimately decrease the payment of inappropriate Medicaid claims.

The MMA directed CMS to use competitive measures to replace the current Medicare fiscal intermediaries and carriers with Medicare administrative contractors (MAC). After setting up the MAC regions, CMS created new entities, called **Zone Program Integrity Contractors (ZPICs)**. The ZPICs serve to audit providers and suppliers of Parts A, B, and C, the Medicare prescription drug benefit (Part D), durable medical equipment (DME), prosthetics, and orthotics supplier (DMEPOS), home health and hospice, and Medicaid services. The objective of ZPICs is to investigate potential fraud in the

Medicare program and ZPICs have the authority to audit the integrity of all Medicare claims for any given provider with comprehensive both pre- and post-pay audits.

With RAC, MIC, MAC, ZPIC, or other CMS program integrity initiatives, the present policy initiatives and statutes mandating adoption and meaningful use of health information technologies and electronic data exchange demands attention to data integrity and content management to manage the audit processes including appeals.

5.2.2.4 Health Insurance Portability and Accountability Act under HITECH

Modifications to the HIPAA Privacy, Security, and Enforcement Rules are mandated under the HITECH Act. The modifications, in final rule making comment periods, are expected to have wide impact on healthcare providers, business associates, contractors, and suppliers as well as disclosure auditing requirements. The American Health Lawyers Association, states that "Virtually every healthcare provider and third-party service provider that stores or accesses individuals' medical information will be affected by this new federal law" (Wieland 2009). A few areas of great impact to management of EHRs under HITECH defined HIPAA are highlighted here. The author recommends seeking legal advice on managing electronically stored information and data exchanges and/or contractual changes with business associates or other suppliers and vendors with access to their patients' PHI.

Business associates are directly subject to the HIPAA security provisions and to sanctions for violation of business associate requirements:

> Sections 164.308, 164.310, 164.312, and 164.316 of title 45, Code of Federal Regulations, shall apply to a business associate of a covered entity in the same manner that such sections apply to the covered entity. The additional requirements of this title that relate to security and that are made applicable with respect to covered entities shall also be applicable to such a business associate and shall be incorporate[d] into the business associate agreement between the business associate and the covered entity. (ARRA 2009)

> . . . A business associate of a covered entity that accesses, maintains, retains, modifies, records, stores, destroys, or otherwise holds, uses, or discloses unsecured protected health information shall, following the discovery of a breach of such information, notify the covered entity of such breach. (ARRA 2009)

Business associates are obligated to report to covered entities breaches of unsecured protected health information:

> The additional requirements of this subtitle that relate to privacy and that are made applicable with respect to covered entities shall also be applicable to such a business associate and shall be incorporated into the business associate agreement between the business associate and the covered entity. (ARRA 2009)

Business associates are directly subject to nearly all of the HIPAA privacy regulations. Pre-HITECH, these obligations for privacy and security matters where subject to contract.

45 CFR Parts 160 and 164RIN 0991–AB62, published in the *Federal Register*, provide significant information for health service organizations on operational impact:

> Section 164.528(a)(1)(i) of the Privacy Rule currently exempts disclosures to carry out treatment, payment, and healthcare operations from these accounting requirements. [The core health care activities of "Treatment," "Payment," and "Health Care Operations" are defined in the Privacy Rule at 45 CFR 164.501.] Covered entities leveraging EHRs are required to provide new details of accounting of disclosures of PHI for treatment, payment, and healthcare operations. Section 13405(c) of the Health Information Technology for Economic and Clinical Health (HITECH) Act, Public Law 111-5, 123 Stat. 265–66, provides that the exemption at § 164.528(a)(1)(i) of the Privacy Rule for disclosures to carry out treatment, payment, and health care operations no longer applies to disclosures "through an electronic health record." Under section 13405(c), an individual has a right to receive an accounting of such disclosures that covers disclosures made during the three years prior to the request. Section 13400 of the statute defines electronic health record as "an electronic record of health-related information on an individual that is created, gathered, managed, and consulted by authorized health care clinicians and staff." (45 CFR Parts 160 and 164RIN 0991–AB62)

The reversal of the treatment payment operations (TPO) accounting exception may require enormous redesign of the auditing and reporting functionalities of EHRs.

> (c) ACCOUNTING OF CERTAIN PROTECTED HEALTH INFORMATION DISCLOSURES REQUIRED IF COVERED ENTITY USES ELECTRONIC

HEALTH RECORD.—(1) IN GENERAL.—In applying section 164.528 of title 45, Code of Federal Regulations, in the case that a covered entity uses or maintains an electronic health record with respect to protected health information—(A) the exception under paragraph (a)(1)(i) of such section shall not apply to disclosures through an electronic health record made by such entity of such information; and (B) an individual shall have a right to receive an accounting of disclosures described in such paragraph of such information made by such covered entity during only the three years prior to the date on which the accounting is requested. (ARRA 2009)

The minimum necessary standard has become the limited data set default under HITECH:

(b) DISCLOSURES REQUIRED TO BE LIMITED TO THE LIMITED DATA SET OR THE MINIMUM NECESSARY.—(1) IN GENERAL.—

(A) IN GENERAL.—Subject to subparagraph (B), a covered entity shall be treated as being in compliance with H. R. 1—151 section 164.502(b) (1) of title 45, Code of Federal Regulations, with respect to the use, disclosure, or request of protected health information described in such section, only if the covered entity limits such protected health information, to the extent practicable, to the limited data set (as defined in section 164.514(e)(2) of such title) or, if needed by such entity, to the minimum necessary to accomplish the intended purpose of such use, disclosure, or request, respectively. (ARRA 2009)

Covered entities utilizing EHRs must provide patient information in electronic form and transmit it to third parties, on the individual's request. The HIT Policy Committee has committed access standards under Stage II meaningful use incentive eligibility.

ACCESS TO CERTAIN INFORMATION IN ELECTRONIC FORMAT.—

In applying section 164.524 of title 45, Code of Federal Regulations, in the case that a covered entity uses or maintains an electronic health record with respect to protected health information of an individual— (1) the individual shall have a right to obtain from such covered entity a copy of such information in an electronic format and, if the individual chooses, to direct the covered entity to transmit such copy directly to an entity or person designated by the individual, provided that any such choice is clear, conspicuous, and specific; and (2) notwithstanding paragraph (c) (4) of such section, any fee that the covered entity may impose for providing such individual with a copy of such information (or a summary or explanation of such information) if such copy (or summary or explanation) is in an electronic form shall not be greater than the entity's labor costs in responding to the request for the copy (or summary or explanation)." (ARRA 2009)

The Health Information Exchanges are recognized and specifically brought within Business Associate requirements:

> Each organization, with respect to a covered entity, that provides data transmission of protected health information to such entity (or its business associate) and that requires access on a routine basis to such protected health information, such as a Health Information Exchange Organization, Regional Health Information Organization, E-prescribing Gateway, or each vendor that contracts with a covered entity to allow that covered entity to offer a personal health record to patients as part of its electronic health record, is required to enter into a written contract (or other written arrangement) described in section 164.502(e)(2) of title 45, Code of Federal Regulations and a written contract (or other arrangement) described in section 164.308(b) of such title, with such entity and shall be treated as a business associate of the covered entity for purposes of the provisions of this subtitle and subparts C and E of part 164 of title 45, Code of Federal Regulations, as such provisions are in effect as of the date of enactment of this title. (ARRA 2009)

In summary, HIPAA compliance is vastly more stringent and complex under HITECH and e-health initiatives. Affectively implementing these new complexities into HIM policy and processes are part of the present and future challenges for compliance experts.

5.2.2.5 Compliance and Healthcare Reform, Affordable Care Act (ACA)

The PPACA of 2010, also known as the Affordable Care Act (ACA), renews the importance of healthcare corporate governance focus on compliance measures. The ACA brings an expectation of clinical integration, and requires that patient information be shared across the continuum of care. This cannot be accomplished without EHRs and electronic data exchange solutions. The expected impact of reform laws, as it relates to health data continuums, includes components such as value-based purchasing, bundled payments, and shared saving from accountable care organizations, and necessitates SOX, GLBA, HIPAA, HITECH, and other compliance standards.

The Office of the Inspector General (OIG) is integrally involved with the **Health Care Fraud Prevention and Enforcement Action Team (HEAT)** in the reform initiatives. The HEAT program is a joint effort by HHS and the US Department of Justice (DOJ) and expects "to leverage resources, expertise, and authorities to prevent fraud and abuse in Medicare and Medicaid" (Levinson 2010). The HHS has three focal points of compliance under reform: transparency, quality, and accountability of healthcare professionals.

- Compliance professionals should be asking questions as they prepare for healthcare reform.
- New payment and delivery models require a fresh examination of fraud and abuse risk.
- OIG is working closely with HHS and DOJ and other law enforcement partners on coordinated efforts to fight fraud and abuse.
- As part of HEAT, OIG is planning to conduct compliance training for providers in selected localities.
- Increasing links between payment and quality further increase boards' responsibilities for ensuring quality of care.
- OIG is committed to assisting boards in meeting their compliance and quality responsibilities.
- OIG is focused on holding responsible corporate officials accountable for healthcare fraud.
- OIG is pursuing those individuals who solicit kickbacks, in addition to the payers of kickbacks.
- Systems are maintained to ensure the independence and integrity of healthcare providers and medical researchers.
- OIG's enforcement and oversight work has addressed conflict-of-interest issues related to payments by pharmaceutical and device manufacturers, continuing medical education, and oversight of HHS-funded and HHS-regulated research.

A comprehensive and consistently applied document retention policy is necessary in healthcare to reduce the risk of being charged with noncompliance spoliation. The appearance of failure to comply with regulatory audit and litigation discovery obligation is not a satisfactory practice. Formalized document retention compliance policies are required from boardroom to bedside in clinical operations. Policies must be consistently enforced. Evaluation of comprehensive document retention policies includes review of management practices related to electronic health data and other electronic PHI.

The court considers the reasonableness of a document retention policy. The failure to keep key business records may be very expensive. If a company can reasonably anticipate litigation based on triggers and either negligently or intentionally destroys relevant documents, the court may assume the missing documents contained harmful information. For the court to determine a failure does not require intentional wrongdoing, consequently governance needs to decide to pay now or pay later when allocating and devoting resources to record and enterprise content management.

5.2.3 Managing Information Throughout Its Lifecycle

Traditional records management focused on a document at the point it became official information with the intent to memorialize it. Computer-generated information challenges that notion because content is generated that must be managed and may never be declared an official record to be retained for business purposes. Figure 5.3 provides a diagram of stages in an information lifecycle from creation through final disposition.

The notion of content versus a record is an important distinction when charged with governing information within an organization because the strategies and tools to manage them may be different. Neil Simons, in an article published in the *Information Management Journal* (2008), defines the differences between content and records:

> Content at its most basic is simply information or data. Some content is electronic, some paper. Some content is transient, some is permanent. Some content is business-critical, some is working content, and much is mere clutter. Some has to be stored and managed according to the strictest compliance and security requirements, other types can be treated casually. Content can exist in multiple forms and multiple stages of completion within its lifecycle. It can be revised and amended according to the needs of users who share it. Only in its completed form does content become a "matter of record" and require different protection throughout its lifecycle as a record rather than as content. More and more content is stored electronically these days, but it's critical to realize that the need to store some information on paper will likely never disappear. Records are a very special type of content. Records represent an organization's "official" version of history. They have different lifecycle requirements than other types of organizational content and may carry different legal and financial consequences if those requirements aren't managed appropriately.

EHR systems provide an excellent example of the need to manage both content and records. EHR systems collect a large amount of content from various sources and applications. A system can receive continuous data from monitoring devices; preliminary results from laboratory systems; clinical notes

Figure 5.3.   Information lifecycle

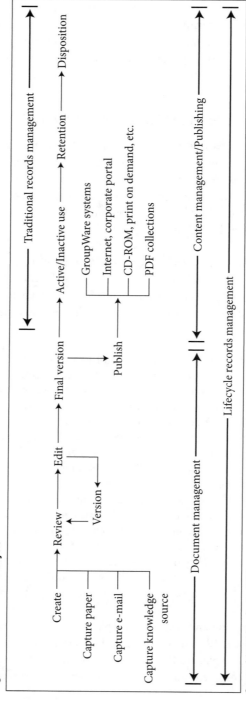

Source: Adapted from Sprehe 2002.

that have been started but not completed; census data on patient admissions, transfers and discharges; clinical decision-support triggers; and much more. All of this information resides in the EHR system (or a data warehouse or registry) and must be managed from creation through final disposition. Healthcare organizations have a regulatory and business need to maintain an official medical record. This means that organizations must declare which records officially represent the episode of care and must be retained for a required period of time. Management and retention requirements will be different for the official medical record versus the content within the EHR system, which means data governance and policies will need to encompass both content and records.

5.2.4 Record Retention

The cornerstone of a viable content and record management program is a working, sound, defensible records management policy that specifies business record categories and retention periods. When retention practices and policies are inconsistent or nonexistent, healthcare organizations risk losing time and money searching for records; evidence may be lost that supports the organization's position in business negotiations or litigation; and the risk of court sanctions, inferences in litigation, and charges of obstruction of justice or contempt of court increases (Weiss 2007). Retention periods are established to comply with both legal and regulatory requirements and business needs. As discussed in chapter 3, from an e-discovery perspective, there is an interrelationship between record retention, litigation hold, and preservation of information. Organizations must have a good handle on the information created and maintained and have an appropriate plan for managing its disposition. The good faith business operations related to record retention and destruction will help distinguish between normal business policies and inappropriate and opportune destruction of potentially relevant information, which could result in challenges and sanctions due to spoliation of evidence.

Healthcare organizations must establish a records retention policy in addition to a retention schedule. Appendix G provides a sample record retention policy created by an AHIMA e-HIM workgroup in 2008. The Sedona Conference, a legal think tank providing leadership on issues related to e-discovery, published guidelines in 2005 that offer a practical, balanced, and authoritative direction for key issues involving record retention policies and scope related to e-discovery. The following five principles from "The Sedona Guidelines: Best Practice Guidelines and Commentary for Managing

Information and Records in the Electronic Age," apply to any type of business, healthcare included:

1. An organization should have reasonable policies and procedures for managing its information and records.
   a. Information and records management is important in the electronic age.
   b. The hallmark of an organization's information and records management policies should be reasonableness.
   c. Defensible policies need not mandate the retention of all information and documents.
2. An organization's information and records management policies and procedures should be realistic, practical and tailored to the circumstances of the organization.
   a. No single standard or model can fully meet an organization's unique needs.
   b. Information and records management requires practical, flexible and scalable solutions that address the differences in an organization's business needs, operations, IT infrastructure and regulatory and legal responsibilities.
   c. An organization must assess its legal requirements for retention and destruction in developing an information and records management policy.
   d. An organization should assess the operational and strategic value of its information and records in developing an information and records management program.
   e. A business continuation or disaster recovery plan has different purposes from those of an information and records management program.
3. An organization need not retain all electronic information ever generated or received.
   a. Destruction is an acceptable stage in the information life cycle; an organization may destroy or delete electronic information when there is no continuing value or need to retain it.
   b. Systematic deletion of electronic information is not synonymous with evidence spoliation.
   c. Absent a legal requirement to the contrary, organizations may adopt programs that routinely delete certain recorded communications, such as electronic mail, instant messaging, text messaging and voice-mail.

d. Absent a legal requirement to the contrary, organizations may recycle or destroy hardware or media that contain data retained for business continuation or disaster recovery purposes.

e. Absent a legal requirement to the contrary, organizations may systematically delete or destroy residual, shadowed or deleted data.

f. Absent a legal requirement to the contrary, organizations are not required to preserve metadata; but may find it useful to do so in some instances.

4. An organization adopting an information and records management policy should also develop procedures that address the creation, identification, retention, retrieval and ultimate disposition or destruction of information and records.

a. Information and records management policies must be put into practice.

b. Information and records management policies and practices should be documented.

c. An organization should define roles and responsibilities for program direction and administration within its information and records management policies.

d. An organization should guide employees regarding how to identify and maintain information that has a business purpose or is required to be maintained by law or regulation.

e. An organization may choose to define separately the roles and responsibilities of content and technology custodians for electronic records management.

f. An organization should consider the impact of technology (including potential benefits) on the creation, retention and destruction of information and records.

g. An organization should recognize the importance of employee education concerning its information and records management program, policies and procedures.

h. An organization should consider conducting periodic compliance reviews of its information and records management policies and procedures, and responding to the findings of those reviews as appropriate.

i. Policies and procedures regarding electronic management and retention should be coordinated and/or integrated with the organization's policies regarding the use of property and information, including applicable privacy rights or obligations.

j. Policies and procedures should be revised as necessary in response to changes in workforce or organizational structure, business practices, legal or regulatory requirements and technology.

5. An organization's policies and procedures must mandate the suspension of ordinary destruction practices and procedures as necessary to comply with preservation obligations related to actual or reasonably anticipated litigation, government investigation or audit.

   a. An organization must recognize that suspending the normal disposition of electronic information and records may be necessary in certain circumstances.

   b. An organization's information and records management program should anticipate circumstances that will trigger the suspension of normal destruction procedures.

   c. An organization should identify persons with authority to suspend normal destruction procedures and impose a legal hold.

   d. An organization's information and records management procedures should recognize and may describe the process for suspending normal records and information destruction and identify the individuals responsible for implementing a legal hold.

   e. Legal holds and procedures should be appropriately tailored to the circumstances.

   f. Effectively communicating notice of a legal hold should be an essential component of an organization's information and records management program.

   g. Documenting the steps taken to implement a legal hold may be beneficial.

   h. If an organization takes reasonable steps to implement a legal hold, it should not be held responsible for the acts of an individual acting outside the scope of authority and/or in a manner inconsistent with the legal hold notice.

   i. Legal holds are exceptions to ordinary retention practices and when the exigency underlying the hold no longer exists (i.e., there is no continuing duty to preserve the information), organizations are free to lift the legal hold.

5.2.4.1 Inventory and Categorizing Records for Retention

The first step in establishing a record retention schedule is to categorize and inventory records and information. Work with departments and business process owners in the healthcare organization to identify a list of records and information, identifying the form and format and where they are retained. The inventory process will be the start of the retention matrix identifying the records maintained, where they are stored, the format in which they are stored, and the record steward or custodian.

The value of categorizing organizational content and records for the retention schedule is to assist in identifying, finding, and managing information over time. Records can be categorized by business/record type, format (paper, electronic, microfilm, and so on), source system, privacy/security classification, or any combination or classification that fits the needs of the organization. For example, records may be classified by both type and format—a healthcare organization may decide to migrate all paper-based logs to digital image files for long-term archiving. The retention schedule can be queried and sorted for categories of records to identify the specific subset.

5.2.4.2 Determining Retention Requirements

Once an inventory is complete, the next step is to understand the legal, regulatory, and business retention requirements for the information. Healthcare organizations will have retention requirements related to both general business records (such as employment records, contracts, financial documents, and such) and health records. To establish retention of health records, healthcare organizations need to determine the applicable federal and state laws and regulations, analyze accreditation and payer requirements, and then analyze the organization's business needs for the information. Table 5.1 identifies the federal regulatory requirements for medical records in various care settings. In addition to the CFR, other federal requirements such as SOX, the Employee Retirement Income Security Act (ERISA), the Fair Labor Standards Act, and GLBA all impose record retention requirements (Daley and Cotton 2005).

The retention requirements established by regulation and law become the baseline for a minimum retention period. Healthcare organizations must also determine their business need for the information. For example, an academic research hospital's mission may provide the overarching business driver for medical records to be retained permanently—their business need for decades and even a century of records for research data may be an overarching requirement.

In addition to medical records, healthcare organizations must identify their business records when establishing their retention schedule. Many records within an organization do not have a required retention period by regulation or law. Table 5.2 provides a list of other business records that should be considered when developing a record retention schedule.

Table 5.1   Federal regulations for retention of health records

Setting	Citation	Requirement
Clinics, rehabilitation agencies, and public health agencies as providers of outpatient physical therapy and speech language pathology services	42 CFR 485.721(d) 42 CFR 486.161(d)	As determined by the respective state statute, or the statute of limitations in the state. In the absence of a state statute, five years after the date of discharge; or in the case of a minor, three years after the patient becomes of age under state law or five years after the date of discharge, whichever is longer.
Comprehensive outpatient rehabilitation facilities (CORFs)	42 CFR 485.60(c)	Five years after patient discharge
Critical access hospitals (CAHs)	42 CFR 485.638(c)	Six years from date of last entry, and longer if required by state statute, or if the records may be needed in any pending proceeding
Home health agency	42 CFR 484.48(a)	Five years after the month the cost report with which the records are associated is filed with the intermediary, unless state law stipulates a longer period of time
Hospice care	42 CFR 418.74	Retention period not specified
Hospital—medical records	42 CFR 482.24(b)(1)	Five years
Hospital—radiology services	42 CFR 482.26(d)	Report copies and printouts, films, scans, and other image records must be retained for five years
Long-term care facilities	42 CFR 483.75(l)(2)	As required by state law; or five years from the date of discharge when there is no requirement in state law; or for a minor, three years after a resident reaches legal age under state law
Psychiatric hospitals	42 CFR 482.61	Five years

Source: Adapted from Rhodes 2002

5.2.5 Record Manager, Custodians, and Stewards

The complexity and volume of information and the increasingly different ways it is stored requires a healthcare organization to define roles and disseminate responsibilities for content and record management. The level of custodianship and stewardship depends on a person or entity's relationship to the data and data system and proximity to the case in litigation. As in traditional paper-based records, HIM should remain the official custodian of the medical

Table 5.2   Other healthcare business records

Record	Suggested Period of Retention	Remarks
Administrative Offices		
Accident/incident reports	6 years	
Annual reports	Permanent	
Appraisal reports	Permanent	
Articles of Incorporation	Permanent	
Birth records	Permanent	
Bylaws	Permanent	
Daily census	5 years	
Communicable disease reports	3 years	
Construction records	Permanent	
Correspondence	5 years	Keep only that of continuing interest. Review annually.
Death records	Permanent	
Endowments, trusts, bequests	Permanent	
Insurance policies	6 years after expiration	
Licenses, permits, contracts	Permanent	
Minutes of board meetings (directors, executive committees, medical staff)	Permanent	
Permits (alcohol and narcotics, etc.)	Life of permit plus 6 years	
Physician personnel records	Permanent	
Policies and procedure manuals	Life of manual plus 6 years	
Property records (deeds, titles)	Permanent	
Property records (leases)	Term of lease plus 6 years	
Reports (departmental)	3 years	Many daily and non-annual reports may be destroyed after year-end statistics are compiled.
Statistics on admissions, services, discharges	Permanent	
Admissions and Discharges		
Listings	6 years	
Register	Permanent	

(continued)

Table 5.2   Other healthcare business records (continued)

Record	Suggested Period of Retention	Remarks
Business Office		
Alien-statement of income paid	As long as contents may be material in the administration of an Internal Revenue law	
Bank deposits	2 years	
Bank statements	6 years	
Budgets	5 years	
Cash receipts	6 years	
Cashier's tapes	6 years	
Charge (slips) to patients	5 years	
Check vouchers	10 years	
Checks (cancelled)	7 years	
Check registers	6 years	

Correspondence
    Credit and collections
    General
    Insurance
	
	7 years
	6 years
	4 years	

Equipment depreciation records	Permanent	
Income (daily summary)	5 years	

Invoices
 	
    Fixed assets
    Accounts receivable
    Accounts payable
	
	Life of asset plus 6 years
	6 years
	6 years	

Journals (general)	Permanent	
Ledgers (general)	Permanent	
Ledger cards (patients)	7 years	

Payroll
    Bonds
    Insurance
    Individual earnings
 	
    Journals
    Rate schedules
    Social security reports
    Withholding tax exemption
      (W-4 forms)
    Witholding tax statements
      (W-2 forms)
	
	10 years
	8 years
	Term of employment plus
	   6 years
	25 years
	6 years
	4 years
	4 years
	
	4 years after taxes paid	

Posting audits	7 years	
Unemployment tax records	4 years	

Record	Suggested Period of Retention	Remarks
Vouchers		
Capital expenditures	Permanent/life of item plus 6 years	
Cash	10 years	
Welfare agency records	7 years	
Clinic		
Appointment books	3 years	
Encounter statistics	1 year	
Patient's name index	Permanent	
Dietary		
Food costs	5 years	
Meal counts	5 years	
Menus	2 years	
Engineering		
Blueprints	Permanent	
Calibration records	6 years	
Equipment records	Life of equipment plus 6 years	
Equipment maintenance records	5 years (6 years for electronic medical records systems)	
Equipment operating records	Life of equipment plus 6 years	
Inspections of buildings/grounds	1 year	
Maintenance log	6 years	
Purchase orders	10 years	
Work orders	2 years	
Laboratory, Therapy, and X-ray		
Appointment books	3 years	
Blood/blood component disposition	5 years	
Refrigeration and blood inspection records	5 years	
Index to patient records	10 years/permanent for unusual cases	
Radioisotopes (receipt, transfer, use, storage delivery, disposal, and reports of over-exposure)	Permanent	
Registers (chronological of tests)	5 years or until statistics are completed	

(continued)

Table 5.2   Other healthcare business records (continued)

Record	Suggested Period of Retention	Remarks
Requests for tests	2 weeks	
Research papers published	Permanent	
Medical Records		
Birth registration copy	Permanent	
Death registration copy	Permanent	
Delivery room log	Permanent	
Disease index	Permanent	
Nursing		
Operation index	Permanent	
Patient records index	Permanent	
Physician index	10 years	
Surgery log	Permanent	
Tumor registry files	Permanent	
Applications (nonemployees)	2 years	
Attendance and time records	2 years	
Minutes of meetings	Permanent	
Personnel records	6 years after termination of employment	
Training (attendance, course outlines, and examinations)	Permanent	
Personnel		
Absence reports	5 years	
Applications (nonemployees)	4 years	
Employee health records	5 years after termination of employment	
Employee history	5 years in full, after 5 years reduce to payroll card rate	
Garnishment records	7 years	
Job classifications	Permanent	
Overtime reports	5 years	
Payroll and time records	5 years	
Pension records	Permanent	
Vacation lists	2 years	
Volunteer service (certification of hospital workers)	Permanent	

Record	Suggested Period of Retention	Remarks
Pharmacy		
Controlled substances (inventory and orders)	2 years	
Controlled substances (dispensed and administered)	2 years	
Methadone	3 years	
Other prescriptions	2 years	
Public Relations		
Clippings (historical)	Permanent	
Contributor records	Permanent	
Marketing materials	6 years	
Photographs (institutional)	Permanent	
Publications (house organs)	Permanent	
Purchasing and Receiving		
Packing slips	3 months	
Purchase orders	2 years	
Purchase requisitions	3 years	
Receiving report	5 years	
Returned goods credit	2 years	

Source: Tomes 2002.

record. The AHIMA e-Discovery Task Force (2008) defined several roles for data management:

- Primary or direct custodians—Those persons who work with the data directly or have direct involvement or knowledge of the events of the case. For example, a staff nurse who has made an entry into the medical record and is knowledgeable about the events of a case in litigation. Primary custodians may be deposed or required to testify because of their direct involvement or knowledge of the case.
- Data owners or stewards—Individuals with responsibility to oversee business process areas may be designated as the data owners or stewards. They have knowledge of the procedures used to create, manage, and preserve specific types of records. Examples of business process areas include finance, radiology, lab, risk management, compliance, and nursing.
- Business associates and third parties—This includes contractors and others who serve a variety of functions associated with a party's information

but who are not parties to the litigation. Examples include Internet service providers, application service providers such as a claims clearinghouse, and other providers who provide services ranging from offsite data storage to complete outsourcing of the IT department.

- Official record and system custodians—The HIM department historically has been the designated official custodian of the overall medical record. The HIM department has played an important role in the processing of subpoenas for the organization, whether or not the organization was named in litigation.
- Enterprise record manager/officer—This person controls and directs the organization's records and information management program and personnel. This role manages, controls, and directs active records systems and centers, records organization and evaluation, and inactive records systems. This manager also controls correspondence, reports and directives, and record retention.

5.2.6 The Importance of Education and Training

One of the most effective compliance tools for a record management program is a well-designed training and education program for staff and applicable third parties. Training should address organizational policies, the importance of record management practices, benefits and risks of not following policies, handling a litigation hold, and retention requirements. Periodic audits or assessments of compliance with record management policies will help identify training and retraining needs.

5.3 Maintaining Documentation of Content and the Records Management Program

Having a comprehensive, legally-sufficient records management program does little good unless the entity can document it. Much like any other governmental requirement, if the entity cannot demonstrate that it has maintained its records properly, the government may assume otherwise and may issue sanctions. Consequently, the entity must maintain documentation supporting the development and implementation of the program. This documentation must include the following:

- Documentation supporting the development of the overall records management program, specifically the governance, officers, policies, and records retention program
- Written procedures, including the procedures in effect each year (rather than just the current procedures)
- Written approval for the records management program

- Signed records retention schedules
- Documentation for the destruction of records under a records retention program
- Audit reports indicating compliance with the program
- A record of legal research performed (for example, statutes and regulations imposing retention periods, statutes of limitations, and authorized media)

Keep records that document the records management program for a reasonable time—long enough to demonstrate a pattern of activity and regular compliance—unless the law specifies a retention period. Ten years is a good starting point, based on the likelihood of litigation or audit and the volume of records involved.

If healthcare organizations consider all records and media when they develop records retention programs, create retention and destruction schedules, manage the program, and document their management, they will likely have legally sufficient and effective records management programs (Tomes 2002).

References

45 CFR 160 and 164RIN 0991–AB62: Request for information. 2010.

AHIMA. 2008. Practice brief: Enterprise content and record management for healthcare. Journal of AHIMA 79(10):91–98.

AHIMA e-Discovery Task Force. 2008. Litigation response planning and policies for e-discovery. Journal of AHIMA 79(2):69–75.

AIIM International and ARMA International. 2006. Revised Framework for Integration of EDMS & ERMS Systems (ANSI/AIIM/ARMA TR48-2006). Silver Spring, MD: AIIM International and ARMA International.

American Recovery and Reinvestment Act of 2009. Public Law 111-5.

Centers for Medicare and Medicaid Services. 2006. Medicaid Integrity Program—General Information. http://www.cms.gov/MedicaidIntegrityProgram.

Centers for Medicare and Medicaid Services. 2010. RAC demonstration. http://www.cms.gov/RAC/02_ExpansionStrategy.asp.

Daley, J., and C.V. Cotton. 2005. Defenders of the faith: In corporate records compliance. Inside Litigation Spring:42–43.

Data Governance Institute. n.d. The DGI Data Governance Framework. http://www.datagovernance.com/dgi_framework.pdf.

Department of Health and Human Services. 2008. Medicare Claim Review Programs: MR, NCCI Edits, MUEs, CERT, and RAC. http://www.decisionhealth.com/dhps/images/MCRP_Booklet.pdf.

Dimick, C. 2009. New records opening to HIM professionals: Wider content and record management initiatives offer new roles. Journal of AHIMA 80(6):48–49, 56.

Electronic Discovery Reference Model. 2010. http://edrm.net.

Gramm-Leach-Bliley Financial Modernization Act. 1999a. Public Law 106-102.

Gramm-Leach-Bliley Financial Modernization Act. 1999b. Public Law 106-102. Title V—Privacy. Subtitle A—Disclosure of Nonpublic Personal Information.

Levinson, D.R. Highlights of the keynote address before the Health Care Compliance Association Annual Compliance Institute. April 19, 2010.

Nunn, S. 2009. Driving compliance through data governance. Journal of AHIMA 80(3):50–51.

Rhodes, H. 2002. Practice brief: Retention of health information (updated). AHIMA. http://library.ahima.org/xpedio/idcplg?IdcService=GET_HIGHLIGHT_INFO&QueryText=%28Tomes%29%3cand%3e%28xPublishSite%3csubstring%3e%60BoK%60%29&SortField=xPubDate&SortOrder=Desc&dDocName=bok1_012545&HighlightType=HtmlHighlight&dWebExtension=hcsp.

Sarbanes-Oxley Act of 2002. Public Law 107-204.

The Sedona Conference. 2007. The Sedona Principles, Second Edition: Best Practices Recommendations & Principles for Addressing Electronic Document Production. http://www.thesedonaconference.org/content/miscFiles/TSC_PRINCP_2nd_ed_607.pdf.

Simons, N. 2008. CMS, RMS? Spelling out the right information management solution. Information Management Journal 42(6):58–62.

Sprehe, T.J. 2002. Enterprise Records Management: Strategies and Solutions. Prepared for Hummingbird Ltd. http://viewer.zoho.com/api/urlview.do?url=http://mimage.hummingbird.com/alt_content/binary/pdf/collateral/wp/rmstrategies.pdf.

Tax Relief and Health Care Act of 2006. Public Law 109-432.

Tomes, J.P. 2002. AHIMA Practice brief: Retaining healthcare business records. Journal of AHIMA 73(3):56A–G.

Weiss, C.N. 2007 (Feb.). Corporate governance: The importance of a compliant record retention program. Corporate Counsel Newsletter. http://www.abanet.org/buslaw/newsletter/0057/materials/pp4.pdf.

Wieland, J.B. 2009. The HITECH Act: Congress includes sweeping expansion of HIPAA and data breach notification requirements in stimulus bill. Health Lawyers Weekly 7(7).

Update: Guidelines for Defining the Legal Health Record for Disclosure Purposes

Historically, the definition of the legal health record was fairly straightforward: the contents of the paper chart (together with radiology films or the results of other imaging studies) formed the healthcare provider's legal business record. Patients had limited interest in or access to the information contained in their records.

However, with the advent of various electronic media, the Internet, and the consumer's enhanced role in compiling their health information, the definition of the legal health record has become more complex. The need to ensure information is accessible for its ultimate purposes, regardless of the technologies employed or users involved, remains. Therefore, the definition of the legal health record must be reassessed in light of new technologies, users, and uses.

Each organization must define the content of the legal health record to best fit its system capabilities and legal environment. Considerations for the content of the legal health record should include ease of access to different components of patient care information, guidance from the medical staff and the organization's legal counsel, community standards of care, federal regulations, state law and regulations, standards of accrediting agencies, and the requirements of third-party payers.

A patient's health record plays many roles in addition to those involved in caring for a patient where documentation of the patient's health history, health status (sickness and wellness), observations, measurements, and prognosis are recorded. This documentation allows the record to serve as the legal record substantiating healthcare services provided to the patient. It also serves as a method of communication among healthcare providers caring for a patient and provides supporting documentation for reimbursement of services provided to a patient.

The legal health record is a subset of the entire patient database, which serves as the legal business record for the organization. The roles of the legal health record are to:

- Support the decisions made in a patient's care
- Support the revenue sought from third-party payers
- Document the services provided as legal testimony regarding the patient's illness or injury, response to treatment, and caregiver decisions

Recognizing the challenges associated with the impact of technology on the legal health record, AHIMA formed a work group of members from provider settings, law practices, information technology vendors, and information systems consultants to develop guidelines to assist organizations in defining their health records for legal applications.

This practice brief discusses the issues involved in ensuring that a health record serves the legal needs of the provider or facility whether in a paper-based, hybrid (a combination of paper and electronic), or fully electronic state. The rules that permit the patient's health record to constitute the legal business record must be taken into account, and the organization must be able to fulfill its obligations with the legal health record regardless of the physical state of the health record.

It is imperative that healthcare organizations define their legal health records. There is no one-size-fits-all definition of the legal health record. Laws and regulations governing the content vary by practice setting and state. However, there are common principles to be followed in creating a definition.

Definition of the Legal Health Record

The legal health record is generated at or for a healthcare organization as its business record and is the record that will be disclosed upon request. It does not affect the discoverability of other information held by the organization. The custodian of the legal health record is the health information manager in collaboration with information technology personnel. HIM professionals oversee the operational functions related to collecting, protecting, and archiving the legal health record, while information technology staff manage the technical infrastructure of the electronic health record.

The legal health record is the documentation of healthcare services provided to an individual during any aspect of healthcare delivery in any type of healthcare organization. It is consumer- or patient-centric. The legal health record contains individually identifiable data, stored on any medium, and collected and directly used in documenting healthcare or health status.

Legal health records must meet accepted standards as defined by applicable Centers for Medicare and Medicaid Services Conditions of Participation, federal regulations, state laws, and standards of accrediting agencies such as the Joint Commission on Accreditation of Healthcare Organizations, as well as the policies of the healthcare provider.[1]

Legal health records are records of care in any health-related setting used by healthcare professionals while providing patient care service or for administrative, business, or payment purposes. Some types of documentation that comprise the legal health record may physically exist in separate and multiple paper-based or electronic or computer-based databases.

The Legal Paper-based Health Record

The 2001 practice brief "Definition of the Health Record for Legal Purposes" defines the legal paper-based health record as "the legal business record generated at or for a healthcare organization. This record would be released upon request."[2]

The Legal Hybrid Health Record

When the legal health record consists of information created as paper documents and information created in electronic media, it is considered to be in a hybrid environment. Organizational policies should document the information that is considered the legal health record and identify the source (paper or electronic) of that information. A matrix can be used for this purpose.[3] Policies should also indicate when the record is considered complete. The hybrid record transition plan and policy should define the "legal source of truth," reflecting whether the legal record is paper, hybrid, or fully electronic. This policy provides for a specific schedule that provides both retrospective and prospective dates wherein the user can identify the source legal record.

The paper portion of the legal health record is collected and archived in paper or plastic folders. Electronic portions of the record are collected and archived in source systems or in electronic folders in the EHR system. There must be a clear indication of the locations where portions of a patient record are located.

Electronic versus Legal Health Records

An electronic health record (EHR) system is generally thought of as the portal through which clinicians access a patient's health record, order treatments or therapy, and document care delivered to patients. Many healthcare providers have eliminated the paper record and use EHR systems as their organizations' legal records (although a paper record may be "published" for release of information purposes). Many other organizations are planning a similar transition. EHR systems allow providers to gather multiple types of data about a patient (e.g., clinical, financial, administrative, and research).

Healthcare informaticists agree that an EHR system is not one or even two or more products. Rather, an EHR system consists of a plethora of integrated component information systems and technologies. The electronic files that make up the EHR system's component information systems and technologies consist of different data types, and the data in the files consist of different data formats. (See "Data Formats of the EHR," below, for a description of format types.)

Data Formats of the EHR

Some data formats are structured and some are unstructured. For example, the data elements in a patient's automated laboratory order, result, or demographic and financial information system are coded and alphanumeric. Their fields are predefined and limited. In other words, the type of data is discrete, and the format of these data is structured. Consequently, when a healthcare professional searches a database for one or more coded, discrete data elements based on the search parameters, the engine can easily find, retrieve, and manipulate the element.

However, the format of the data contained in a patient's transcribed radiology or pathology result, history and physical, or clinical note system using word-processing technology is unstructured. Free-text data, as opposed to discrete, structured data, are generated by word processors, and their fields are not predefined and limited. Consequently, when a healthcare professional searches unstructured text, the search engine cannot easily find, retrieve, and manipulate one or more data elements embedded in the text.

Likewise, the format of the data contained in a patient's dictated radiology or pathology result, history and physical, or clinical note system using speech recognition technology (real-time speech in, text out) is unstructured. However, the speech recognition technology's engine takes the unstructured, free-text speech data and codifies the data, often with the help of templates.

Hence, the format of the outputted text data becomes structured, with pre-defined and limited fields. Search engines then easily can find, retrieve, and manipulate one or more data elements embedded in the text.

Diagnostic image data stored in a diagnostic image management system, such as a picture archiving and communications system, represent a different type of data: bit-mapped data. However, the format of bit-mapped data is also unstructured. Saving each bit of the original image creates the image file. In other words, the image is a raster image, the smallest unit of which is a picture element or pixel. Together, hundreds of pixels simulate the image. Examples of digital modalities that generate digital diagnostic image data are digitized x-rays or computed radiography and computed tomography, magnetic resonance, and nuclear medicine scans. Most diagnostic image data remain based on analog, photographic films, such as analog x-rays. To digitize these data, these analog films must be digitally scanned, using film digitizers.

Document image data are yet another type of data; document image data are bit-mapped, and the format is unstructured. These data are stored in an electronic document management system. These data are based on analog paper documents or on analog photographic film documents. Most often, analog paper-based documents contain handwritten notes, marks, or signatures. However, such documents can include preprinted documents (such as forms), photocopies of original documents, or computer-generated documents available only in hard copy. Analog photographic film-based documents are processed using an analog camera and film, similar to analog x-rays. Therefore, both the analog paper-based and the photographic film-based documents must be digitally scanned, using scanning devices that are similar to fax machines.

The EHR system's component information systems and technologies consist of additional data types, the formats of which also are unstructured.

Real audio data consist of sound bytes, such as digital heart sounds.

Motion or streaming video or frame data, such as cardiac catheterizations (cine), consist of digitized film attributes, such as fast-forwarding.

The files that consist of vector graphic (or signal-tracing) data are created by saving lines plotted between a series of points, accounting for the familiar ECGs, EEGs, and fetal traces.

As such, portions of the legal EHR may be located in various electronic systems. These input systems may include laboratory information systems, pharmacy information systems, picture archiving and communications systems (PACS), cardiology information systems, results reporting systems, computerized provider order entry systems, nurse care planning systems, word-processing systems, and fetal trace monitoring systems.

Depending on their size and structure, healthcare providers may store structured clinical and administrative data in a database or clinical data repository. In addition, healthcare providers may store unstructured patient clinical data in separate databases or repositories (e.g., PACS archive, fetal trace archive) and provide pointers from the clinical portal to these various repositories. In this manner, architecturally, these databases are logically but not physically linked.

Defining the Subset of Data that Constitutes the Legal EHR

The challenge for HIM professionals in defining a legal health record in an EHR system is to determine which data elements, electronic-structured documents, images, audio files, and video files become part of the legal electronic health record. The first step is to determine what legal entities enforce regulations, guidelines, standards, or laws to the healthcare organization defining its legal health record. Although these various entities may have defined a legal record in paper terms (e.g., requiring a medication sheet rather than an electronic medication administration record), these entities' definitions must become the basis for the legal health record definition at the organization.

The second step is to determine whether the records are created in the ordinary course of business of the healthcare provider or entity.

The third step is creating a matrix (or other document) that defines each element in the legal health record. Such a matrix could include a column indicating whether that particular element would be released on first request or subpoena.

HIPAA and the Legal Health Record

The HIPAA privacy rule requires that organizations identify their "designated record set," which is defined as "a group of records maintained by or for a covered entity that is: (i) the medical records and billing records about individuals maintained by or for a covered health care provider; (ii) the enrollment, payment, claims adjudication or case or medical management record systems maintained by or for a health plan; or (iii) used, in whole or part, by or for the covered entity to make decisions about individuals."[4] Healthcare providers are required to define the data or documents that meet this definition. The legal health record will be a subset of this designated record set that meets the requirements for a business record used for legal purposes. Organizations must list those specific data elements and documents within the designated record set that comprise its legal health record. Source media (paper versus electronic) should be defined. If electronic, the source system should also be defined. The owners of these differential source data should be reflected in the designated record set policy and should also be documented. This matrix or document can include the column suggested above as to whether it is released on first request or subpoena.

Information from the legal health record is disclosed in response to authorized requests for copies of a patient health record. Electronic records should be transmitted in a method that minimizes the risk of a breach of security and protects the patient's privacy as defined in the HIPAA privacy and security standards and by the privacy and security policies of the healthcare provider. HIPAA does not define a preferred method of electronic transmission. However, some states require that copies of medical records provided to patients be in "human-perceptible form," which might limit the ability of the provider to transmit the electronic portions of the legal health record directly to third parties (such as a personal health record vendor, for example).

Facility policies should also address copying paper records, printing copies of electronic documents, and transmitting protected health information to authorized requestors via courier, mail, fax, e-mail, and other processes. In addition, facility policies must address, in accordance with HIPAA privacy standards, the method for documenting errors, corrections, or addendums in both paper and electronic documents and ensure that original and amended versions of a document are available and produced for official (or certified) copies of health records.

Considerations for Defining the Legal Health Record for Legal Purposes

As stated previously, there is no one-size-fits-all definition of the legal record because laws and regulations governing the content vary by practice setting and by state. However, there are common principles to be followed in creating a definition. This section addresses health record issues to assist healthcare organizations in defining the content of their legal records. Final definition of the legal health record rests with individual healthcare organizations and their legal counsels.

Alerts, Reminders, and Pop-Ups

Alerts, reminders, pop-ups, and similar tools are used as aides in the clinical decision-making process. The tools themselves are not considered part of the legal health record; however, associated documentation is considered a component. For example, a provider is alerted to perform a diabetic foot exam on a diabetic patient. The initial alert that prompts the provider is not part of the legal health record, but the subsequent action taken by the provider, including the condition acted upon and the associated note detailing the exam, is considered part of the record.

Similarly, any annotations, notes, and results created by the provider as a result of an alert, reminder, or pop-up are also considered part of the legal health record. Once the documentation, results, and graphs have been entered in an electronic manner, those alerts acted upon and results become a permanent part of the record and are maintained in a manner similar to any other information contained within the legal health record.

Continuing Care Records

Continuing care records are records received from another healthcare provider. Historically, these records were generally not considered part of the legal health record unless they were used in the provision of patient care. In the electronic health record it may be difficult to determine if information was viewed or used in delivering healthcare. It may be necessary to define such information as part of the legal health record. Policies should reflect the proper disposition of health records from external sources (e.g., other healthcare providers) if they are not integrated into the electronic and legal health record.

Data and Documents to Be Considered Part of the Record

- Advance directives
- Allergy records
- Alerts and reminders (see "Alerts, Reminders, and Pop-Ups," above)
- Analog and digital patient photographs for identification purposes only
- Anesthesia records
- Care plans
- Consent forms for care, treatment, and research
- Consultation reports

- Diagnostic images
- Discharge instructions
- Discharge summaries
- E-mail messages containing patient-provider or provider-provider communications regarding care or treatment of specific patients[5]
- Emergency department records
- Fetal monitoring strips from which interpretations are derived
- Functional status assessments
- Graphic records
- History and physical examination records
- Immunization records
- Instant messages containing patient-provider or provider-provider communications regarding care or treatment of specific patients[6]
- Intake and output records
- Medication administration records
- Medication orders
- Medication profiles
- Minimum data sets (MDS, OASIS, IRF PAI)
- Nursing assessments
- Operative and procedure reports
- Orders for treatment including diagnostic tests for laboratory and radiology
- Pathology reports
- Patient-submitted documentation
- Patient education or teaching documents
- Patient identifiers (medical record number)
- Photographs (digital and analog)
- Post-it notes and annotations containing patient-provider or provider-provider communications regarding care or treatment of specific patients
- Practice guidelines or protocols and clinical pathways that imbed patient data
- Problem lists
- Progress notes and documentation (multidisciplinary, excluding psychotherapy notes)
- Psychology and psychiatric assessments and summaries (excluding psychotherapy notes)
- Records received from another healthcare provider if they were relied on to provide healthcare to the patient (see "Continuing Care Records," above)
- Research records of tests and treatments[7]
- Respiratory therapy, physical therapy, speech therapy, and occupational therapy records

- Results of tests and studies from laboratory and radiology
- Standing orders
- Telephone messages containing patient-provider or provider-provider communications regarding care or treatment of specific patients
- Telephone orders
- Trauma tapes
- Verbal orders
- Wave forms such as ECGs and EMGs from which interpretations are derived
- Any other information required by the Medicare Conditions of Participation, state provider licensure statutes or rules, or any third-party payer as a condition of reimbursement

Data from Source Systems

Source-system data are the data from which interpretations, summaries, and notes are derived. They may be designated part of the legal health record, whether or not they are integrated into a single system or maintained as part of the source system.

Records from source systems may be considered part of the legal health record, based on the content of the source system's record. Historically, reports or findings upon which clinical decision making is based are parts of the legal health record. For example, the written result of a test such as an x-ray, an ECG, or other similar procedures are always part of the record, whether these reports are integrated into a single system or part of a source system.

Working notes used by a provider in completing a final report are not considered part of the legal health record unless they are made available to others providing care to a patient. However, documents that are kept in a separate system of record (such as notes from a particular area of specialty that are kept separately but are final products) are always considered part of the record.

The determining factor in whether something is to be considered part of the legal health record is not where the information resides or the format of the information, but rather how the information is used and whether it is reasonable to expect the information to be routinely released when a request for a complete medical record is received.

The legal health record excludes health records that are not official business records of a healthcare organization.

Downtime Procedure Documents

In the event that the EHR system is unavailable, a process must be implemented to continue with documentation of patient care and responses to that care. For most facilities, this process will be paper-based.

Once the EHR system is restored, the information from the downtime documents must be made part of the EHR, which may incorporate data entry, scanning, or re-creating documents in various subsystems.

Emerging Issues

As EHR technology evolves, a number of challenges to the definition of the legal health record are emerging. Organizations must resolve these challenges with their legal counsel and information technology departments. Many of these items have not historically been included in the legal health record and will entail new storage and retrieval costs if they are defined as part of the record. Some examples of documents and data that should be evaluated for inclusion or exclusion include:

- Audio files of dictation
- Audio files of patient telephone calls
- Nursing shift-to-shift reports (handwritten or audio)
- Telephone consultation audio files
- Videos of office visits
- Videos of procedures
- Videos of telemedicine consultations

Personal Health Records

Organizational policy should address how personal health information will or will not be incorporated into the patient's health record. Copies of personal health records that are created, owned, and managed by the patient and are provided to a healthcare organization should be considered part of the legal health record, if so defined by the organization and if the information is used to provide patient care services, review patient data, or document observations, actions, or instructions. This includes patient-owned, -managed, and -populated tracking records, such as medication tracking records and glucose and insulin tracking records. (See "Personal Health Record Formats," below, for an outline of formats.)

Personal Health Record Formats

PHRs electronically may include subsets of personal health information from provider organization databases into the electronic records of authorized patients, their families, other providers, and sometimes health payers and employers. A range of people and groups maintain the records, including the patients, their families, and other providers.

PHRs come in a variety of forms and formats, with no single sign or sponsorship model yet to emerge. Currently, the most common PHR variations and models include:

Shared data record: The shared data record model consumes the largest number of PHRs and is the most effective. Here, both provider (or employer or health plan) and patient maintain the record. In addition, the provider (or employer or health plan) supports the record. As such, the patient receives and adds information over time. The focus of this model is to keep track of health events, medications, or specific physiological indicators, such as exercise and nutrition.

EHR extensions: The EHR extension model extends the EHR into cyberspace so that an authorized patient can access the provider's record and check on the record's content. Often this model also allows an authorized patient to extract data from the healthcare provider's record. The record is still maintained by the provider but is available to the patient in an online format.

Provider-sponsored information management: The provider-sponsored information management model represents provider-sponsored information management by creating communication vehicles between patient and provider. Such vehicles can include reminders for immunizations or flu shots, appointment scheduling, prescription refill capabilities, and monitoring tools for disease management in which regular collection of data from the patient is required.

Documents Not Included in the Legal Health Record

Administrative Data and Documents

Administrative data and documents should be provided the same level of confidentiality as the legal health record. However, administrative data should not be considered part of the legal health record and would not be produced in response to a subpoena for the medical record. Healthcare organizations might more appropriately consider some administrative data and documents as working documents.

Administrative data are patient-identifiable data used for administrative, regulatory, healthcare operation, and payment (financial) purposes. Examples of administrative data include:

- Abbreviation and do-not-use abbreviation lists
- Audit trails related to the EHR
- Authorization forms for release of information
- Birth and death certificate worksheets
- Correspondence concerning requests for records
- Databases containing patient information
- Event history and audit trails
- Financial and insurance forms
- Incident or patient safety reports
- Indices (disease, operation, death)
- Institutional review board lists
- Logs
- Notice of privacy practices acknowledgments (unless the organization chooses to classify them as part of the health record)
- Patient-identifiable claims
- Patient-identifiable data reviewed for quality assurance or utilization management
- Protocols and clinical pathways, practice guidelines, and other knowledge sources that do not embed patient data
- Psychotherapy notes
- Registries
- Staff roles and access rights
- Work lists and works-in-progress

Derived Data and Documents

Derived or administrative data are derived from the primary healthcare record and contain selected data elements to aid in the provision, support, evaluation, or advancement of patient care. Derived data and documents should be provided the same level of confidentiality as the legal health record. However, derived data should not be considered part of the record and would not be produced in response to a subpoena for the medical record.

Derived data consist of information aggregated or summarized from patient records so that there are no means to identify patients. Examples of derived data are:

- Accreditation reports
- Anonymous patient data for research purposes
- Best-practice guidelines created from aggregate patient data
- OASIS reports
- ORYX, Quality Indicator, Quality Measure, or other reports
- Public health reports that do not contain patient-identifiable data
- Statistical reports
- Transmission reports for MDS, OASIS, and IRF PAI

Notes

1. For example, as defined by the Centers for Medicare and Medicaid Services for hospitals found in Condition of Participation 482.24, the medical record includes "at least written documents, computerized electronic information, radiology film and scans, laboratory reports and pathology slides, videos, audio recordings, and other forms of information regarding the condition of a patient."
2. Amatayakul, Margret, et al. "Definition of the Health Record for Legal Purposes." *Journal of AHIMA* 72, no. 9 (2001): 88A–H.
3. AHIMA e-HIMTM Work Group on Health Information Management in a Hybrid Environment. "The Complete Medical Record in a Hybrid EHR Environment," parts I–III. October 2003. Available online in the FORE Library: HIM Body of Knowledge at www.ahima.org.
4. "Standards for Privacy of Individually Identifiable Health Information; Final Rule." 45 CFR Parts 160 and 164. *Federal Register* 65, no. 250 (2000). Available online at http://aspe.hhs.gov/admnsimp.
5. In the paper world, conversations between a provider and patient or between providers (e.g., hallway consultations) are not always recorded and made part of the medical record. With many EHR systems, such conversations can occur electronically via e-mail and instant messaging. In other systems, records or portions of records can be forwarded to another provider's work queue for review and comment. HIM professionals need to work with counsel and leaders of the medical staff to determine if such e-mails and notations are to be included as part of the legal health record.
6. Ibid.

7. Organizational policies should differentiate whether research records are part of the legal health record or if the research center maintains its own records. This should be verified with the institutional review board, since this may influence whether they are part of the legal health record.

References

Centers for Medicare and Medicaid Services. "Conditions of Participation for Hospitals." Available online at www.cms.hhs.gov/manuals/107_som/som107ap_a_hospitals.pdf.

HIMSS. "HIMSS Electronic Health Record Definitional Model, Version 1.1." Available online at www.himss.org/content/files/ehrattributes070703.pdf.

Health Level Seven. "The Legal Aspects of the Electronic Health Record." Unpublished work product of the HL7 work group on legal aspects of the EHR. May 2005.

"Standards for Privacy of Individually Identifiable Health Information; Final Rule." 45 CFR Part 164.501. *Federal Register* 65, no. 250 (2003). Available online at www.hhs.gov/ocr/hipaa.

Prepared by

Kathleen Addison, CCHRA(C)
James H. Braden, MBA
Jacqueline E. Cupp, RHIA
Darla Emmert, RHIT
Lois A. Hall, RHIT
Terri Hall, MHA, RHIT, CPC
Barbara Hess, MBA, CHP, PAHM
Deborah Kohn, RHIA, CHE, CPHIMS
Michele T. Kruse, MBA, RHIA
Kelly McLendon, RHIA
Julie McQueary, RHIA
Debra Musa, RHIT
Keith L. Olenik, MA, RHIA, CHP
Carol Ann Quinsey, RHIA, CHPS
Rebecca Reynolds, MHA, RHIA
Cheryl Servais, MPH, RHIA
Amy Watters, RHIA
Lou Ann Wiedemann, MS, RHIA

Melinda Wilkins, MEd, RHIA
Michele Wills, RHIA
Nancy E. Vogt, RHIT, CHP

Acknowledgments

Mary D. Brandt, MBA, RHIA, CHE, CHPS
Jill Callahan Dennis, JD, RHIA
Michelle Dougherty, RHIA, CHP
Kathy Giannangelo, RHIA, CCS
Karen G. Grant, RHIA, CHP
Matthew J. Greene, RHIA, CCS
Kathleen A. Frawley, JD, MS, RHIA
Barry S. Herrin, CHE, Esq.
Godwin O. Odia, MBA, RHIA
Donald Simborg
Andrea B. Thomas, MBA, RHIA, CPHS
Lydia M. Washington, MS, RHIA, CPHIMS
Carolann M. Weishar, RHIA

This work group was supported by a grant to FORE from Precyse Solutions, Inc.

Article citation:

AHIMA e-HIM Work Group on the Legal Health Record. "Update: Guidelines for Defining the Legal Health Record for Disclosure Purposes." *Journal of AHIMA* 76, no. 8 (September 2005): 64A–G.

The Legal Process and Electronic Health Records

The custodian of an electronic health record (EHR) has the same concerns as the custodian of a paper health record when the record becomes involved in the legal process. Most often this occurs in some form of lawsuit in which a party seeks to discover and introduce evidence from the record. The custodian must determine whether to release the record, what portions of the record should be released, and whether the record is admissible as evidence.

However, the custodian of an EHR has several additional concerns when an EHR is involved in litigation. These include whether any difference exists between releasing patient data maintained electronically from that maintained on paper, what parts of the EHR should be released, and whether printouts of electronic data qualify as admissible evidence. This practice brief will review the EHR custodian's responsibilities in the legal process.

Definition of the Legal Health Record

AHIMA defines the legal health record as "generated at or for a healthcare organization as its business record and is the record that would be released upon request. It does not affect the discoverability of other information held by the organization. The custodian of the legal health record is the health information manager in collaboration with information technology personnel. HIM professionals oversee the operational functions related to collecting, protecting, and archiving the legal health record, while information technology staff manage the technical infrastructure of the electronic health record."[1]

Who Is the Custodian of the EHR?

The health information custodian is the person who has been designated responsible for the care, custody, and control of the health record for such persons or institutions that prepare and maintain records of healthcare. The official custodian or designee should be authorized to certify records and supervise all inspections and copying or duplication of records. The HIM professional or designee is often considered the custodian of the health record and may be called to testify to the admissibility of the record. He or she may be asked to verify the timeliness and normal business practices used to develop and maintain the health record.[2]

Authentication for Legal Processes

Authentication is an attestation that something, such as a medical record, is genuine. The purpose of authentication is to show authorship and assign responsibility for an act, event, condition, opinion, or diagnosis.[3] Every entry in the health record should be authenticated and traceable to the author of the entry. The Rules of Evidence indicate that the author of the entry is the only one who has knowledge of the entry. The Federal Regulations/Interpretive Guidelines for Hospitals (482.24(c)(1)(i)) require that there be a method for determining that the author did, in fact, authenticate the entry.[4] This process should be defined in HIM written policies and procedures and substantiates the authentication of an entry in a legal process.

If allowed by state, federal, and reimbursement regulations, electronic signatures are acceptable as authentication. Electronic signature technology should provide verification of the identity of the author.[5]

Certifying Health Records When Requested for the Legal Process

The certification process verifies that the copy provided is an exact duplicate of the original. Certification may be provided using a written certification letter stating that the copy provided is an exact copy of the original. State laws may differ in requirements for certification. Generally, a statement and signature of the record custodian are sufficient; however, some states may require a witness or notary signature as well.

There are some simple steps you can take when responding to requests for EHRs for legal process:

1. **Determine if the request is valid**—verify identity and authority of the requestor. Request legal picture identification, such as a driver's license or passport.
2. **Validate that the format of the request meets state legal requirements** for a valid subpoena or court order. Check state law for specific requirements.
3. **Determine the legal power of the document:**
    a. Patient or legal guardian request via phone—information may not be disclosed without written authorization.
    b. Patient or legal guardian request via e-mail—these requests are difficult to authenticate. Organizations should outline a policy to deal with these requests in accordance with state laws.

    c. Patient or legal guardian request via formal HIPAA-appropriate written authorization—information may be disclosed according to patient or legal guardian wishes.

    d. Patient or legal guardian request via fax—same as formal authorization, if state law allows.

    e. Legal request from a lawyer with authorization attached—information may be disclosed.

    f. Subpoena—information may be disclosed depending on state law and hospital or clinic policy.

    g. Court order—information may be disclosed.

    h. In accordance with Health Care Proxy—information may be disclosed to the proxy if the patient is deemed incompetent.

    i. Workers' compensation—information may be disclosed depending on state policy.

4. **Disclose the information to the designated recipient.** The information should be disclosed to the intended recipient according to the patient or legal guardian, court, or lawyer designated on the subpoena or court order or as outlined in number 1, above.

Determining if Healthcare Information May Be Disclosed

Having reviewed and established that the request is HIPAA compliant, determine if the information may be disclosed based on the context of the request received. Be sure to review and verify that federal rules and regulations have been met and that a conflict does not exist with state-specific statute(s). Confirm that state law does not require a subpoena or court order prior to disclosing the information. Verify compliance with pertinent state statutes prior to disclosing the requested information.

If state and federal laws have been satisfied, conduct the appropriate analysis to determine if a signed consent by the patient is required or if the request requires that protected health information be de-identified prior to disclosure. If so, obtain the appropriate authorization from the patient or refer to the disclosure of minimum necessary information to comply with law enforcement type requests.

At this time, paper is generally an acceptable means to submit copies; however, organizations may want to refer to specific state law for the availability of alternative methods, if applicable. Examples of electronic disclosures include the creation of media such as electronic faxing, CD, DVD, PC-to-PC transmissions, and digital images.

Since federal and state laws will be challenged with the need to address the electronic disclosure of protected health information, routine assessment of acceptable alternative options to comply with such disclosures is recommended. If conflict exists, guidance should be sought from legal counsel for further clarification. The HIPAA security rule should be referenced if the information is released electronically. Appropriate safeguards must be in place if the transaction is covered by the security rule.

Unless otherwise directed, a response in a paper format as the certified copy is considered acceptable. State law should be evaluated to ensure that information is not required in a format other than paper. If submission of the information is recommended or required in another format, confirm whether it is possible to meet these terms based on hospital policy and procedure.

Information that May Be Disclosed for the Discovery Process

Healthcare organizations involved in a lawsuit are subject to the discovery phase of the legal process. Parties involved in a lawsuit can obtain or discover any nonprivileged matters including EHRs that are relevant to the lawsuit. Information or documentation is discoverable even if inadmissible at trial if it is "reasonably calculated" to lead to discovery of admissible evidence.

Processes used in discovery include subpoenas, depositions, interrogatories, requests for admission, and production of documents. The electronic era has changed the way discovery is conducted. Paper is no longer the only source of documentation to be disclosed. Computer files, erased files, and e-mail can also be subpoenaed. The most common discovery method to discover EHRs is to serve the healthcare organization with a subpoena duces tecum.

Every state has established time frames to comply with the discovery request. It is vital that organizations adhere to these dates. The custodian should consult with the organization's attorney for advice on disclosure of healthcare information. The attorney may authorize disclosure or seek protective relief from a court.

Admissibility of Health Records

Historically, health records were considered hearsay and inadmissible in legal proceedings. However, the Federal Rules of Evidence and the Uniform Rules of Evidence codified the business records exception to the hearsay rule, thereby allowing health records to be used at trial.[6]

The key to admissibility of business records at trial is that they are prepared and maintained in accordance with the Federal Rules of Evidence (803(6)). The person testifying or certifying the records for trial must be conversant with the policies and the processes used to ensure accuracy of the records.[7]

Printing Documents

The HIM department should promulgate a policy that provides for a consensus-driven schedule and migration path for the transition of each record set (e.g., diagnostic reports from laboratory and radiology and transcribed reports) from paper through hybrid to an EHR system. This transition schedule must include time frames to stop or disable printing of these record sets predicated on agreed-upon criteria being met (e.g., EHR access, EHR uptime, and availability).

The printed document policy must include the formal processes for review and (if warranted) approval-control over new requests for access and printing from the EHR. Additionally, the policy should designate where copies of an EHR may be printed in an organization coupled with methods to control or dispose of paper copies immediately following authorized use.

The printing of electronic health record sets by authorized users should include a watermark or automated label with the following information:

- Confidential health information
- Instructions for use, such as "do not file in patient record," "do not remove from facility," or "discard copy in designated disposal area"
- For all unauthenticated reports, indication that the report has not been reviewed for accuracy or authenticated

If the EHR system allows, standard sets for release types should be predefined in the system. If this is not possible, a printing matrix must be developed that coincides with the organization's EHR migration and transition plan.

Information such as data released from the nursing units for patient transfers must be generated from the published features of the electronic software and should not include screen prints.

As custodian of the medical record and EHR, HIM professionals should have control over subsequent printing of paper versions of the medical record or EHR pursuant to authorized release of protected health information. HIM professionals should ensure that there are defined policies, audit trails, and controls over the printing of the medical record.

Advocacy for Uniform Legislation

It is clear from the variation in state laws that HIM professionals have an opportunity to be advocates for consistent, comprehensive federal regulations.

Becoming an advocate is as easy as phoning, writing, or e-mailing your elected representatives about the need for consistent, comprehensive federal regulations regarding the release of health information. AHIMA's Advocacy Assistant helps identify elected officials, information on how to contact them, and provides sample letters (log on at www.ahima.org/dc). Check with your component state association to determine which activities it is involved in and become a volunteer. Support AHIMA's Hill Day activities. Read local newspapers and carry the message to your community and work setting.

Notes

1. AHIMA. "Update: Guidelines for Defining the Health Record for Disclosure Purposes." *Journal of AHIMA* 76, no. 8 (2005): insert.
2. AHIMA. "Maintaining a Legally Sound Health Record." *Journal of AHIMA* 73, no. 2 (2002): insert.
3. Ibid.
4. Ibid.
5. Ibid.
6. Skupsky, Donald S., and John C. Montana. *Law Records and Information Management: The Court Cases.* Denver, CO: Information Requirements Clearinghouse, 1994, 40.
7. Ibid.

Legal Process Glossary of Terms

Abstract   a condensation of a record.

Administrative agency   created by statute or the Constitution. They may hear disputes arising from administrative law. A common example would be a case dealing with workmen's compensation.

Administrative law   rules and regulations developed by various administrative bodies empowered by Congress. This falls under the umbrella of public law.

Administrative regulation   a rule issued by an administrative agency to regulate the area in which Congress created the agency to execute governmental policy. Courts rank regulations below statutes when they conflict, but otherwise regulations have the force of law.

Arbitration   a dispute that is submitted to a third party or panel of experts outside the judicial trial system. All parties involved in the dispute must agree to have their differences heard and settled by an arbitrator or arbitration panel and agree that the settlement will be binding.

Authentication   an attestation that something, such as a medical record, is genuine. Authentication refers to both verifying a computer user's identity and professional responsibility for the entries in the medical record.

The purpose of authentication is to show authorship and assign responsibility for an act, event, condition, opinion, or diagnosis. Entries in the healthcare record should be authenticated by the author.[1]

Verification of the identity of a user or other entity is a prerequisite to allowing access to information systems.[2]

Business records   an exception to the hearsay rule that permits the court to receive into evidence records prepared and kept in the regular course of business. Medical records fall under this exception provided that the method of record keeping conforms to certain established guidelines:

- The record was made in the regular course of business.
- The entries in the record are made promptly.
- The entries were made by the individual within the enterprise with firsthand knowledge of the acts, events, conditions, and opinions.
- Process controls and checks exist to ensure the reliability and accuracy of the record.
- Policies and procedures exist to protect the record from alteration and tampering.
- Policies and procedures exist to prevent loss of stored data.

Case law   law originating from court decisions where no applicable statutes exist; also known as common law.

Confidentiality   protection given to health records and other patient information to guard personal, private information about patients and their care.

Consent to use and disclose information   written permissions given by a patient to a healthcare provider to use and disclose healthcare information for the purpose of treatment, payment, or healthcare operations.

Court order   the power of a court jurisdiction, whether state or federal, to order the production of medical records without the patient's informed consent, as opposed to a subpoena, which may be signed by a lawyer.

(continued)

Custodian of records (aka record custodian)   a person who has charge or custody of an institution's records whether stored in paper or electronic format.

Data   basic facts about people, processes, measurements, and conditions represented in dates, numerical statistics, images, and symbols. An unprocessed collection or representation of raw facts, concepts, or instructions in a manner suitable for communication, interpretation, or processing by humans or automatic means.

Database   a collection of data organized for rapid search and retrieval.

Data element   a combination of one or more data entities that forms a unit or a piece of information, such as a patient identifier, a diagnosis, or treatment.

Data entity   a discrete form of data, such as a number or a word.

Data integrity   state of data being complete, accurate, consistent, and up to date.

Defendant   individual or company that is the object of a lawsuit.

Deposition   a discovery device under which an attorney questions a witness under oath to learn about matters in the case and to preserve testimony for use at a subsequent testimony.

Digital signature   a block of data that is appended to a message in such a way that the recipient of the message can verify the contents and verify the originator of the message.

Digital signatures apply an algorithm to an electronic document, yielding a unique string of characters known as a message digest. The digest uses private key encryption, and the signature is placed on the electronic document.

Discovery   stage in the litigation process during which both parties use strategies to discover information about a case, the primary focus of which is to determine the strength of the opposing party's case. Discovery may involve requests for admissions, interrogatories, subpoenas, and other methods of discovering potential evidence.

Discovery process   compulsory disclosure of pertinent facts or documents to the opposing party in a civil action, usually before a trial begins.

Duplicate one of two or more documents that are the same. Many state and federal laws provide that certain duplicates are duplicate originals and admissible in evidence to the same extent as an original. A common example of a duplicate is an imaged record.

Electronic health record (EHR) medical information compiled in a data-gathering format for retention and transferal of protected information via a secured, encrypted communication line. The information can be readily stored onto an acceptable storage medium, such as a compact disk.

Electronic medical record (EMR) an electronic system to automate paper-based medical records.

Electronic signature technology that uses a unique personal identification number, electronic identification, or biometric scans to place a signature on an electronic document.

Emancipated minor an individual not of the age of majority but who is given adult status due to life events in accordance with the applicable statutes (e.g., high school graduate, not cohabitating with a parent or legal guardian, member of the US military, is or has been legally married or divorced, is or has been pregnant).

Enumeration to count off or designate one by one; to list.

Encryption method of scrambling data so that they cannot be read unless uncoded. A method of securing data by transforming data into a coded format that cannot be accessed without the appropriate decoding mechanism.

Evidence information that a fact-finder may use to decide an issue. Information that makes a fact or issue before a court or other hearing more or less probable.

Health information in HIPAA privacy provisions, any information (oral or recorded) that is created or received by a healthcare provider, health plan, public health authority, employer, life insurer, school or university, or healthcare clearinghouse and relates to the physical or mental health of an individual, the provision of healthcare to an individual, or payment for the provision of healthcare.

Hearsay general statements made outside of court not admissible as evidence in a court proceeding.

(continued)

Individually identifiable health information   under HIPAA, a subset of health information (see above), including demographic information collected from an individual. The information:

- Is created or received by a healthcare provider, health plan, public health authority, employer, life insurer, school or university, or healthcare clearinghouse
- Relates to past, present, or future physical or mental health or condition of an individual, the provision of healthcare to an individual, or the past, present, or future payment for the provision of healthcare to an individual
- Identifies the individual
- Is a reasonable basis to believe the information can be used to identify the individual

Integrity   correctness. Verification that information remains in its original form and has not been altered, manipulated, or modified in an unauthorized manner.

Interrogatories   a discovery device in which one party asks written questions of another, such as the name of the individual responsible for the proper maintenance of your medical records.

Law enforcement   the detection and punishment of violations of the law.

Legal process   all of the summons or writs that are issued by a court during a legal action, or by an attorney in the name of the court but without court review.

Legal representatives   a parent, guardian, or other person who has authority to act on behalf of a minor patient in making decisions related to healthcare unless the minor patient can legally consent to healthcare services without the consent of an adult. For adult patients, legal representative means the legal guardian of an incompetent patient, the healthcare agent designated in an incapacitated patient's healthcare power of attorney, or the personal representative or spouse of a deceased patient. If no spouse survives a deceased patient, legal representative also means an adult member of the deceased patient's immediate family.

Liability   legal responsibility, often with financial repercussions, for any adverse occurrence. Enforceable by civil remedy or criminal punishment.

Media   the materials upon which information is stored, such as microfilm or optical disk. Any physical places that store or have the capacity to store information.[3]

Medical record a record that identifies the patient and documents the diagnosis and care the patient received.

Microfilm a photographic storage medium on which documents can be greatly reduced in size.

Minor a person who has not yet reached the age of majority so as to be considered an adult by law.

Motion to quash the procedural device used to challenge the validity and seeking to nullify a subpoena.

Original document an authentic writing as opposed to a copy.

Peer review scrutiny of a healthcare professional by other such professionals to determine whether he or she is qualified to practice his or her profession in a facility and to identify and remedy patterns of unacceptable behavior.

Plaintiff individual who brings a lawsuit.

Protected health information according to HIPAA, any information, whether oral or recorded in any form or medium, that (1) is created or received by a healthcare provider, health plan, public health authority, employer, life insurer, school or university, or healthcare clearinghouse; and (2) relates to past, present, or future physical or mental health or condition of an individual, the provision of healthcare to an individual, or the past, present, or future payment for the provision of healthcare to an individual.

Psychotherapy notes under the HIPAA privacy rule, notes recorded (in any medium) by a healthcare provider who is a mental health professional documenting or analyzing the content of conversation during a private counseling session or a group, joint, or family counseling session and that are separated from the rest of the individuals' medical record. Notes exclude medication prescription and monitoring, counseling session start or stop times, the modalities and frequencies of treatment furnished, results of clinical tests, and any summary of diagnosis, functional status, the treatment plan, symptoms, prognosis, and progress to date. The privacy rule gives such notes extra protection, as may state law.

Record the preservation of information or data on some storage medium so that it may be read at some future time.

Record custodian (aka custodian of records) a person who has charge or custody of the institution's records whether stored in paper or electronic format.

(continued)

Record retention program   a facility's plan that specifies how long the facility keeps its records in accordance with the applicable regulatory statutes.

Regular course of business   doing business in accordance with your normal practice and custom, as opposed to doing it differently because you may be sued or are being sued.

Regulation   a rule issued by a government agency other than the legislature. Unless a regulation conflicts with a constitution or a statute, it has the force of law.

Request for admissions   a pretrial discovery device in which one party requests the other to admit, deny, or object to certain facts, such as that a medical record was kept in the regular course of business.

Res ipsa loquitor   an exception to the general principle that a patient must prove negligence in order to establish liability. The thing speaks for itself. The doctrine is applicable where a court determines, as a matter of law, that the occurrence is such as in the ordinary course of things would not have happened if the party exercising control or management had exercised proper care.

Res judicata   a doctrine that courts follow to avoid duplicate litigation and conflicting decisions, which means an issue that has been settled by a judgment.

Respondeat superior   the doctrine holding an employer or principal liable for the employee's wrongful acts. Let the superior make the answer.

Retention schedule   a document specifying which records an entity will maintain and for how long. Generally a retention schedule is drawn up in conjunction with state and federal retention requirements.

Risk management   oversight of the medical, legal, and administrative operations within a healthcare organization to minimize its exposure to liability.

Rules of evidence   court or administrative agency rules that specify what evidence a fact-finder may consider and under what circumstances.

Signature   with respect to an electronic health record, the verification by a user generated by a private key.

Spoliation (of evidence)   the intentional destruction, alteration, or concealment of potential evidence. Spoliation may have such adverse consequences as a court order instructing the jury that they may presume the document was adverse; discovery sanctions, such as fines; or even a separate lawsuit.

Subpoena ad testificandum   a written order commanding a person to appear and to give testimony at a trial or other judicial or investigative proceeding.

Subpoena duces tecum   a written order commanding a person to appear, give testimony, and bring all documents, papers, books, and records described in the subpoena. The devices are used to obtain documents during pretrial discovery and to obtain testimony during trial.

Subpoena validity   those authorized to issue a subpoena vary from state to state. A subpoena usually contains the following:

- Name of the court (or other official body in which the proceeding is being held)
- Names of the plaintiff and the defendant
- Docket number of the case
- Date, time, and place of the requested appearance
- Specific documents sought (if a subpoena duces tecum)
- Name and telephone number of the attorney who caused the subpoena to be issued
- Signature or stamp and seal of the official empowered to issue the subpoena

Notes

1. AHIMA. "Maintaining a Legally Sound Health Record." *Journal of AHIMA* 73, no. 2 (2002): insert.
2. Amatayakul, Margret, Steven Lazarus, Tom Walsh, and Carolyn Hartley. *Handbook for HIPAA Security Implementation*. Chicago, IL: AMA Press, 2004.
3. Ibid.

Prepared by

Wanda Bartschat, MSA, RHIA
Alicia Blevins, RHIA
Lauren Burnette, RHIA
Kerry Costa, RHIA
Michele D'Ambrosio, MBA, RHIA
Gladys Glowacki, CCHRA(C)
Karen B. Griffin
Marina Katrompas
Frances LaPrad, RHIT, CPHQ

Susan Manning
Meg McElroy, RHIA
Randall L. Patton, RHIA
Carol Ann Quinsey, RHIA, CHPS
Barbara J. Riesser, RN, CCS, CCS-P, CPC
Joseph J. Russo, JD, Esq.
Janet Sayer, JD, MS, RHIA
Kathleen Schleis, RHIA, CHP
Rita Scichilone, MHSA, RHIA, CCS, CCS-P, CHC
Barbara Ann Thompson, RHIT
Jonathan P. Tomes, JD

Acknowledgments

AHIMA e-HIM Work Group on Defining the Legal Health Record

Kathleen A. Frawley, JD, MS, RHIA

Andrea B. Thomas, MBA, RHIA, CHPS

This work group was supported by a grant to the Foundation of Research and Education of AHIMA (FORE) from Precyse Solutions, Inc.

Article citation:

AHIMA e-HIM Work Group on Defining the Legal Health Record. "The Legal Process and Electronic Health Records." *Journal of AHIMA* 76, no. 9 (October 2005): 96A–D. [expanded online version]

Update: Maintaining a Legally Sound Health Record—Paper and Electronic

The health record is the legal business record for a healthcare organization. As such, it must be maintained in a manner that follows applicable regulations, accreditation standards, professional practice standards, and legal standards. The standards may vary based on practice setting, state statutes, and applicable case law. An attorney should review policies related to legal documentation issues to ensure adherence to the most current standards and case law.

HIM professionals should fully understand the principles of maintaining a legally sound health record and the potential ramifications when the record's legal integrity is questioned. This practice brief will review the legal documentation guidelines for entries in and maintenance of the health record—both paper and electronic. Many of the guidelines that originally applied to paper-based health records translate to documentation in electronic health records (EHRs). In addition, new guidelines and functionalities have emerged specific to maintaining legally sound EHRs. It is of the utmost importance to maintain EHRs in a manner that will support a facility's business and legal processes; otherwise duplicate paper processes will need to be maintained.

AHIMA convened an e-HIM® work group to re-evaluate and update the 2002 practice brief "Maintaining a Legally Sound Health Record" to address the transition many organizations face in the migration from paper to hybrid to fully electronic health records. Issues unique to EHRs are addressed specifically if they are different or require expansion. Many organizations use a hybrid record (which includes both paper and electronic documentation), scanning paper documents into an electronic document management system. Even though a scanned document ends up in an electronic state, the documentation principles for paper-based records still apply. If there are unique issues for scanned records, they are specified in this brief.

Authentication for Legal Admissibility

Generally, statements made outside the court by a party in a lawsuit are considered hearsay and not admissible as evidence. Documentation in the health record is technically hearsay; however, Federal Rules of Evidence (803(6)) and the Uniform Business and Public Records Act adopted by most states allow exception to the hearsay rule for records maintained in the regular course of business, including health records. All records must be identified and authenticated prior to admissibility in court.

Four basic principles must be met for the health record to be authenticated or deemed admissible as evidence. The record must have been:

- Documented in the normal course of business (following normal routines)
- Kept in the regular course of business
- Made at or near the time of the matter recorded
- Made by a person within the business with knowledge of the acts, events, conditions, opinions, or diagnoses appearing in it

EHRs are admissible if the system that produced them is shown to be accurate and trustworthy. The Comprehensive Guide to Electronic Health Records outlines the following facts to support accuracy and trustworthiness:

- Type of computer used and its acceptance as standard and efficient equipment
- The record's method of operation
- The method and circumstances of preparation of the record, including:
  - The sources of information on which it is based
  - The procedures for entering information into and retrieving information from the computer
  - The controls and checks used as well as the tests made to ensure the accuracy and reliability of the record
  - The information has not been altered[1]

As EHRs become more commonplace, the federal courts are beginning to differentiate the standards to be applied to authenticate EHRs, based on the type of information stored. For example, when a computer record contains the assertions of a person, such as a progress note or dictated report, the record must fit within the hearsay exception to be admissible. These records are referred to as computer-stored.

In contrast, computer-generated records contain the output of computer programs, untouched by human hands. Examples may include decision-support alerts and machine-generated test results. The admissibility issue here is not whether the information in the record is hearsay, but whether the computer program that generated the record was reliable and functioning properly (a question of authenticity). In most cases, the reliability of a computer program can be established by showing that users of the program actually do rely on it on a regular basis, such as in the ordinary course of business.

Testifying about Admissibility

Typically, the health record custodian is called upon to authenticate records by providing testimony about the process or system that produced the records. An organization's record-keeping program should consist of policies, procedures, and methods that support the creation and maintenance of reliable, accurate records. If so, the records will be admissible into evidence.

Electronic and imaged health records. Case law and the Federal Rules of Evidence provide support to allow the output of an EHR system to be admissible in court. The rule states, "If data are stored in a computer or similar device, any printout or other output readable by sight, shown to reflect the data accurately, is an 'original.'"[2] As a result, an accurate printout of computer data satisfies the best evidence rule, which ordinarily requires the production of an original to prove the content of a writing, recording, or photograph. Organizations that maintain EHRs should clearly define those systems that contain the legal EHR or portions of the EHR. Each of these systems should be configured and maintained, ensuring that entries originated in a manner consistent with HIM principles and their business rules, content, and output meet all standards of admissibility.

An important component of this effort is to establish methods to authenticate the electronic data stored in the EHR, namely to verify that data has not been altered or improperly modified consistent with Federal Rules of Evidence. HIPAA security implementation standards require organizations to authenticate protected electronic health information as a means of ensuring data integrity, including data at rest and transmitted data. Cryptographic applications commonly used to authenticate include message authentication codes and digital signatures.

Authorship

Authorship is the origination of recorded information. This is an action attributed to a specific individual or entity, acting at a particular time. Authors are responsible for the completeness and accuracy of their entries in the health record.

AHIMA recommends that anyone documenting in the health record (regardless of media) have the authority and right to document as defined by the organization's policies and procedures. Individuals must be trained and competent in the fundamental documentation practices of the organization and legal documentation standards. Organizations should define the level of record documentation expected of their practitioners based on the practitioners' licensure, certification, and professional experience.

Authentication of Entries

Authentication shows authorship and assigns responsibility for an act, event, condition, opinion, or diagnosis. Health Level Seven (HL7) has defined a legally authenticated document or entry as "a status in which a document or entry has been signed manually or electronically by the individual who is legally responsible for that document or entry."[3] Each organization should establish a definition of a legally authenticated entry and establish rules to promptly authenticate every entry in the health record by the author responsible for ordering, providing, or evaluating the service furnished.

Many states have regulations or rules of evidence that speak to specific characteristics required for authenticating entries. Before adopting any authentication method other than written signature, the organization should consult state statutes and regulations regarding authentication of entries. The medical staff bylaws (where applicable) or organizational policies should also approve computer authentication and authentication of scanned entries and specify the rules for use. Organizations automating health records in a state that does not expressly permit the use of computer keys to authenticate should seek permission from the applicable state agency.

Types of Signatures

For paper-based records, acceptable methods to identify the author generally include written signature, rubber stamp signature, or initials combined with a signature legend on the same document. Acceptable methods of identifying the author in EHRs generally include electronic or digital signatures or computer key. Acceptable methods for authenticating a scanned document may follow paper or electronic guidelines.

Signatures are the usual method to authenticate entries in a paper-based record. The Centers for Medicare and Medicaid Services (CMS) Interpretive Guidelines for Hospitals 482.24(c)(1) require name and discipline at a minimum. A healthcare organization can choose a more stringent standard requiring the author's full name with title or credential to assist in proper identification of the writer. Healthcare organization policies should define the acceptable format for signatures in the health record.

A **countersignature** requires a professional to review and, if appropriate, approve action taken by another practitioner. Countersignatures should be used as required by state licensing or certification statutes related to professional scope of practice. The entries of individuals who are required to practice under the direct supervision of another professional should be countersigned by the individual who has authority to evaluate the entry. Once countersigned, the entry is legally adopted by the supervising professional as his or her own entry. For example, licensed nurses who do not have the authority to supervise should not countersign an entry for a graduate nurse who is not yet licensed. Practitioners who are asked to countersign should do so carefully. The CMS Interpretive Guidelines for Hospitals (482.24(c)(1)(I)) require that medical staff rules and regulations identify the types of documents or entries nonphysicians may complete that require a countersignature by a supervisor or attending medical staff member.

Rubber stamp signatures are acceptable if allowed by state, federal, and reimbursement regulations. From a reimbursement perspective, some fiscal intermediaries have local policies prohibiting the use of rubber stamp signatures in the health record even though federal regulation allows their use. Healthcare organization policies should state if rubber stamp signatures are acceptable and define the circumstances for their use after review of state regulations and payer policies.

When rubber stamp signatures are used, a list of signatures should be maintained to cross-reference each signature to an individual author. The individual whose signature the stamp represents should sign a statement that he or she is the only one who has the stamp and uses it. There can be no delegation to another individual for use of the stamp. Sanctions should be established for unauthorized or inappropriate use of signature stamps.

Initials can be used to authenticate entries such as flow sheets, medication records, or treatment records. They should not be used for such entries as narrative notes or assessments. Initials should never be used for entries where a signature is required by law. Authentication of entries by only initials should be avoided because of the difficulty in positively identifying the author of an entry based on initials alone and distinguishing that individual from others having the same initials.

If a healthcare organization chooses to use initials in any part of the record for authentication of an entry, there should be corresponding full identification of the initials on the same form or on a signature legend. A signature legend may be used to identify the author and full signature when initials are used to authenticate entries. Each author who initials an entry must have a corresponding full signature on record. For EHRs, apply recommendations for computer key signatures.

Fax signatures. The acceptance of fax documents and signatures is dependent on state, federal, and reimbursement regulations. Unless specifically prohibited by state regulations or healthcare organization policy, fax signatures are acceptable. The Federal Rules of Evidence and the Uniform Rules of Evidence allow for reproduced records used during the course of business to be admissible as evidence unless there is a genuine question about their authenticity or circumstances dictate that the originals be admissible rather than the reproductions. Some states have adopted the Uniform Photographic Copies of Business and Public Records Act, which allows for the admissibility of a reproduced business record without the original. The Uniform Business Records as Evidence Act also addresses the admissibility of reproductions. When a fax document or signature is included in the health record, the document with the original signature should be retrievable from the original source.

Electronic signatures are acceptable if allowed by state, federal, and reimbursement regulations. In 2000 the US government passed the Electronic Signatures in Global National Commerce Act, which gives electronic signatures the same legality as handwritten signatures for interstate commerce. State regulations and payer policies must be reviewed to ensure acceptability of electronic signatures when developing healthcare organization policies. ASTM and HL7 have standards for electronic signatures. Electronic signature software binds a signature or other mark to a specific electronic document. It requires user authentication such as a unique code, biometric, or password that verifies the identity of the signer in the system.

If electronic signatures are used in the EHR, the software program or technology should provide message integrity—assurance that the message sent or entry made by a user is the same as the one received or maintained by the system. If electronic signatures are used in the EHR, the software program or technology should also provide for nonrepudiation—assurance that the entry or message came from a particular user. It will be difficult for a party to deny the content of an entry or having created it.

A **digital signature** provides a digital guarantee that information has not been modified, as if it were protected by a tamper-proof seal that is broken if the content is altered.[4]

A **computer key** or other code is an acceptable method to authenticate entries in an EHR if allowed by state, federal, and reimbursement regulations. When computer codes are used, a list of codes should be maintained that links each code to an individual author. Authorized users should sign a statement ensuring that they alone will use the computer key. Sanctions should be established for unauthorized or inappropriate use of computer keys.

Digital ink or digitized signatures differ from electronic signatures in that they use handwritten signatures on a pen pad. The actual written signature is converted into an electronic image. Digitized signatures are acceptable if allowed by state, federal, and reimbursement regulations. State regulations and payer policies must be reviewed to ensure acceptability of digitized signatures when developing healthcare organization policies.

Specific Authentication Issues

There are a number of unique authentication scenarios and issues that organizations must address.

Auto-authentication. The author of each entry should take specific action to verify that the entry is his or her entry or that he or she is responsible for the entry and that the entry is accurate. Computer technology has provided opportunities to improve the speed and accuracy of the authentication process. However, authentication standards still require that the author attest to the accuracy of the entry. As a result, any auto-authentication technique that does not require the author to review the entry is likely to fall short of federal and state authentication requirements and place the organization at legal risk.

Failure to disapprove an entry within a specific time period is not an acceptable method of authentication. A method should be in place to ensure that authors authenticate dictated documents after they are transcribed. Auto-authentication methods where the dictator is deemed to have authenticated a transcribed document if no corrections are requested within a specified period of time are not recommended.

Authenticating documents with multiple sections or completed by multiple individuals. Some documentation tools, particularly assessments, are set up to be completed by multiple staff members at different times. As with any entry, there must be a mechanism to determine who completed information on the document. At a minimum, there should be a signature area at the end of the document for staff to sign and date. Staff who have completed sections of the assessment should either indicate the sections they completed at the signature line or initial the sections they completed.

Some EHR documentation tools, particularly assessments, are also intended to be completed by multiple staff members at different times. Here too there must be a mechanism to determine who completed information in the document.

Documenting care provided by a colleague. Individuals providing care are responsible for documenting that care. Documentation must reflect who performed the action. Patient care carried out by another provider, as well as clinical information supplied by another person to the writer of the entry, should be clearly attributed to the source.

Some EHR systems provide the capability to indicate differences between the person who enters information and the author of a document. In either case, documentation must reflect who performed the action. If documentation of care is entered for another provider, at a minimum the document should contain the identification of the person who entered the information along with the date the entry was made and authentication by the actual provider of care with the corresponding date of authentication.

Documentation Principles

Regardless of the format, text entries, canned phrases, or templates should follow fundamental principles for the quality of the entry. Content should be specific, objective, and complete.

Use **specific** language and avoid vague or generalized language. Do not speculate. The record should always reflect factual information (what is known versus what is thought or presumed), and it should be written using factual statements. Examples of generalizations and vague words include patient doing well, appears to be, confused, anxious, status quo, stable, as usual. If an author must speculate (i.e., diagnosis is undetermined), the documentation should clearly identify speculation versus factual information.

Chart **objective** facts and avoid using personal opinions. By documenting what can be seen, heard, touched, and smelled, entries will be specific and objective. Describe signs and symptoms, use quotation marks when quoting the patient, and document the patient's response to care.

Document the **complete** facts and pertinent information related to an event, course of treatment, patient condition, response to care, and deviation from standard treatment (including the reason for it). Make sure the entry is complete and contains all significant information. If the original entry is incomplete, follow guidelines for making a late entry, addendum, or clarification.

Other Documentation Issues

Organizational policies must address the use of approved abbreviations in the health record. A second emerging documentation issue is the cut and paste functionality in EHRs. Organizations must consider whether they will allow cutting and pasting and how they will handle cut-and-paste content from one entry to another.

Use of abbreviations. Every healthcare organization should have a goal to limit or eliminate the use of abbreviations in medical record documentation as part of its patient safety efforts. Healthcare organizations should set a standard for acceptable abbreviations to be used in the health record and develop an organization-specific abbreviation list. Only those abbreviations approved by the organization should be used in the health record. When there is more than one meaning for an approved abbreviation, choose one meaning or identify the context in which the abbreviation is to be used. Every organization should have a list of abbreviations, acronyms, and symbols that should not be used.

EHRs. Abbreviations should be eliminated as information is formatted for the EHR. Electronic order sets, document templates for point-and-click or direct charting, voice recognition, or transcribed documents can be formatted or programmed to eliminate abbreviations.

Cut, copy, and paste functionality is not generally regarded as legitimately available in the paper record. Analogous functions in paper records include photocopying a note, cropping it, and pasting or gluing it into the record.

The primary issue with the cut, copy, and paste functionality in the EHR is one of authorship—who is the author and what is the date of origination for a copied entry?

Cutting and pasting saves time; however, it also poses several risks:

- Cutting and pasting the note to the wrong encounter or the wrong patient record
- Lack of identification of the original author and date
- The acceptability of cutting and pasting the original author's note without his or her knowledge or permission

Organizations should develop policy and procedures related to cutting, copying, and pasting documentation in their EHR systems. By following these guidelines and training clinical staff, providers can allow cutting and pasting within certain boundaries.

- In general, the original source author and date must be evidenced in copied information. If users are allowed to copy forward from a previous entry by another person, an attribution statement referring to the original document, date, and author should be attached or incorporated where applicable.
- Cutting, copying, and pasting must not be perceived as "OK unless proven otherwise" but instead should be considered "not OK until proven otherwise."
- Each potential function must be evaluated for policy or procedure acceptance or rejection by a practice.
- In some settings, copy and paste may be acceptable for legal record purposes but not for others (clinical trials data, quality assurance data, pay-for-performance data).
- In the hybrid environment, audit tracking of copy and paste may not be available because it involves different systems.
- In some contexts, it is never legitimate, including settings where the actual function takes personal health information outside the security environment.
- Some systems have an intermediate step allowing information to be brought forward but require another validation step.
- As a mitigation step, boilerplate text or libraries may be devised to describe common or routine information as agreed upon by the organizational standards.

Linking Each Patient to a Record

Every page in the health record or computerized record screen must identify patients by name and health record number. Patient name and number must be on both sides of every page as well as on every form and computerized printout. Paper and computer-generated forms with multiple pages must have the patient name and number on all pages.

EHRs. Each data field in the health record must be linked to the patient's name and health record number. Patient name and number must be on every page of printed, viewed, or otherwise transmitted information. The system in use must have a means of authenticating information reported from other systems.

Referencing another patient in the paper record. If it is necessary to refer to another patient to describe an event, the patient's name should not be used—the record number should be referenced in its place.

Timeliness and Chronology of Entries

Timeliness of an entry is critical to the admissibility of a health record in court as required by the Uniform Rules of Evidence. Entries should be made as soon as possible after an event or observation is made. An entry shall never be made in advance. If it is necessary to summarize events that occurred over a period of time (such as a shift), the notation shall indicate the actual time the entry was made with the narrative documentation identifying the time events occurred, if time is pertinent to the situation.

Timeliness of an entry presumes that the medium to which the entry is made is accessible. The principle of availability has been recognized as also consistent with timeliness, with the understanding that an entry would be made as soon as the record or system is available.

EHRs. Facilities must define what constitutes the legal health record in their organizational policies. Procedures must be in place to define timeliness for each component of the EHR system where there are no real-time automated links between subsystems.

Chronology

The record must reflect the continuous chronology of the patient's healthcare. Tools should be provided for caregivers to view episode-based information.

The chronology must be readily apparent in any given view. It is recommended that organizations have a facility-wide standard view. EHR systems should have the capability of producing an output that chronicles the individual's encounter.

Date and Time

Every entry in the health record must include a complete date (including month, day, and year) and a time. Time must be included in all types of narrative notes even if it may not seem important to the type of entry.

Charting time as a block (e.g., 7 a.m.–3 p.m.) is not advised, especially for narrative notes. Narrative documentation should reflect the actual time the entry was made. For certain types of flow sheets, such as a treatment record, recording time as a block could be acceptable. For example, a treatment that can be delivered any time during a shift could have a block of time identified on the treatment record with staff signing that they delivered the treatment during that shift. For assessment forms where multiple individuals are completing sections, the date and time of completion should be indicated as well as who has completed each section (time is not required on standardized data sets such as the MDS and OASIS).

EHR systems must have the ability to date- and time-stamp each entry as the entry is made. Every entry in the health record must have a system-generated date and time based on current date and time. Date and time stamps must be associated with the signature at the time the documentation is finalized. For businesses operating across time zones, the time zone must be included in the date and time stamp. The date and time of entry must be accessible by the reviewer. Systems must have the ability for the documenter to enter date and time of occurrence for late entries.

Imaged records. The same standards for paper records apply to imaged records. Additionally, all scanned documents must be date- and time-stamped with the date scanned.

Legibility and Display

All entries to the record should be legible. If an entry cannot be read, the author should rewrite the entry on the next available line, define what the entry is for, referring back to the original documentation, and legibly rewrite the entry. For example: "Clarified entry of [date]" and rewrite entry, date, and sign. The rewritten entry must be the same as the original. All entries to the record should be made in black ink to facilitate legible photocopying of records. Entries should not be made in pencil.

Labels should be procured from a specific vendor to ensure adhesiveness and not placed over documentation. Organizations should review written documents as detailed in the practice brief "Ensuring Legibility of Patient Records."[5]

EHRs. Graphic user interface display options should accommodate ergonomic needs of all users (e.g., visual acuity). Critical results should not rely on color due to consideration for color-blind users. Asterisks or labels can be used as additional visual cues. Screen resolution should be adjustable for individual user preference. Imaged documents incorporated in the system should require a minimal number of clicks and keystrokes to open. Devices such as bar codes should be part of an organization's quality check protocol. If data are used in multiple organizational systems, legibility should be a shared quality check between applications. Free-text entries should be spellchecked to ensure the legibility requirement of ability to understand.

Imaged records. All entries to be scanned into the record should be made in black ink to facilitate legible reproduction of records. Entries should not be made in pencil. Paper records as well as corresponding microfilm should be retained for the period defined by facility policy.

Legibility of all records, including scanned records, should be included in an organization's quality control processes.

Computer screens must be of sufficient size and resolution to display information appropriate for the intended use and intended users. Displays must support viewing information in its entirety without scrolling. PACS images, especially scanned documents, require close attention to display support of required legibility.

Corrections, Errors, Amendments, and Other Documentation Problems

There will be times when documentation problems or mistakes occur, and changes or clarifications will be necessary. Proper procedures must be followed in handling these situations. ASTM and HL7 have standards that apply to error correction.

Error Correction Process

When an error is made in a health record entry, proper error correction procedures must be followed:

- Draw a line through the entry. Make sure that the inaccurate information is still legible.
- Write "error" by the incorrect entry and state the reason for the error in the margin or above the note if room.
- Sign and date the entry.
- Document the correct information. If the error is in a narrative note, it may be necessary to enter the correct information on the next available line, documenting the current date and time and referring back to the incorrect entry.

Do not obliterate or otherwise alter the original entry by blacking out with marker, using whiteout, or writing over an entry.

EHRs. Correcting an error in an electronic or computerized health record system should follow the same basic principles. The system must have the ability to track corrections or changes to the entry once the entry has been entered or authenticated. When correcting or making a change to an entry in a computerized health record system, the original entry should be viewable, the current date and time should be entered, the person making the change should be identified, and the reason should be noted. In situations where a hard copy is printed from the EHR, the hard copy must also be corrected.

Every entry should be date-, time-, and author-stamped by the system. A symbol that indicates a new or additional entry that has resulted in an additional version should be viewable. It must be clear to the user that there are additional versions of the data being viewed. A preferred method is to apply a strikethrough for error with commentary and date-, time-, and author-stamp or equivalent functionality to retain original versions linked to the corrected version.

Hybrid records. Organizational policy must define how errors are corrected in imaged documents while preserving in a readable form the original document or image. The practice brief "Electronic Document Management as a Component of the Electronic Health Record" provides guidelines for retraction, resequencing, and reassignment:

- **Retraction** involves removing a document for standard view, removing it from one record, and posting it to another within the electronic document management system. In the record from which the document was removed, the document would not be considered part of the designated record set or visible to anyone. Someone should be designated by the organization to view or print the retracted documents. An annotation should be viewable to the clinical staff so that the retracted document can be consulted if needed.
- **Resequencing** involves moving a document from one place to another within the same episode of care. No annotation of this action is necessary.
- **Reassignment** (synonymous with misfiles) involves moving the document from one episode of care to a different episode of care within the same patient record. As with retractions, someone in the organization should be designated to view or print the reassigned document. An annotation should be viewable to the clinical staff so that the reassigned document can be consulted if needed.[6]

Late Entry

When a pertinent entry was missed or not written in a timely manner, a late entry should be used to record the information in the health record.

- Identify the new entry as "late entry."
- Enter the current date and time. Do not try to give the appearance that the entry was made on a previous date or time.
- Identify or refer to the date and incident for which the late entry is written.
- If the late entry is used to document an omission, validate the source of additional information as much as possible (e.g., where you obtained the information to write the late entry).
- When using late entries, document as soon as possible. There is no time limit to writing a late entry; however, the more time that passes, the less reliable the entry becomes.

Amendments

An addendum is another type of late entry that is used to provide additional information in conjunction with a previous entry. With this type of correction, a previous note has been made and the addendum provides additional information to address a specific situation or incident. When making an addendum:

- Document the current date and time.
- Write "addendum" and state the reason for the addendum, referring back to the original entry.
- Identify any sources of information used to support the addendum.
- When writing an addendum, complete it as soon after the original note as possible.
- In an electronic system it is recommended that organizations have a link to the original entry or a symbol by the original entry to indicate the amendment. ASTM and HL7 have standards related to amendments.

Healthcare organizations should have policies to address how a patient or his or her representative can enter amendments into the record. The HIPAA privacy rule requires specific procedures and time frames be followed for processing an amendment. A separate entry (progress note, form, typed letter) can be used for patient amendment documentation. The amendment should refer back to the information questioned, date, and time. The amendment should document the information believed to be inaccurate and the information the patient or legal representative believes to be correct. The entry in question should be flagged to indicate a related amendment or correction (in both a paper and electronic system). At no time should the documentation in question be removed from the chart or obliterated in any way. The patient cannot require that the records be removed or deleted.

Version Management

An organization must address management of document versions. Once documentation has been made available for patient care, it must be retained and managed regardless of whether the document was authenticated (if authentication applies). Organizations must decide whether all versions of a document will be displayed or just the final, who has access to the various versions of a document, and how the availability of versions will be flagged in the health record.

It is acceptable for a draft of a dictated and transcribed note or report to be changed before authentication unless there is a reason to believe the changes are suspect and would not reflect actual events or actions. Facility policy should define the acceptable period of time allowed for a document to remain in draft form before the author reviews and approves it (e.g., 24 to 72 hours).

Once a document is no longer considered a draft or has been authenticated, any changes or alterations should be made following the procedures for a late entry or amendment. The original document must be maintained along with the new revised document.

Chart Content

Organizations must define the content of their legal health records based on regulations and standards of practice. This step is critical in determining the information disclosed upon request that documents clinical encounters and the documentation that must be retained and protected for required periods of time. The practice brief "Update: Guidelines for Defining the Legal Health Record for Disclosure Purposes" provides information on determining the health record content.[7] The following topics address unique content issues.

Decision Support

Decision support, including system-generated notifications, prompts, and alerts, should be evidence-based, validated, and accepted by the organization. The patient health record should include documentation of the clinician's actions in response to decision support. This documentation is evidence of the clinician's decision to follow or disregard decision support. The organization should define the extent of exception documentation required (e.g., what does no documentation mean).

Notification and Communication with Patients or Family

If notification of the patient's physician or family is required or a discussion with the patient's family occurs regarding care of the patient, all such communications (including attempts at notification) should be documented. Include the time and method of all communications or attempts. The entry should include any orders received or responses, the implementation of such orders, and the patient's response. Messages left on answering machines should be limited to a request to return call and are not considered a valid form of notification. An organization should determine whether copies of letters to patients are retained as part of the legal patient record, if they should be disclosed to others, and their retention period.

Informed Consent

Informed consent entries include explanation of the risks and benefits of a treatment or procedure, alternatives to the treatment or procedure, and evidence that the patient or appropriate legal surrogate understands and consents to undergo the treatment or procedure. This type of information should be carefully documented. Laws, regulations, and organization policy define the format of informed consent (e.g., must it be a distinct form or a documented discussion).

EHRs. With electronic consent, the patient views the consent and electronically signs it. An organization should verify that the electronic signature or authentication protocol meets all legal and regulatory requirements. The informed consent shall contain enough information for the patient to clearly choose various options of care and treatment during the episode of care. The informed consent should not allow for any "striking out" or deleting, but should provide for standard inclusions or exclusions.

Imaged records. When imaging, regulations, laws, or organization policies should define whether the original paper form or the patient's original ink signature is retained, the retention period, and the retrieval expectation. Policy should define if the legal medical record and a legal signature include a scanned image of the document or signature. Storage and retention should be consistent with the organization's policy for all other contents of the legal patient record.

Managing Data from Other Facilities or the Patient

Clinical information received from other facilities or from the patient should be evaluated by the clinician. The organization's policy should define whether the data in its entirety or just the data abstracted and transferred by the clinician is incorporated into the patient's health record. The source of the clinical data should be documented.

EHRs. If medical images are received from outside healthcare organizations or the patient, the images may be uploaded into the core clinical system. Retain attribution detail of source organization, author, and date.

Hybrid records. Organizations should define the procedure for the transfer of clinical information received on CD or DVD into the hybrid record. Options may include print to paper then image or upload into EHR or interface with the hybrid record. It must be determined whether laws, regulations, or organization policy requires retention of the original media or a photocopy.

Customized Clinical Views

If the EHR system can provide customized clinical views, the organization should determine who is authorized to create and maintain the customized views. When clinical data are pulled into a customized view and used for clinical decision making, the logic or programming should be retained and made retrievable by the organization. The organization is encouraged to retain the methods and logic of customized clinical views; however, the system logic is not considered part of the legal health record.

Templates, Boilerplates, Canned Text

Care must be taken that these methods support clinical care and accurate documentation and not simply expedite the process. Creation and periodic review of these tools should be based on clinically appropriate, standards-based protocol for common or routine information. Documentation by this method should require an active choice in response to the interaction between the patient and provider. When a clinician reviews and authenticates, the author is indicating he or she reviewed and completed the documentation and accepted the accuracy as his or her own.

Flowsheets

Organization policy should establish form design and documentation standards, including frequency of documentation. All entries are date-, time-, and author-stamped. The policy should define the frequency and standard time frame for documentation of clinical observations and assessments. In paper, if initials identify author only, full signature should be elsewhere on the form for easy reference.

EHRs. Organization policy should outline the frequency of data entry or capture and standard intervals for display of information (e.g., exact time, every five seconds, every 10 minutes, every 30 minutes, every hour). Policy should define the frequency of data captured directly from clinical monitoring systems, machine to machine (e.g., continuous, every five seconds, every 15 minutes). All data are date- and timed-stamped with the author noted. The standard frequency for view or print of archived flowsheet data should be defined. The system should provide views of archived data by date, time, author, or data field.

Output Format

Organization policy should determine whether the record must be complete before output is generated and who has the authority to generate output from the EHR. The EHR system must have the capability of providing a chronological record of the patient's encounter. When the EHR output is generated for disclosure, the organization must define the standardized forms, formats, and order based on user needs (e.g., different views, formats, and order for lawyers, insurance companies, patients, or healthcare providers). Organizations must also decide what versions of documents will be provided.

The organization should define a standard technology for output according to the information system capability, privacy and security standards, and user need and capability to use the format chosen.

Printing Guidelines

The organization must define the standard form and format of the paper health record and define who can reproduce paper documents for internal or external disclosure. The organization must also define the scope and reasons for printing paper internally. Printing can be a legal challenge if clinicians print from the EHR and then document on the printouts rather than in the system. Strict control of printing policies should be in place.

EHRs. Organizations must decide if they will reproduce the EHR in paper format. If printing from the EHR system is allowed, organization policies should define who has the authority to print and under what circumstances. Printing should be tracked in the audit trail and information on user and location available if needed. Policies should also define the form and format of documents that print from the EHR. For example, is it a screen print of the clinician view or a form that mimics the traditional paper record forms? What interval of time is printed as a standard—by encounter, date ranges, any point in time, or at discharge?

Organizations must decide which version is printed—only the most current version of a document or other versions as well. If other versions are printed, determine under what circumstances previous archived versions are printed. Organizations must decide whether to print the traditional final lab results report versus all the preliminary results and whether lab result trends are printed. When separate covered entities share a clinical data repository and use shared information for clinical decision making, the organization should define what information from the repository can be printed. An organization should also determine if preliminary, unauthenticated reports can be printed and under what circumstances.

Permanency

All entries in the health record, regardless of form or format, must be permanent (manual or computerized records). The Rules of Evidence require policies and procedures be in place to prevent alteration, tampering, or loss. The organization must consider the issue of permanency of records in its records management policies. In a paper system, permanency is affected by lifespan of the actual paper or microfilm that health information is recorded on. Retention policies and schedules developed by the organization determine the permanency of the information.

EHRs. The organization must consider the issue of permanency of records in its electronic records management policies. In an electronic system, permanency is affected by the digital nature of data, which may be more readily subject to change or technology obsolescence than is information recorded on paper. This includes changes to the actual data itself or changes that occur over time in data formats and storage devices. Use of standard file formats and clinical nomenclatures may facilitate data conversion as technology changes and are a major consideration for permanency. Procedures to protect against data degradation and loss of integrity during system conversions must be addressed.

Other Permanency Issues

Ink color. For hard-copy paper records, blue or black ink is preferred to ensure readability when records are copied. The ink should be permanent (no erasable or water-soluble ink should be used). Never use a pencil to document in the health record. Black ink is preferred for records that will be imaged.

Printer. When documentation is printed from a computer for entry in the health record or retention as the permanent record, the print must be permanent. For example, a laser printer should be used rather than an ink-jet printer, because the latter ink is water soluble.

Fax copies. When fax records are maintained in the health record, assurance must be made that the record will maintain its integrity over time. For example, if thermal paper is used, a copy must be made for filing in the health record because the print on thermal paper fades over time. (See section on fax signatures for admissibility as evidence.)

Photocopies. The health record should contain original documents whenever possible. There are times when it is acceptable to have copies of records and signatures, particularly when records are sent from another provider.

Carbon copy paper. If there is a question about the permanency of the paper (e.g., NCR or carbon paper), a photocopy should be made. Policy should indicate when items are copied and how the original is disposed. At times, carbon copies of documents may be used on a temporary basis and the original will replace the carbon.

Use of labels. Labels and label paper (adhesive-backed paper) are used for a variety of reasons including patient demographics, transcription of dictated progress notes, printing of physician orders for telephone orders, medication, or treatment records. When labels are used in the record, a number of issues or concerns must be considered and addressed before implementation. Organization policies and practices should address how and where labels will be placed. Information may not be obscured by the label, and the adhesiveness of the label must be adequate for the retention period of the document.

Retention

Organizations must establish retention schedules for the content of the legal health record that comply with federal and state regulations and the needs for patient care, research, and administrative purposes (e.g., legal and compliance).

EHRs. Electronic storage media such as magnetic and optical formats must meet the organization's retention schedule and include retention of all types of data including discrete data, text, audio, video, and images. Policies should address backup procedures to ensure retention and protect against data loss.

Organizations should also address retention of data and information associated with the EHR but which may not be strictly part of the EHR—items such as audit trails, alerts and reminders, and metadata associated with structured as well as unstructured data. This may be important in certifying the integrity of the information for risk management and legal purposes.

Retention policies should comply with accreditation standards and federal and state law and regulations. Information life cycle management should be built into EHR systems in the development phase. If an EHR crosses multiple disparate information systems, retention policies must be applied to each component. EHR systems must include a function or feature that allows for litigation holds that exempt specific records from the retention policy due to legal, compliance, or other business needs.

Imaged records. With imaged documents, an organization needs to decide how long to retain the paper after scanning. Considerations include provisions for quality assurance in the scanning process, the organization's definition of its legal record (paper, electronic, or both), and the frequency and timing of backups of the scanned images.

Other considerations in retention of paper may include state regulations, requirements of the organization's malpractice risk carrier, and in the case of organizations that conduct research, FDA regulations. When paper is retained after scanning, there must be an established cataloguing and indexing method so that it can be retrieved. Schedules or guidelines for conversion of document images from magnetic to optical storage should be addressed.

Depending on the organization's need for longevity of scanned images, it may also wish to consider converting scanned images to microfilm for longer retention periods. Occupational health records, for example, must be retained for 30 years.

Storage

An organization must store health records in a way that prevents loss, destruction, or unauthorized use. Traditional methods for storing paper records include open-space shelving for active files and off-site box storage for archived records.

EHRs. Organizations must ensure that EHR systems provide basic database storage standards, including appropriate security measures. Major considerations include how to store information in order to convey it to an external user in an acceptable medium and the volume of records to be stored (e.g., what types must be included).

Obsolescence of Technology

Stored records must be accessible for the length of the retention period regardless of the technology used. When records are stored as microfilm and microfiche, an organization must retain hardware to access or reproduce the records for the length of the retention period.

EHRs. Organizations require a plan to access or reproduce EHR data. As technology changes, consideration must include "backwards compatibility" or some type of access to previous systems from the new or upgraded system.

Purging and Destruction

Records should be purged and destroyed in a consistent manner based on an established retention schedule, plan, and procedure. Destruction is acceptable unless there is a concern that certain records or documents were selected for destruction. When this happens, behavior is considered suspect, and it can appear that information that was harmful to the organization was destroyed. Plans should include method of destruction (e.g., shredding, burning) and should consider security of the destruction process.

EHRs. The organization should have a plan for destruction of storage media, including hard drives and portable media such as diskettes and USB drives. Consideration should be given to determining if an EHR system can indicate records to be purged based on the organization's policy. The organization should have a policy that defines purging versus archiving and how the system will support the policy.

Data Integrity: Access, Audit Trail, and Security

Integrity is defined as the accuracy, consistency, and reliability of information content, processes, and systems. Information integrity is the dependability or trustworthiness of information, which is an important concept in a legal proceeding. Integrity of the health record is maintained through access, network security, audit trail, security, and disaster recovery processes.

To protect the integrity of the paper legal health record, organizations should define the policy and procedures regarding the content and reconciliation processes to ensure accuracy and completeness of the health record.

EHRs. To protect the integrity of the electronic legal health record, policies and procedures must be in place:

- Regarding the reconciliation of electronic processes (e.g., process for checking individual data elements, reports, files)
- To assess potential data corruption, data mismatches, and extraneous data
- Regarding managing different iterations of documents (version control), with clear indication of when each version is viewable by caregivers for use in making clinical decisions

- To define when the record is complete and permanently filed (locking the record with view-only access), including temporary locking of high-risk charts by certain users
- Regarding downtime processes and ability to capture data following downtime through direct entry or scanning

Performance criteria and functionality should define and minimize the intrinsic risks by appropriate design, deployment, development, and detection of the EHR. Performance criteria and functionality should also define and minimize the extrinsic risks by appropriate test conversion planning, testing and data validation, and minimization of system downtime.

Access Control

Access control is the process that determines who is authorized to access patient information in the health record. Controlling access is an important aspect of maintaining the legal integrity of the health record. In the paper world this is controlled through physical security safeguards, chart tracking, and out guide systems.

EHRs. Access control and validation procedures must be in place to validate a person's access to the system based on role or function. Access should be terminated automatically after a predetermined period of inactivity. Organizations must also define access to information for emergency situations (break-the-glass access). Policies must address facility access controls to meet the HIPAA security rule.

Audit Trail

An audit trail is a business record of all transactions and activities, including access, associated with the medical record. Elements of an audit trail may include date, time, nature of transaction or activity, and the individual or automated system linked to the transaction or activity. Transactions may include additions or edits to the medical record. Activities may include access to view or read, filing, and data mining. Audit trail functionality is important to support the legal integrity of the record. The purpose of an audit trail is to create a system control to establish accountability for transactions and activities as well as compliance with facility policies, procedures, and protocols related to medical record access and maintenance.

For the paper medical record, an audit trail may include a sign-out sheet, a manual or electronic chart tracking system (e.g., flagging devices or software), or a log book.

EHRs. Audit trails are critical legal functionality for EHR systems because they record key information on data creation, access, and revision. An audit trail may be one of the following types of business records:

- Electronic file of transactions and activities (data creation, access, revision along with date and time)
- Hard-copy report of transactions and activities
- Batch file processing report
- Information system data transmission or interface report
- Exception report of unauthorized access attempts

Special Considerations for an EHR Audit Trail

Teaching environment—academic medical centers. The high turnover of students, interns, and residents in an academic facility or a specific clinical department may necessitate the need to maintain a large file of unique EHR access codes or requirements. Timely activation and deactivation of identification and authentication tools may affect the reliability of audit trail data and must be addressed by organization policies to prevent negative impact on legal integrity of the record.

Health systems—mergers, acquisitions, and divestitures. Physicians and other clinicians who provide direct patient care at multiple locations or facility management and staff who work at other institutions may have more than one EHR access code or level of access when facilities merge or acquire other patient care sites with similar EHR software.

EHR Audit Trail Performance Criteria and Functionalities

- Make sure audit trail functionality is turned on in EHR applications.
- Include date and time stamps on all transactions.
- Do not allow back-door access by a staff member (e.g., system administrator) to make alterations in the EHR without an audit trail record. If back-door access is possible, have the software vendor fix the problem to ensure the EHR retains integrity in a legal proceeding.

Network Security

Electronic network security protects EHR data from unauthorized internal or remote access or illegitimate internal or remote transactions. The purpose of an electronic network security protocol is to preserve the integrity of EHR data and to protect patient privacy, consistent with facility and regulatory requirement, as well as accreditation standards. Electronic network security protocols must address the following access mechanisms:

- Remote access through virtual private network
- Remote access through a local area network
- Remote access through wireless network
- Remote access through a workstation
- Internal access through a workstation

Disaster Recovery and Business Continuity

An important aspect of maintaining a legally sound health record is securing the record to prevent loss, tampering, or unauthorized use. Rules of evidence require an organization to have policies and procedures in place to protect against alterations, tampering, and loss. Systems and procedures should also be in place to prevent loss (such as tracking and sign-out procedures), establish secure record storage areas or systems, and limit access to only authorized users.

Organizations should develop and implement controls to safeguard data and information, including the clinical record, against loss, destruction, and tampering. Organizations should:

- Develop and implement policies when removal of records is permitted
- Protect data and information against unauthorized intrusion, corruption, or damage
- Prevent falsification of data and information
- Develop and implement guidelines to prevent the destruction of records
- Develop and implement guidelines for destroying copies of records
- Protect records in a manner that minimizes the possibility of damage from fire and water

EHRs. Establish (and implement as needed) policies and procedures for responding to an emergency such as fire, vandalism, system failure, and natural disaster that damages systems containing electronic protected health information. Organizations must address and develop the following to adequately prepare for a disaster and prevent loss or destruction of information:

- Data backup plan
- Disaster recovery plan
- Emergency mode operation plan
- Testing and revision procedures
- Applications and data criticality analysis

Business Continuity

Disaster recovery planning includes information and plans on how operations are to continue in the event of a disaster. If a department, business unit, or system is unavailable, a plan must be in place to continue operations. To develop a plan consider the following:

- List all departments that are directly or indirectly affected by extended system downtime
- List all daily procedures that must be followed to maintain acceptable levels of operations
- List actions (manual procedures) completed during downtimes for each department
- Expand the process to plan for the system if it were unavailable for an extended period of time
- Outline specific details steps to integrate backlogged data maintained during the downtime
- List additional procedures to be followed after recovery activities are complete

Conclusion

Maintaining a legally sound health record covers a vast territory from the content of the health record and how entries are recorded to the functionality in the system to access, audit trails, and security. While the electronic age brings new variables to an old and complex problem, the foundation remains the same: health records must be maintained in a manner that follows applicable regulations, accreditation standards, professional practice standards, and legal standards. HIM professionals play a critical role in the transition from paper to electronic records and must partner with clinical, legal, and information technology to adequately address the legal business issues for the health record.

Notes

1. *Comprehensive Guide to Electronic Health Records*, 2000 ed. New York, NY: Faulkner and Gray, 2000.
2. Department of Justice Bulletin on Computer Records and the Federal Rules of Evidence. March 2001.
3. Health Level Seven. "Glossary of Terms." Available online at www.hl7. org.au/Docs/HL7%20Glossary%20-%202001.pdf.
4. Tech Encyclopedia. "Digital Signature." Available online at www.tech web.com/encyclopedia.

5. Glondys, Barbara. "Ensuring Legibility of Patient Records." *Journal of AHIMA* 74, no. 5 (2003): 64A–D.
6. AHIMA. "Electronic Document Mangement as a Component of the Electronic Health Record." October 2003. Available online in the FORE Library: HIM Body of Knowledge at www.ahima.org.
7. AHIMA. "Update: Guidelines for Defining the Legal Health Record for Disclosure Purposes." *Journal of AHIMA* 76, no. 8 (2005): 64A–G.

References

AHIMA. *Health Information Management Practice Standards: Tools for Assessing Your Organization.* Chicago, IL: AHIMA, 1998.

AHIMA. "E-mail as a Provider-Patient Electronic Communication Medium and Its Impact on the Electronic Health Record." October 2003. Available online in the FORE Library: HIM Body of Knowledge at www.ahima.org.

AHIMA. "Implementing Electronic Signatures." October 2003. Available online in the FORE Library: HIM Body of Knowledge at www.ahima.org.

AHIMA. "The Strategic Importance of Electronic Health Records Management." *Journal of AHIMA* 75, no. 9 (2004): 80A–B.

Amatayakul, Margret. "Access Controls: Striking the Right Balance." *Journal of AHIMA* 76, no. 1 (2005): 56–57.

Anderson, Ellen Miller. "Online Clinical Documentation in the Electronic Legal Medical Record." 2004 IFHRO Congress and AHIMA Convention Proceedings. October 2004. Available online in the FORE Library: HIM Body of Knowledge at www.ahima.org.

ASTM. *Annual Book of ASTM Standards.* Volume 14.01, Healthcare Informatics, Section 8, Signature Attributes. West Conshohocken, PA: ASTM, 2000.

Centers for Medicare and Medicaid Services. Interpretive Guidelines for Hospitals. Available online at www.cms.hhs.gov/manuals/107_som/som107ap_a_hospitals.pdf.

Dougherty, Michelle. "Maintaining a Legally Sound Health Record." *Journal of AHIMA* 73, no. 8 (2002): 64A–G.

Fox, Leslie, and Walter Imbiorski. *The Record That Defends Its Friends,* 6th ed. Chicago, IL: Care Communications, 1994.

"Health Insurance Reform: Security Standards; Final Rule." 45 CFR Parts 160, 162, and 164. Federal Register 68, no. 34 (2003). Available online at www.cms.hhs.gov/hipaa/hipaa2/regulations/security/03-3877.pdf.

Health Level Seven. Ann Arbor, MI: Health Level Seven, 1997, Sections 9.4.5–9.4.11, 9.5.5–9.5.10.

Hirsh, Harold L. "Will Your Medical Records Get You into Trouble?" *Legal Aspects of Medical Practice* 6, no. 9 (1978): 46–51.

Huffman, Edna K. *Health Information Management,* 10th ed. Berwyn, IL: Physicians' Record Co., 1994.

Joint Commission on Accreditation of Healthcare Organizations. *2005 Comprehensive Accreditation Manual for Hospitals, Update 3.* Oakbrook Terrace, IL: Joint Commission, 2005.

Murer, Cherilyn G., Michael A. Murer, and Lyndean Lenhoff Brick. *The Complete Legal Guide to Healthcare Records Management.* Washington, DC: Healthcare Financial Management Association, 2000.

National Institute of Standards and Technology. Security Considerations in Information System Development Life Cycle. Revised 2004. Available online at http://csrc.nist.gov/publications/nistpubs.

Quinsey, Carol Ann. "A HIPAA Security Overview." *Journal of AHIMA* 75, no. 4 (2004): 56A–C.

Roach, William H. Jr., and the Aspen Health Law and Compliance Center. *Medical Records and the Law,* 3d ed. Chicago, IL: Aspen Publishers, 1998.

Rollins, Gina. "The Prompt, the Alert, and the Legal Record: Documenting Clinical Decision Support Systems." *Journal of AHIMA* 76, no. 2 (2005): 24–28.

Scott, Ronald W. *Legal Aspects of Documenting Patient Care.* Annville, PA: Aspen Publishers, 1994.

"Standards for Privacy of Individually Identifiable Health Information; Final Rule." 45 CFR Parts 160 and 164. *Federal Register* 65, no. 250 (2000). Available online at www.hhs.gov/ocr/hipaa/finalreg.html.

Waller, Adele, and Oscar Alcantara. "Ownership of Health Information in the Information Age." *Journal of AHIMA* 69, no. 3 (1998): 28–38.

Acknowledgments

AHIMA e-HIM Work Group on Maintaining the Legal EHR:

Deborah Adair, MPH, MS, RHIA
Sharon Baigent, BA, CCHRA(A)
Joyce Booker, RHIT

Melanie Brighton, RHIT
Michelle Dougherty, RHIA, CHP
William French, MBA, RHIA, CPHQ
Marie Gardenier, RHIA, CHPS
Reed Gelzer, MD, MPH, CHCC
Marge Klasa, DC, APRN, BC
Nancy Korn-Smith, RHIT
Karanne Lambton, CCHRA(C)
Richard Leboutillier, MPA, CPHQ
Marlie Nunes, CMT
Suzanne Reviere, RHIA
Melissa Swanfeldt
Anne Tegan, MHA, RHIA, HRM
Andrea Thomas, MBA, RHIA
Lydia Washington, MS, RHIA, CPHIMS
Shelley Weems, RHIA, CCS
Kathy Westhafer, RHIA, CHPS

This work group was supported by a grant to the Foundation of Education and Research of AHIMA (FORE) from Precyse Solutions, Inc.

Article citation:

AHIMA e-HIM Work Group on Maintaining the Legal EHR. "Update: Maintaining a Legally Sound Health Record—Paper and Electronic." *Journal of AHIMA* 76, no. 10 (November–December 2005): 64A–L.

Litigation Response Planning and Policies for e-Discovery

With the enactment of the Federal Rules of Civil Procedure (FRCP), the legal discovery process in healthcare is beginning a radical transformation. The rules governing the discovery of electronic information and the legal process will vary by court jurisdiction (federal, state, or local) as well as the nature, size, and type of case under litigation (civil, criminal, or class action). To prepare for these new changes, healthcare organizations must revisit how they manage information stored electronically.

To successfully manage e-discovery, health organizations must develop a well-defined structure and process to understand, manage, and prepare for litigation. Legal counsel and HIM and IT professionals should work together to successfully manage the electronic discovery (e-discovery) process, implement a litigation response plan, and develop or update organizational policies.

This practice brief outlines five key steps in developing a litigation response plan and process. It uses the FRCP as the foundation for its recommendations.

HIM and IT professionals should seek the opinion of their organization's legal counsel in the final development, review, and approval of the e-discovery plan, policies, and procedures.

How to Develop a Litigation Response Plan

1. Conduct an Evaluation of Applicable Rules

Legal counsel plays a crucial role in e-discovery preparation. As a first step, organizational legal counsel conducts a thorough evaluation of all e-discovery rules applicable at the federal, state, and local levels.

Following this evaluation, legal counsel should educate the governing board, senior and middle management, and other departments with whom it works closely (e.g., risk management, compliance, HIM, and IT) about these rules and regulations and how they expect they will be applied to the organization.

Within the organization, the actual process by which the discovery of electronic information will occur will depend on the jurisdiction of the court and the type and complexity of the case to be litigated. The process may also depend on the scope and complexity of the organization's business and state of operations.

2. Identify a Litigation Response Team

Fundamental to the management and administration of e-discovery is a group of interdisciplinary professionals who serve as the organization's litigation response team. This team is responsible for implementation and ongoing review of the e-discovery process.

The litigation response team should conduct an assessment of the organization's current practices against the e-discovery rules that are applicable to the organization and jurisdiction.

It should then implement new policy and procedures necessary to successfully manage the e-discovery process. This step includes discussion and analysis of e-discovery issues and development of organizational resources such as enterprise retention and destruction schedules and IT system diagrams.

The litigation response team should also oversee the identification, preservation, search, retrieval, and production of responsive electronic and other potentially relevant information related to pending and current litigation. It should provide input to legal counsel about the forms, formats, methods, status, costs, location, and burden of production of potentially responsive information. The team should also oversee the ongoing review, monitoring, and evaluation of e-discovery processes within the organization.

Litigation Response Team Roles

The litigation response team should be comprised, at a minimum, of individuals from the legal counsel or risk management, HIM, and IT departments. Depending on its type, structure, and complexity, the organization may choose to appoint other members to the team, which may include, but are not limited to:

- Chief medical information officer
- Compliance officer
- Executive management (chief operating officer, chief information officer)
- Executive nursing management (vice president of nursing)

- Financial officer
- Other designated department or business process area managers (business office, radiology, laboratory/pathology, emergency services, or other designated management)

Their roles are outlined in the following descriptions.

The governing board should maintain ultimate responsibility for the oversight of e-discovery within the organization. It should also approve the organization's operational plan for e-discovery if appropriate.

The CEO or his or her designee should work closely with legal counsel or risk management in the ongoing review of e-discovery litigation. The status of e-discovery litigation should be reported to the governing board on a regular basis. The litigation response team and planning process should be supported by an executive sponsor.

Depending on the size and structure of the organization, legal counsel and risk management may operate as a single department or separately. Legal counsel may be involved in one or a number of "meet and confer conferences" with opposing counsel and the court early in the litigation process. Because of this, legal counsel must play an integral role in oversight of the e-discovery process while working collaboratively with IT and HIM to ensure relevant information is identified, preserved, and produced in the face of pending litigation.

The IT department should provide the technical support for the organization's hardware and software systems. The IT department will be a valuable resource for legal counsel. The IT department can assist in describing to a court how the organization's technical systems are structured, maintained, and operated. IT should also be able to detail how data are accessed, stored, retrieved, and destroyed.

The IT department can play an integral role in development of the organization's information management plan and its ongoing maintenance and update. It should work closely with the HIM department to understand and articulate the organization's records management requirements.

The HIM department should provide authoritative and technical knowledge about the management of both paper and electronic health information within the organization. The HIM department traditionally has been recognized as the official custodian of the patient's medical records. Because of this, in most organizations, the HIM department accepts and processes subpoenas for patient medical records. HIM should work closely with legal counsel in the identification, preservation, and production of all information (electronic and paper) relevant to litigation.

The HIM director should be knowledgeable about the flow, forms, formats, and location of information and records maintained by the organization, including maintenance and management of the retention and destruction schedules. The HIM department should work closely with IT and be involved in the development of the organization's information management plan and its ongoing maintenance and update.

Depending on the structure of the organization, management from ancillary departments may support the IT and HIM departments in ensuring relevant information is identified, preserved, and retained in the face of pending litigation. The organization should establish the role of ancillary department management in an e-discovery team and organizational response to e-discovery requests for information. Each ancillary department should develop its own specific policies to describe the methods by which entries are made into the medical record and organizational process for ensuring the quality and integrity of the data.

The organization must also define the role of the medical staff in an e-discovery team and organizational response to an e-discovery request for information. Many healthcare organizations designate a member of their medical staff or an individual with extensive clinical background to function as the chief medical information officer. This person can be a valuable resource to legal counsel in understanding the applications and functionality of the organization's information systems and the impact they have on the delivery of a patient's care. Medical staff rules, regulations, and bylaws should specify the practices for documentation in the medical record.

Depending on the structure and complexity of the organization, the compliance officer may or may not be designated as an active member of the organization's e-discovery team. Regardless of structure, the potential involvement of compliance in e-discovery cannot be overlooked. The compliance office should work closely with the litigation response team to ensure adherence with e-discovery organization policies and procedures.

Depending on the structure of the organization, the nursing office may support the IT and HIM departments in ensuring relevant information is identified, preserved, and retained in the face of pending litigation. The role of the nursing office on the e-discovery team and organizational response to an e-discovery request for information should be established by the organization. The nursing office should also develop its own specific policies that describe the methods by which nursing personnel make entries into the medical record and organizational process for ensuring the quality and integrity of the data.

> **E-discovery** is the pretrial legal process used to describe the method by which parties will obtain and review electronically stored information. Amendments to the Federal Rules of Civil Procedure in December 2006 place electronically stored information on equal footing with paper documents in the court.
>
> Electronic data of any kind can serve as evidence. This may cover data or devices including, but not limited to, text, images, voice, databases, spreadsheets, legacy systems, tape, PDAs, instant messages, e-mail, calendar files, and Web sites.

3. Analyze Issues, Risks, and Challenges

Prior to developing organizational policies and procedures, the litigation response team must analyze the new issues, risks, and challenges resulting from e-discovery. This analysis will shape policy and procedure. It will also identify gaps in organizational resources.

The topics below highlight the emerging challenges. Direct questions are provided for the litigation response team to use as discussion starters.

Characteristics of electronically stored information (ESI). ESI is information created, manipulated, communicated, stored, and best used in digital form. It requires the use of computer hardware and software. Organizations should distinguish ESI from conventional media such as paper documents, photographs, microfilm, and analog recordings in their e-discovery processes. The volume of ESI is significantly greater than that of paper documents.

Questions to answer:
- Where is ESI located within the organization?
- What will be the standard procedures and method(s) by which the organization will identify and disclose relevant ESI?

Preparing for a meet and confer pretrial conference. A judge, magistrate, or special master will oversee the e-discovery litigation between parties. Prior to trial, the parties' legal counsel will meet and confer with the judge, magistrate, or special master to discuss and agree upon matters and the approach to be taken with regard to the discovery of electronic information.

The meet and confer sessions could be conducted in one session or several. The actual number of sessions will depend on a multitude of factors affecting the case, including size, scope, and complexity of the case as well as the knowledge, education, and experience of the judge, magistrate, special master, and attorneys involved in the e-discovery litigation.

Given the expansive amounts of electronic information that exist within information systems today, e-discovery can be an intricate, time-consuming, and costly undertaking. Therefore, before an e-discovery meet and confer conference takes place, it is important that legal counsel is educated and knowledgeable about the organization's information systems and records management policies.

Questions to answer:
- In response to a request for ESI, how will the organization locate, index, cull, search, classify, and produce all potentially responsive information?
- What benefit (if any) would there be to an enterprise content and records management system?
- How will the organization determine its true costs to index, classify, store, cull, search, retrieve, and produce ESI?
- If asked, how would the organization describe the "good faith operation" of its information management systems?
- Is there a resource that identifies all information operating systems that are in existence within the organization, including the type, nature, and location of all information systems, as well as the voice, back-up, legacy, and orphan systems?
- Have all record custodians been identified?
- What are the organizational policies and procedure related to records storage, management, and destruction?
- Does counsel have a current copy of the organization's information management plan?
- Does counsel have a current copy of the organization's information technology operating procedures?

Four Levels of Custodianship

Electronically stored information presents organizations with four levels of record custodianship. These depend on a person or entity's relationship to the data and data system and proximity to the case in litigation. As in traditional paper-based records, HIM should remain the official custodian of the record.

Level 1: Primary or Direct Custodians. Those persons who work with the data directly or have direct involvement or knowledge of the events of the case. For example, a staff nurse who has made an entry into the medical record and is knowledgeable about the events of a case in litigation. Primary custodians may be deposed or required to testify because of their direct involvement or knowledge of the case.

Level 2: Data Owners or Stewards. Individuals with responsibility to oversee business process areas may be designated as the data owners or stewards. They have knowledge of the procedures used to create, manage, and preserve specific types of records. Examples of business process areas include finance, radiology, lab, risk management, compliance, and nursing.

Level 3: Business Associates and Third Parties. Contractors and others who serve a variety of functions associated with a party's information but who are not parties to the litigation. Examples include Internet service providers, application service providers such as a claims clearinghouse, and other providers who provide services ranging from off-site data storage to complete outsourcing of the IT department.

Level 4: Official Record and System Custodians. The HIM department historically has been the designated official custodian of the overall medical record. The HIM department has played an important role in the processing of subpoenas for the organization, whether or not the organization was named in litigation.

Definition of official custodian of the record. In the traditional, paper-based realm of healthcare discovery, designation of the "official custodian" of the medical record was clear. In most healthcare organizations the HIM department served in this capacity. The mechanics of the traditional paper-based discovery process have been tied closely with the identification of the official custodian of the medical record.

In today's ESI realm, the role of official custodian is not nearly as clear. The loss of a clear designation will generate issues with the retention, preservation, and production of electronically stored information.

ESI presents four basic levels of custodianship, described in the sidebar above.

In today's new realm of electronic discovery, the HIM department should be designated to maintain the administrative and technical knowledge about how ESI is managed and used within the organization. It should remain the official custodian of the record. The HIM department should be responsible for content and compliance responsibilities associated with the management of electronic information. It should be knowledgeable about the forms, format, and location of potentially responsive ESI.

Staff within the IT department may serve as the official custodian of the information system. Examples of this include the computers, servers, back-up and legacy systems, communications and voice systems, and near-line media. The IT staff who serve in this capacity will play an essential role in the discovery of ESI.

These personnel run the technical infrastructure of the organization's information management systems on a day-to-day basis. They understand the overall relationships between the different files, structure, and storage mechanisms of the organizations' information management systems. Generally, IT staff aren't experts on the specific content or the related managed policies; instead they understand how the organization's systems operate on a technical level.

Questions for discussion:
- How will the organization define and delineate "official custodianship" of its health and business records?
- Have data owners and stewards and the records they manage been identified?
- How will the organization communicate to its data owners and stewards and business associates a potential need to identify, preserve, and produce potentially responsive information for e-discovery litigation?

Preservation and legal holds. The organization has a legal duty to preserve all potentially responsive information in the face of threatened or impending litigation. The scope of that duty encompasses all potential evidence related to those identifiable facts and may shift as litigation develops.

Questions for discussion:

- Has the organization completed a comprehensive retention and destruction schedule that identifies all enterprise records (both paper and electronic) as well as the data owners?
- What potential "triggers" will initiate a potential litigation investigation and possible legal hold?
- Who within the organization will be responsible for establishing a litigation hold?
- How will all potential evidence be assimilated, indexed, and produced?
- Who will monitor the legal hold and reissue or lift it as pertinent facts change over time?
- At what point in the process should legal counsel negotiate a stipulated plan for the preservation of data to make sure the opposing side understands its obligations and to limit its own potential liability?
- Will the organization need special technology to index, classify, store, cull, search, retrieve, and produce ESI?

Form(s) of production. In traditional paper-based discovery, the physical form of production occurs generally only through paper. Documents were entered into evidence by one of the following ways:

1. Admission under the Business Records Rule (Federal Rule of Evidence 803(6) ([Medical Records])
2. Authenticated and admitted under the Best Evidence Rules (Federal Rules of Evidence 1001 and 1001[3])
3. Authenticated, Bates stamped (sequentially numbered or date and time marked), indexed, and labeled to correspond to the categories of a document request

The FRCP provide that legal counsel meet and confer early in litigation and agree upon the form(s) and manner of production of ESI.

Questions for discussion:

- At what point in litigation involving production of ESI will legal counsel meet with HIM and IT to discuss the forms, format, and location of all potentially responsive information?
- How will legal counsel, HIM, and IT work together to identify the most cost-efficient and effective means to produce potentially responsive information?

Reasonably accessible information versus not reasonably accessible information. The FRCP contain provisions for two-tiered discovery. The management of ESI provides for some unique challenges not presented by paper-based and other traditional media. All ESI must be rendered usable through technology—computer, operating system, or application software.

ESI that is readily available through appropriate technology and able to be used and read is considered "accessible." Much of the electronic information subject to discovery is not easily rendered usable without appropriate technologies. This usually involves significant cost and burden. This type of ESI is considered "not reasonably accessible."

Questions for discussion:

- How will the organization produce ESI from the EHR system that is accessible to a plaintiff party if required?
- How will the organization account for and determine its true costs to search, cull, and produce data that are "reasonably accessible" versus data that are "not reasonably accessible"?

Cost shifting. In traditional paper-based document discovery an organization's costs were generally associated with locating responsive documents, assembling them into proper order, Bates stamping them, and presenting them to the requesting party for inspection and copying. With e-discovery the costs to cull, search, retrieve, and produce ESI can be very expensive and will depend greatly on the location, form, accessibility, and format of the information.

The FRCP contain provisions to balance ESI discovery costs between the parties. If a party shows good cause, the court can order the search, retrieval, or testing and sampling of inaccessible information. An organization without appropriate technologies or methods to index, classify, store, cull, search, retrieve, and produce potentially responsive information could face escalating costs, burdens, and potentially sanctions.

Questions for discussion:

- How will the organization determine its true costs to index, classify, store, cull, search, retrieve, and produce ESI?
- How will the organization respond to third-party subpoenas for ESI?
- What measures will the organization take to determine the burden and cost of production of third-party ESI?

E-mail management. The effects resulting from the mismanagement of company e-mail relevant to litigation can have a negative impact on the organization. Through the persistent efforts of legal counsel, coupled with court opinion and enactment of the FRCP, e-mail has become a proverbial "cache to the cash" for a savvy litigant.

Questions for discussion:

- What systems and processes are in place for the classification, management, storage, and retention of company e-mail?
- What is the organization's policy with regard to the use and transmission of protected health information in company e-mail?
- What are the organization's current policies and practices with regard to the screening and monitoring of company e-mail?
- How will e-mail be searched, indexed, reviewed, retained, and produced if relevant to litigation?

The litigation response team must also analyze issues, risks, and challenges surrounding nonapparent and ancillary ESI.

The role, use, and retention of metadata and ephemeral data. Operating system and application software require that electronic files be labeled so that the information can be stored, retrieved, viewed, and communicated. This process creates bits of information about the data known as metadata.

Metadata can be a useful way to authenticate the integrity of data. Recent court opinion suggests that short-lived data (such as RAM) are potentially discoverable and should be preserved if the information does not exist in any other form or cannot be obtained through any other means or source. The potential for the discovery of ephemeral data could pose a significant burden upon the organization.

Questions for discussion:

- How will the organization identify, store, retain, and manage its metadata when required for e-discovery?
- Under what possible circumstances (if any) could the organization be ordered to preserve and produce ephemeral data for a legal proceeding?
- What are the locations, sources, and types of ephemeral data that exist within the organization?

Legacy data systems. In certain cases, the retrieval or restoration of ESI that is contained on legacy systems may be warranted. Access could solely depend on the availability of a retired operating system and application software. ESI that is not migrated and inaccessible places significant burden on the organization when that ESI is needed for business or legal purposes.

Questions for discussion:

- What provisions will the organization establish to provide for the efficient and effective migration of legacy data?
- How long will legacy data not needed for business and legal purposes be retained?
- What will be the mechanism for destruction of legacy data?

Back-up media. One of the biggest problems facing organizations today is the common practice of replicating ESI wholesale, in mirror image, as a precaution against data loss in the event of a disaster. While mirror image back-up tapes may be good procedure for the short-term, the long-term implications of retaining them may be detrimental in litigation. It is important to remember that routine maintenance of back-up tapes makes information on the tape potentially discoverable. The organization could be ordered to search and restore its back-up tapes for a legal proceeding.

Questions for discussion:

- What is and should be organizational practice with regard to the disposition and processing of its back-up tapes and other media?
- Have retention and destruction schedules been established for back-up media?

Screening ESI for privilege. One of the greatest costs associated with the discovery of ESI is the potential waiver of privilege that could result from the inadvertent production of privileged material. The tremendous costs to screen ESI for privilege must be borne by the organization. In a healthcare organization, counsel will need to take added measure to ensure that no unauthorized protected health information is inadvertently produced to a requesting party.

Question for discussion:

- What will be the organization's policy and procedure with regard to screening for privilege?

Preparing for e-Discovery

E-discovery is a complex process that will require a multidisciplinary approach to successfully implement and manage. Developing a litigation response team, a plan, and policies are critical steps in the process. Healthcare organizations should complete the following 10 activities to prepare for e-discovery.

1. Establish a litigation response team with a designee from the legal, HIM, and IT departments
2. Review, revise, or develop an organizational information management plan and provide legal counsel with any and all previous plans developed by the organization
3. Identify the data owners or stewards within the organization
4. Review, revise, or develop an enterprise records retention schedule
5. Conduct thorough assessment of the locations, forms, and business and legal use for all legacy systems, back-up media, and orphaned data in existence
6. Review, revise, or develop organizational policies related to e-discovery
7. Review, revise, or develop organizational policy on e-mail management
8. Develop established approach and methodology to determine burdens and costs of producing electronically stored information
9. Identify designated person(s) responsible for establishing a legal hold within the organization and establish a process for communication and review of existing holds
10. Establish an organizational program to educate and train all management and staff on e-discovery compliance

AHIMA has a variety of resources on e-discovery available in the FORE Library: HIM Body of Knowledge at www.ahima.org. The September 2006 practice brief "The New Electronic Discovery Rule" provides a summary of key components of the FRCP and the impact on HIM and IT.

4. Develop Organizational Policy and Procedures

The next step in litigation response planning is development or updating of the organizational policies and procedures related to e-discovery. Organizations should have the following policy and procedures in place.

Preparation for a pretrial conference. This policy outlines the steps to complete prior to legal counsel attending a pretrial conference. The goal of this policy is to ensure that the organization adequately prepares for the pretrial conference, has researched key issues that will be addressed with the judge and plaintiff attorney during the conference, and understands what it is agreeing to in the discovery plan and the impact on pretrial activities.

Preservation and legal hold for health records and information. This policy outlines the process for preserving paper and electronic health records and related information when there is a reasonable anticipation of litigation. The policy guards against spoliation of evidence.

Retention, storage, and destruction of paper and electronic health information and records. This policy establishes the conditions and time periods for which paper-based and electronic health records will be stored, retained, and destroyed after they are no longer active for patient care or business purposes and to ensure appropriate availability of inactive records.

An enterprise record retention and destruction schedule should accompany this policy to provide a complete and accurate accounting of all relevant records within the organization.

Production and disclosure of electronic health information and records. This policy outlines the steps in the disclosure process for electronic and information records related to a legal proceeding. Many of these procedures would be managed through the release of information process within an HIM department.

5. Develop a System for Ongoing Monitoring and Evaluation

The response team's responsibilities extend to evaluating the efficacy of the organization's policies and procedures after implementation. This includes developing and regularly reviewing staff orientation and annual training materials and creating an ongoing audit and monitoring process.

Audit and monitoring activities can include audits of business process areas to determine compliance with e-discovery policies, as well as random audits of human resource files to verify staff training on e-discovery. The litigation response team should work with the compliance office to establish triggers and monitors to assess adherence to e-discovery policies throughout the organization.

References

AHIMA e-HIM Work Group on e-discovery. "New Electronic Discovery Civil Rule." *Journal of AHIMA* 77, no. 8 (Sept. 2006): 68A–H.

Allman, T. "Ruling Offers Lessons for Counsel on Electronic Discovery Abuse." *Washington Legal Foundation* 19 (October 2004).

Allman, T. "Fostering a Compliance Culture: The Role of the Sedona Guidelines." *The Information Management Journal* (March/April 2005): 54–61.

Baldwin-Stried, Kimberly. "e-discovery and HIM: How Amendments to the Federal Rules of Civil Procedure Will Affect HIM Professionals." *Journal of AHIMA* 77, no. 9 (Oct. 2006): 58–60.

Dimick, Chris. "e-discovery: Preparing for the Coming Rise in Electronic Discovery Requests." *Journal of AHIMA* 78, no. 5 (May 2007): 24–29.

Jurevic, A. "When Technology and Health Care Collide: Issues with Electronic Medical Records and Electronic Mail." University of Missouri Kansas City Law Review, Health Law Symposium, 1998.

Logan, D., J. Bace, and M. Gilbert. "Understanding e-discovery Technology." Gartner Research (ID Number: G00133224), 2005.

Marchand, L. "Discovery of Electronic Medical Records." American Trial Lawyers Association Annual Convention Reference Materials, 2001.

Patzakis, J. "How the New Federal Rules Will Likely Change e-discovery Practice." *The Metropolitan Corporate Counsel* 38 (June 2006).

Patzakis, J., and B. Murphy. "The New Federal e-discovery Rules and Their Impact." Guidance Software audio seminar, June 2006.

Pooley, J., and D. Shaw. "Finding Out What's There: Technical and Legal Aspects of Discovery." *Texas Intellectual Property Law Journal* 4 (Fall 1995).

Solomon, S. "The Ever-Increasing Legal Challenge of Change Precipitated by Technology, Compliance and Law." Paper presented at the 15th National Conference on Managing Electronic Records, May 2007, Chicago, IL.

US Courts. "Summary of the Report of the Judicial Conference Committee in Rules of Practice and Procedure." September 2005. Available online at www.uscourts.gov/rules.

Prepared by

AHIMA e-discovery Task Force:

Kim Baldwin-Stried Reich, MBA, MJ, RHIA, CHC, CPHQ
Deborah Beezley, RHIT
Michelle Dougherty, RHIA, CHP
Sandra Nunn, MA, RHIA, CHP
Lydia Washington, MS, RHIA, CPHIMS

Acknowledgments

Katherine Ball, MD
Jill Callahan Dennis, JD, RHIA
Neil Puller, MBA, MD

Article citation:

AHIMA e-discovery Task Force. "Litigation Response Planning and Policies for e-discovery." *Journal of AHIMA* 79, no. 2 (February 2008): 69–75

AHIMA Model e-Discovery Policies

Preparing for Pretrial Conference

AHIMA Model e-Discovery Policies			
Subject/Title	Preparing for Pretrial Conference		
		Revision History	
		Effective Date:	
Departments	Legal Services	*Original Issue Date:*	
Affected:	Health Information Management	*Last Reviewed:*	
	Information Technology	*Last Revision:*	

PURPOSE: The purpose of this policy is to outline the steps that must be taken prior to legal counsel attending a pretrial conference for a potential legal action. The goal of this policy is to ensure that the organization adequately prepares for the pretrial conference, has researched key issues that will be addressed with the Judge and plaintiff attorney during the conference, and understands what it is agreeing to in the discovery plan/Form 35 and the impact on pretrial activities.

SCOPE: This policy addresses the operational steps that must be taken after receiving notice of a legal action, which require participation in a pretrial conference as outlined in the Federal Rules of Civil Procedures. It does not address the steps that an organization must go through in order to plan for implementation of the e-discovery rule. This model policy addresses the Federal Rules of Civil Procedures that apply to proceedings in the federal court system. Organizations must research and tailor the policy to address state and local rules on e-discovery and legal process.

POLICY: It is the policy of this organization to comply with the Federal Rules of Civil Procedures and the e-discovery amendment. The organization will take steps to prepare for the pretrial conference to ensure that all information relevant to a case is identified, retained, and communicated appropriately. It is the policy to enter into an accurate discovery plan/Form 35 outlining the discovery plan and information.

PROCEDURE:

Notification of Pretrial Conference:

Responsible	Action
Legal	Upon notification that a legal proceeding has been filed with the court, the legal department will notify the litigation response team of the scheduling of a pretrial conference and schedule a meeting of the team.
Litigation Response Team	The team will meet to discuss the case and legal proceeding. If discussed as potential litigation or when subpoena received provide an update of the legal proceeding filed with the court. The team should discuss the following to outline information for the discovery plan/Form 35, which will be negotiated when the parties to the legal action meet and confer: • The type of information that is relevant to the case (including location, format, etc.) and the pertinent retention period • Implement steps to apply legal hold procedures if not in place • Identify privileged information • Review and update if applicable the organization's quick peek and cull back language • Review expected costs and other information that will be negotiated during the pretrial conference

Identifying Potential Sources of Relevant Information:

Responsible	Action
Litigation Response Team/ Data Owners/HIM	The litigation response team/data owners/HIM will identify the potential sources of information that may hold potentially relevant information. • Legal health record/EHR system, including source information systems (nursing, ED, lab, radiology, etc.) • Local area server for the office • Personal share or personal folders on server • Dedicated server for organization • Laptop and/or department computer • Home computer, Blackberry, and/or PDA • E-mail including archived e-mail and sent e-mail • E-mail trash bin, desktop recycle bin • Text/instant message archives • Removable storage media (e.g., disks, CDs, DVDs, memory sticks, and thumb drives) • Department/office files such as financial records • Personal desk files • Files of administrative personnel in department/office • Files located in department/office staff home • Web site archives

Responsible	Action
HIM and Data Owners	HIM and data owners will establish search parameters (patient identifiers, search terms, key words, etc.) and conduct the search process for information relevant to the case. They will also maintain a record of the systems searched, search parameters (terms), and search results.
IT	IT will provide assistance to HIM in the search and retrieval process for various systems and data sources.
HIM	HIM will screen or filter the search results, eliminating information that is not appropriate (wrong patient, not relevant, etc.).
Legal	Legal will review the content of the data/data sets found to determine relevancy to the proceeding and identify information that is considered privileged.
Legal and HIM	Legal and HIM will determine the final list of relevant data/data sets, location, and search parameters used to locate.
HIM and IT	HIM and IT will determine the format, the information will be disclosed, such as: • Print • ASCII • PDF • TIF • Screen shot • Mirror copy of data file • Review of material online
HIM, IT, and Legal	HIM, IT, and legal will calculate the costs for search, retrieval, and disclosure methods using the organization's established formula.

Identification of Privileged Information and Inadvertent Production:

Responsible	Action
Litigation Response Team	The team will identify the types of information that are considered privileged.
Legal	When reviewing the information identified through searches, legal will flag and pull information that is considered privileged and would not be disclosed.
HIM, IT, or Legal	If it is discovered that information considered privileged was inadvertently provided to the opposing party, the organization will notify the opposing party. The discovery plan/Form 35 should address the process and handling of electronic information inadvertently produced to the opposing party through the quick peek and cull-back agreement/language.

Providing Information for Discovery Plan/Form 35:

Responsible	Action
Legal	During the pretrial conference the parties to the litigation meet with the judge and agree to a discovery plan (documented on Form 35). It is important that the organization's attorney have accurate information in preparation for that meeting. Legal counsel should have accurate information on the data that is relevant to the case, the format, the forms of production, and the costs.
Legal and Litigation Response Team	Legal will update the litigation response team with the terms of the discovery response plan/Form 35 agreement that the organization must follow.

APPROVALS:

Legal Department Approval:		Date:	
HIM Department Approval:		Date:	
IT Department Approval:		Date:	
Specify Other Department		Date:	

Article citation:

AHIMA e-discovery Task Force. "AHIMA Model e-discovery Policies: Preparing for Pretrial Conference." *Journal of AHIMA* 79, no. 2 (February 2008): BoK Extras

AHIMA Model e-Discovery Policies

Preservation and Legal Hold for Health Information and Records

AHIMA Model e-Discovery Policies			
Subject/Title	Preservation and Legal Hold for Health Information and Records		Page __ of __
		Revision History:	
		Effective Date:	
Departments	Health Information Management	*Original Issue Date:*	
Affected:	Information Technology	*Last Reviewed:*	
	Legal Services and Compliance Services	*Last Revision:*	

PURPOSE: The purpose of this policy is to outline the process for preserving paper and electronic health records and related information when there is a reasonable anticipation of litigation to prevent spoliation of evidence.

SCOPE: This policy addresses the operational steps and communication process when litigation is anticipated and identifies the process to preserve and apply a legal hold on health information and records, whether paper-based or electronic. It applies to any health information/record regardless of whether it is maintained in the Health Information Management department or by the clinical, ancillary, or financial department that created it.

POLICY: It is the policy of the organization to preserve health information and records (paper and electronic) and related information that are or will potentially be utilized in litigation. It is the policy of the organization to place relevant records under a legal hold and suspend normal destruction practices to prevent against spoliation.

PROCEDURE:

Trigger Events and Application of a Legal Hold

Responsible	Action
Litigation Response Team	The team will identify the trigger events that may indicate the potential threat of litigation (such as receipt of a subpoena, unexpected negative care outcome, verbal communication of pending litigation, etc). Develop the communication process when a trigger event occurs between departments/individuals and the litigation response team. The following are examples of trigger events: • Any notice of a lawsuit • Charge of discrimination • Notice of claim • Demand letter from a lawyer • Meeting at which someone brings a lawyer • Challenge to a corrective action (if the employee alleges a violation of state/federal law such as discrimination, harassment, whistleblower, etc.) • Any person verbally telling the department that they intend to sue
Litigation Response Team	The team will receive communication about trigger event and evaluate situation. If there is a reasonable anticipation that litigation will follow, the team will review the potential issue and make a determination on whether to apply a legal hold to relevant information. The team will develop and define the process and decision making for deciding when to apply a legal hold. The Sedona Conference Commentary on Legal Holds provides the following list of factors to consider in making a decision: • The nature and specificity of the complaint or threat • The party making the claim • The position of the party making the claim • The business relationship between the accused and accusing parties • Whether the threat is direct, implied, or inferred • Whether the party making the claim is aware of the claim • The strength, scope, or value of a potential claim • The likelihood that data relating to a claim will be lost or destroyed • The significance of the data to the known or reasonably anticipated issues • Whether the company has learned of similar claims • The experience of the industry • Whether the relevant records are being retained for some other reason • Press and/or industry coverage of the issue directly pertaining to the client or of complaints brought against someone similarly situated in the industry
Litigation Response Team	The team will document the facts used at the time to decide whether there is a duty to preserve information.
Litigation Response Team	If determined that a legal hold is warranted the team will begin the preservation and legal hold processes.

Obligation to Identify, Locate, and Maintain Relevant Information

Responsible	Action
Litigation Response Team	Once litigation or potential litigation is identified, the response team must engage appropriate individuals to assist in identifying, locating, and maintaining relevant information (IT, Records Manager/HIM, and data owners/stewards of potentially relevant information). A legal hold team (a subset of the litigation response team) could be formed to follow through with appropriate departments and data owners/stewards. Note: To assist with this process consider developing a list of applications and the data owner/steward. This will streamline the process of identifying where potential information may be found, who to contact to search relevant databases, and who to contact to interview.
Legal Hold Team	Meet or communicate with applicable departments/data owners to determine the information available and identify the relevant information to be preserved (in all sources and formats) including information held by business associates. The following examples of potential sources to search are provided by The Sedona Conference Commentary on Legal Holds: • Local area server for the office • Personal share or personal folders on server • Dedicated server for organization • Laptop and/or department computer • Home computer, Blackberry, and/or PDA • E-mail including archived e-mail and sent e-mail • E-mail trash bin, desktop recycle bin • Removable storage media (e.g., disks, CDs, DVDs, memory sticks, and thumb drives) • Department/office files • Personal desk files • Files of administrative personnel in department/office • Files located in department/office staff home
Legal Hold Team and Data Owners/Stewards	The team will implement a process to suspend normal destruction and maintain relevant information in conformance with the legal hold notice.
IT/Security Manager/HIM (data center, server, and server manager, EDMS manager)	IT/Security Manager/HIM will preserve relevant information. The optimal method of preservation will be determined by the type of data and/or agreements made during a pretrial conference. Examples of preservation methods include: • Making a mirror of image of a hard drive • Sequestering or archiving information/records • Retain back-up media to prevent destruction • Take a "snapshot" of information at a point of time and retain on separate media onto something else • For e-mail and voicemail files sequester an account and transfer files for a specific span of time • For paper records make photocopy. If originals requested, sequester files to protect from loss, destruction or alteration.

Preservation/ Legal Hold Notice

Responsible	Action
Legal Hold Team	Once relevant information is identified provide a written notice of a legal hold to the department/data owner and identify the relevant information.
Legal Hold Team	Review the legal hold notices in effect. Periodically reissue or amend as needed.
Legal Hold Team Representative	Designate an individual to oversee legal hold notices and answer questions (e.g., someone from legal department who is part of the legal hold team).

Monitoring Legal Holds

Responsible	Action
Litigation Response Team	The team will implement a process to monitor legal holds to track compliance.
Legal Hold Team	The team will periodically query data owners to ensure they are complying with notice requirements.
Data Owners	Data owners will respond to query with confirmation that relevant information outlined in the legal hold notice continues to be maintained.
Compliance Officer	The compliance officer will periodically audit for compliance with legal hold notice and maintenance of relevant information.

Release of a Legal Hold

Responsible	Action
Litigation Response Team	Once it is determined that the legal hold is no longer necessary, the litigation response team will release the legal hold.
Legal Hold Team	The legal hold team will review other legal holds to ensure there isn't an overlap before notifying the data owners/departments of the release.
Legal Hold Team	The team will provide written notice that the legal hold has been lifted and resume normal retention and destruction processes. Include in the notice to the departments/data owners a list of applicable records that were under legal hold. Require a sign-off by the department/data owner.
HIM, IS. and Data Owners	If information was scheduled for destruction during the litigation hold period proceed with destruction process.
Compliance	Audit to ensure that information is not unnecessarily retained after the legal hold is lifted.

APPROVALS:

Legal Department Approval:		Date:	
HIM Department Approval:		Date:	
IT Department Approval:		Date:	
Specify Other Department		Date:	

Article citation:

AHIMA e-discovery Task Force. "AHIMA Model e-discovery Policies: Preservation and Legal Hold for Health Information and Records." *Journal of AHIMA* 79, no. 2 (February 2008): BoK Extras

AHIMA Model e-Discovery Policies

Retention, Storage, and Destruction of Paper and Electronic Health Information and Records

AHIMA Model e-Discovery Policy			
Subject/Title	Retention, Storage, and Destruction of Paper and Electronic Health Information and Records		Page __ of __
		Revision History	
		Effective Date:	
Departments Affected	Health Information Management, Information Technology, Legal Services Departments/Data Owners	*Original Issue Date:*	
		Last Reviewed:	
		Last Revision:	

PURPOSE: The purpose of this policy is to achieve a complete and accurate accounting of all relevant records within the organization; to establish the conditions and time periods for which paper-based and electronic health information and records will be stored, retained, and destroyed after they are no longer active for patient care or business purposes; and to ensure appropriate availability of inactive records.

SCOPE: This policy applies to all enterprise health information and records whether the information is paper-based or electronic. It applies to any health record, regardless of whether it is maintained in the Health Information Management Department or by the clinical or ancillary department that created it.

POLICY: It is the policy of this organization to maintain and retain enterprise health information and records in compliance with applicable governmental and regulatory requirements. The organization will adhere to retention schedules and destruction procedures in compliance with regulatory, business, and legal requirements.

Data Owners: Each department or unit that maintains patient health records, either in electronic or paper form, is required to designate a records management coordinator who will ensure that records in his or her area are preserved, maintained, and retained in compliance with records management policies and retention schedules established by the Health Information Management Department *[or other designated authority]*.

Property Rights: All enterprise health information and records generated and received are the property of the organization. No employee, by virtue of his or her position, has any personal or property right to such records even though he or she may have developed or compiled them.

Workforce Responsibility: All employees and agents are responsible for ensuring that enterprise health information and records are created, used, maintained, preserved, and destroyed in accordance with this policy.

Destruction of Enterprise Health Information and Records: At the end of the designated retention period for each type of health record and information, it will be destroyed in accordance with the procedures in this policy unless a legal hold/preservation order exists or is anticipated.

Unauthorized Destruction: The unauthorized destruction, removal, alteration, or use of health information and records is prohibited.

PROCEDURE:

Responsible	Action
Data Owner/ Departments	Data owners/departments will designate records coordinator for their areas and report that designation to the Records Committee and Litigation Response Team.
Record Committee	*[Note: This may be an existing committee, such as the Medical Record Committee, that has membership representing Legal, Compliance, IS/IT, Information Security, HIM, Clinical, and others as appropriate]* The record committee's role is to authorize any changes to the Retention, Storage, and Destruction policy and procedures; review and approve retention schedules and revisions to current retention schedules; address compliance audit finding; and review and approve control forms relating to business records.
HIM	HIM will convene the Record Committee as needed *[or at regular intervals]* and maintain responsibility for the following: • Review, maintain, publish, and distribute retention schedules and records management policies. • Audit compliance with records management (both electronic and paper) policies and retention schedules and report findings to Record Committee. • Serve as point of contact for Records Coordinators. • Provide training for Records Coordinators. Training will be provided on an individual basis to Records Coordinators and any individual or department that needs assistance. • Oversee operation of designated offsite record storage center(s) for archival storage of paper health records and information or serve as contract administrator for such services. • Contract for destruction of paper and electronic records and certification thereof.

Responsible	Action
IT/HIM/ Data Owners	IT/HIM/Data Owners will ensure that electronic storage of enterprise health information and records is carried out in conjunction with archiving and retention policies.
Records Coordinators	Records coordinators are responsible for implementing and maintaining records management programs for their designated areas. They will organize and manage online records management control forms relating to enterprise records and information in their areas of responsibility to accomplish the following: • Transfer records to storage • Identify, control, and maintain records in storage • Retrieve and/or return records from/to storage • Document the destruction of records and the deletion of records from the records inventory • Monitor the records management process Record coordinators will obtain (if not already trained) and maintain records management skills.
Legal Services	Legal Services serves as subject matter expert and provides counsel regarding records designations and legal and statutory requirements for records retention and pending legal matters. It ensures that access to or ownership of records is appropriately protected in all divestitures of property or lines of business or facility closures.

Guidelines for Retention of Records/Information and Schedules:

Responsible	Action
Record Retention	Unless otherwise stipulated, retention schedules apply to all records. Records will only be discarded when the maximum specified retention period has expired, the record is approved for destruction by the record owner, and a Certificate of Destruction is executed.
Non-record Retention	Non-records are maintained for as long as administratively needed, and retention schedules do not apply. Non-records may and should be discarded when the business use has terminated. For example, when the non-record information, such as an employee's personal notes, is transferred to a record, such as an incident report, the notes are no longer useful and should be discarded. Preliminary working papers and superseded drafts should be discarded, particularly after subsequent versions are finalized. Instances where an author or recipient of a document is unsure whether a document is a record as covered or described in this policy should be referred to the Compliance Officer for determination of its status and retention period.

(continued)

Responsible	Action
E-mail Communication Retention	Depending on content, e-mail messages between clinicians and between patients and clinicians and documents transmitted by e-mail may be considered records and are subject to this policy. If an e-mail message would be considered a record based on its content, the retention period for that e-mail message would be the same for similar content in any other format. The originator/sender of the e-mail message (or the recipient of a message if the sender is outside Organization) is the person responsible for retaining the message if that message is considered a record. Users must save e-mail messages in a manner consistent with departmental procedures for retaining other information of similar content. Users should be aware of *Messaging Policies* that establish disposal schedules for e-mail and manage their e-mail accordingly.
Development of Records Retention Schedules	Retention Schedule Determined by Law: All records will be maintained and retained in accordance with Federal and state laws and regulations. *[Note: attach minimum retention schedules to this policy]*. Electronic records must follow the same retention schedule as physical records, acknowledging the format and consolidated nature of records within an application or database. Changes to Retention Schedule: Proposed changes to the record retention schedules will be submitted to the Records Committee for initial review. The Records Committee, in consultation with the Legal Services Department, will research the legal, fiscal, administrative, and historical value of the records to determine the appropriate length of time the records will be maintained and provide an identifying code. The proposed revisions will be submitted to the Records Committee for review and approval. The approved changes will be published and communicated to the designated Records Coordinators. Retention of Related Computer Programs: Retention of records implies the inherent ability to retrieve and view a record within a reasonable time. Retained electronic data must have retained with it the programs required to view the data. Where not economically feasible to pay for maintenance costs on retired or obsolescent software only for the purpose of reading archived or retained data, then data may be converted to a more supportable format, as long as it can be demonstrated that integrity of the information is not degraded by the conversion. Data Owners should work closely with IT personnel in order to comply with this section. Retention of Records in Large Applications: Retention of data for large-scale applications, typically those that reside in the data center and are accessed by a larger audience, shall be the responsibility of the IT department. The Data Owner shall establish policy for the systems and format for the retained data consistent with the requirements of the Data Ownership policy *[reference policy]*.

Responsible	Action
Development of Records Retention Schedules *(continued)*	Retention of Records on Individual Workstations: Primary responsibility for retention of data created at the desktop level—typically with e-mail, Microsoft "Office" applications such as Word, Excel, PowerPoint, Access, or other specialized but locally run and saved computer applications—shall be with the user/author. The user/author will ensure that the documents are properly named and saved to be recognizable by the user in the future, and physically saved to a "shared drive." By saving a copy in this manner, IT will create an archive version of the saved document for a specified number of years after the user deletes the copy from the shared drive. Records with retention periods in excess of this period will require an alternative means of retention. Users are responsible for the security of any confidential information and/or protected health information created or maintained on their workstations.

Storage and Destruction Guidelines

Responsible	Action
Active/Inactive Records	Records are to be reviewed periodically by the Data Owner to determine if they are in the active, inactive, or destruction stage. Records that are no longer active will be stored in the designated off-site storage facility. Active stage is that period when reference is frequent and immediate access is important. Records should be retained in the office or close to the users. Data Owners, through their Records Coordinator, are responsible for maintaining the records in an orderly, secure, and auditable manner throughout this phase of the record life-cycle. Inactive stage is that period when records are retained for occasional reference and for legal reasons. Inactive records for which scheduled retention periods have not expired or records scheduled for permanent retention will be cataloged and moved to the designated off-site storage facility. Destruction stage is that period after records have served their full purpose, their mandated retention period, and finally are no longer needed.
Storage of Inactive Records	All inactive records identified for storage will be delivered with the appropriate Records Management Forms to the designated off-site storage facility where the records will be protected and stored and will remain accessible and cataloged for easy retrieval. Except for emergencies, the designated off-site storage facility will provide access to records during normal business hours.

(continued)

Responsible	Action
Records Destruction	General Rule: Records that have satisfied their legal, fiscal, administrative, and archival requirements may be destroyed in accordance with the Records Retention Schedules.
	Permanent Records: Records that cannot be destroyed include records of matters in litigation or records with a permanent retention. In the event of a lawsuit or government investigation, the applicable records that are not permanent cannot be destroyed until the lawsuit or investigation has been finalized. Once the litigation/investigation has been finalized, the record may be destroyed in accordance with the Records Retention Schedules but in no case shall records used in evidence to litigation be destroyed earlier than a specified number of years from the date of the settlement of litigation.
	Destruction of Records Containing Confidential Information: Records must be destroyed in a manner that ensures the confidentiality of the records and renders the information unrecognizable. The approved methods to destroy records include: *[Note: specify based on local, state, and federal rule; these could potentially include recycling, shredding, burning, pulping, pulverizing, and magnetizing.]* A Certificate of Destruction form must be approved and signed by the appropriate management staff prior to the destruction of records. The Certificate of Destruction shall be retained by the off-site storage facility manager.
	Destruction of Non-Records Containing Confidential Information: Destruction Non-Records containing personal health information or other forms of confidential corporate, employee, member, or patient information of any kind shall be rendered unrecognizable for both source and content by means of shredding, pulping, etc., regardless of media. This material shall be deposited in on-site, locked shred collection bins or boxed, sealed, and marked for destruction.
	Disposal of Electronic Storage Media: Electronic storage media must be assumed to contain confidential or other sensitive information and must not leave the possession of the organization until confirmation that the media is unreadable or until the media is physically destroyed.
	Disposal of Electronic Media: Electronic storage media such as CD-ROMS, tape reels, or floppy disks containing confidential or sensitive information may only be disposed of by approved destruction methods. These methods include: *[Note: specify based on local, state, and federal rules; these could potentially include: burning, shredding, or some other approach which renders the media unusable; degaussing, which uses electro-magnetic fields to erase data; or, preferred for magnetic media when media will not be physically destroyed, "zeroization" programs (a process of writing repeated sequences of ones and zeros over the information].* CD-ROMs, magneto-optical cartridges and other storage media that do not use traditional magnetic recording approaches must be physically destroyed.

Responsible	Action
Records Destruction *(continued)*	Disposal of IT Assets: Department managers must coordinate with the IT Department on disposing surplus property that is no longer needed for business activities according to Disposal of IT Assets Policy. Disposal of information system equipment, including the irreversible removal of information and software, must occur in accordance with approved procedures and will be coordinated by IT personnel.

APPROVALS:

Legal Department Approval:		Date:	
HIM Department Approval:		Date:	
IT Department Approval:		Date:	
[Specify Other Department]		Date:	

Article citation:

AHIMA e-discovery Task Force. "AHIMA Model e-discovery Policies: Retention, Storage, and Destruction of Paper and Electronic Health Information and Records." *Journal of AHIMA* 79, no. 2 (February 2008): BoK Extras

AHIMA Model e-Discovery Policies

Production and Disclosure of Health Information and Records for e-Discovery

AHIMA Model e-Discovery Policy			
Subject/Title	Production and Disclosure of Health Information and Records for e-Discovery		Page __ of __
		Revision History	
		Effective Date:	
Departments Affected	Health Information Management Information Technology Legal Services	*Original Issue Date:*	
		Last Reviewed:	
		Last Revision:	

PURPOSE: The purpose of this policy is to outline the steps in the production and disclosure process for health information and records related to e-discovery for pending litigation.

SCOPE: This policy addresses e-discovery production and disclosure procedures related to the Federal Rules of Civil Procedures. Health information and records include both paper and electronic data related to relevant patient medical records and enterprise sources.

POLICY: It is the policy of this organization to produce and disclose relevant information and records in compliance with applicable laws, court procedures, and agreements made during the litigation process.

PROCEDURE:

Accurate Patient Identification

Responsible	Action
HIM	For litigation involving an individual's medical records, verify the patient's identity in the master patient index, including demographic information and identifiers including the medical record number. *[Note: When conducting searches, it is critical to accurately identify the correct patient and relevant information.]*
HIM	Note multiple medical record numbers, identifiers, aliases, etc., that will be used during the search process to find relevant information.

Subpoena Receipt and Response

Responsible	Action
Litigation Response Team	Upon receipt, subpoenas should be reviewed to determine that all elements are contained, the parties and the purpose are clearly identified, and the scope of information requested is clear. • Validate the served subpoenas before official acceptance. The validation process includes at a minimum: • Verification of appropriate service of the subpoena and that the organization is under legal obligation to comply with it • Verification that seal and clerk of the court signature are present and valid Review of the venue and jurisdiction of court of the case and verification that the court is located within legal distance/mileage requirements.
HIM	Notify the Litigation Response Team that subpoena has been received and determine if a legal hold is in place. If not, the Litigation Response Team should determine whether a legal hold should be applied.
HIM	If the subpoena requests "any and all records," HIM and/or Legal Services should work with the judge and/or plaintiff attorney to clarify the scope and type of information being requested. *[Note: The e-discovery process will identify vast volumes of data, which can overwhelm a case; the parties should identify information that is necessary and relevant rather than providing all information.]*
Litigation Response Team/ Legal Services	Provide direction to HIM in the processing of the subpoena, including the specific information to produce, agreed-upon file formats and forms of production, whether an objection will be filed, timeframe to produce and disclose. and whether on-site testing/sampling will be conducted by requesting party.

Search and Retrieve Process

Responsible	Action
Litigation Response Team	Identify the sources of information that may hold potentially relevant information, such as: • Legal Health Record/EHR System (including source information systems such as nursing, ED, lab, radiology, etc.) • Local area server for the office • Personal share or personal folders on server • Dedicated server for organization • Laptop and/or department computer • Home computer, PDA • E-mail, including archived e-mail and sent e-mail • E-mail trash bin, desktop recycle bin • Text/instant message archives

Responsible	Action
Litigation Response Team *(continued)*	• Removable storage media (e.g., disks, CDs, DVDs, memory sticks, and thumb drives) • Department/office files such as financial records • Personal desk files • Files of administrative personnel in department/office • Files located in department/office staff home • Web site archives
HIM, Data Owners	Based on direction from the litigation response team on the potential locations of relevant information and the information agreed upon in the discovery plan and/or subpoena, establish search parameters (patient identifiers, search terms, key words, etc.) and conduct the search process. Maintain a record of the systems searched, search methodology, search parameters (terms), and search results.
IT	Provide assistance to HIM and Data Owners in the search and retrieval process for various systems and data sources.
HIM, Data Owners	Screen or filter the search results, eliminating inappropriate information (e.g., wrong patient, outside the timeframe, not relevant to the proceeding, etc.).
Legal Services	Review the content of the data/data sets found to determine relevancy to the proceeding and identify information that is considered privileged.
Legal Services, HIM, Data Owners	Determine the final list of relevant data/data sets, location, and search methodology.

Production of Records/Data

Responsible	Action
HIM, Data Owners, IT	Determine the format in which the information will be disclosed, such as: paper, ASCII, PDF, TIF, screen shot, mirror copy of data file, or review of material on-line. The format will vary depending on data, source, and agreement made in the Discovery Plan/Form 35.
HIM, Data Owners, IT	Produce the information in the agreed-upon format as outlined in the discovery plan/Form 35.
Legal Services, HIM, Data Owners, IT	Mask, redact, or retract non-relevant, privileged, or confidential information (such as on a different patient) as appropriate.
Legal Services	Conduct final review of information before disclosing to requesting party.
Legal Services	Retain a duplicate of information disclosed to requesting party.

Charges for Copying and Disclosure

Responsible	Action
HIM, Data Owners, IT	For the information searched and disclosed, calculate the costs for search, retrieval, and disclosure methods using the organization's established formula and governmental formulas for reproduction charges.
HIM	Invoice requesting parties for allowable charges related to reproduction of health information and records.
Legal Services	Determine whether other expenses may be charged in accordance with the discovery plan or negotiation with litigants and/or judge.

Testing and Sampling

Responsible	Action
Legal Services	A party to the legal proceeding may request to test and sample the search and retrieve methodology. Testing and sampling should be discussed and agreed upon during the pretrial conference and part of the discovery plan, including whether an external party will test and sample the search and retrieve methodologies. The costs and charges should also be determined and negotiated.
HIM, Data Owners	Retain information on all of the searches, including methodology, key words, and systems in case the methodology has to be recreated for testing purposes and to determine if sample was statistically valid.
Litigation Response Team, HIM	Assign a monitor for the outside party during their testing protocols.

Attorney/Third Party Request to Review Electronic Data

Responsible	Action
Litigation Response Team	Determine the procedures for allowing an attorney or third party to review the electronic records and search results on-line. This includes where the review will occur, system access controls, monitoring during the review session, and the charges, if any.
Legal Services, IT, HIM, Data Owners	Mask, redact, or retract non-relevant, privileged, or confidential information (such as on a different patient) as appropriate.
HIM, Data Owners	Verify the outside party is allowed access to the record and systems by reviewing all supporting documentation (e.g., signed consent, credentials from retained firm, etc.).
HIM, Data Owners	Prepare for access by identifying the types of information that party is allowed to access. If an authorization has been signed by patient or legal representative, allow access to legal medical record and/or other information as outlined in the authorization. If other types of information will be reviewed, access is allowed based on the subpoena, court order, state/federal statutes, or agreed-upon discovery plan.

Responding to Interrogatories, Deposition, Court Procedures

Responsible	Action
Legal Services	Legal Services manages the process for completion of the interrogatories and will coordinate processes related to a deposition and testifying in court.
HIM (official record custodian)	HIM may provide information for an interrogatory, be deposed, or testify in court. HIM is the official custodian of the record and can testify whether the records were kept in the normal course of business and the authenticity of the records. In addition, HIM also addresses the good faith operations related to records management, retention/destruction, and the search and retrieval process/parameters.
IT (official system custodian)	IT may provide information for an interrogatory, be deposed, or testify in court. IT is the official custodian of the information system and may testify about the technical infrastructure, system architecture, security practices, source applications, and the good faith operations from a technical infrastructure perspective.
Data Owners	Data owners may provide information for an interrogatory, be deposed, or testify in court. The data owners may testify about the specific issues related to their department/business process area.
Primary/Direct Custodian	Primary/direct custodians may provide information for an interrogatory, be deposed, or testify in court. The primary/direct custodians are those person(s) who work with the data directly or have direct involvement/ knowledge of the events the litigation. For example, a staff nurse who has made an entry into the medical record and is knowledgeable about the events of a case in litigation.
Business Associates/ Third Parties	Business Associates/Third Parties may provide information for an interrogatory, be deposed, or testify in court. These include contractors and others who serve a variety of functions associated with a party's information but who themselves are not parties to the litigation. Examples include Internet service providers, application service providers such as a claims clearinghouse, and other providers who provide services ranging from off-site data storage to complete outsourcing of the IT Department.

APPROVALS:

Legal Department Approval:		Date:	
HIM Department Approval:		Date:	
IT Department Approval:		Date:	
[Specify Other Department]		Date:	

Article citation:

AHIMA e-discovery Task Force. "AHIMA Model e-discovery Policies: Production and Disclosure of Health Information and Records for e-discovery." *Journal of AHIMA* 79, no. 2 (February 2008): BoK Extras

Developing a Legal Health Record Policy

Health records serve a variety of purposes. Their primary purpose is to document the care and services provided to patients. However, health records must also be maintained for business and evidentiary purposes.

In order to serve as business records, health records must be maintained in a manner that complies with applicable regulations, accreditation standards, professional practice standards, and legal standards. These standards may vary based on care setting, legal jurisdiction, and location.

Therefore, an organization must identify the content required for its legal health record as well as the standards for maintaining the integrity of that content. This applies regardless of the media used to create and store health records—paper, electronic, or hybrid.

This practice brief guides healthcare organizations in creating a legal health record policy for business and disclosure purposes. It provides considerations and questions that organizations transitioning to electronic health records (EHRs) should address. (Additional considerations for specialty institutions and specialty records such as behavioral health are not addressed in this article.)

This practice brief is not intended as legal advice. Organizations should consult with their legal counsel to develop their legal health record policy.

Legal Health Record Policy Template

Policy Name: The Health Record for Legal and Business Purposes

Effective Date:

Departments Affected: HIM, Information Systems, Legal Services, *[any additional departments affected]*

(continued)

Purpose: This policy identifies the health record of *[organization]* for business and legal purposes and to ensure that the integrity of the health record is maintained so that it can support business and legal needs.

Scope: This policy applies to all uses and disclosures of the health record for administrative, business, or evidentiary purposes. It encompasses records that may be kept in a variety of media including, but not limited to, electronic, paper, digital images, video, and audio. It excludes those health records not normally made and kept in the regular course of the business of *[organization]*.

Note: The determining factor in whether a document is considered part of the legal health record is not where the information resides or its format, but rather how the information is used and whether it is reasonable to expect the information to be routinely released when a request for a complete health record is received. The legal health record excludes health records that are not official business records of a healthcare provider. Organizations should seek legal counsel when deciding what constitutes the organization's legal health record.

Policy: It is the policy of *[organization]* to create and maintain health records that, in addition to their primary intended purpose of clinical and patient care use, will also serve the business and legal needs of *[organization]*.

It is the policy of *[organization]* to maintain health records that will not be compromised and will support the business and legal needs of *[organization]*.

Responsibilities

It is the responsibility of *[the health records manager or other designated position]* to:

- Work in conjunction with information services, legal services, and *[other stakeholders]* to create and maintain a matrix or other document that tracks the source, location, and media of each component of the health record. *[Reference an addendum or other source where the health record information is found.]*
- Identify any content that may be used in decision making and care of the patient that may be external to the organization (outside records and reports, PHRs, e-mail, etc.) that is not included as part of the

legal record because it was not made or kept in the regular course of business.

- Develop, coordinate, and administer a plan that manages all information content, regardless of location or form that comprises the legal health record of *[organization]*.
- Develop, coordinate, and administer the process of disclosure of health information.
- Devise and administer a health record retention schedule that complies with applicable regulatory and business needs.
- *[Other responsibilities]*

It is the responsibility of the information services department *[or other appropriate department(s)]* to:

- Ensure appropriate access to information systems containing components of the health record
- Execute the archiving and retention schedule pursuant to the established retention schedule
- *[Other responsibilities]*

[Additional responsibilities for other individuals or departments]

Maintaining EHR Integrity

As EHR systems become more prevalent, more healthcare organizations need to redefine their legal health record policy. Many EHR systems have limitations that may affect their use for legal purposes. However, regardless of the media they use, organizations must have a single set of health information that forms their legal health record.

Organizations that have transitioned to or are in the process of transitioning to EHRs must consider the following issues to maintain the integrity of the legal health record. These issues will need to be addressed procedurally. They can be addressed either as part of the legal health record policy or in separate policies.

During the transition to electronic health records, organizations should document the information that comprises the health record for business and legal purposes, the various sources and location of the information, and the media in which the information are maintained. This document can then be used to identify the information that will be disclosed upon receipt of an authorized request for health records.

Health information exchange. Healthcare organizations should develop policies and procedures addressing acceptance and retention of documents, images, waveforms, and other information received from external facilities. Generally physicians should determine the efficacy of the information received. The decision on whether to include the information in the legal health record should be based on its content and clarity. If acceptance is not possible, the policy should further address the retention or destruction of non-compatible information.

Downtime documentation. To ensure an accurate legal record, organizations should develop a procedure addressing documentation when EHR systems are unavailable due to planned or unplanned downtime. All clinical staff should be instructed to immediately begin documenting patient care on downtime health record forms according to the policy. The start and stop times of the downtime should be documented in the health record to ensure accuracy of the legal record.

The documentation process should account for the length of downtime. For example, if the system is unavailable for less than 30 minutes, an organization may decide that the information documented on paper will be entered into the EHR once the system becomes available.

The pros and cons of transferring downtime documentation into the EHR must be fully evaluated. For example, one benefit is having all information in one location with no need to maintain two systems. However, long downtimes could result in large amounts of paper documentation, and it may not be feasible to enter this information at a later date.

A multidisciplinary group of individuals representing physicians, nurses, allied health, HIM, compliance, and IT should be included in this discussion. Organizations may want to seek input from their vendors to ensure that the EHR application meets the organization's requirements for entering information after the fact. Vendors can also advise if their systems can indicate the existence of a separate paper record, if one exists.

Critical data to enter into the EHR post-downtime might include those elements that the EHR uses to calculate totals (e.g., intake and output) and data that have patient safety rules and alerts (e.g., medications, height, and weight).

The policy should address the timeliness of data entry post-downtime, staff responsible for entry, and how original paper documents will be retained, entered into the EHR, or scanned.

Document completion (lockdown). Organizations must determine when users can no longer create or make changes to electronic documentation. Organizations with several source systems (i.e., systems that do not automatically record the date and time of entries and systems that allow editing documents without tracking changes) should consider locking down documents at some determined time after a patient encounter. This will help ensure health records are accurate and meet spoliation expectations.

Because EHRs allow users to access the information from anywhere access is allowed, the EHR documentation function must control when an individual can document in an EHR. There may be limitations with how the EHR handles this function, which organizations will need to factor into their policies. Organizations must determine how long the documentation function will be available. The multidisciplinary group should be included in discussions to determine when electronic documentation will be considered complete.

Amendments and corrections. Procedures should address how amendments and corrections should be made to the EHR. Amendments and corrections should be in chronological order and included with the original document both online and in printed format. If possible, the system should clearly identify amendments including date, time, and author. Corrections to the EHR should be visible to anyone with access. Identification and tracking of corrections should not be limited to a background or back-end program visible only to IT staff.

Authentication. The person entering the data should authenticate individual health record entries. Electronic entry should automatically record the person documenting the care with his or her full name and credentials, the date, and time. Consideration should also be given to situations where multiple individuals are responsible for creating documentation. An admission assessment, for example, may contain sections requiring input from a variety of caregivers. An organization's policy should address how this is accomplished in coordination with the functionality within the EHR application.

There may be times when an individual forgets to enter documentation at the time of care delivery and another individual makes entries on his or her behalf. Policy must indicate when this is appropriate and how it will be handled based on functionality within the EHR. To ensure adherence to state regulatory requirements, organizations should also review state-specific guidelines on authenticating orders.

Documents prepared outside the EHR (e.g., transcribed documents and scanned images) should be assigned an electronic signature that is automatically date- and time-stamped. This type of authentication should clearly state "electronically signed" to identify the source of the document. Authentication of each health record entry should be visible to anyone with access. Authentication should not be limited to a background or back-end program visible only to IT staff. Authentications should be readable when EHR documents are printed.

Organizations should also define their cosignature policy and procedures including the positions that require cosignatures. The policy and procedures should outline how and where cosignatures should be documented (e.g., whether the cosignature occurs in the designated EHR, the source system, or the scanning system). The cosignature method should be evaluated to determine whether documentation will be considered legal if two people need to authenticate the same documentation.

If digital signatures are used in the EHR, staff will not be able to cosign, as the second signature will invalidate the first signature along with the documentation. Organizations may need to consider allowing the first author to indicate that they have reviewed the documentation and the second person to actually authenticate the information. If the EHR does not include digital signatures for authentication, the process of cosigning done on paper should be imitated in the EHR.

Timing of cosignatures should be addressed in policy as well. Some states regulate the timing of cosignatures on verbal orders. The Centers for Medicare and Medicaid Services' guidelines for physicians at teaching hospitals state that "the teaching physicians must review with each resident during or immediately after each visit the beneficiary's medical history, physical exam, diagnosis, and record of tests and therapies."[1] From a legal perspective, cosignatures should not be done once a shift while supervising students as it appears that oversight might not be managed in a timely manner.

Versioning. Organizations must address management of document versions. This will relate primarily to transcribed reports that are made available for viewing prior to authentication or review by the author. Organizations must decide whether all versions of a document will be displayed or just the final version; who has access to the various versions of a document; and how the availability of versions will be flagged in the EHR. A multidisciplinary group of physicians, risk management, HIM, and IT professionals should be included in the discussion.

An organization risks severe legal implications if it is unable to produce the original report after information was initially distributed or made available in the EHR and then later changed or updated. It is acceptable for a draft of a dictated and transcribed note or report to be changed before authentication unless there is reason to believe the changes are suspect and don't reflect actual events or actions.

Organization policy should define the acceptable period of time allowed for a document to remain in draft form before the author reviews and approves it (e.g., 24 to 72 hours). Once a document is no longer considered a draft or has been authenticated, any changes or alterations should be made following the procedures for a correction, late entry, or amendment. The original document must be maintained along with the new revised document.

Metadata. Organizations need to be aware of the metadata stored in their EHR systems. Metadata will not be routinely disclosed as part of the legal health record, but this information could be requested for legal purposes as part of electronic discovery. Organizations should determine how long this information must be kept. Data retention policies should include metadata.

Clinical decision support. Currently there are no generally accepted rules on including decision support such as system-generated notifications, prompts, and alerts as part of the legal record. The decision is up to individual organizations, with input from physicians, legal counsel, risk management, and administration.

At a minimum the EHR should include documentation of the clinician's actions in response to decision support. This documentation is evidence of the clinician's decision to follow or disregard decision support. The organization should define the extent of exception documentation required (e.g., what no documentation means).

Definitions

Organizations may also find it helpful to include the following definitions in their legal health record policy. Other key terms included in the organization's final policy should be defined and added to this list.

Business record: "a recording/record made or received in conjunction with a business purpose and preserved as evidence or because the information has value. Because this information is created, received, and maintained as evidence and information by an organization or person, in pursuance of legal obligation or in the transaction of business, it must consistently deliver a full and accurate record with no gaps or additions."[2]

Data: basic facts about people, processes, measurements, and conditions represented in dates, numerical statistics, images, and symbols. An unprocessed collection or representation of raw facts, concepts, or instructions in a manner suitable for communication, interpretation, or processing by humans or automatic means.[3]

Data element: a combination of one or more data entities that forms a unit or piece of information, such as patient identifier, a diagnosis, or treatment.[4]

Electronic health record: medical information compiled in a data-gathering format for retention and transferral of protected information via secured, encrypted communication line. The information can be readily stored on an acceptable storage medium such as compact disc.[5]

Evidence: information that a fact finder may use to decide an issue. Information that makes a fact or issue before court or other hearing more or less probable.[6]

Legal health record: AHIMA defines the legal health record as "generated at or for a healthcare organization as its business record and is the record that would be released upon request. It does not affect the discoverability of other information held by the organization. The custodian of the legal health record is the health information manager in collaboration with information technology personnel. HIM professionals oversee the operational functions related to collecting, protecting, and archiving the legal health record, while information technology staff manage the technical infrastructure of the electronic health record."[7]

The legal health record is a formally defined legal business record for a healthcare organization. It includes documentation of healthcare services provided to an individual in any aspect of healthcare delivery by a healthcare organization.[8, 9] The health record is individually identifiable data in any medium, collected and directly used in documenting healthcare or health status. The term also includes records of care in any health-related setting used by healthcare professionals while providing patient care services, reviewing patient data, or documenting observations, actions, or instructions.[10]

Metadata: descriptive data that characterize other data to create a clearer understanding of their meaning and to achieve greater reliability and quality of information. Metadata consist of both indexing terms and attributes.[11]

Original document: an authentic writing as opposed to a copy.[12]

Personal health record: an electronic, universally available, lifelong resource of health information needed by individuals to make health decisions. Individuals own and manage the information in the PHR, which comes from healthcare providers and the individual. The PHR is maintained in a secure private environment, with the individual determining access rights. The PHR is separate from and does not replace the legal health record of any provider.[13]

Regular course of business: doing business in accordance with the normal practice of business and custom, as opposed to doing it differently because an organization may be or is being sued.[14]

Source systems: the systems in which data were originally created.

- **Primary source system:** an information system that is part of the overall clinical information system in which documentation is most commonly first entered or generated.
- **Source of legal health record:** the permanent storage system where the documentation for the legal health record is held.

Appendix A: Developing a Legal Health Record Policy

Notes

1. Centers for Medicare and Medicaid Services. "Documentation Guidelines for E&M Services." Available online at www.cms.hhs.gov/MLNEdWebGuide/25_EMDOC.asp.
2. AHIMA e-HIM Work Group on e-discovery. "New Electronic Discovery Civil Rule." *Journal of AHIMA* 77, no. 8 (Sept. 2006): 68A–H.
3. AHIMA e-HIM Work Group on the Legal Health Record. "Update: Guidelines for Defining the Legal Health Record for Disclosure Purposes." *Journal of AHIMA* 76, no. 8 (Sept. 2005): 64A–G.
4. Ibid.
5. Ibid.
6. Ibid.
7. Ibid.

8. Amatayakul, Margret, et al. "Definition of the Health Record for Legal Purposes." *Journal of AHIMA 72,* no. 9 (Oct. 2001): 88A–H.
9. AHIMA e-HIM Work Group on the Legal Health Record. "Update: Guidelines for Defining the Legal Health Record for Disclosure Purposes."
10. Ibid.
11. Fenton, Susan, Kathy Giannangelo, Crystal Kallem, et al. "Data Standards, Data Quality, and Interoperability." *Journal of AHIMA 78,* no. 2 (Feb. 2007): 65–68.
12. AHIMA e-HIM Work Group on the Legal Health Record. "Update: Guidelines for Defining the Legal Health Record for Disclosure Purposes."
13. AHIMA e-HIM Personal Health Record Work Group. "The Role of the Personal Health Record in the EHR." *Journal of AHIMA 76,* no. 7 (Jul.–Aug. 2005): 64A–D.
14. AHIMA e-HIM Work Group on the Legal Health Record. "Update: Guidelines for Defining the Legal Health Record for Disclosure Purposes."

References and Resources

Relevant State and Federal Laws and Regulations

California Civil Discovery Law. Available online at http://californiadiscovery.findlaw.com/index.htm.

Discovery Resources. Available online at www.discoveryresources.org.

"Federal Rules of Civil Procedure." December 1, 2006. Available online at http://judiciary.house.gov/media/pdfs/printers/109th/31308.pdf.

Findlaw. Available online at http://findlaw.com.

The Library of Congress. Thomas. Available online at http://thomas.loc.gov.

LexisNexis. Law Library. Available online at www.lexisnexis.com/applieddiscovery/lawLibrary/default.asp.

National Conference of State Legislatures. Available online at www.ncsl.org.

US Courts. Available online at www.uscourts.gov/rules.

US Courts. "Summary of the Report of the Judicial Conference Committee on Rules of Practice and Procedure." Available online at www.uscourts.gov/rules/jc09-2000/Summ.htm.

Accreditation Standards

Joint Commission. "The Joint Commission Standards." Available online at www.jointcommission.org/Standards.

Practice Standards

AHIMA Electronic Health Record Practice Council. "Resolution on the Legal Health Record." 2006. Available online in the FORE Library: HIM Body of Knowledge at www.ahima.org.

AHIMA e-HIM Work Group on the Legal Health Record. "Update: Maintaining a Legally Sound Health Record—Paper and Electronic." *Journal of AHIMA* 76, no. 10 (Nov.–Dec. 2005): 64A–L.

AHIMA e-HIM Work Group on the Legal Health Record. "The Legal Process and Electronic Health Records." *Journal of AHIMA* 76, no. 9 (Oct. 2005): 96A–C.

AHIMA Work Group on Electronic Health Records Management. "The Strategic Importance of Electronic Health Records Management." Appendix A: Issues in Electronic Health Records Management. *Journal of AHIMA* 75, no. 9 (Oct. 2004): Web extra.

Black's Law Dictionary 8th ed. 2004. See Hannah v. Heeter, 213 W.Va. 704, 584 S.E.2d 560 (W.Va. 2003).

Cottrell, Carlton. "Legal Health Record: A Component of Overall EHR Strategy." *Journal of AHIMA* 78, no. 3 (Mar. 2007): 56–57, 66.

Kohn, Deborah. "When the Writ Hits the Fan." *Journal of AHIMA* 75, no. 8 (Sept. 2004): 40–44.

McWay, Dana C. Legal Aspects of Health Information Management. Albany, NY: Delmar Publishers, 1997.

Patzakis, John. "How the New Federal Rules Will Likely Change eDiscovery Practice." The Metropolitan Corporate Counsel, June 2006. Available online at www.metrocorpcounsel.com.

Quinsey, Carol Ann. "Is 'Legal EHR' a Redundancy?" *Journal of AHIMA* 78, no. 2 (Feb. 2007): 56–57.

The Sedona Conference Working Group Series. "The Sedona Conference Glossary for e-discovery of Digital Information Management." May 2005. Available online at www.sedonaconference.org.

The Sedona Conference Working Group Series. "The Sedona Principles Addressing Electronic Document Production." July 2005. Available online at www.sedonaconference.org.

The Sedona Conference Working Group Series. "The Sedona Guidelines for Managing Information and Records in the Electronic Age." September 2005. Available online at www.sedonaconference.org.

Tomes, Jonathan P. "Spoliation of Medical Evidence." *Journal of AHIMA* 76, no. 9 (Oct. 2005): 68–72.

University of Sydney. "Records Management Services." Available online at www. usyd.edu.au/arms/rms/body.htm.

Withers, Kenneth J., Esq. Federal Judicial Center and Sedona Conference Observer, MER Conference, Chicago, IL, May 24, 2006.

Prepared by

Members of the AHIMA EHR Practice Council:

> Kathleen Addison
> Barbara Demster, RHIA
> Terri Hall, RHIT
> Beth Liette, RHIA
> Keith Olenik, MA, RHIA, CHP
> Mary Ellen Mahoney, MS, RHIA
> Ann Tegen
> Lydia Washington, MS, RHIA, CPHIMS
> Victoria Weaver, RHIA
> Lou Ann Wiedemann, MS, RHIA

Article citation:

AHIMA EHR Practice Council. "Developing a Legal Health Record Policy." *Journal of AHIMA* 78, no. 9 (October 2007): 93–97.

Developing a Legal Health Record Policy: Appendix A

The tables below provide examples of a matrix tool that can help organizations identify and track the paper and electronic portions of the legal health record during and up to the full implementation of a paperless environment. Items for special consideration as to whether to include on the matrix may include those listed below. It is up to each individual organization to determine what health information is considered a part of its legal health record.

- **Alerts, reminders, pop-ups**
- **Continuing Care Records** (unless used in the provision of patient care)
- **Administrative data/documents:** patient-identifiable data used for administrative, regulatory, healthcare operations, and payment (financial) purposes
- **Derived data/documents:** information aggregated or summarized from patient records so that there are no means to identify patients.
- **Data/documents:** documentation of patient care that took place in the ordinary course of business by all healthcare providers.
- **Data from source systems:** written results of tests. Data from which interpretations, summaries, notes, flowcharts, etc., are derived.
- **New technologies:** audio files of dictation or patient telephone calls, handwritten nursing shift-to-shift reports, telephone consultation audio files, videos of office visits, and videos of procedures or telemedicine consultation.
- **Personal health records (PHRs):** copies of PHRs that are created, owned, and managed by the patient and are provided to a healthcare organization (s) might be considered part of the legal health record if so defined by the organization.
- **Research records:** organizational policy should differentiate whether research records are part of the legal health record and how these records will be kept.
- **Discrete structured data.** Laboratory orders/refills, orders/medication orders/MARs, online charting and documentation, and any detailed charges.
- **Diagnostic image data:** CT, MRI, ultrasound, nuclear medicine, etc.
- **Signal tracing data:** EKG, EEG, fetal monitoring signal tracings, etc.

- **Audio data:** heart sounds, voice dictations, annotations, etc.
- **Video data:** ultrasound, cardiac catheterization examinations, etc.
- **Text data:** radiology reports, transcribed reports, UBS, itemized bills, etc.
- **Original analog document—document image data:** signed patient consent forms, handwritten notes, drawings, etc.

Legal Health Record Matrix

Type of Document	Media Type: Paper (P) or Electronic (E)*	Primary Source System Application (non-paper)	Source of the Legal Health Record	Electronic Storage Start Date	Stop Printing Start Date	Fully Electronic Record (drill down composition)
History and physical	P/E	Transcription system	EHR	1/2/2007	3/2/2007	12/17/2007
Physician orders	E	CPOE system	EHR	1/2/2007	3/2/2007	12/17/2007
EKG	P					

*Includes scanned images

Maintaining the Legal EHR: Verification Legend Document Principles

Report/Document Type	Audit	Authentication	Authorship	Copy/ Paste	Amend	Correct	Clarify
Encounter history	0*	0	0	X*	0	0	0
Encounter physical	0	0	0	X	0	0	0
Medical history	0	0	0	X	0	0	0

0* Allowed and monitored—based on reported and randomized audits to determine adherence to policies and procedures for accurate, timely, and complete documentation principles.
X* Prohibited and monitored—based on reported and randomized audits to determine prohibited use of copy and past, pull forward, etc.

Article citation:

"Developing a Legal Health Record Policy: Appendix A." *Journal of AHIMA* 78, no. 9 (October 2007): web extra.

Electronic Signature, Attestation, and Authorship (Updated)

Editor's note: This update supplants the October 2003 practice brief "Implementing Electronic Signatures."

Electronic health record (EHR) systems provide the ability to sign entries electronically; however, implementing and using e-signatures is complex. This practice brief provides insight into the technology used to implement e-signatures, the related health IT standards, the regulatory environment, and recommendations on best practices.

This online version of the practice brief provides additional e-signature resources, tools, a glossary, and best practices to assist HIM professionals with EHR implementation and policy development.

While this practice brief addresses an organization's internal approach to determining e-signature policy and procedures, the foundational principles should extend beyond an organization's operations to external health information exchange efforts and participation agreements with HIE partners. As the healthcare industry evolves, an HIE's business plan and supporting functions must include valid, legal, consistent, and agreed-upon e-signature methods of nonrepudiation for use by all participants.

An Evolving Definition of E-Signature

The EHR has changed certain concepts and terms related to signatures. In the past, HIM professionals identified the act of signing an entry as authentication. However, this definition has evolved.

In EHRs, **authentication** is the security process of verifying a user's identity that authorizes the individual to access the system (e.g., the sign-on process). Authentication is important because it assigns responsibility to the user for entries he or she creates, modifies, or views. Attestation, on the other hand, is the act of applying an e-signature to the content, showing authorship and legal responsibility for a particular unit of information.[1]

Signatures, like medical records, can be either **analog** (e.g., stored on paper and unable to be read by a computer) or **digital** (e.g., stored on electronic media such as disks that can be read by a computer). The term *electronic signature* is frequently used in references and regulations in reference to signatures in a digital format. However, an **electronic signature** is a generic, technology-neutral term for the various ways that an electronic record can be signed (attested). It can include a digitized image of a signature, a biometric identifier, a secret code or PIN, or a digital signature.

Regardless of the type used, a signature serves three main purposes:

- **Intent:** an electronic signature is a symbol that signifies intent such as an approval of terms, confirmation that the signer reviewed and approved the content, or the signer authored the document and approves the content.
- **Identity:** the signature identifies the person signing.
- **Integrity:** a signature guards the integrity of the document against repudiation (the signer claiming the entry is invalid) or alteration.[2]

In EHRs, e-signatures encompass a broad range of technologies and methods, ranging from an "I agree" button in a clickthrough agreement, to an electronic tablet that accepts a handwritten signature, to a digital signature cryptographically tied to a digital ID or certificate.

Signature mechanisms that are typically found in EHRs today are listed in the sidebar at right. In today's environment, the type of individual software application drives the production of clinical documentation in the medical record, therein also driving the method and applicability of e-signatures. Limitations of an individual system's requirements and the flexibility of how those signatures are applied will continue to depend on system specifics for these applications.

Laws, Regulations, and Electronic Signature Acts

Since the advent of fax machines, handwritten signatures have been accepted electronically. With the rise in technology, there has been an influx of laws and regulatory agencies providing standards for use of e-signatures.

However, there is no single overwhelmingly accepted standard, law, or regulation, and organizations must access individual resources to review existing language specific to e-signatures, attestation, and authorship of medical record documents in an EHR. Unfortunately, these sources may contradict one another, making it even more difficult for the organization to determine its policy.

Typical E-Signature Mechanisms

Signature mechanisms typically found in EHRs today are listed below in order of their strength—level 1 is the weakest and level 3 the strongest.

Level 1—Digitized Signature: an electronic representation (applied image) of a handwritten signature. The image may be created by various methods, such as a signature pad, scanning a wet signature, or digital photography. The signature may be captured in real time (at the time the user applies the signature), or a previously saved image may be applied. A digitized signature is the weakest form of e-signature because someone could acquire a copy of the image of the handwritten signature and forge an electronic document.

Digitized signatures are often used for documents such as patient consents, agreements, and authorizations. They may also be used or preferred for documents that are printed and shared with physicians outside the healthcare organization, particularly for transcribed documents such as consultations and letters that are distributed to referring physicians. Organizations should develop policies to ensure readability and identification of the signer of digitized signatures.

Level 2—Button, PIN, Biometric, or Token: a frequently used e-signature methodology in EHR systems includes clicking a button or entering a unique personal identification number (PIN), electronic identification, token, or biometric scan at the completion of an entry for the signature process. EHR systems and organization policy should require some action that represents this signing process, such as pushing an attest button.

To strengthen the signature (which in turn strengthens the integrity of the record), healthcare organizations can add more tiers of security to the signature, such as a unique PIN, biometric, or digital signature. Strengthening the signature process minimizes the risk that an individual can refute the validity of the entry.

Level 3—Digital Signature: a digital signature is a cryptographic signature (a digital key) that authenticates the user, provides nonrepudiation, and ensures message integrity. This is the strongest signature because it protects the signature by a type of tamper-proof seal that breaks if the message content were to be altered.

Nonrepudiation serves to protect the integrity of the document. It guarantees that the source of the medical record documentation cannot later deny that he or she was the author. Nonrepudiation may be achieved through the use of a digital signature, which serves as a unique identifier for an individual (much like a written signature on a paper document); confirmation service, which uses a message transfer agent to create a digital receipt (providing confirmation that a message was sent or received); and time stamp, which proves that a document existed at a certain date and time.

A digital certificate may be implemented as part of a digital signature. A digital certificate is an electronic credit card with attendant end-to-end security safeguards that establish a user's credentials when doing business or other transactions on the Web. It is issued by a certification authority and contains the user's name, a serial number, expiration dates, a copy of the certificate holder's public key (used for encrypting messages and digital signatures), and the digital signature of the certificate-issuing authority so that a recipient can verify that the certificate is real.

Some digital certificates conform to the X.509 standard, published by the International Telecommunication Union. Digital certificates can be kept in registries so that authenticating users can look up other users' public keys.

Joint Commission Accreditation Standards

The Joint Commission accepts the use of e-signatures in hospitals and ambulatory care facilities, according to standard RC.01.02.01 in the *2009 Accreditation Manual for Hospitals and Ambulatory Care Facilities.*[3] The elements of performance require that:

- Only authorized individuals make entries in the medical record.
- The hospital or organization defines the types of entries in the health record made by nonindependent practitioners that require countersigning, in accordance with law and regulation.
- The author of each medical or clinical record entry is identified in the health record.

- Entries in the health record are authenticated by the author. Information introduced into the medical record through transcription or dictation is authenticated by the author.
- The individual identified by the signature stamp or method of electronic authentication is the only individual who uses it.

The Joint Commission also accepts the use of e-signatures in home care, long-term care, and mental health, subject to the requirements outlined above.

Payer and Health Plan Requirements

In addition to regulations, laws, and accreditation standards, payers and health plans may also require the use of e-signatures. Organizations should check payer requirements, local policies, and transmittals to determine the acceptability of e-signatures, technology requirements (such as digital signature technology), and specifications or limitations of use.

Health IT Standards for E-Signatures

Since there is no single overarching accepted standard for e-signatures, organizations must access individual health IT standards, regulations, and laws to review existing language specific to e-signatures, attestation, and authorship of medical record documents in an EHR. As general interoperability of systems improves over time, consistent standards will also be developed that can be applied to e-signatures.

Consistency and standardization are necessary. Users should be cognizant of the variability of existing standards, the ever-changing nature of such standards, and the various standard groups to remain up to date on current protocols and best practices.

Some of the standards that organizations can reference include:

- HL7 EHR-System Records Management and Evidentiary Support Functional Profile Standard. Health Level Seven developed the EHR-System Records Management and Evidentiary Support Functional Profile Standard, which identifies system functionality and conformance criteria related to authentication, attestation, pending records, amendments, and version management. Highlights from this standard for attestation include the need to link content to the authors, identify all authors or contributors of an entry, and display the name and credentials of authors.

- ASTM E1762–95(2003)–Standard Guide for Electronic Authentication of Health Care Information. ASTM International developed a standard in 2003 that outlines the appropriate process for applying an electronic signature, which involves securely identifying the individual's identity and frequency, creating a logical manifestation of a signature, and ensuring the integrity of the signed document. The standard provides guidance on handling multiple signatures and signature attributes (e.g., time stamp, signature purpose, and signer's role).
- ISO/IEC 14888-3 Information Technology–Security Techniques–Digital Signatures with Appendix. This ISO standard specifies principles and technical requirements for digital signatures and the related cryptographic techniques including integer factoring, discrete logarithm, and constructing the message.
- Certification Commission for Healthcare Information Technology. Although not a standards organization, CCHIT develops certification criteria for EHR applications that draw from existing health IT standards. The 2009 ambulatory care EHR certification criteria require that systems have the ability to finalize a note and change the status of the note to complete so subsequent changes are recorded as such; record the identity of the user finalizing the note and the date and time; handle cosignatures; addend or correct a finalized note; provide the full content of the original and modified note; and identify the author of the change.

Workflow Process for E-Signatures

It is equally important to understand the workflow process related to e-signatures. The diagram on the next page identifies the recommended process flow for e-signatures, including the need to collect all authors and complete a new version of the document or entry if there is a change after signature.

Implementation of E-Signatures in EHR, Electronic Document Management, and Transcription Systems

Healthcare organizations may implement e-signature functionality in a number of electronic record systems that include EHR applications, electronic document management systems, and transcription systems.

The different application of e-signatures has been a source of confusion for HIM professionals because implementation issues, workflow, and procedures differ between systems commonly used for EHRs. If an organization uses different types of systems, HIM professionals must understand the application of e-signatures in each of them. Policies and procedures should specify the application and applicable processes because e-signatures must be appropriately applied in all systems.

E-Signature Workflow Process

The diagram below identifies the recommended process flow for e-signatures, including the need to collect all authors and complete a new version of the document or entry if there is a change after signature. It follows the process from document creation through the various e-signature processes and to document completion. Solid lines represent the workflow. Dotted lines indicate system activity behind the scenes.

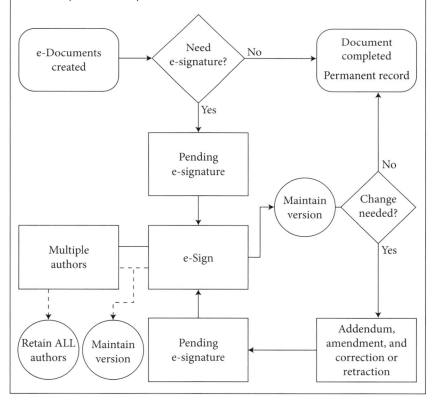

Authorship and Signature Special Considerations

Authorship attributes the origination or creation of a particular unit of information to a specific individual or entity acting at a particular time. While this concept seems fairly straightforward, authorship issues can arise in certain situations. Organizations should consider the following issues when developing their e-signature policies.

Multiple, dual, co-, and counter signatures. When there are multiple authors or contributors to a document, all signatures should be retained so that each individual's contribution is unambiguously identified. Care should be taken not to overwrite any author signatures on a document. Each signature should be complete and retained according to the organization's legal health record policy. Transcribed reports must show the name of the dictator and display the names of all electronic signers. The order of application of each signature must be provable via date and time stamps or other unambiguous means.

Entries made on behalf of another. Organizations must consider what procedures they will take when authors cannot or do not attest a document because they are no longer available to sign (e.g., resignation, sabbatical, or death). In the event a physician or other clinical provider is gone for an extended absence, leaving unsigned electronic documents or entries, the organization requires a process to identify qualified alternate signers for purposes of record closure. A qualified alternate signer is one who is able to uphold the purpose of attestation, is familiar with the clinical case, and can validate the accuracy of the documentation.

When entries must be left unsigned due to unfamiliarity by other caregivers and a lack of alternate signers, explanatory documentation should be included in the EHR to indicate the reason for record closure with e-signature validation gaps. Organizations should develop clear policies and procedures or medical staff bylaws on how to authenticate unsigned documents. The e-signature statement should indicate who signed and who the alternate signer signed for.

Proxy signatures (alternate or group signatures). Organizations also require processes by which a provider is authorized to electronically sign documentation on behalf of the original author. The proxy accepts responsibility for the content of the original documentation. Organizational policy should outline monitoring practices to detect inappropriate electronic proxy signature practices, whether from ignorance, negligence, or overt policy abuse.

Auto-attestation (also known as auto-authentication). Auto-attestation is the process by which an entry is implicitly signed (attested) through the user authentication process at sign-on. It is also the process by which a physician or other practitioner attests an entry that he or she cannot or has not reviewed because it has not yet been transcribed or the electronic entry cannot be displayed.

Healthcare organizations must consult legal counsel if they choose to pursue this approach. Federal regulations (both the Uniform Electronic Transactions

Act and Medicare Conditions of Participation for Hospitals) require that each author take a specific action to verify and attest an entry. In general, auto-attestation is not a recommended practice.

Batch signing. Batch signing is the process of applying a signature to multiple entries at one time. Batch signing of entries or physician orders may be acceptable if the following criteria can be met:

- All entries or orders can be viewed.
- Each entry or order can be acted upon individually, including editing the content.
- The entry or order can be removed from the batch.

Scribes. Some providers use scribes or assistants to type entries into the system for subsequent authorization. In some situations, the physician or other provider gives his or her access code to the assistant to allow direct entry of the notes. The system recognizes the author as the physician or the other authorized provider of care, instead of the assistant.

Organizations must put checks and balances in place to ensure that the physician or other legally responsible individual has reviewed the health record entries and authenticated them.[4] Organizations can consider assigning scribes unique user IDs to identify them as the authors of the entries and require the authorized providers or physicians to attest to the accuracy of the entries.

Data Elements for Display of E-Signatures

The full printed name of the author should appear at the end of an entry or document with the date and time, the digitized signature, or a signature statement with the author's credentials. For example, "Electronically signed by Dr. John Doe on 6/1/09 at 01:15am" or an abbreviation such as "/es/Dr. John Doe, 6/1/09; 01:15am."

The following are examples of statements that should be readable and viewable as part of the electronic record, output, or printed report. The statements may vary across healthcare entities, but should be based on the intent of the signature:

- Electronically signed by
- Signed by
- Authenticated by

- Sealed by
- Data entered by
- Approved by
- Completed by
- Verified by
- Finalized by
- Validated by
- Generated by
- Confirmed by
- Reviewed by

In the event of an addendum to a transcribed record, the addendum should be added to the top or bottom of the report and a second e-signature applied that includes the date and time the addendum was electronically signed. For example:

- Electronically signed by John Doe, M.D. on 6/1/09 at 01:15am
- Electronically signed by John Doe, M.D. on 6/2/09 at 03:45pm

When more than one signature is required, such as in the case of a resident or physician assistant dictating under the supervision of a physician, both signatures should appear on the bottom of the report similar to the sample format above.

For those systems that do not support dual signature functionality, an alternative is to have a statement on the bottom of the report that reads, "Dictated by Mary Smith, PA, under the supervision of Dr. John Smith," with the electronic signature affixed by the supervising physician. The process for handling multiple signatures should be addressed in organizational policy.

If initials are displayed on a screen or printed view of a document, such as on a flowsheet, the full signature should be referenced on the document.

Additional guidance on signatures related to billing for residents, certified nurse practitioners, and the attending can be found in the AHIMA practice brief "Applying the Teaching Physician Guidelines." [*J AHIMA*, August 2009]

Preliminary (Pending) Entries and Documents

A preliminary entry is documentation that is available for viewing but has not been authenticated or attested. This is not to be confused with an incomplete entry or documentation, where an entry or dictation is started but never completed.

Some systems may not allow preliminary entries and may require a signature in order for the document to be displayed in the EHR. In these cases, versioning should be used. This guidance applies to entries in the EHR as well as transcribed documents. Where applicable, these entries and documents should display a header or watermark stating the document has not yet been authenticated, such as "Draft Copy," "Pending," "Preliminary," or similar language. Organizations will need to determine the viewing ability of unsigned documents.

Organizations should also develop a policy outlining the process to clean up unsigned documents. Without such a policy, documents could remain in the system for long periods of time, hindering patient care. A regular process for monitoring pending notes also should be implemented.

Amendments, Corrections, Retractions, and Deletions in the EHR

Handling amendments, corrections, retractions, and deletions in the EHR is complex and varies based on the system. The process flow diagram illustrates the proper way to handle changes to EHR records. The signature event closes the record, and any subsequent changes are handled as a new version. All versions are retained.

Organizations must evaluate the proper handling of these situations in all clinical applications that are part of the EHR. Along with proper system functionality, organizational policies should address handling of each change.

The AHIMA toolkits "Amendments, Corrections, and Deletions in the Electronic Health Record Toolkit" and "Amendments, Corrections, and Deletions in Transcribed Reports Toolkit" assist with proper implementation of these complex issues. They are available online at www.ahima.org/infocenter/practice_tools.asp.

Version Management and Retention

If policy allows signed documents to be edited, all signed versions must be available for medico-legal purposes. There must be a procedure for accessing each version. If documents in the e-signature application are the legal medical record copy, no signed documents can be deleted permanently from the system.

If documents are printed and maintained as part of a hard-copy record or are transferred to another system or repository, this is not an issue.

If a document or note is available for use before it is finalized and signed, a version of the unsigned record must be retained for medico-legal purposes if changes were made.

E-Signature Lifecycle

When evaluating EHR systems and electronic document management systems it is important to determine whether the e-signature functionality is part of the electronic system or another piece of software attached to the system for authentication purposes. In either case the signature must be retained the same length of time as the record to which it is appended.

As the custodians of the record, HIM professionals bear the responsibility of ensuring that the EHR and the electronic document management system maintain the signature tied to the content for the required length of time. This applies to all clinical applications that are sources for the legal health record.

Security of Passwords and PINs

Secure e-signature methods have become more readily available over the last decade as technology has advanced. However, many facilities have been hesitant to implement these options for fear of disrupting clinicians' preferred workflow. The recommended best practice for e-signatures is authentication and a second level of identification to attest to authorship through use of a PIN, biometric scan, secure ID card, or digital signature.

Passwords or other personal identifiers must be controlled carefully to ensure that only the authorized individual can access the EHR system and apply a specific e-signature. Each individual who accesses the EHR and signs records must have his or her own identifier. Use of an administrative log-in or shared log-in will contaminate the integrity of the legal health record. If the system allows administrative sign-on, there is no guarantee that the correct author has signed the entry, thus compromising the integrity of the record and creating legal concerns.

Since the e-signature password is tied to the system log-on process, unencoded passwords should not be sent across networks. For organizations that use passwords, the following password or PIN characteristics are recommended to strengthen password security and simplify password management for the end user:

- Passwords should be a minimum of six to eight characters.
- Characters should be case sensitive and contain at least one alpha and one numeric character and special characters.
- Users should be unable to reuse passwords for at least three password change cycles.
- Users should be able to change their own passwords or PINs for increased flexibility and control.
- Passwords should be set to automatically expire after a set elapsed time with user prompts to set new password at next log-on.
- Organizations should prohibit group or shared passwords, overuse of administrative passwords, or group passwords. Attestation, access controls, audit records, and other security features are all dependent on the accurate identification and authorization of the user; use of group and shared passwords will cause catastrophic failure of security protocols and render the legal health record useless.

Finally, practitioners authorized to use e-signatures should be required to sign a statement acknowledging their responsibility and accountability for the use of their e-signature stating that they are the only one who has access to and will use their specific signature code. Organizational policy should define appropriate disciplinary actions for inappropriate use or sharing of unique identifiers.

HIM Operations

Allowing clinician access to the EHR does not come without challenges. Every electronic signature location—nursing unit, HIM department, personal office, or home—has to be carefully considered to ensure patient health information is protected. Therefore, deciding which clinicians will be able to electronically sign charts, as well as what, where, and how they may sign, is imperative.

Determining who will support the system is equally important. Organizations will need to provide ongoing support. To minimize confusion, clinicians should be given one number to call for assistance; if possible, an existing help desk system in the facility.

Staff familiar with the application can provide a backup to the help desk staff when needed. Super users or staff familiar with the application in the HIM department or other departments can support staff changes over time.

The application should be available at all times. However, organizations will need to analyze whether access issues of availability are different on and off site. Policies need to address availability while backups are performed or system updates or upgrades are installed. If the network has routine or extended downtimes, procedures for notifying users must be clear. In addition, organizations must negotiate support agreements that support around-the-clock access.

It is important that policies address the need to monitor or review all documents and documentation to ensure e-signatures are affixed and recorded in a timely manner. Periodic audits are recommended to confirm display of e-signatures and that interfaces between systems work as intended.

HIM departments should maintain a list of physicians or other healthcare practitioners who are authorized to use e-signatures. Organizations in the midst of migrating to a full EHR require a way to distinguish among documents to be manually signed and those that are electronically signed.

It is important for HIM professionals to identify what information is available from the application and evaluate its usefulness as a monitoring tool to ascertain whether a user viewed, edited, or printed any documents or pages. Policy and procedures should include assigning responsibility for evaluating exception reports, audit trails, and other access reports.

Finally, it is best to confirm the application has a method to ensure content completion and the validity of a signature by allowing the author to individually review and attest each entry one at a time.

Staff will require written procedures to follow if the application is unavailable. It is recommended that staff wait for restoration of the application rather than revert to manual signatures. A decision to revert to paper must not be made lightly. It is nearly impossible for HIM staff to reconcile documents that were signed manually with those waiting for electronic signature while the application was unavailable. Any difference in procedures depending on the duration of the downtime, or if the downtime is planned or unplanned, should be clear.

Organizational policy must address system access and monitoring, handling of authorship issues and data elements, changes to records, security and handling of passwords, support, and disciplinary action.

Documents signed electronically must be retained in conformity with the organization's definition of the legal health record and retention policy.

E-signatures are complex by nature, yet they are critically important to support the organization's legal health record. Proper attention to system functionality, regulatory requirements, and organizational policies is required for successful implementation and ongoing management.

Appendixes

Appendix A: HL7 EHR-System Records Management and Evidentiary Support Functional Profile Standard Excerpt
Appendix B: Laws, Regulations, and E-Signature Acts
Appendix C: E-Signature Model Policy Considerations [MS Word version]
Appendix D: Glossary of Terms
Appendix E: Amendments, Corrections, and Deletions in Transcribed Reports Toolkit

Notes

1. Health Level Seven. HL7 EHR System Records Management and Evidentiary Support Functional Profile 2009. Available online at www.hl7.org.
2. Smedinghoff, Thomas, and Ruth Hill Bro. "Electronic Signature Legislation." FindLaw Library. January 1999. Available online at http://library.findlaw.com/1999/Jan/1/241481.html.
3. Joint Commission. *2009 Comprehensive Accreditation Manual for Hospitals (CAMH): The Official Handbook.* Oak Brook, IL: Joint Commission Resources, 2008.
4. AHIMA. "Guidelines for EHR Documentation to Prevent Fraud." *Journal of AHIMA* 78, no. 1 (Jan. 2007): 65–68.

Resources

AHIMA. "Update: Maintaining a Legally Sound Health Record—Paper and Electronic." *Journal of AHIMA* 76, no. 10 (Nov/Dec 2005): 64A–L.

American Bar Association. "Digital Signature Guidelines." Available online at www.abanet.org/scitech/ec/isc/dsgfree.html.

ASTM International. ASTM E1762-95(2003) Standard Guide for Electronic Authentication of Health Care Information. Available online at www.astm.org/Standards/E1762.htm.

Certification Commission for Healthcare Information Technology. "Criteria and Test Scripts." 2009 Final Ambulatory EHR Criteria and Test Scripts plus Child Health and Cardiovascular Medicine Options. Available online at www.cchit.org/participate/cts.

Colorado Secretary of State. Uniform Electronic Transactions Act (UETA) Program. Available online at www.sos.state.co.us/pubs/UETA/UETA_Home_Page.htm.

E-HIM Work Group on Implementing Electronic Signatures. "Implementing Electronic Signatures." October 2003. Available online in the AHIMA Body of Knowledge at www.ahima.org.

Federal Information Processing Standards Publication 186. May 19, 1994. Available online at www.itl.nist.gov/fipspubs/fip186.htm.

International Law and Policy Forum. "An Analysis of International Electronic and Digital Signature Implementation Initiatives." September 2000. Available online at www.ilpf.org/groups/analysis_IEDSII.htm.

International Organization for Standardization. ISO/IEC 14888-3 Information Technology–Security Techniques–Digital Signatures with Appendix. Available online at www.iso.org.

International Telecommunication Union. Available online at www.itu.int/en/pages/default.aspx.

IsSolutions, LLC. Available online at www.goissolutions.com.

Nunn, Sandra. "Enterprise E-Signature: Managing Flourishing E-Signatures at the Organizational Level." *Journal of AHIMA* 80, no. 5 (May 2009): 48–49.

Prepared By

Donna Barron, BA, RHIT
Lauren Blumenthal, RHIA, PMP
Suzonne Bourque, RHIA, CCS
Natasha Brovarny, RHIT
Jennifer Childress, RHIT
Jill S. Clark, MBA, RHIA
Dawn L. Criswell, MS, RHIA, FAHIMA
Julie Dillard, MHA, RHIA

Michelle Dougherty, MA, RHIA, CHP
Marie Gardenier, MBA, RHIA, CHPS
Darice Gryzbowski, MA, RHIA, FAHIMA
Terri Hall, MHA, RHIT, CPC, CAC
Marla Hardison, CCS-P
Janice Hecht, MBA, RHIA
Beth Hjort, RHIA, CHPS
Kim Jackson, RHIT, CHP
Mary Johnson, RHIT, CCS-P
Diane M. Lerch, RHIA, CHPS, CCS, CHA
Dorothy W. Maxim, MS, RHIA
David Ike Mozie, PhD, RHIA
Indra Osi, RHIA, CHP
Deanna Panzarella
Janis L. Pavlick, RHIA
Ulkar Qazen, MSJ, RHIA
Sharron Ray, MHA, RHIA, MT, ASCP
Linda Spurrell, LPN, RHIT, CHP
Dolores Stephens, MS, RHIT
Susan Sugg, MSA, RHIA, PMP
Vicky Turner-Howe, RHIT, CCS
Kim Vernon, RHIA
Traci E. Waugh, RHIA
Lou Ann Wiedemann, MS, RHIA, CPEHR

Acknowledgments

Beth Acker, RHIA
Rhonda L. Anderson, RHIA
Mark S. Dietz, RHIA
Angela K. Dinh, MHA, RHIA
Sheila Green-Shook, MHA, RHIA, CHP
Tracy G. Hickey, MBA, RHIA
Deborah Kohn, MPH, RHIA, CHE, FACHE, CPHIMS, FHIMSS
Kelly McLendon, RHIA
Mary Meysenburg, MPA, RHIA, CCS
Debra Musa-Cross, RHIT, CHP
Kimberly Baldwin-Stried Reich, MBA, MJ, RHIA, CHC, CPHQ
Heather Black Shea, JD
Monica Tormey, RHIA

The information contained in this practice brief reflects the consensus opinion of the professionals who developed it. It has not been validated through scientific research.

Article citation:

AHIMA e-HIM Workgroup: Best Practices for Electronic Signature and Attestation. "Electronic Signature, Attestation, and Authorship (Updated)." *Journal of AHIMA* 80, no. 11 (November–December 2009): expanded online edition.

Enterprise Content and Record Management for Healthcare

It is estimated that more than 90 percent of all information created and used in organizations today is electronic.[1] While the current rate of electronic health record (EHR) adoption may lower this figure in some healthcare organizations, the trend is clearly toward an increase in electronic information. The requirement to better manage electronic health information and the dearth of management strategies to help the healthcare industry meet demands such as e-discovery and compliance has highlighted the need for an overarching strategy to aggressively manage records and content.

To avoid fragmented, chaotic information processes, healthcare organizations must adopt an integrated set of strategies, standards, best practices, and technologies for managing patient-centric and organizational information. This practice brief explores the emerging requirements for enterprise records and content management in healthcare organizations.

A Broadening Role for HIM Professionals

Traditionally, HIM professionals have managed the health record, whether it is paper-based, hybrid, or electronic. However, an increasing number of HIM professionals are expanding their role to manage all types of clinical content, including PACS images, voice, text, and speech files, e-mail, and software versions, regardless of whether it is officially part of the health record.

A broader role for HIM professionals is now emerging in the form of the enterprise records manager. The position oversees all of a healthcare organization's records and content, including financial, administrative, and clinical data.

Depending on job description and expertise, HIM professionals may be responsible for record and content management on a number of different levels (see "Levels of Content and Records HIM May Manage," on the following page). However, this role involves enterprise content and records management (ECRM).

ECRM combines two concepts: electronic records management and enterprise content management. At the foundational level, the two main components are defined as follows:

Electronic records management is the electronic management of digital and analog records contained in IT systems using computer equipment and software according to accepted principles and practices of records management. *Records management* is the field of management "responsible for the efficient and systematic control of the creation, receipt, maintenance, use, and disposition of analog and digital records, including processes for capturing and maintaining evidence of and information about business activities and transactions in the form of records."[2]

Enterprise content management includes the technologies, tools, and methods used to capture, manage, store, preserve, and deliver content across an enterprise.[3]

Briefly described, content is generally considered the intellectual substance of a document. A record is defined as information created or received in the transaction of business and maintained as evidence in pursuance of legal obligations. Appendix A, "ECRM Concepts, Terms, and Definitions," offers key concepts and definitions of the various aspects of ECRM. All appendixes are included in the online version of this brief, available in the FORE Library: HIM Body of Knowledge at www.ahima.org.

ECRM principles outlined here can and should be applied to all types and levels of information from the health record to all the organization's business records.

Levels of Content and Records HIM May Manage

Depending on job description and expertise, HIM professionals may be responsible for content and record management of varying scope, from traditional management of health records to a wide range of clinical content and organizational records.

Many healthcare organizations are learning the unique challenges associated with managing electronic health information. According to Gartner, "Organizations need to recognize information as a business asset and manage it effectively in order to increase value, reduce risk, and improve operational efficiency."[4] ECRM strategies applied to health records, health information, and organizational information provide value to the entire enterprise by facilitating the location and use of information and effectively managing it throughout its lifecycle.

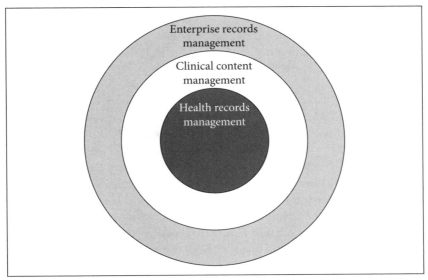

The Case for ECRM

Business drivers for ECRM in healthcare organizations include the following functions.

User efficiency. The facilitation of patient care and associated processes is a common driver for ECRM in healthcare. Clinicians are frequently concerned with the vast amounts of information they must sift through in order to render patient care.

ECRM initiatives respond to the need to organize this vast amount of information so that it can be accessed easily during the patient care process. In this way, ECRM supports patient safety and quality of care. However, its application is not limited to direct patient health information. It may also be applied to policies and procedures, workflow processes, and business documents such as contracts and directories that support patient care and the organization's business needs.

Ideally included in an organization's overall information governance and management plan, ECRM initiatives provide fast, efficient access for multiple purposes, including patient care.

Legal and regulatory compliance. Healthcare organizations must ensure compliance with a plethora of legal and regulatory mandates, including those related to billing, state licensures and certifications, and federal and state privacy and security regulations. They must also be able to appropriately locate and access information in order to compile a complete legal health record.

Due to the prospect of e-discovery, the massive growth of unstructured content and potential for its loss if not properly managed contribute to risk and legal exposure. The appropriate application of ECRM strategies and tools is critical in mitigating these risks.

Any information that could be relevant evidence in a lawsuit is discoverable. In the absence of ECRM, an organization's ability to collect, review, and preserve electronically stored information can be onerous and costly.[5]

Effective record control policies and procedures regarding retention and disposal requirements can reduce costs associated with e-discovery by decreasing the amount of information that needs to be retrieved if records are appropriately destroyed at the termination of their required retention period. These policies and procedures can also reduce the cost associated with restoration of content maintained on media that is difficult to reproduce or that has become obsolete.

An organization's failure to produce relevant requested electronically stored data can potentially result in significant fines or sanctions.

Accreditation and regulatory standards. When components of an EHR are housed in various systems, viewing a patient's complete health record can be difficult, and an inability to present complete and current information can pose a patient safety issue. Accreditation and regulatory bodies may have standards that address this issue. For example, the Joint Commission's accreditation standards require timely and easy access to complete information throughout the healthcare organization, whether paper-based systems, electronic systems, or hybrid systems.[6]

Accredited organizations must have processes in place to effectively manage information, including its capture, reporting, processing, storing, retrieving, disseminating, and display of clinical/service and nonclinical data and information. In addition, the healthcare organization is required to have a complete and accurate health record for each patient assessed, cared for, treated, or served. ECRM is an important strategy for complying with information management and health record standards and regulations.

Business continuity. ECRM involves identifying the organization's mission-critical records and content and planning for management during manmade or natural disasters, making it a critical part of business continuity planning.

Lifecycle Records Management

Content and records, regardless of how they are created and maintained, must be managed throughout their lifecycle, from creation through final disposition. The illustration on the next page identifies the major phases in the records management lifecycle.

Records Management Lifecycle

The record lifecycle is the foundation of ECRM principles. The figure "Lifecycle Records Management" (on the following page) illustrates the record lifecycle from creation through final disposition. The cycle applies to all types of enterprise records, including health records.

The following stages of a record's lifecycle explore the elements of the records management lifecycle and address common components of records management and expand the descriptions for each phase of the lifecycle.

Record creation, capture, or receipt. This phase includes creating, editing, and reviewing work in process as well as capture of content (e.g., through document imaging technology) or receipt of content (e.g., through a health information exchange).

Every organization must establish business rules for determining when content or documents become records. For example, a clinical document must be authenticated or signed in order to be considered a record, or diagnostic results designated as "preliminary" are not considered to be a record until they are designated as "final."

Examples of content that are not considered to be records may include items such as the initial versions of a document, preliminary results, drafts, working documents, and informal communications. The organization decides whether and when this content may be disposed of.

Record maintenance and use. Once records are created they must be maintained in such a way that they are accessible and retrievable. Components of this phase include functions, rules, and protocols for indexing, searching, retrieving, processing, routing, and distributing.

Record classification and metadata. Classification is a critical component of records management. Though not a unique point in the lifecycle, it does support

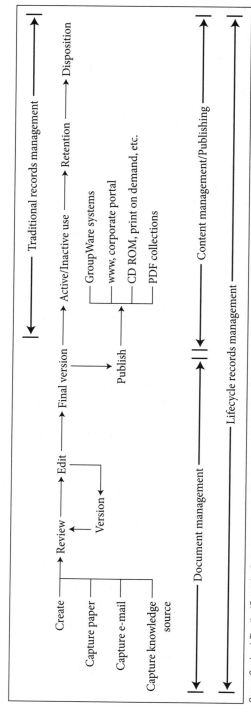

Source: Sprehe, J. Timothy. "Enterprise Records Management: Strategies and Solutions." White paper. September 2002. Available online at www.hummingbird.com/alt_content/binary/pdf/collateral/wp/rmstrategies.pdf.

the other phases. Record classification creates categories or groups of records necessary for access, search, retrieval, retention, and disposition of records.

Metadata are generated at various points in the records management lifecycle, providing underlying data to describe the document, specify access controls and rights, provide retention and disposition instructions, and maintain the record history and audit trail.

Record audit and data controls. Controls and audits support a variety of phases in the record lifecycle. Functions and processes in this component of records management may include edit checks at the data level, decision support tools, identification of classes of records that require auditing, and checks for record completeness.

Record preservation and retention. Preservation is synonymous with storage. Issues associated with preservation include: technology and media obsolescence, media degradation, media in an archival system, conversion over time, and conversion of standards over time.

Closely associated with preservation is retention or the identification of periods of times after which records and content will no longer be kept and are subject to destruction. Planning for preservation and retention should also include strategies to identify and prevent modification or destruction of records that are needed for legal purposes or so-called legal hold.

Record disposal encompasses the destruction process for data and records including the various media types and documentation of destruction.

ECRM Tools and Technologies

Enterprise content and record management is accomplished through a combination of organizational policies, tools, and technologies. The healthcare industry, like other vertical market industries (e.g., finance, energy, insurance, and transportation), has developed a plethora of information systems to meet its own specific business needs, such as EHR systems, patient financial systems, and picture archive and communications systems. However, as in other industries, the technology is focused on the unique transactional and database needs to support healthcare processes and does not usually include functionality to help manage records and content.

The IT industry has developed a multitude of systems to improve the content, documentation, and record management processes common to all industries. These information systems collectively are referred to as enterprise content management (ECM) information systems. ECM system component tools and technology help organizations manage content stored in documents and records to achieve business goals.

Common ECM system tools and technologies include, but are not limited to:

Automatic identification and character recognition technologies, including bar coding, intelligent character recognition, optical character recognition, and optical mark recognition, allow large amounts of analog data to be converted into digital data without manual data input.

Categorization or classification tools automate the placement of content into categories or classes for future retrieval based on the taxonomy.

Computer output to laser disk and enterprise report management technology stores and indexes computer output (primarily computer reports with report-formatted data) on magnetic disks, optical disks, and magnetic tape. Once stored, the reports can be retrieved, viewed, printed, faxed, or distributed to the Internet.

Collaboration technologies enable individual employees or business partners to easily create and maintain project teams regardless of geographic location. As such, they facilitate team-based content creation and decision making.

Document management technology controls and organizes documents. Electronic features and functions specific to document management technology include:

- Document assembly, whereby health record documents can be automatically retrieved in the correct order, based on predefined, user-specific rules and table.
- Document version (or revision) control, whereby health record documents can be automatically assigned version numbers. For example, daily laboratory test result reports (version 1) versus cumulative summary laboratory test result reports (version 2); preliminary radiology procedure result reports (version 1) versus final radiology procedure result reports (version 2); and transcribed operative reports (versions 1, 2) versus signed transcribed operative reports (version 3) versus amended transcribed

operative reports (version 4). Typically, only the most recent or last document version is accessible for view purposes.

- Document check-in and check-out services, whereby users can collaboratively view, review, and edit shared documents without concern about who might be simultaneously updating the document. Clinical teams that author progress notes are an example of document sharing using check-in/check-out capabilities.

- Document security consists of all the technical document tools to protect, control, and monitor document access (e.g., unique user identification or authentication, audit trails, automatic log-offs, and biometric identifiers) and to prevent unauthorized access to documents transmitted over a network.

Electronic document imaging technology captures data via scanning, faxing, or automatic identification. It also stores and retrieves documents regardless of original format.

E-mail management technology classifies, stores, and destroys e-mail messages consistent with organization standards, just like any other document or record.

Forms processing technology accepts scanned forms and extracts data from boxes and lines on forms to populate databases.

Records management technology electronically identifies records and retains them in a secured repository. It also provides controlled access to records and destroys records in accordance with predetermined retention schedules based on either outside regulations or internal business practices.

Electronic features and functions specific to records management technology include:

- Record capture, where a predefined set of metadata are established supporting accurate representation of the record with disciplined disposition and retention actions
- Record preservation format, where a format, such as eXtensible markup language (XML) or portable document format (PDF), is established for retrieval and cross-departmental interchange
- Record retention calculation, where "triggers" automatically save electronic documents or Web content as records according to pre-established business rules

- Record disposition control, where rules provide electronic notifications to managers that certain records or documents have met their retention dates and require manual confirmation to delete, save, or destroy
- Record deletion and destruction and suspension of record deletion and destruction to support litigation

Search/Retrieval technologies allow users to get out of the system what users put into the system.

Taxonomy tools provide a formal structure for information based on an organization's individual needs.

Web content management technology addresses Web-based content creation, review, approval, and publishing processes.

Workflow automation and business process management technology automate business processes, in whole or in part, where documents, information, or tasks are passed from one participant to another for action according to a set of rules. A business process is a logically related set of workflows, work steps, and tasks that provide a product or service to customers.

Desired Functionality

As discussed, some EHR and health IT systems contain few ECM component tools and technologies. Healthcare organizations typically acquire and implement separate ECM systems that complement the acquired and implemented EHR and related systems.

In addition, few ECM information systems contain all the above-mentioned component tools and technologies, and many are provided as toolkits, allowing an organization to develop the required information system based on its unique needs.

The following identifies the most desired functionality to help manage health records and other types of content in a healthcare environment:

- **Declaration of records:** Software can assist with the process of proclaiming documents and content as official records and support organizational policies related to the official legal health record and designated record set.
- **Taxonomy management** provides a shared vocabulary that an enterprise can use to organize and find information.

- **Version/revision** control facilitates the management of multiple revisions of the same unit of information. Changes are usually identified by incrementing an associated number or letter code, termed the revision number, revision level, or simply revision, and associated historically with the person making the change. Revision control allows organizations to revert to a previous revision, which is critical for allowing legitimate users to correct mistakes and to allow groups of editors to track each other's edits. Each version is associated with its own set of metadata.

- **Workflow automation**/business process management products allow a company to create a workflow model and components, such as online forms, and then use this product to manage and enforce the consistent handling of work.

- **Audit logs and trails** are used to monitor individual use of computer systems, security, reconstruction of problem events, problem monitoring, and intrusion detection.

- **Search engines** are retrieval systems that quickly locate information stored on computers. Users enter specific criteria about an item and the engine locates matching items in a short amount of time. An electronic master patient index uses a search engine to locate specific patients within its data repository.

- **Preservation and legal hold:** The 2006 changes to the Federal Rules of Civil Procedure identify the need to preserve and place litigation holds on electronically stored information. Once litigation is reasonably anticipated, the organization has the obligation to suspend routine record destruction activities and place litigation holds on data and information until the legal matter is resolved. Health Level Seven's Record Management and Evidentiary Support Profile addresses EHR requirements that pertain to preservation, retention, litigation hold, and destruction of electronically stored health information.

System Selection and Governance

An organization's system selection process should follow standards. These standards should include a process that identifies the needs and a plan to meet the specific business objectives as well as a comprehensive method for system selection.

Healthcare organizations frequently select "best of breed" health information systems and use varying implementation strategies to manage the transition to these systems while ensuring that users have the features and functions necessary to perform specialized tasks. This almost always affects HIM functions and requires process changes in the HIM department.

Implementing an enterprise record and content management program requires significant organization, process, and changes to job responsibilities. The organization must determine how ECRM will be integrated throughout all departments. It must implement a governance plan that identifies policies and procedures, enabling technologies, assignments of accountability, and ownership of various program aspects.[7]

To effectively address, manage, and communicate the myriad policies, the organization must establish an oversight committee to bring decision makers and data stewards to the table. For example, an enterprise records committee should provide monitoring and oversight of ECRM strategies and be the approval authority for the designated subcommittees.

Appendixes Available Online

Definitions, selection tools, and sample staffing models are available in five appendixes included in the online version of this practice brief. It is available in the FORE Library: HIM Body of Knowledge at www.ahima.org and through www.ahima.org/infocenter/briefs.asp.

- Appendix A: "ECRM Concepts, Terms, and Definitions"
- Appendix B: "ECRM System Selection Techniques and Tools"
- Appendix C: "Health Information Records and Content Management Scenarios"
- Appendix D: "Enterprise Records Committee: Suggested Staffing Model, Subcommittee Structure, and Responsibilities"
- Appendix E: "ECRM Sample Job Description"

ECRM Roles

Achieving a fully implemented enterprise-wide content and record management program may take several years. Starting the process with business units that already recognize the importance of data and compliance with regulatory standards (e.g., HIM, finance, human resources, and internal audit) may help expedite the early phases of the project. Additionally, integrating roles and responsibilities into existing departments, functions, and committee structures with related responsibilities (e.g., information security or litigation response team) may be beneficial.

Records and content management applies to everyone and every business unit within the organization that creates, maintains, or uses electronic or paper-based records.[8] Therefore, various roles and responsibilities need to be clarified. The following section expounds on these various roles for units and individuals.

Business Unit and Department Roles

Records are created as a result of an organization's business needs and processes; however, they are typically created at the business unit level. Roles and responsibilities at the business unit (or department) level need to be identified for the frontline staff and knowledge workers, the record custodian, and the business unit manager.

It is the frontline staff and knowledge workers that often create, retrieve, and use content. This group should be aware of the rationale for the records management program and their responsibilities within it. The group must be proficient in distinguishing records from nonrecords, using appropriate security measures, and classifying documents.

Subject matter expertise about record content and maintenance requirements tends to be domain-specific. For example, human resource staff is most familiar with the requirements for managing human resource records. For this reason, many ECRM programs use a model in which a record custodian is identified as a subject matter expert for a given domain for each business unit.

The record custodian is responsible for records maintenance procedures including indexing electronic and paper records, purging records for storage and destruction, using ECRM technologies, and outlining documentation destruction and related procedures.

Managers of business units or departments are responsible for ensuring that staff create and maintain records according to established policies and procedures. Business unit managers are also responsible for maintaining record integrity. They do so by identifying record classification methods and retention schedules for various record types, ensuring compliance with retention schedules, and placing a hold on record destruction for specific cases. Overall, the business unit manager is seen as the data steward for content and records created and used by the unit.

Finally, business unit managers' awareness and commitment is essential to the success of any ECRM program.

HIM Department Roles

The HIM business unit manager serves a dual ECRM role. As the organization's subject matter expert in health record content and management, the first role of the HIM manager is custodian for the organization's legal health record.

Healthcare organizations should identify the components of their legal health records and how they will ensure that the integrity of the legal health record and its various components are assembled and maintained.[11] Because sections of a health record often originate in different business units within a facility (e.g., radiology department creates an MRI report and nurse creates a pressure ulcer assessment), consideration needs to be given to both the operational needs of the various business units as well as requirements for ensuring a sound legal document.

This requires that the business unit managers, the data stewards, and the HIM managers (the legal health record custodians) collaborate to ensure that the record meets all organizational needs.

The second role of the HIM manager is that of steward for records created and used by HIM staff that are not part of the health record. This role is similar to the role of other business unit managers.

HIM managers also often serve on committees with responsibility for ECRM oversight.

Organizational Oversight for ECRM

Oversight for the ECRM program is established by assigning executive responsibility with operations managed through an enterprise records and content manager in collaboration with the information technology manager (see appendix E in the online version for sample job descriptions).

Organizations may designate executive responsibility and oversight for the enterprise records and content management program. A top-level executive officer is the principal decision maker with the responsibility of ensuring that the organization leverages information for maximum effectiveness enterprise-wide.

The officer also ensures that staff protect information from a variety of threats, monitor the use of information to ensure consistency in information practices, quantify the value of information, and forecast information that will be needed in order to make business units successful. The executive may be the chief information officer, chief operating officer, compliance officer, general counsel, or chief records officer.

The **enterprise content and records manager** is responsible for the organization's records and information management program and personnel. This role manages, controls, and directs active records systems and centers, records organization and evaluation, and inactive records systems. This manager also controls correspondence, reports and directives, and record retention.

The enterprise manager ensures that processes fully support and implement the organization's records and content management policies. He or she may also be responsible for the organization's film- or computer-based imaging operations and personnel.

The **information technology manager** is responsible for managing all organization technologies and provides technology support and training. The manager's primary duties include analyzing systems and processes; maintaining workstations and networks; and designing, developing, and maintaining Web-based applications.

Healthcare organizations must recognize the importance of their information assets and implement a coordinated process to manage their records and content. It will require new thinking, a new approach, and effective use of technology. HIM professionals have a unique skill set in managing health records—paper, hybrid, and electronic—that provides new roles and opportunities.

HIM professionals must actively step up to manage EHRs and clinical content. HIM professionals who wish to push beyond the boundaries of the HIM department have an opportunity to move into an enterprise role to oversee the overarching processes and challenges associated with managing the organization's documents, content, records, and business processes.

Notes

1. Sedona Conference. *The Sedona Principles Addressing Electronic Document Production.* 2nd edition. June 2007. Available online at www.sedonaconference.org.
2. Sprehe, J. Timothy. "Enterprise Records Management: Strategies and Solutions." White paper. September 2002. Available online at www.hummingbird.com/alt_content/binary/pdf/collateral/wp/rmstrategies.pdf.
3. AIIM International and ARMA International. Revised Framework for Integration of EDMS & ERMS Systems (ANSI/AIIM ARMA TR48-2006). AIIM International and ARMA International, 2006.
4. Gartner. "Organizing for Information Management." White paper. 2008.
5. Strong, Karen. "Enterprise Content and Records Management." *Journal of AHIMA* 79, no. 2 (Feb. 2008): 38–42.
6. The Joint Commission. *The Comprehensive Accreditation Manual for Hospitals: The Official Handbook.* Oakbrook Terrace, IL: Joint Commission, 2007.
7. National Institute of Standards and Technology. *An Introduction to Computer Security: The NIST Handbook.* Available online at http://csrc.nist.gov/publications/nistpubs/800-12/handbook.pdf.
8. Gartner. "Organizing for Enterprise Information Management."
9. Daum, P. "From Ad-Hoc to Adherence." *The Information Management Journal* (May/June 2007): 43–49.
10. The International Organization for Standardization. "Information and Documentation—Records Management: Part 2. Guidelines." 2001. Available online at www.iso.org/iso/catalogue_detail?csnumber=35845.
11. Dougherty, Michelle. "How Legal Is Your EHR? Identifying Key Functions That Support a Legal Record." *Journal of AHIMA* 79, no. 2 (Feb. 2008): 24–30.

References

Pearce-Moses, Richard. *A Glossary of Archival and Records Terminology.* Chicago, IL: The Society of American Archivists, 2005.

VA Northern California Health Care System. Policy Statement 00-11 Appendix 30. September 21, 2004.

Appendixes

Definitions, selection tools, and sample staffing models are available in five appendixes included in the online version of this practice brief. It is available in the FORE Library: HIM Body of Knowledge at www.ahima.org.

Appendix A: "ECRM Concepts, Terms, and Definitions"
Appendix B: "ECRM System Selection Techniques and Tools"
Appendix C: "Health Information Records and Content Management Scenarios"
Appendix D: "Enterprise Records Committee: Suggested Staffing Model, Subcommittee Structure, and Responsibilities"
Appendix E: "ECRM Sample Job Descriptions"

Prepared by

Carol Coots, CPC, CPC-H
Kevin Joerling, CRM
Michelle Dougherty, MA, RHIA, CPS
Wannetta Edwards, MS, RHIA
Margaret M. Foley, PhD, RHIA, CCS
Deborah Kohn, MPH, RHIA, FACHE, CPHIMS
Alison Nicklas, RHIA
Jesseca Olsen, RHIA
Amy Richardson, RHIA
Jennifer Teal, RHIA, CPC
Lydia Washington, MS, RHIA, CPHIMS

Acknowledgments

Dawn Criswell, MS, RHIA
Laura Debs, RHIT, CCS-P
Chris Meyers, RHIA
D'Arcy Myjer, PhD, RHIA, FAHIMA
David Sweet, MLS
Lilly Timon, RHIA
Carl Weise, CCRM, ERM

This work was supported by a grant to FORE from Meta Health Technology.

The information contained in this practice brief reflects the consensus opinion of the professionals who developed it. It has not been validated through scientific research.

Article citation:

AHIMA. "Enterprise Content and Record Management for Healthcare" *Journal of AHIMA* 79, no. 10 (October 2008): 91–98.

e-Discovery
Glossary of Terms and Acronyms

This glossary is an amalgamation of terms and vocabulary from HIM, IT, legal, compliance, medical, and other related fields. It is designed to serve as a reference and resource for HIM, IT, and legal professionals. The intention of this Glossary of Terms and Acronyms is to provide a basis for understanding the jargon of professions outside of the reader's experience. The websites provided in this and in the Glossary of Websites offer additional resources and lists of vocabulary terms that may be helpful to healthcare discovery.

Numbers

4G Fourth Generation—An International Telecommunications Union (ITU) standard, replacing the previous 3G standard, that provides Internet access for both mobile and stationary devices, such as phones.

4010A1 X12N HIPAA Transaction Standards   The electronic data interchange (EDI) originally adopted under the Administrative Simplification subtitle of the Health Insurance Portability and Accountability Act of 1996 (HIPAA). 4010A1 is the current electronic data interchange (EDI) change standard for the processing of healthcare claims. On January 1, 2012, providers, payers, and clearinghouses must be using the new HIPAA 5010 standards for electronic claims processing. See also EDI X12.

30(b) (6) Deposition   A procedure by which a subpoenaed or noticed entity designates one or more persons to testify at a deposition on designated topics and whose testimony is intended to bind the entity. See also 30(b)(6) Witness.

30(b) (6) Witness   A witness who is called to testify on behalf of the organization under the Federal Rule of Civil Procedure Rule 30(b)(6).

3D-API   3 Dimensional Application Programming Interface.

3G   Third Generation—An International Telecommunications Union (ITU) standard for mobile phones replacing the previous 2G and 2.5G standards.

26(f) Session   An e-discovery term used interchangeably with the meet and confer session. In a 26(f) session, legal, IT, and records management meet and confer to discuss strategy for litigation hold and the e-discovery process.

A

AACN   **American Association of Critical-Care Nurses**—The largest specialty nursing organization in the world, representing the interests of more than 500,000 nurses who are charged with the responsibility of caring for acutely and critically ill patients. http://www.aacn.org

AAHomecare   **American Association for Homecare**—An industry association created through a merger between the Health Industry Distributors Association Home Care Division, the Home Health Services and Staffing Association, and the National Association for Medical Equipment Services, for home care, such as home IV therapy, home medical services, and home health providers. http://www.aahomecare.org

AAMA   **American Alternative Medical Association**—The American Alternative Medical Association is a division of the American Association of Drugless Practitioners Certification & Accreditation Board, established in 1990. The AAMA is dedicated to promoting an enhanced professional image and prestige among doctors of traditional and nontraditional therapies and methodologies. The national and international membership body is made up of NDs, NMDs, DNs, DOs, DCs, PhDs, MDs, DDSs, AyDs, DDs, OMDs, and other alternative healthcare doctors. http://www.joinaama.com

AANP   **American Association of Naturopathic Physicians**—Founded in 1985, the American Association of Naturopathic Physicians (AANP) is the national professional society representing licensed or licensable naturopathic physicians who are graduates of four-year residential graduate programs. http://www.naturopathic.org

AAO-HNS   **American Academy of Otolaryngology—Head and Neck Surgery**—The world's largest organization representing specialists who treat the ear, nose, throat, and related structures of the head and neck. The Academy represents more than 12,000 otolaryngologists—head and neck surgeons who diagnose and treat disorders of those areas. http://www.ent.net.org

AAOS   **American Academy of Orthopaedic Surgeons**—Founded in 1933, AAOS engages in health policy and advocacy activities on behalf of musculoskeletal patients and the profession of orthopaedic surgery and is the preeminent provider of musculoskeletal education to orthopaedic surgeons and others in the world. http://www.aaos.org

AAP   **American Academy of Pediatrics**—A professional member organization of 60,000 pediatricians committed to the attainment of optimal physical, mental, and social health and well-being for all infants, children, adolescents, and young adults. http://www.aap.org

AAPPO   **American Association of Preferred Provider Organizations**—A national association composed of preferred provider organizations (PPOs) and affiliate organizations, which advocates for consumer awareness of healthcare benefits and advocates for greater access, choice, and flexibility. http://www.aappo.org

ABA   **American Bar Association**—A voluntary professional organization with over 400,000 members, the ABA provides law school accreditation, continuing legal education, information about the law, programs to assist lawyers and judges in their work, and initiatives to improve the legal system for the public. http://www.abanet.org

Abandonment   In law, the improper withdrawal from the care of a patient after establishment of a physician-patient relationship. To avoid charges of abandonment, the provider should provide adequate notice and opportunity for the patient to obtain substitute care. Generally, the duty of care continues until such time that the provider's services are no longer needed; there is mutual consent to termination; the patient dismisses the provider; or the provider discontinues care after providing appropriate notification and opportunity for the patient to seek alternative care.

ABC   **Activity-Based Costing**—An analysis of healthcare costs based upon a review of the healthcare organization's processes or activities. The costs are then associated with significant activities or events. It relies on the following three-step process: 1. activity mapping, which involves mapping activities in an illustrated sequence; 2. activity analysis, which involves defining and assigning a time value to activities; and 3. activity billing, which involves generating a cost for each main activity.

Aberrancy   Services in medicine that deviate from what is typical in comparison to the national norm.

ABMS   **American Board of Medical Specialties**—A not-for-profit organization that assists 24 approved medical specialty boards in the development and use of standards in the ongoing evaluation and certification of physicians. ABMS, recognized as the "gold standard" in physician certification, believes higher standards for physicians means better care for patients. http://www.abms.org

ABN   **Advance Beneficiary Notice**—A letter given to a Medicare beneficiary when the provider believes that Medicare will deny payment for a service that is not reasonable and/or medically necessary.

ABU   **American Board of Urology**—The ABU is organized to encourage study, improve standards, and promote competency in the practice of urology.

ABU certifies urologic physicians who meet its educational, professional standing, and examination criteria. To become certified, a urologist must have core competencies in all domains of urology, including but not limited to pediatric urology, endourology, female urology, andrology, oncology, urolithiasis, and general urology. All certified urologists are trained to evaluate and treat all patients with urological disorders. http://www.abu.org

Abuse   Incidents or practices that, although not usually considered fraudulent, are inconsistent with accepted sound medical, business, or fiscal practices of physicians or suppliers of equipment.

AC   Affiliated Contractor—A Medicare carrier, Fiscal Intermediary (FI), or other contractor such as a Durable Medical Equipment Medicare Administrative Contractor (DME MAC) that shares some or all of the Program Safeguard Contractor's (PSC's) jurisdiction; Affiliated Contractors perform non-PSC Medicare functions such as claims processing.

ACA   American Counseling Association—Founded in 1952, the 45,000-member not-for-profit professional and educational organization is dedicated to the growth and enhancement of the counseling profession. ACA is the world's largest association exclusively representing professional counselors in various practice settings and helps counseling professionals develop their skills and expand their knowledge base. http://www.counseling.org

ACAM   American College for Advancement in Medicine—ACAM is the voice of integrative medicine. Integrative medicine combines conventional care with alternative medicine to improve patient care. http://www.acam.org

Accreditation   An evaluative process to determine that an entity meets certain predetermined standards and levels of quality.

Accrete   The term used by Medicare regarding the process of adding new members to a health plan.

Accrual   An amount of money set aside to cover expenses. In the managed care setting accruals are based upon a combination of data from the health plan's authorization system, claims system, lag reports, and prior historical data.

ACF   Administration for Children and Families—One of 11 federal agencies that are part of the Department of Health and Human Services. ACF is responsible for approximately 60 programs that promote the economic and social well-being of children, families, and communities such as providing services and assistance to needy children and families, including Temporary

Assistance to Needy Families (TANF), child support enforcement, Head Start, child care, and foster care and adoption assistance. http://www.acf.hhs.gov

ACF   **Ambulatory Care Facility**—A medical center that provides a wide range of healthcare services including wellness services, acute care, ambulatory surgery, and outpatient care in one central location. Also known as a clinic or outpatient medical center.

ACFAOM   **American College of Foot & Ankle Orthopedics & Medicine**— Founded in the late 1940s as the American College of Foot Orthopedists and incorporated in 1951 as an Illinois nonprofit corporation, ACFAOM has approximately 900 members. It is the only specialty organization affiliated with the American Podiatric Medical Association (APMA) that represents the medical, orthopedic, and biomechanical aspects of podiatric practice. http://www.acfaom.org

ACG   **Ambulatory Care Group**—A method to classify and categorize outpatient care services.

ACH   **Automated Clearinghouse**—An electronic network for the processing of financial transactions.

ACID Properties   **Atomicity, Consistency, Isolation, Durable Properties**— Properties essential to an online transaction processing (OLTP) system.

ACLS   **Advanced Cardiac Life Support**—A set of clinical interventions for the urgent and emergent treatment of cardiac arrest and other life-threatening medical emergencies.

ACO   **Accountable Care Organization**—A provider group that accepts responsibility for the cost and quality of care delivered to a specific population of patients cared for by the group's clinicians. The ACO has been a model for healthcare reform, and has taken on far greater significance with passage of the Patient Protection and Affordable Care Act of 2010 (PPACA).

ACOG   **American College of Obstetricians and Gynecologists**—A not-for-profit member organization composed of over 52,000 professionals that advocates for women's health, provides education to professionals, and publishes clinical practice guidelines. http://www.acog.org

ACR   **American College of Rheumatology**—A professional membership organization that provides professional education for its members through several venues. The mission of the ACR is advancing rheumatology. http://www.rheumatology.org

ACR   Adjusted Community Rating—A community rating that is influenced by certain group demographics. This represents the estimated payment rates that health plans with Medicare risk contracts would have received for their Medicare enrollees if paid their private market premiums, adjusted for differences in benefit packages and service use. Health plans estimate their ACRs annually and adjust subsequent-year supplemental benefits or premiums to return any excess Medicare revenue above the ACR to enrollees.

ACRO   American College of Radiation Oncology—A professional medical college managed by a volunteer board of chancellors, ACRO strives to ensure the highest quality care for radiation therapy patients and promote success in the practice of radiation oncology through education, responsible socio-economic advocacy, and integration of science and technology into clinical practice. http://www.acro.org

Action   A lawsuit or legal demand to assert rights in a courtroom.

Action Ex Delicto   In law, an action to recover damages for a breach of a duty existing by reason of general law.

Action in Personam   A lawsuit against a person on the basis of personal liability.

Action Transmittal   A federal issuance that conveys program guidance information to grantees of actions they are expected or required to take. They clarify and explain procedures and methods for establishment of program policies and add details to program regulations or policy guide requirements.

Active Concealment   In law, the concealment by words or acts of something one is legally bound to disclose.

Active Data   Information (data or computer files) residing on the direct access storage media of a computer that can be accessed and used without any restoration process.

Actively at Work   An insurance policy requirement that stipulates coverage will not go into effect until the employee's first day of work on or after the effective date of coverage or if a dependent is disabled on the effective date.

Active Management   A current concept in litigation that contends executive decision makers conduct an ongoing review of the discovery process and hold the discovery team accountable for management of the documents, budget, and compliance with standards.

Active Records   Records residing in native application format related to current and ongoing business activities that are referred to on a regular basis in operational activities.

Actuarial   Refers to statistical calculations that were used to determine a managed care organization's rates and premiums charged to customers based on projections of utilization and cost for a defined population.

Actuary   A professionally trained individual, usually with experience or education in insurance, responsible for preparing statistical studies such as determining insurance policy rates, dividend reserves, and dividends, as well as conducting various other statistical studies.

Acute Care   Treatments used to either reduce or eliminate the symptoms of an illness of a nonchronic nature and restore function.

ADA   **Americans with Disabilities Act**—Legislation that was enacted to provide people with disabilities equal protection and opportunity in employment, public accommodations, and telecommunications. http://www.access-board. gov/about/laws/ada.htm

ADA   **American Dental Association**—A professional member organization for dentists that maintains hardcopy dental claim forms and the associated claim submission specifications as well as the current dental terminology code set. http://www.ada.org

ADA   **American Dietetic Association**—The world's largest organization of food and nutrition professionals. ADA is committed to improving the nation's health and advancing the profession of dietetics through research, education, and advocacy. http://www.eatright.org

ADC   **Average Daily Census**—The mean number of patients per day during a specified time (for example, over a month or year) in a hospital, which is measured at a selected time, usually midnight.

ADEA   **Age Discrimination in Employment Act**—The federal law that prohibits employment discrimination of businesses with 20 or more employees based on an employee or applicant's age. This law is aimed primarily at persons over the age of 40.

Adherence to Professional Standards   A term used in healthcare quality management that refers to the evaluation and measurement of a patient's care or clinical circumstance.

Adjudication of a Claim   Processing a claim to determine the appropriate payment with regard to the terms of a contract based on the information and benefits available.

Adjusted Admissions   A measure of all patient care in a hospital (inpatient and outpatient). This estimate is calculated by multiplying outpatient visits by the ratio of outpatient charges per visit to inpatient charges per admission.

Adjustment   Additional payment or correction of records on a previously processed claim.

ADL   **Activities of Daily Living**—A qualitative measure of a patient's ability to independently follow a daily routine of basic activities such as dressing, eating, bathing, and getting out of bed.

Administrative Agency   A federal, state, or local government agency with responsibility for the administration of a particular body of law; for example, the Department of Health and Human Services.

Administrative Code Sets   The term under HIPAA that refers to nonclinical or nonmedical code sets. The codes are used to characterize a business transaction rather than describe or classify a medical condition.

Administrative Costs/Load   The amount added to the prospective actuarial cost of healthcare services for administrative expenses. Examples of administrative expenses include quality/risk management, utilization review, maintenance of facilities, and so on.

Administrative Law   The body of law that deals with the operations and duties of the administrative agency. Also refers to the body of law on a particular subject created by an administrative agency through regulations and decisions.

Administrative Services Only   A business agreement between a provider and an outside contractor in which the client bears all the financial risk for claims. Administrative services–only contracts include health plans, hospitals, independent practice associations (IPAs), healthcare delivery networks, etc. Insurance companies or other management entities and a self-funded health plan or group of providers contract for administrative services such as billing, practice management, marketing, etc. Administrative services–only agreements are a form of professional outsourcing.

Administrative Simplification   The mandate for standardization of healthcare information systems as promulgated under Title II, Subpart F of HIPAA that authorizes the Department of Health and Human Services (HHS) to: 1. adopt standards for transactions and code sets that are used to exchange health data; 2. adopt standard identifiers for health plans, healthcare providers, employers, and individuals; and 3. adopt standards to protect the security and privacy of personally identifiable health information.

Administrative Supervision   In insurance, refers to a situation in which a health plan's operations are placed under the direction and control of the state commissioner of insurance or a person appointed by the commissioner.

Administrative Tribunal   Refers to the officer or officers who conduct trial-like hearings for administrative agencies.

Admissibility   Refers to the legal standards under which evidence is admitted in certain hearings and trials.

Admission   A term that is commonly used in both the healthcare and legal settings with two different and distinct meanings: 1. healthcare—entry into a hospital or other healthcare entity as a patient; and 2. legal—a writing or statement made by a party that admits the truth of a matter.

Admissions per 1,000   The number of patients admitted to a hospital or hospitals per 1,000 health plan members. In the managed care setting, the indicator is calculated by taking the total number of inpatient and/or outpatient admissions from a specific group—for example, the employer group or HMO population at risk—for a specific period of time (usually one year) and dividing it by the average number of covered members in that group during the same period, and multiplying the result by 1,000.

Adobe Acrobat   An Adobe software program designed to create, view, and manipulate PDF files.

ADR   Alternative Dispute Resolution—A legal procedure for the resolution of a dispute by a means other than litigation, such as arbitration, mediation, or mini-trial.

Advance Directive   A written instruction that is recognized under law as expressing a patient's wishes concerning future medical treatment in the event that the patient becomes incompetent. Examples include living wills or durable power of attorney for healthcare.

Adverse Action   A term used to refer to an action taken against a practitioner's clinical privileges or medical staff membership in a healthcare organization. Also known as a licensure disciplinary action.

Adverse Event   The occurrence of an unplanned or undesirable event that has a temporary or permanent negative outcome. An adverse event may or may not be related to error or poor quality of care. Expected adverse drug reactions and negative events that occurred due to error are both adverse events.

Adverse Inference Instruction   A sanction imposed on a party in civil litigation that invites a jury to find a fact unfavorable to that party.

Adverse Selection   The tendency for individuals with an impaired health status, or who are prone to higher than average utilization of benefits, to enroll in disproportionate numbers in lower-deductible plans, resulting in the premiums not covering costs. Some populations, due to age or health status of the individuals, have a great potential for high utilization and tend to be sicker than the general population.

Advisory Committee on Civil Rules   The Advisory Committee on Civil Rules (Advisory Committee) was established by the Judicial Conference Committee of Rules and Practice of the United States. The function of the Advisory Committee is to "carry on a continuous study of the operation and effect of the general rules of practice and procedure now or hereafter in use" in its particular field taking into consideration suggestions and recommendations received from any source, new statutes, court decisions affecting the rules, and legal commentary. The Advisory Committee was responsible for drafting what became the December 1, 2006, Amendments to the Federal Rules of Civil Procedure. http://www.uscourts.gov/RulesAndPolicies.aspx

Advocacy   To speak or write in favor of or to support or urge by argument.

Advocate   An individual who pleads for the cause of another and defends that cause.

AEP   **Annual Election Period**—The time in which Medicare Advantage Managed Care and Medicare Part D members may change prescription drug plans, change Medicare Advantage plans, return to Original Medicare, or enroll in a Medicare Advantage plan for the first time. This time period runs from November 15 through December 31 each year. Enrollment changes take effect on January 1. This is the only period during which most people with Medicare can change prescription drug plans.

AES   **Advanced Encryption Standard**—Symmetric cipher. The official United States Federal Information Processing Standard (FIPS) Number 197 established in 2001 for federal government approved encryption algorithms.

AFEHCT   **Association for Electronic Healthcare Transactions**—A membership group that promotes the interchange of electronic healthcare information in an open and secure environment. Improves and reduces the cost of healthcare through the use of EDI. Furthers the use of standards and the application of healthcare information technology to the delivery, financing, and administration of healthcare.

Affidavit   A voluntary statement of facts, or a voluntary declaration in writing of the facts or authenticity of a document that a person swears to be true for an official, such as a notary public, authorized to administer an oath.

Affiliation   A form, joint venture, or cooperation characterized by the coordination and integration of activities without a merger or formal consolidation.

Affiliation Agreement   A written agreement between two or more otherwise independent entities or individuals that defines how they will do business with one another. Affiliation agreements between hospitals may specify procedures for referring or transferring patients. Agreements between providers may include joint managed care contracting.

Affirm   To uphold a statement as true. Also meaning to uphold the judgment of a lower tribunal court. For example, the district court affirmed the ILBA's decision.

Affirmative Defense   A response to allegations in a complaint that constitutes a defense of the claim, even if all the allegations are true.

Aftercare   Services following hospitalization or rehabilitation, individualized for the patient's needs.

Agency   A relationship whereby one entrusts the performance of an act to another who assumes the duty to so act. An agency relationship may exist by agreement of the parties or be implied to exist under certain circumstances.

Age/Sex Factor   An insurance underwriting measurement that represents the medical risk costs of one population compared to another based on age and sex factors.

Age/Sex Rates   An actuarial table that rates each grouping by age and sex; each group has its own rates. Age/sex rates are used to calculate premiums for group billing, and demographic changes are adjusted automatically in the group.

Aggregate Data   Data combined from several measurements or a combination of other, more individual data.

Aggrieved Party   Defined in the Uniform Computer Transactions Information Act (UCTIA) 102(a)(3) as a "party entitled to a remedy for breach of contract."

AHA   **American Hospital Association**—Composed of almost 5,000 hospitals, healthcare systems, networks, and other providers and 37,000 individuals, the AHA represents and serves all types of hospitals, healthcare networks, and their patients and communities. AHA provides representation and advocacy activities for its members and assists in ensuring member voices are heard in national health policy development, legislative, and regulatory debates, and judicial matters. http://www.aha.org

AHIC   **American Health Information Community**—A former federal advisory body that made recommendations to the Secretary of the US Department of Health and Human Services (HHS) on how to accelerate the development and adoption of health information technology.

The AHIC advanced more than 200 recommendations over the course of 25 meetings from the time of its charter in 2005 until it concluded business on November 12, 2008. AHIC recommendations typically addressed a wide variety of enablers and barriers, such as:

- Standards and certification—for priority areas or use cases
- Business case—includes public- and private-sector reimbursement policy
- Business processes—necessary to integrate health IT into healthcare or consumer management of health
- Social and cultural issues—includes public awareness and consumer engagement
- Privacy and security—includes a long list of complex interrelated issues
- Medical-legal issues—includes liability and licensure of clinicians

AHIC makes recommendations to the HHS that are focused on consumer/patient needs, population health needs, and the technology/interoperability necessary to advance the use of health information technology.

AHIC Workgroups   Seven workgroups formed between November 2005 and October 2007 to discuss topics, present their findings periodically at AHIC community meetings, and make recommendations to the AHIC. The AHIC workgroups were:

- Biosurveillance Data Steering
- Population and Clinical Care Connections
- Consumer Empowerment
- Chronic Care
- Electronic Health Records
- Confidentiality, Privacy, and Security
- Quality
- Personalized Healthcare

The American Health Information Community (AHIC) successfully concluded its operations at its final meeting on November 12, 2008.

AHIMA   American Health Information Management Association—The premier member association composed of over 51,000 healthcare professionals dedicated to the management of health information. http://www.ahima.org

AHIP   America's Health Insurance Plans—A national association representing nearly 1,300 member companies providing health insurance coverage to more than 200 million Americans. Member companies offer medical insurance, long-term care insurance, disability income insurance, dental insurance, supplemental insurance, stop-loss insurance, and reinsurance to consumers, employers, and public purchasers. http://www.ahip.org

AHLA **American Health Lawyers Association**—A 501(c)(3) corporation composed of more than 10,000 members, the AHLA is the nation's largest nonpartisan membership and educational organization devoted to legal issues in the healthcare field. http://www.healthlawyers.org

AHMA **American Holistic Medical Association**—A professional membership organization founded in 1978 to unite licensed physicians who practice holistic medicine. http://www.holisticmedicine.org

AHRQ **Agency for Healthcare Research and Quality**—One of 11 agencies that are part of the Department of Health and Human Services. The mission of the AHRQ is to improve the quality, safety, efficiency, and effectiveness of healthcare for all Americans. http://www.ahrq.gov

AIIM **Association for Information and Image Management**—A not-for-profit organization that helps users of Enterprise Content Management technologies to understand the challenges associated with document management, content, records, and business processes within the organization. http://www.aiim.org

Algorithm A set of rules for solving a problem in a defined and limited number of steps.

ALI **American Law Institute**—A national member organization composed of judges, attorneys, and professors to promote clarification, simplification, and improvement in law. http://www.ali.org

ALJ **Administrative Law Judge**—A state or federal official who presides over hearings and appeals involving governmental agencies. Matters heard by an ALJ generally relate to a particular subject matter within the jurisdiction of the agency involved in the hearing. ALJs conduct evidentiary hearings on appeals of Medicare Part A and Medicare Part B determinations.

ALJ Hearing A quasi-judicial hearing before a federal ALJ that results in a new decision from an independent reviewer.

Allegation In law, statements made by a litigant that describe the litigant's position and what the litigant intends to prove.

Allied Health Professionals Licensed healthcare professionals other than physicians, nurse practitioners, physical therapists, podiatrists, psychologists, dentists, and chiropractors. Also known as nonphysician clinicians.

Allowable Charge   The maximum fee that a third party will reimburse the provider for a given service or supply.

Allowable Costs or Expenses   Any medically necessary healthcare expense, in part or all furnished by a healthcare provider that qualifies as a covered expense.

ALS   Advanced Life Support—A level of care provided by emergency medical technicians (EMTs) that consists of invasive life-saving procedures including the placement of advanced airway adjuncts, intravenous infusions, manual defibrillation, electrocardiogram interpretations, and other clinical interventions.

ALS   Automated Litigation Support—The application of specialized computer software and processes to aid in the collection, review, production, and presentation of documentary evidence. Automated litigation support technologies are routinely utilized in electronic discovery proceedings.

ALS   Amyotrophic Lateral Sclerosis—A progressive and chronic motor neuron disease of the nerves that come from the spinal cord and are responsible for supplying electrical stimulation to the muscles. Also known as Lou Gehrig's Disease.

Alternate Delivery Systems   A healthcare service provided in a setting other than an acute inpatient or private practice, designed to provide needed services in a more cost-effective manner. The term is also used to describe all forms of healthcare delivery except traditional fee-for-service private practices, such as HMOs, PPOs, IPAs, and other systems of providing healthcare.

AMA   American Medical Association—A professional membership organization composed exclusively of medical students and practicing and retired physicians. The AMA unites physicians nationwide to work on important professional and public health issues. The AMA is also the owner and publisher of the CPT and HCPCS data coding and classifications schemes. http://www.ama-assn.org

Ambient Data   Files or data stored in nontraditional computer storage areas or formats, such as unallocated space or file slack.

Ambulatory Care   Those healthcare services rendered in a clinic, outpatient facility, physician's office, or other outpatient site. Also known as outpatient care.

Ambulatory Surgical Center   A public or private entity that provides surgical services to individuals on an outpatient basis.

AMDIS **Association of Medical Directors of Information Systems**—A professional membership organization for physicians interested in and responsible for healthcare information technology. AMDIS members are the thought leaders, decision makers, and opinion influencers dedicated to advancing the field of applied medical informatics and thereby improving the practice of medicine. http://www.amdis.org

American Academy of Allergy, Asthma & Immunology The American Academy of Allergy, Asthma & Immunology is the largest professional medical organization in the United States devoted to the allergy/immunology specialty. http://www.aaaai.org

American Academy of Dermatology The largest, most influential and most representative of all dermatologic associations, composed of over 16,000 professionals, it represents virtually all practicing dermatologists in the United States. http://www.aad.org

American Academy of Family Physicians One of the largest national medical organizations, representing more than 94,700 family physicians, family medicine residents, and medical students nationwide. Founded in 1947, its mission has been to preserve and promote the science and art of family medicine and to ensure high-quality, cost-effective healthcare for patients of all ages. http://www.aafp.org

American Academy of Neurology An international professional association established in 1948, composed of 22,500 neurologists and neuroscience professionals dedicated to promoting the highest quality patient-centered neurological care. http://www.aan.com

American Academy of Nurse Practitioners A professional membership organization formed in 1985 to provide nurse practitioners with a unified way to network and advocate for nurse practitioner issues. It was the first national organization created for nurse practitioners of all specialties. http://www.aanp.org

American Academy of Ophthalmology A national professional membership association of eye MDs. Eye MDs are ophthalmologists and medical and osteopathic doctors who provide comprehensive eye care, including medical, surgical, and optical care. More than 90 percent of practicing US eye MDs are Academy members, and the Academy has more than 7,000 international members. http://www.aao.org

American Academy of Periodontology An 8,000-member association of dental professionals specializing in the prevention, diagnosis, and treatment of diseases affecting the gums and supporting structures of the teeth and in the placement and maintenance of dental implants. http://www.perio.org

American Association of Neurological Surgeons   The professional membership organization that speaks for all of neurosurgery. The AANS is dedicated to advancing the specialty of neurological surgery in order to promote the highest quality of patient care. http://www.aans.org

American Board of Dermatology   One of 24 medical specialty boards that make up the American Board of Medical Specialties (ABMS). http://www.abderm.org

American Board of Internal Medicine   An independent evaluation body that enhances the quality of healthcare by certifying internists and subspecialists who demonstrate the knowledge, skills, and attitudes essential for excellent patient care. http://www.abim.org

American Board of Otolaryngology   Founded and incorporated in 1924, the American Board of Otolaryngology is a member of the American Board of Medical Specialties. Its mission is to ensure that at the time of certification and recertification, diplomates have met the professional standards of training and knowledge in otolaryngology—head and neck surgery. http://www.aboto.org

American Board of Radiology   One of 24 medical specialty boards that make up the American Board of Medical Specialties (ABMS). The mission of the American Board of Radiology is to serve patients, the public, and the medical profession by certifying that its diplomates have acquired, demonstrated, and maintained a requisite standard of knowledge, skill, and understanding essential to the practice of diagnostic radiology, radiation oncology, and radiologic physics. http://www.theabr.org

American Chiropractic Association   The largest professional association in the United States representing doctors of chiropractic. ACA promotes the highest standards of ethics and patient care, contributing to the health and well-being of millions of chiropractic patients. http://www.acatoday.org

American College of Cardiology   A nonprofit medical society composed of physicians, nurses, nurse practitioners, physician assistants, pharmacists, and practice managers that bestows credentials upon cardiovascular specialists who meet its stringent qualifications. http://www.acc.org

American College of Gastroenterology   A professional membership organization established to advance the medical treatment and scientific study of gastrointestinal disorders. The College will strive to serve the evolving needs of physicians in the delivery of high-quality scientific, humanistic, clinical, ethical, and cost-effective healthcare to gastroenterology patients. http://www.acg.gi.org

American College of Physicians   A national organization of physicians who specialize in the prevention, detection, and treatment of illnesses in adults. ACP is the largest medical-specialty organization and second largest physician group in the United States. Its membership of 130,000 includes internists, internal medicine subspecialists, and medical students, residents, and fellows. http://www.acponline.org

American Gastroenterological Association   The trusted voice of the gastrointestinal community. Founded in 1897, the AGA has grown to include 17,000 members from around the globe who are involved in all aspects of the science, practice, and advancement of gastroenterology. http://www.gastro.org

American Neurological Association   A professional member society of academic neurologists and neuroscientists devoted to advancing the goals of academic neurology; to training and educating neurologists and other physicians in the neurologic sciences; and to expanding both understanding of diseases of the nervous system and the ability to treat them. http://www.aneuroa.org

American Nurses Association   A full-service professional organization representing the interests of the nation's 3.1 million registered nurses through its constituent member nurses associations and its organizational affiliates. The ANA advances the nursing profession by fostering high standards of nursing practice, promoting the rights of nurses in the workplace, projecting a positive and realistic view of nursing, and lobbying Congress and regulatory agencies on healthcare issues affecting nurses and the public. http://www.nursingworld.org

American Orthopaedic Association   Founded in 1887, the American Orthopaedic Association (AOA) is the oldest and most distinguished orthopaedic association in the world. It is the only orthopaedic organization that so strongly emphasizes a single theme of purpose: leadership in orthopaedics. http://aoassn.org

American Recovery and Reinvestment Act of 2009   (Pub. L. 111-5) Signed into law on February 17, 2009, this legislation was enacted to stimulate the US economy. The act contains provisions for federal tax relief and investment in education, healthcare, energy, and infrastructure, and expansion of unemployment benefits and other social welfare programs. The act also contains provisions designed to improve healthcare within the United States, such as the adoption of certified electronic health records and a study of the effectiveness of medical treatments, as well as congressional mandates, such as limitations on executive compensation in federally aided banks. http://frwebgate.access. gpo.gov/cgi-bin/getdoc.cgi?dbname=111_cong_bills&docid=f:h1enr.pdf

American Society of Anesthesiologists   The largest professional society for anesthesiologists, the ASA is dedicated to giving its members the education, research, and practice tools they need to serve their patients and their profession. http://www.asahq.org

American Society of Bariatric Physicians   A professional medical association for physicians, nurse practitioners, and physician assistants who are focused on the treatment and management of overweight and obese patients and their related conditions and comorbidities. http://www.asbp.org

American Society of Colon and Rectal Surgeons   The premier society for colon and rectal surgeons and other surgeons dedicated to advancing and promoting the science and practice of the treatment of patients with diseases and disorders affecting the colon, rectum, and anus. http://www.fascrs.org

American Society of Dermatology   A nonpartisan professional association of dermatologists across the country. The mission of this organization is to facilitate optimal dermatologic care being available to all citizens of this country by preserving, promoting, and enhancing the private practice of dermatology. http://www.asd.org

American Society of Nephrology   A professional membership organization that leads the fight against kidney disease by educating health professionals, sharing new knowledge, advancing research, and advocating the highest quality care for patients. http://www.asn-online.org

Americans with Disabilities Act   (Pub. L.110-325) Signed into law on July 26, 1990, this legislation was enacted to provide people with disabilities equal protection and opportunity in employment, public accommodations, and telecommunications. See ADA.

AMHCA   **American Mental Health Counselors Association**—A professional membership organization of almost 6,000 mental health counselors. AMHCA's mission is to enhance the profession of mental health counseling through licensing, advocacy, education, and professional development. http://www.amhca.org

AMIA   **American Medical Informatics Association**—A member organization that advances the informatics professions related to health and disease. The AMIA plays a pivotal role in the transformation of the US health system through the continued improvement, development, and implementation of health information technology. AMIA is an integrating force that strengthens the nation's ability to create and manage the science and knowledge base of healthcare. AMIA is active in the development of global health information policy and technology with particular emphasis on using health information technology to meet the health needs of underserved populations. http://www.amia.org

Amicus Curiae   Latin term meaning "friend of the court." An organization or person who is not a party in a given civil action but is permitted by the court to file a brief and/or participate in oral argument.

Amount in Controversy   The damages claimed by the injured party in a lawsuit.

Analog   Electronic mathematical representation in the form of a set of continuous values as opposed to a series of discrete quantities (digital).

Analysis of Rights   The ethical approach to a case based on consideration of whether an action affirms or violates basic human rights.

Ancillary Services   Additional services provided in conjunction with medical care, such as radiology, physical therapy, or laboratory tests.

Anonymized Data   Data that were previously identifiable data. For data to be truly anonymized, any provider, third party, or investigator must not be able to link deidentified data back to an individual. Also known as deidentified data.

ANOVA   **Analysis of Variance**—A statistical method for determining whether significant differences exist between two or more sample means.

ANPA   **American Neuropsychiatric Association**—Established in 1988, the ANPA is a nonprofit organization of professionals in neuropsychiatry, behavioral neurology, neuropsychology, and the clinical neurosciences. http://www.anpaonline.org

ANS   **American National Standards**—Standards developed, approved, and maintained by organizations accredited by the American National Standards Institute (ANSI).

ANSI   **American National Standards Institute**—A voluntary membership organization composed of businesses from all sectors that coordinates development and use of voluntary consensus standards and conformity assessments.

ANSI Standard   A set of rules that governs the structure of data in a message format for the exchange of business and operational information. Each ANSI standard is developed by an ASC X12 committee and adopted by the full X12 committee through public process announcement and review.

Answer   A written pleading filed by a defendant in response to a complaint filed against the defendant. The purpose of the answer is to respond to each allegation in the complaint by admitting or denying the allegation in whole or in part. The answer must be typewritten, follow specific pleading rules, and be served on the defendant within a specific statutory time as defined by law and the courts.

Anti-Kickback Statute   The federal law that prohibits the offer or receipt of certain remuneration in return for referrals for or recommending purchase of supplies and services reimbursable under government healthcare programs. Anti-kickback is a component of the Medicare and Medicaid Patient Protection Act of 1987 and provides for criminal penalties for certain acts impacting Medicare and state healthcare (for example, Medicaid) reimbursable services. Enforcement actions have resulted in principals being liable for the acts of their agents.

Antitrust   Term used to define the laws to protect trade and commerce from monopolies, unlawful restraints, or unfair business practices.

AoA   Administration on Aging—One of 11 federal agencies that are part of the Department of Health and Human Services.

AOA   American Osteopathic Association—A member association representing more than 64,000 osteopathic physicians (DOs). The AOA serves as the primary certifying body for DOs and is the accrediting agency for all osteopathic medical colleges and healthcare facilities. http://www.osteopathic.org

AOTA   American Occupational Therapy Association—A national professional association established in 1917 to represent the interests and concerns of occupational therapy practitioners and students of occupational therapy and to improve the quality of occupational therapy services. http://www.aota.org

APA   American Psychiatric Association—A professional medical specialty society representing more than 38,000 psychiatric physicians from the United States and around the world. APA members are primarily medical specialists who are psychiatrists or in the process of becoming psychiatrists. Founded in 1844, APA is the world's largest psychiatric organization. APA physicians work together to ensure humane care and effective treatment for all persons with mental disorders, including intellectual disability and substance-related disorders. APA is the voice and conscience of modern psychiatry. http://psych.org

APACHE   Acute Physiologic and Chronic Health Evaluation—A proprietary scoring system that generates a severity score for such health factors as underlying disease and chronic health status.

APC   Ambulatory Payment Classification—The method for payment of Medicare claims for outpatient care.

APDRG   **All Patient Diagnosis-Related Groups**—An enhancement to the original DRGs classification methodology, designed to apply to a population broader than that of Medicare beneficiaries, who are predominately older individuals. The APDRG set includes groupings for pediatric and maternity cases as well as for services for HIV-related conditions and other special cases.

APDU   **Advance Planning Document Update**—A regular supplement to an Advance Planning Document (APD) submitted by the states to the federal government that describes ongoing systems development. Generally, this document is submitted annually, but it may be submitted more frequently if major project changes occur.

APHA   **American Public Health Association**—Founded in 1872, the APHA aims to protect all Americans, their families, and their communities from preventable, serious health threats and strives to ensure community-based health promotion and disease prevention activities and preventive health services are universally accessible in the United States. APHA represents a broad array of health professionals and others who care about their own health and the health of their communities. http://www.apha.org

APHSA   **American Public Human Services Association**—A nonprofit, bipartisan organization of individuals and agencies concerned with human services. http://www.aphsa.org

API   **Application Programming Interface**—A computer code that is a set of instructions or services used to standardize an application.

APL   **A Programming Language**—A symbolic programming language that uses mathematical notations with particular terminology associated. It is particularly suited to interactive programming and mathematics and is noted for both power and brevity.

APMA   **American Podiatric Medical Association**—Founded in 1912, APMA is the leading resource for foot and ankle health information. The organization represents a vast majority of the estimated 15,000 podiatrists in the country. http://www.apma.org

Apparent Agency   A legal doctrine by which one actor may be deemed to operate on behalf of another.

Apparent Authority   The legal doctrine based on Section 429 of the Second Restatement of Torts of 1965, which provides: "One who employs an independent contractor to perform services for another which are accepted in the reasonable belief that the services are being rendered by the employer or by his servants, is subject to liability for physical harm caused by the negligence of the contractor in supplying such services, to the same extent as though the employer were supplying them himself or by his servants." Also known as ostensible agency.

Appeal—Legal   The process of seeking review from a lower court decision by a higher court.

Appeal—Insurance   A complaint filed by a health plan member when the member is in disagreement with a decision about healthcare services. All health plans maintain formal processes for the member to follow when filing an appeal.

Appellant   A party who appeals the decision of a lower court and brings it to a higher jurisdiction; or the party who takes an appeal from one court or jurisdiction to a different one.

Appellate Court   A court to which the judgment reached in a trial court is appealed.

Application   Software or a computer program designed to perform one specific task.

Apportionment of Damages   Proration of an award determined by verdict among those entitled to receive its benefit or against those obligated to pay.

Apportionment of Fault   Proration of responsibility for damages among those whose acts contributed to the injuries or loss.

Appropriate Care   A diagnostic or treatment measure whose expected health benefits exceed its expected health risks by a wide enough margin to justify the measure.

Appropriateness of Care   A term used in healthcare quality management that refers to the evaluation of the medical necessity and clinical outcome of a patient's care.

Approved Amount   The amount Medicare determines to be reasonable for a service that is covered under Medicare Part B. Medicare Part B will pay for 80 percent of these approved amounts and no more. If a doctor does not accept the approved amount, by law she or he can charge no more than 15 percent above this amount. The approved amount is sometimes called the approved charge or allowable amount.

APTA   American Physical Therapy Association—A national professional organization representing more than 74,000 members. Its goal is to foster advancements in physical therapy practice, research, and education. http://www.apta.org

Arbitration   Alternative process to resolve a dispute without resorting to the courts.

Archival Data   Information not directly accessible to a computer user that is maintained by an organization for recordkeeping purposes. Archival data are often written on removable media.

Archive   The term used to describe a repository of documents and other artifacts that are maintained in long-term storage for future access. An archive may or may not include electronically stored information (ESI).

Arden Syntex   An ANSI-approved specification that covers sharing of computerized health knowledge bases among personnel, information systems, and institutions. The scope has been limited to discrete clinical knowledge base modules known as Medical Logic Modules (MLM) that contain sufficient health knowledge to make a single decision. Examples include contraindication alerts, management suggestions, data interpretations, treatment protocols, and diagnosis scores.

ARM   Assured Records Management—A rational approach to realigning an organization's continuum of technical and nontechnical capabilities to improve corporate control over electronic information assets at the records level.

ARMA   Association of Records Managers and Administrators—ARMA, now known as ARMA International, is a not-for-profit professional association and the authority on managing records and information—paper and electronic. http://www.arma.org

ARRA   American Recovery and Reinvestment Act of 2009 (Pub. L. 111-5)—ARRA was enacted to provide stimulus for the US economy and establish an infrastructure to support industry adoption of electronic health records (EHRs). See American Recovery and Reinvestment Act of 2009.

Artificial Intelligence   A branch of computer science that seeks to develop computers that either emulate or surpass human intelligence and reasoning.

ASA   American Surgical Association—Founded in 1880, the ASA is the nation's oldest and most prestigious surgical organization. The association's mission is to be the premier organization for surgical science and scholarship and to provide a national forum for presenting the developing state of the art and science of general and subspecialty surgery and the elevation of the standards of the medical/surgical profession. http://www.americansurgical.info

ASC   Ambulatory Surgery Center—A freestanding surgical center that is certified by Medicare to provide surgical services outside of the hospital.

ASC   **Accredited Standards Committee**—An organization that has been accredited by the American National Standards Institute (ANSI) for the development of American National Standards (ANS).

ASCII   **American Code for Information Interchange**—ASCII is text code that assigns a number to each key on the keyboard. The text does not include special formatting features; it can be easily exchanged and read by most computer systems.

ASCO   **American Society of Clinical Oncology**—A nonprofit organization founded in 1964 with the overarching goals of improving cancer care and prevention. Nearly 30,000 oncology practitioners belong to ASCO, representing all oncology disciplines and subspecialties. Members include physicians and healthcare professionals in all levels of the practice of oncology. http://www.asco.org

ASC X12   **Accredited Standards Committee X12**—An ANSI chartered committee that develops, maintains, interprets, publishes, and promotes the proper use of electronic data interchange (EDI) standards and related documents for national and global markets.

ASHA   **American Speech-Language-Hearing Association**—The professional, scientific, and credentialing association for 140,000 members and affiliates who are speech-language pathologists, audiologists, and speech, language, and hearing scientists in the United States and internationally. The mission of ASHA is making effective communication—a human right—accessible and achievable for all. http://www.asha.org

ASHRM   **American Society for Healthcare Risk Management**—A membership subgroup of the American Hospital Association (AHA) composed of more than 5,300 members representing healthcare, insurance, law, and other related professions. http://www.ashrm.org

ASO   **Administrative Services Only**—A HIPAA term that signifies an arrangement in which a self-insured patient contracts with a third-party administrator to administer a health plan.

ASO   **Administrative Services Organization**—An entity with a self-funded health plan that contracts with an insurance company to perform its administrative services only; the self-funded entity assumes all risk.

ASP   **Application Service Provider**—A provider of computer-based services over a network or on the Internet.

ASPR   **Assistant Secretary for Preparedness and Response Programs**—The principal advisor to the Secretary of Health and Human Services on matters relating to public health and medical emergencies, whether resulting from acts of nature, accidents, or terrorism. The ASPR coordinates interagency interfaces between HHS; the Homeland Security Council; the National Security Council; other federal departments and agencies; state, local, and tribal public health; and private healthcare sectors. The Office of the ASPR is composed of five suboffices summarized as follows:

- BARDA—Biomedical Advanced Research and Development Authority
- OPEO—Office of Preparedness and Emergency Operations
- OMSPH—Office of Medicine, Science, and Public Health
- OPSP—Office of Policy and Strategic Planning
- RPE—Office of Resources, Planning, and Evaluation

ASPS   American Society of Plastic Surgeons—The largest plastic surgery specialty organization in the world. Founded in 1931, the society is composed of board-certified plastic surgeons who perform cosmetic and reconstructive surgery. http://www.plasticsurgery.org

Assault   The threat or use of force against someone that causes that person to have apprehension of danger or offensive contact. An attempt to commit battery with the intent to cause physical injury.

Assessment   The systematic process of collecting and analyzing data involving multiple sources and elements.

Assignment   An agreement made by the provider to accept reimbursement from a third-party payer as payment in full for services.

Assistant-At-Surgery   A surgeon who supports the primary surgeon during a procedure.

Assisted Living Facility   Extended care for patients who are independent, but need assistance with daily living activities.

Assumption of Risk   In law, the plaintiff's acceptance, either express or implied, depending on the situation, of the risk that he or she has reason to anticipate.

ASTM International   American Society for Testing and Materials—An organization formed by technical experts, engineers, and scientists, originally to deal with rail breaks in the railroad system. http://www.astm.org

ASTRO   American Society for Radiation Oncology—A professional medical society for radiation oncologists and other members of the radiation therapy treatment team. More than 10,000 radiation oncologists, radiation oncology nurses, medical physicists, radiation therapists, dosimetrists, and biologists are part of ASTRO's membership, making it the largest radiation oncology organization of its kind. http://astro.org

Asymmetric Cryptosystem   A generic term used for a cryptosystem that performs encryption and decryption (or signature and verification) using two keys in such a way that knowledge of one key does not provide information about the other. A computer algorithm or series of algorithms that utilize two different keys with the following characteristics: 1. one key signs a given message; 2. one key verifies a given message; and 3. the keys have the property that, knowing one key, it is computationally infeasible to discover the other key.

ATIS   Alliance for Telecommunications Industry Solutions—Formerly known as ECSA, ATIS is a US-based body committed to the rapid development and promotion of technical and operations standards for the communications and related information technologies industry worldwide and is accredited by the American National Standards Institute (ANSI). ATIS is composed of over 1,100 industry professionals from more than 350 communications companies. ATIS prioritizes the industry's most pressing technical and operational issues, and creates solutions that support the rollout of new products and services into the communications marketplace. Its standardization activities for wireless and wire line networks include interconnection standards, number portability, improved data transmission, Internet telephony, toll-free access, telecom fraud, and order and billing issues, among others. http://www.atis.org

At Risk   Any contractual or financial agreement in which a provider or health plan assumes financial liability for the costs of services needed by the population of members. The hospital or the medical group assumes the risk for the financial burdens of overutilization or adverse selection, rather than the insurance firm.

ATSDR   Agency for Toxic Substances and Disease Registry—One of 11 federal agencies that are part of the Department of Health and Human Services.

Attachment   A file associated with another record for purposes of transfer or storage. Attachments are often processed and managed as a single unit with their parent files.

Attorney-Client Privilege   The term that denotes the professional obligation of legal counsel not to reveal any communications, conversations, or correspondence between the attorney and his/her client. Attorney-client privilege stems from the legal theory that a person should be able to speak honestly and openly to his/her attorney without fear the information will be revealed. Documents prepared by a client in preparation for a legal proceeding or other legal matters are generally considered to be privileged and fall under the attorney-client work product doctrine.

Attribute   A characteristic of information or data that sets it apart from other data through location, length, or type.

AUA   **American Urological Association**—Founded in 1902, the AUA is a professional member association for the advancement of urologic patient care, and works to ensure that its more than 16,000 members are current on the latest research and practices in urology. The mission of the AUA is to promote the highest standards of urological clinical care through education and research, and in the formulation of healthcare policy. http://www.auanet.org

Audit   The formal examination of an organization's accounts, information systems, or financial situation. An audit may also include examination of the organization's compliance with applicable standards, laws, and regulatory requirements.

Audit Trail   A chronological sequence of audit records, such as communications or transactions by individuals or accounts, each of which contains evidence directly relating to and resulting from the execution of a business process or system function.

Authentication   The process by which the healthcare provider (physician and/ or other practitioner) signs entries into the medical record to attest to the information. Legally acceptable methods of authentication include: 1. handwritten signature, 2. electronic signature, and 3. rubber stamp. Organizational policy should dictate under what conditions/terms it is acceptable for a healthcare provider to authenticate an entry of another provider or utilize a rubber stamp signature.

Authenticity   The ability of a record to communicate its original message.

Authentic Record   A concept that guarantees a record that remains as reliable as the day it was created. An authentic record is one that can be accurately identified and relied upon as true and correct.

Author   The person or office responsible for a file's creation. Also called the originator.

Authorized Official   An appointed individual of status equal to president, chief financial officer, or general partner who has been granted the legal authority to enroll, make changes of status, and commit a provider/supplier to abide by the laws of Medicare.

Authorized Representative   A person who has the legal right to make healthcare decisions on another individual's behalf (for example, through a power of attorney).

Avoidable Consequences   A legal term used to refer to the failure of a party that claims damages to minimize those damages. A party that fails to mitigate damages may not be able to recover for those damages.

Award   A term that generally refers to the monies given to a party to a lawsuit, arbitration case, or administrative claim. The term is also used to describe the decision of an arbitrator or commissioner.

AWP   **Average Wholesale Price**—The standard cost of a pharmaceutical drug, calculated by averaging the cost of an undiscounted version to a pharmacy provider by a large number of wholesale suppliers.

<hr>

B

Backup   Generally, a copy of electronically stored information on a medium apart from the primary hard drive.

Backup Data   Data that are not currently in use by an organization and are stored on portable media to free computer space and facilitate disaster recovery, if necessary.

Backup Tape   Portable media used to store backup data.

Balance Billing   A bill to the responsible party for the difference between the provider's charge and the amount of payment from a third-party payer. Medicare rules stipulate the excess amount cannot be more than 15 percent above the approved charge.

Balancing Test   A judicial doctrine based on constitutional law, whereby the court measures competing interests (state vs. federal) and decides which interest should prevail.

Bandwidth   The gross measurement of the amount of information that can be transmitted over a connection. Bandwidth is usually given as bits per second, or sometimes as larger denomination of bits, such as megabits per second.

Bankruptcy Court   A separate unit of the federal court system. Bankruptcy cases are filed and heard only at the federal level.

BAR   **Billing Account Record**—An HL7 messaging term used to denote additions or changes to the patient's billing account information.

BARDA   **Biomedical Advanced Research and Development Authority**—An office of the Assistant Secretary for Preparedness and Response (ASPR) responsible for providing coordination and expert advice regarding public health, medical countermeasures, late-stage advanced development, and procurement.

Base Capitation   The stipulated monetary amount to cover the cost of health-care per person covered, generally minus mental health and substance abuse services.

BASIC   Beginner's All-Purpose Symbolic Instruction Code—A computer language that uses words instead of symbols, developed in the 1960s at Dartmouth College. It is the language of most microcomputers.

Basic Benefits   A set of federal- or state-required health services specified in an enrollee's certificate of coverage.

Basic Hospitalization Plan   Benefits for hospitalization with a ceiling or limited coverage after which coverage goes into effect.

Basic Medical/Surgical Insurance   Benefits for services in conjunction with basic hospitalization plans and major medical coverage.

Bates Stamping   In law, a process by which documents are stamped with unique numbers. Bates numbers today are affixed electronically to a document image, either as an overlay or burned in permanently.

Battery   The use of force against another person resulting in harmful or offensive contact.

Bayesian Approach   A quality measurement application that applies probabilistic reasoning to clinical information (such as test results, history, and physical exam, or any aspect of the diagnostic process) with prior beliefs about the probability of a particular disease.

BBA   Balanced Budget Act—A 1997 law enacted to cut the costs of Medicare.

BBRA   Balanced Budget Refinement Act—A 1999 act created to address the flawed policy and excessive payment reductions resulting from the Balanced Budget Act (BBA).

BCBSA   Blue Cross Blue Shield Association—The national coordinating agency for all Blue Cross Blue Shield health insurance organizations. http://www.bcbs.com

BCNF   Boyce Codd Normal Form—A method of normalization of data in a relational database.

Beacon Community   A community cooperative agreement program with the Office of the National Coordinator for Health Information Technology (ONC) that provides funding to selected communities to strengthen their health information technology (health IT) infrastructure and exchange capabilities.

Benchmark   A point of reference by which something can be measured.

Beneficiary   A person, member, or enrollee designated by an insuring organization as eligible to receive benefits provided in the member's Certificate of Coverage.

Benefit Limitations   An insurance term used to denote any provision, other than an exclusion, that restricts coverage as outlined in the patient's scope of benefits, regardless of medical necessity.

BestCrypt   A commercial disk encryption system that supports Linux and Windows.

BHM   Behavioral Health Medicine—The interdisciplinary field of medicine that stresses individual responsibility in the application of behavioral and biomedical science, knowledge, and techniques to maintain health and prevent illness and dysfunction or rehabilitate the individual.

Billed Amount   The amount charged for each service performed by the provider.

Bill of Particulars   A pleading device that predates deposition and interrogatory in discovery. Deriving from common law practice, it is a written statement of the particulars of a claim for which an action is brought, set out in response to a demand by the defendant in the action. The plaintiff's response must be detailed enough to put the defendant on notice as to the nature of the claims made against him.

Binary Computing   A low-level system of computing in which just two numbers, 0 and 1, are used.

Bing   A Microsoft decision engine.

Biomedical Engineering   The application of engineering principles and techniques to the medical field.

Biometric Authentication   The verification of an individual's identity through a biometric trait that cannot be duplicated by a hacker. A secure form of authentication.

Biometrics   The various methods for uniquely recognizing humans based on one or more physical or behavioral traits. Among physiological biometrics are fingerprints, DNA, and face recognition. Behavioral biometrics, called behaviometrics, include gait, vocal inflection, and rhythm.

BIOS   Basic Input/Output System—The BIOS manages the interface between hardware and software. It is the lowest level of software interface.

Bit   A binary digit with a value of 0 or 1. A bit is the basic unit of digital information storage and communication.

Bitstream   The term used to describe a time series of bits of information. When these bits of information are stored on a computer, a computer file is created and can be used in a legal proceeding. Bitstream data are also sometimes known as the residual data. Bitstream data are generally not produced to the court unless questions exist about the authenticity and/or creation of the information.

Blanket Authorization   A form, which patients sign once, consenting to the release of all information to Medicare or another insurance organization.

BLBA   Black Lung Benefits Act—The federal worker's compensation law that provides cash payments and medical benefits to disabled coal miners suffering from pneumoconiosis (black lung disease).

Block Cipher   One of two interdependent categories of cipher used in classical cryptography. The other cipher category is known as a stream cipher. Block and stream ciphers differ in how large a piece of the message is processed in an encryption.

Blog   An online website typically arranged in chronological order that journals and shares the personal thoughts and ideas of an individual or group of individuals for post and publication.

Blowfish   A block-ciphering algorithm that uses a 32- to 448-variable key length symmetric cipher.

BMP   Bitmap—A type of image file format used to store digital images. Also known as pixmap.

Board Certified   A physician who has qualified for and passed an examination given by a medical-specialty board and is certified as a specialist in that specific area of practice.

Board Eligible   A doctor who is eligible to take a board certification exam.

Board of Medical Examiners   A body or subdivision of such body that is designated by a state for licensing, monitoring, and disciplining physicians, dentists, or boards of allopathic or osteopathic examiners or an equivalent body.

Bookmark   A term used to describe the saving of an address or a shortcut to an Internet site; also denotes the marking of a document or specific place within the document for later retrieval.

Boolean Search   A commonly used database search methodology named for British-born Irish mathematician George Boole. Using any combination of full-text and document metadata, Boolean searching examines the logical relationships among search terms contained within a computer database.

Borrowed Servant Doctrine   A legal status that results when an employer loans an employee to another. It generally requires that the employee come under the direct control and supervision of the party to whom he or she is loaned.

Boycott   Planned action by competing entities to prevent another competitor from accessing a particular service, product, or market in such a way that there is a desired anticompetitive effect.

BPM   Business Process Management—A concept used to denote an analysis of a multistep business process or work items. Items are identified and tracked as they move through each step, with either specified people or applications processing the information. The process flow is determined by process logic, and the applications (or processes) play virtually no role in determining where the messages are sent.

Breach   A violation of a legal duty or wrongful conduct that serves as the basis for a civil remedy.

Breach Notification Requirement   The requirement under the HITECH Act that mandates that HIPAA-covered entities and/or their business associates provide written notice to an individual or to the HIPAA-covered entity when a breach occurs that compromises the security or privacy of an individual's protected health information (PHI). In addition to providing written notice to the individual, HIPAA-covered entities and their business associates must also provide notice of the breach to the Secretary of Health and Human Service (HHS) and, in some instances, the media.

Breach of Confidentiality   A failure to keep confidential information protected from disclosure by law or contract. A breach of confidentiality may give rise to a cause of action by, for example, a patient against the person and/or entity that committed the breach.

Break the Glass   The term used to describe the emergent situation in which an authorized user of an information system is given access to information he/she could not normally access given his or her specific role or job function.

Brief A written argument submitted to a court citing the facts and legal authorities on which a party relies in a case. A brief is also a digest of judicial opinion. Paralegals or junior attorneys usually draft briefs.

Broker An entity who obtains orders for insurance and places business with more than one company with no exclusive contract.

Browser Any commercial software used for viewing the World Wide Web resources. Examples of commercial browsers include Netscape's Navigator, Microsoft's Internet Explorer, and Mozilla's Firefox.

Brute Force Attack A term used in data security to denote an attempt of trying every possible code, combination, or password until the right one is found.

Bundled Payment A term that refers to the establishment of an inclusive package price or global payment for all of the services required for a specific episode of care, usually related to a procedure such as open heart surgery.

Burden A legal term denoting the obligation imposed on a particular party to prove a fact; in common parlance, a cost imposed in undertaking a certain act. For example, in e-discovery, the cost that may be imposed on a party in responding to discovery requests.

Burden of Proof In law, the responsibility in a legal proceeding of presenting sufficient evidence to prove a matter.

Burn The activity of copying files onto a removable media.

Business Associate Under HIPAA, the term is used to refer to a person or organization that performs a function or activity, but is not part of the entity's organization or workforce. A business associate may or may not be a covered entity for purposes of HIPAA. The regulations governing business associate agreements under HIPAA can be found at 45 CFR section 160.103. Also referred to as Part II of HIPAA.

Business Coalition An employer-sponsored organization that explores healthcare options, often acting as a change agent. For example, the Leapfrog Group.

Business Record A record that is made in the regular course of business. It is recorded at the time an event occurred or is made within a reasonable time thereafter and not made in preparation for trial. The purpose of the entry is to accurately record events that occurred. Medical records, although hearsay, are generally admissible into evidence under the Business Records Rule.

Business Transaction In the business setting, the term is used in to denote a business interaction between people and legal entities.

Bylaws   Rules for governance of a business or staff that affect the rights and duties of members of the organization but not outsiders.

Byte   A basic unit of measurement of information storage in computer science, made up of 8 or 16 bits. Through the arrangement of bits, 0 and 1 values, a byte can express any of 256 characters.

C

C   The programming middle-level language of choice for most software development that is fast, efficient, and portable due to a small vocabulary of only 30 words.

C++   **C Plus Plus**—A general-purpose programming language, C++ is an enhancement made to the original C programming language that includes classes, templates, operator overloading, and exception handling, among other improvements. C++ and C are highly compatible.

CAH   **Critical Access Hospital**—A rural facility designated by the Centers for Medicare and Medicaid Services (CMS) as meeting the applicable requirements as defined under Section 1820c of the Social Security Act and Part 42 CFR Part 485. Among the requirements are that the hospital maintains no more than 25 inpatient beds and that it is at least 35 miles away from any other hospital or CAH.

CAHPS   **Consumer Assessment of Healthcare Providers and Systems**— An initiative of the Agency for Healthcare Research and Quality (AHRQ). CAHPS is a public-private program that surveys patients' experiences with ambulatory and facility-level care. CAHPS maintains a national repository of data from health plan and hospital surveys.

CALEA   **Communications Assistance for Law Enforcement Act**—A federal law that enables the government, when necessary to protect national security, to intercept wire and electronic communications and call-identifying information.

Canada Health Infoway   A not-for-profit Canadian organization that collaborates with provinces and territories, healthcare providers, and technology solution providers to accelerate the use of electronic health records (EHRs). The Canada Health Infoway is an active participant in AHIMA EHR workgroups. http://www.infoway-inforoute.ca

Capitated   A common term used in managed care to refer to a payment system in which managed care plans pay healthcare providers a fixed amount to care for a patient over a given period regardless of quantity of services rendered. The amount is determined by assessing a payment on a per-member/per-month basis or per covered life. The method of payment in which the provider is paid a fixed amount for each person served no matter what the actual number or nature of services delivered. The rate may be fixed for all members or it can be adjusted for the age and gender of the member, based on actuarial projections of medical utilization.

Cap on Damages   In law, a term used to denote the upper limit, such a legislative mandate on the amount of civil damages that can be recovered in a tort action.

CAPTA   Child Abuse Prevention and Treatment Act—An act that provides federal funding to states in support of assessment, prevention, prosecution, investigation, and treatment activities of child abuse. This act also provides grants to public agencies and nonprofit organizations for demonstration programs and projects. It also sets forth a minimum definition of child abuse and neglect.

Captain of the Ship Doctrine   In law, a common doctrine that established that a physician can be held liable for the actions of subordinates present during the event, based on the doctor's functioning as "the captain of the ship," and controlling and directing the actions of those in assistance. Often used in reference to operating room situations; that is, the surgeon is the "captain of the ship."

CAQH   Council for Affordable Quality Healthcare—A not-for-profit, collaborative alliance of the nation's leading health plans and networks, with a mission to improve healthcare access and quality for patients and reduce administrative burdens for healthcare providers and their office staff. http://www.caqh.org

CARF   Commission on Accreditation of Rehabilitation Facilities—An independent not-for-profit organization that reviews and grants accreditation services nationally and internationally for those facilities or programs desiring accreditation. http://www.carf.org/home

Carrier   A health insurance company under contract with the federal government to handle claims processing for Medicare Part B services. See also Fiscal Intermediary and Medicare Administrative Contractor.

Case Law   Reported, aggregate decisions of cases on a particular legal subject.

Case Management—Healthcare   The process of clinical monitoring and coordination of a patient's treatment and discharge plan. Case management services are used for hospitalized patients or other selected health plan members with chronic, medically complex conditions requiring high-cost or extensive services.

Case Management—Litigation   The process by which litigation is controlled in the civil justice system. It may be aided by electronic information systems.

Case Management Process   The way in which case management tasks are performed, including assessment, problem identification, outcome identification, planning, monitoring, and evaluation.

Case Management Software—Litigation   Support software that assists lawyers in preparation for litigation, usually installed and run through a firm's LAN.

Case Mix   The clinical composition (diagnosis, age, sex, and other characteristics) of a patient population related to the probable intensity and frequency of services.

Case Sensitive   A technical term used to distinguish between uppercase and lowercase letters.

CAT Scanner   A Computer Axial Topography scanner device consisting of a bundled x-ray machine, computer processor, and application software.

Causation   An essential element to be proven in many kinds of cases, such as recovery of damages in a tort or contract action. A plaintiff must prove that a certain action or event caused a certain result that harmed or injured the plaintiff.

Cause of Action   In law, a set of facts that are enough to justify the right to sue an individual, party, or organization.

Caveat Emptor   In law, the Latin term that means let the buyer beware. The premise of this doctrine is that the buyer is purchasing a product at his/her own risk and should examine it for obvious defects, nonperformance, and/or imperfections.

CBO   **Congressional Budget Office.**

CCD   **Continuity of Care Document**—An XML-based standard developed through a collaborative effort between ASTM and HL7, designed to specify the encoding, structure, and semantics of a patient summary clinical document for exchange.

CCHIT   **Certification Commission for Healthcare Information Technology**—Formed through a partnership between the American Health Information Management Association (AHIMA), the Healthcare Information Management Systems Society (HIMSS), and the National Alliance for Health Information Technology (the Alliance), the CCHIT is a voluntary and independent private-sector HHS initiative for the certification of electronic health records and their networks. A primary goal of CCHIT is to accelerate the adoption of healthcare information technology and provide confidence to purchasers and users of healthcare technologies. On August 30, 2010, CCHIT was officially designated as an Authorized Testing and Certification Body (ONC-ATCB) by the Office of the National Coordinator. Scope of ONC-ATCB authorization: Complete EHR and EHR Modules. http://www.cchit.org

CCN   **CMS Certification Number**—A unique Medicare/Medicaid provider number used in survey and certification, assessment-related activities, and communications. In order to distinguish its role from that of the National Provider Identifier (NPI), in March 2007, the Centers for Medicare and Medicaid Services (CMS) renamed the Medicare/Medicaid Provider Number to CMS Certification Number (CCN).

CCOW   **Clinical Context Object Workgroup**—An ANSI-approved, end-user-focused standard that complements HL7's traditional emphasis on data interchange and enterprise workflow. CCOW is an HL7 standard protocol that enables disparate applications to synchronize in real time at both the user and interface levels.

CCPAHC   **Center for Cell Phone Applications in Healthcare**—An initiative of the Medical Records Institute (MRI) that will concentrate on the dialogue and study of the capabilities of modern cell phones, smart phones, PDAs, and other mobile devices for healthcare.

CCR   **Continuity of Care Record**—The CCR is rooted in peer-to-peer data transmission. The CCR is a standard for the transmission of patient summaries developed by ASTM International.

CDA   **Clinical Document Architecture**—An HL7 standard based on XML designed to specify the encoding, structure, and semantics of clinical documents for exchange.

CDAC   **Clinical Data Abstraction Center**—An organization chosen by the CMS to perform the reabstraction of and to identify any discrepancies in medical records and medical records systems. CMS conducts a quarterly retrospective validation for all hospitals submitting data to the CDAC. Once the data are submitted, they will be subject to sampling and a validation process, complete with an appeals process for hospitals scoring less than 80 percent.

CDAr2   **Clinical Document Architecture Release 2**—An HL7 model standard for the exchange of clinical documents, such as histories and physicals, discharge summaries, and progress notes. The CDAr2 leverages XML, coded vocabularies, and the HL7 Reference Information Model (RIM). CDAr2 documents are both machine-readable for electronic parsing and processing and human-readable for human review and retrieval by authorized users.

CDC   Centers for Disease Control and Prevention—The CDC is one of 11 federal agencies that are part of the Department of Health and Human Services. The mission of the CDC is to collaborate with partners within the United States and internationally to monitor health, detect and investigate health problems, conduct research to enhance prevention, develop and advocate sound public health policies, implement prevention strategies, promote healthy behaviors, foster safe and healthful environments, and provide leadership and training. http://www.cdc.gov

CD-ROM   Compact Disc Read-Only Memory—A form of computer storage that uses laser discs that can hold billions of bytes of data.

CDS   Clinical Decision Support—A term used to denote the capability of an information system, clinical application, or process that utilizes system alerts or triggers to help health professionals make clinical decisions to enhance patient care.

Census   In healthcare, the term is used to refer to the number of patients hospitalized at a given time.

Center of Excellence   A healthcare facility selected to provide specific services based on criteria such as experience, outcomes, efficiency, and effectiveness. Tertiary and academic medical centers are often designated as centers of excellence for one or more services such as organ transplantation.

Certificate   A message from a certificate authority (CA) that binds a public key to a name. The CA signs the certificate using its own private key. All recipients of a certificate must trust the issuing CA and own its public key in order to read its certificates.

Certificate Authority   A public key infrastructure entity whose core purpose is the issuance of digital certificates to use by other parties. It exemplifies a trusted third party. Some certification authorities charge fees for their service while other certificate authorities are free. It is also not uncommon for government and other institutions to have their own certificate authorities.

Certificate of Confidentiality   A certificate that helps researchers protect the privacy of subjects in research projects against any compulsory legal demands that might seek the names or other identifying characteristics of a research subject.

Certificate of Coverage   A written description of benefits included in a health plan, required by state law.

Certificate of Destruction   A certificate (paper or electronic) that verifies the destruction of documents. Many public health and governmental organizations require approval in advance before documents can be destroyed.

Certificate Validity   The timeframe between the date a certificate was issued and the date when it will expire.

Certification   The process by which an agency (government or nongovernment) grants recognition to those who have met a set of qualifications as determined by a credentialing body.

Certiorari   A writ that commands a lower court to certify proceedings for review by a higher court.

CERT Program   **Comprehensive Error Rate Testing Program**—A program established by CMS to produce a national Medicare fee-for-service (FFS) error rate compliant with the Improper Payments Elimination and Recovery Act of 2010. CERT randomly selects a sample of Medicare FFS claims, requests medical records from providers who submitted the claims, and reviews the claims and medical records for compliance with Medicare coverage, coding, and billing rules. The results of the reviews are published in an annual report. More information about the CERT program and the annual report are available at http://www.cms.hhs.gov/cert.

CFR   **Code of Federal Regulations**—The official compilation of rules and regulations issued by federal agencies.

CGD   **Certification Guidance Document**—A document issued by the ONC that outlines the process by which the Secretary of HHS recognizes one or more bodies comply with the criteria and standards set forth for the certification of EHR technology.

Chain-of-Custody   In law, a concept that applies to handling of evidence in such way as to maintain its integrity. Chain-of-custody is the document or paper trail showing the seizure, custody, control, transfer, analysis, and disposition of physical and electronic evidence.

CHAMPUS   **Civilian Health and Medical Program of the Uniformed Services**—A federal government healthcare program for dependents of active duty or retired members of the armed forces.

Chance of Survival Doctrine   In law, the principle that a wrongful-death plaintiff need only prove that the defendant's conduct was a substantial factor in contributing to the plaintiff's death; that is, the plaintiff might have survived if not for the actions of the defendant.

Change of Venue   The transfer of a case from the court in which it was commenced to a court located elsewhere for reasons of fairness or convenience.

Character   A configuration of a fixed number of bits in the core storage of a computer. Also the basic element or symbol from which words and language are constructed.

Charge   The asking price for a service.

Charitable Immunity   The case in which a hospital that is primarily maintained as a charitable institution is not liable for the negligence of its employees unless it fails to exercise ordinary care in the selection or retention of said employees.

Chattel   A term used to refer to all property that is not real property. For example, automobiles or stock certificates.

Child Document   The term used to refer to documents that are attached to other documents. See also Parent Document.

CHIME   **College of Healthcare Information Management Executives**— Composed of more than 1,100 members, CHIME is a professional membership organization dedicated to serving the professional development needs of healthcare CIOs and advocating more effective use of information management in healthcare. http://www.cio-chime.org

CHIN   **Community Health Information Network**—A secure, integrated, electronic communication network that permits multiple providers, payers, employers, and related entities to share information and communicate information within the network.

Chip   An integrated circuit made of silicon containing a large amount of electrical circuitry. Chips are used in the basic construction of computers.

CHIP   **Children's Health Insurance Program**—A jointly financed (federal and state) program administered by the US Department of Health and Human Services (HHS) that provides matching funds to states for health insurance to families with children. The CHIP program was designed to provide health insurance to families with modest incomes that do not qualify for Medicaid funding. Also known as the State Children's Health Insurance Program (SCHIP).

CHIPRA   **Children's Health Insurance Program Reauthorization Act of 2009**—An act that expands and reauthorizes the Children's Health Insurance Program (CHIP) through 2013.

Chiropractic Services   Care within the scope of training for a licensed chiropractor, including adjustments of the spine to treat pain.

Chosen Plaintext Attack   A term used to describe the process where a cryptanalyst is able to define his own plaintext, feed it into the cipher, and analyze the resulting ciphertext.

Chronic Care Healthcare that is provided over a prolonged period of time, as defined by contract, usually greater than 90 days.

Chronic Illness An illness or disease that is persistent over time, cannot be cured, involves one or more organ systems, produces symptoms regularly, and typically worsens over time, often leading to disability and death.

Churning The practice of providing a service more than necessary to increase revenue or meet quotas.

CI Clinical Informatics—A term used to describe a specialized body of science and knowledge. Informatics is an intersection of science, medicine, and healthcare.

Many subdomains of informatics exist including bioengineering and healthcare clinical informatics, which includes: nursing informatics, imaging informatics, consumer health informatics, public health informatics, dental informatics, clinical research informatics, bioinformatics, and pharmacy informatics. Clinical informatics is also known as health informatics (HI) or medical informatics (MI).

CIA Corporate Integrity Agreement—A unique written agreement between the Office of the Inspector General of the Department of Health and Human Services and a healthcare provider or other entity as part of a settlement for alleged civil wrongdoing relating to federal health laws. The government may enter into a CIA with an entity instead of seeking to exclude the entity from Medicare, Medicaid, or other federal healthcare programs.

Cipher The mathematical method used to encrypt data to protect the privacy and security of data.

Ciphertext or Cyphertext Data Ciphertext data are encrypted data; also known as cyphertext data.

Circuit Court or Court of Appeals The appellate court within the federal judicial system. There are 11 geographical circuit courts and one special court. Generally speaking, courts of appeals hear appeals from US bankruptcy and district courts and final rulings of federal administrative agencies.

Circumstantial Evidence Testimony based on deductions an ordinary intelligent person might infer rather than on personal observation.

Citation A reference to a judicial decision, statute, or other authority for a fact or legal proposition. A citation is also a written notice requiring one to appear in court to answer a charge, such as in a traffic ticket.

Civil   Pertaining to all aspects of law other than those that are criminal or military.

Civil Action   Legal action brought for any purpose other than the punishment of a crime.

Claim—Healthcare   An itemized statement of services (a bill) provided by a healthcare provider for an individual patient, usually for a single episode of care.

Claim—Legal   The aggregation of operative facts that give rise to a right that is enforceable in a court of law.

Claim Adjustment Reason Codes   In HIPAA, a national administrative code set used to identify the reasons for differences between the original provider charge for a claim and the payer's payment for it.

Claim Attachment   Hardcopy forms or electronic records that are needed to process a claim in HIPAA.

Claim Lag   The period of time between when a claim is incurred and payment, required for a review process.

Claims Processing Edits   Global or payer-specific business rules. (Example: HIPAA transaction standards.) All electronic transactions will run against these specific rules. If an error is detected, the claim is rejected.

Claim Status Category Codes   HIPAA's national administrative code set that indicates the category of the status of healthcare claims.

Claim Status Codes   HIPAA's national administrative code set, used in the X12 277 Claim Status Notification transaction, which indicates the category of the status of healthcare claims.

Clawback   The act of taking something back. Often used to denote the recovery of tax allowances by additional forms of taxation.

Clawback Agreement   An agreement between parties to a case by which they exchange information that has been subject to a reasonable privilege review and by which privileged information inadvertently turned over is returned to the producing party. Terms of any such agreement may vary.

Clayton Act   A federal antitrust law that prohibits a range of business activities that may substantially lessen competition, such as a corporate merger of two businesses with the effect of substantially eliminating the competition between them.

Clearinghouse   An entity that performs high-level edits and electronically routes both paper and electronic transactions to a receiving party, occasionally performing data translations in the process. A clearinghouse may or may not offer translation services of nonstandard electronic transactions.

Cleartext   Cleartext data are useable, unencrypted data; also known as plaintext data. See Plaintext.

Clerk of the Court   The court official charged with overall court operations or with some aspect of administration, particularly the processing of court records and documents, such as a subpoena, summons, and so on.

CLIA   **Clinical Laboratory Improvement Amendments**—Congress passed the Clinical Laboratory Improvement Amendments in 1988 and established quality standards for all laboratory testing to ensure the accuracy, reliability, and timeliness of test results regardless of where the test was performed. See also Clinical Laboratory.

Clinical Data Repository   A database that consolidates information from a variety of clinical sources to present a unified view of a single patient in real time.

Clinical Information System   A comprehensive and integrated information system used in healthcare organizations designed to manage all administrative, financial, and clinical aspects of a hospital, both electronically and on paper.

Clinical Integration   A term used to describe the operational integration of a variety of healthcare services from the same healthcare organization with the purpose of streamlining administrative processes and increasing potential for improved clinical outcomes for the benefit of the patient.

Clinical Laboratory   Under CLIA, a laboratory is defined as a facility that performs testing on materials derived from the human body for the purpose of providing information for the diagnosis, prevention, or treatment of any disease or impairment, or the assessment of the health of human beings.

Cloud Computing   An indefinite term. Essentially, it refers to data and services hosted on the Internet by third parties, thus making it unnecessary to maintain the data or services within an organization. These may include Web 2.0 technologies. See Web 2.0.

CMI   **Case Mix Index**—The average DRG weight for all cases paid under prospective payment, the case mix measures the relative cost of care for a given population.

CMIO   **Chief Medical Informatics Officer or Chief Medical Information Officer**—The CMIO is a person with a clinical background who "speaks the language of the clinicians." In many healthcare organizations, the CMIO oversees the selection, development, and implementation of computerized patient record systems. The CMIO focuses on issues of quality, safety, usability, and process improvement and seeks to ensure that clinicians are fully engaged in the entire process and may be a valuable resource for legal counsel in matters pertaining to the applications, functions, and usage of the organization's information systems and the impact they have on the care of the patient.

CMN Certificate of Medical Necessity—A certificate required by the CMS to prove the medical necessity of an item of medical equipment given to a Medicare beneficiary.

CMP Civil Monetary Penalty—The amount of money assessed by a judge in a legal proceeding for nonperformance or other contractual matters.

CMR Comprehensive Medical Review—Analysis of a sample of claims and all important data for selected providers in a specific time period.

CMS Centers for Medicare and Medicaid Services—One of 11 federal agencies that are part of the Department of Health and Human Services. The role of CMS is to administer the Medicare and Medicaid health insurance programs to ensure effective, up-to-date healthcare coverage and to promote quality care for beneficiaries. http://www.cms.hhs.gov

CMSA Case Management Society of America—An international not-for-profit organization dedicated to supporting and developing case management and professional collaboration across the healthcare continuum to advocate for the well-being of and improved health outcomes for patients. http://cmsa.org

CMSDC Centers for Medicare and Medicaid Services Data Center—A central data repository of claims data.

CMYK Cyan, Magenta, Yellow, and Black—Refers to the subtractive method used in four-color printing and desktop publishing.

COACH Canada's Health Informatics Association—A professional membership organization composed of more than 1,500 multidisciplinary members dedicated to the advancement of health informatics. https://secure.coachorg.com

Coalesce In information technology, an SQL function that accepts a list of parameters, returning the first nonnull value from the list.

COB Coordination of Benefits Contractor—The agency responsible for consolidating the activities that support the collection, management, and reporting of other insurance coverage for Medicare beneficiaries.

COBOL   Common Business Oriented Language—This is a high-level language designed primarily to handle business computer applications such as inventory or payroll.

COBRA   Consolidated Omnibus Budget Reconciliation Act (Pub. L. 99-272)—Amends the Employee Retirement Income Security Act (ERISA), the Internal Revenue Code (IRC), and the Public Health Service Act to provide continuation of group health coverage that otherwise might be terminated. COBRA provides certain former employees, retirees, spouses, former spouses, and dependent children the right to temporary continuation of health coverage at group rates. See also Consolidated Omnibus Budget Reconciliation Act of 1985.

CODASYL   Conference on Data Systems Languages—A computer industry consortium effort that led to the development of COBOL computer language.

Code—IT   A generic term used for language and symbols in programming at all levels.

Code—HIM   A number or alphanumeric classification assigned to every diagnosis, description of symptoms, task, and/or service a medical practitioner may provide to a patient including medical, surgical, and diagnostic services. Commonly used healthcare code sets include CPT, ICD, HCPCS, SNOMED, and/or LOINC classification methodologies.

Code—Legal   A collection or compilation of the statutes passed by the legislative body of a state, often annotated with citations of cases decided by the state supreme court.

Code Set   Title II of the Health Insurance Portability and Accountability Act (HIPAA) specifies that every provider who does business electronically must utilize the same healthcare transactions, code sets, and identifiers. Code sets are used to identify specific diagnosis and clinical procedures on claims and encounter forms. The HCPCS, CPT-4, and ICD-9 codes are the standard code sets utilized by providers for diagnostic and procedural data classification.

Code Set Maintaining Organization   In HIPAA, an organization that creates and maintains the code sets taken up by the Secretary of HHS for use in the transactions for which standards are adopted.

Codicil   A term used to refer to an addition or change to an executed last will and testament that becomes part of the original will.

Codification   The process of arranging, compiling, and systematizing the laws of a given jurisdiction or a discrete brand of the law into an ordered code.

Codify   To enact a statute or regulation that embodies a principle of common law or a particular judicial interpretation of the law. Also referred to as the organization of existing statutes or a body of law into a code.

Coding   Refers to the automated or human process by which documents are examined and evaluated using predetermined code sets. Coded data may be objective (name of the sender or date) or subjective (evaluation of the clinical data). HIM coding professionals utilize ICD and CPT and other coding classification schemes in the analysis, abstraction, and reporting of clinical data.

Coinsurance   A fixed or variable cost-sharing ratio between an enrollee of a health plan and the insurer. The percentage of costs paid by the member.

Coinsurance   Insurance that is provided jointly by two or more insurers.

Collaborative Decision Making   An approach to decision making that brings together all stake-holding parties in the outcome to contribute their input on what they want, why they want it, and how to handle conflicts.

Common Knowledge   A rare exception from expert testimony that recognizes that certain medical matters are so routine that a nonmedical juror is capable of understanding the applicable standard of care simply from prior experience.

Common Law   The body of law derived from prior judicial decisions as opposed to statutes or regulations.

Common Rule   A rule of medical ethics concerning human research and testing governed by the Institutional Review Boards.

Communication Protocol   The technical term used to describe the method by which two computers coordinate their communications.

Comparative Fault   In law, a term that refers to situations in which a plaintiff may have been at least partly responsible for a wrongful act. It may result in a lower damage award for the plaintiff.

Comparative Negligence   In law, a term that refers to situations in which a plaintiff may have been at least partly negligent. It may result in a lower damage award for the plaintiff. See Comparative Fault.

Comparative Performance Report   A report to monitor and profile a physician's billing patterns and/or clinical performance within an area or locality for the purpose of providing comparative data related to the physician's utilization patterns and clinical outcomes.

Compensable Injury In law, a term used to denote an accidental injury arising from employment or during the course of employment for which the employee is statutorily entitled to compensation.

Competency Having the necessary knowledge or technical skill to perform a given procedure within the bounds of success and failure deemed compatible with acceptable care.

Compiler A computer program that translates computer language source code into another language, generally from a high-level language to a low-level language.

Complaint The document by which, on filing, a civil action is commenced in the federal judicial system. The party filing the complaint is the plaintiff and the party against whom the complaint is filed is the defendant.

Compliance The measure of conformity and/or acting in accordance to accepted standards in a regulatory context.

Compliance Date The date by which a covered person must obey a standard, an implementation specification, or a modification under HIPAA.

Compliance Guidance A written document generated by Office of the Inspector General (OIG) that enables hospitals, home healthcare, nursing homes, thirty-party billing companies, and physician practices to establish compliance programs.

Compliance Officer A professional, who may or may not be an attorney, responsible for conformance and adherence to regulatory requirements. The compliance officer may be a potential 30(b)(6) witness for the organization.

Compliance Program A healthcare organization's program that enforces internal control and monitors conduct to prevent and correct improper activity.

Comprehensive Alcohol Abuse, Alcoholism Prevention and Rehabilitation Act An act passed in 1970 that established the National Institute on Alcohol Abuse and Alcoholism (NIAAA) as part of the National Institute of Mental Health (NIMH), that recognized alcohol abuse and alcoholism as major public health problems.

Comprehensive Drug Abuse Prevention and Control Act of 1970 (Pub. L. No. 91-513) A federal law enacted by Congress on October 29, 1970, that requires the pharmaceutical industry to maintain physical security and strict record-keeping for certain types of drugs. The Controlled Substances Act of 1970 is a component piece of this legislation and provided for establishment of the Drug Enforcement Administration and provides the legal basis for the US government to fight the ongoing war against illicit drugs.

Compromise—IT   An intrusion into a computer system where unauthorized disclosure, modification, or destruction of data is suspected.

Compromise—Legal   An agreement between two or more parties to settle a dispute amongst themselves.

Compurgation   Latin for "together" and "purge." In law, a term used to describe a trial in which a defendant could have as many as 11 supporters to testify they thought the defendant was telling the truth.

Compurgator   In law, a person who appears in court and makes an oath in support of a civil or criminal defendant.

CompuSec   A fast Microsoft Windows Advanced Encryption Standard (AES) disk encryption algorithm.

Computer Forensic Expert   A specialist well versed in computer forensics who is often called upon to testify in a court of law about applications and data contained on a computer system.

Computer Forensics   The application of the scientific method to digital media in order to establish factual information to be used by a court of law.

Computer Fraud   A fraud carried out through the use of the Internet or through the use of computers.

Computer Fraud and Abuse Act   (18 USC. § 1030) Enacted by Congress in 1984 to reduce computer hacking, this law governs cases primarily with federal interest when federal computers are involved or there is hacking crosses state lines.

Computer Information Transaction   Defined in the UCITA 102(a)(11) as an "agreement or the performance of it to create, modify, transfer, or license computer information or informational rights in computer information." The term includes a support contract under Section 612. The term does not include a transaction merely because the parties' agreement provides that their communications about the transaction will be in the form of computer information.

Computer Language   A rigidly structured method of creating or arranging instructions in a computer program.

Computer Program   A set of instructions, statements, or related data that cause a computer to perform a specified function, which is automatically executed in actual or modified form in a computer system.

CON   Certificate of Need—A certificate issued to a healthcare entity by a governmental body that proposes to construct or modify a healthcare facility, offer new or different services, or acquire new medical equipment.

Concealment   In law, the act of refraining to disclose information or an act, which prevents or hinders the discovery of something.

Concealment   A term used within the insurance industry to refer to the intentional withholding by an insured individual from an insurer of material facts or information that in good faith ought to be disclosed.

Concealment Rule   In law, the principle that a defendant's conduct prevented a plaintiff from discovering the existence of a claim, tolling the statute of limitations to the point in time when the plaintiff discovered or should have discovered the claim.

Concept Search   Searching for grouped bundles of words, phrases, and properties in electronically stored information (ESI).

Concerted Action   In law, an action that was arranged, planned, and agreed upon by parties acting together to further some scheme or cause, so that all involved are liable for the actions of each other.

Concordance   A commonly used e-discovery technology used by the legal profession to search, retrieve, and organize documents.

Conditional (C)   A data element requirement designator that indicates the presence of a specified data element that is dependent on the value or presence of other data elements in the segment.

Confess   In law, to admit to an allegation as true; to make a confession.

Confession   In law, a statement acknowledging guilt by a suspect. Confessions are usually in writing and made by a criminal suspect to acknowledge guilt and details of a crime.

Confession and Avoidance   In law, a plea in which a defendant admits allegations but pleads additional facts that deprive the admitted facts from having an adverse legal effect.

Confidentiality   A term used to refer to the act of ensuring an individual's health information is maintained as confidential and is disclosed and accessible only to those authorized to have access in accordance with law.

Conflict of Laws   In law, the term used to denote a difference between laws from different states or countries in a case in which a transaction or occurrence took place that is central to the case or has a connection to two or more jurisdictions. The conflict of laws doctrine may have relevance in matters related to the exchange of health information between states.

Conformance Criteria   A term used to denote information system functionality required of an automated information systems vendor.

Connectathon   A unique, vendor-neutral forum for testing software and hardware, first sponsored by Sun Microsystems in 1986. It is a network allowing vendors to test their interoperability solutions, with a special emphasis on NFS and Internet protocols.

Consent   To acquiesce to a course of treatment or action.

Consequential Damages   Losses or injuries that are consequences of an act but are not the direct and immediate result of that act. Also known as special damages.

Consideration   In contract law, that which is given or promised by the other in exchange for something.

Consolidated Health Informatics Initiative   An e-government initiative designed to help adopt vocabulary and message standards to facilitate the communication of clinical information across the federal health enterprise.

Consolidated Omnibus Budget Reconciliation Act of 1985   (Pub. L. 99-272) Signed into law on April 7, 1986, this federal legislation was enacted to make changes in spending and revenue provisions for purposes of deficit reduction and program improvement consistent with the budget process. This law requires employers who offer group health coverage to continue to do so for a prescribed period of time (usually 18 to 36 months) after employment has been terminated so that the employee can continue to benefit from group health rates until becoming a member of another health insurance plan. See COBRA.

Conspiracy   A concerted activity of expressed, written, implied, or tacit agreements between or among separate economic entities.

Consultation   A review and report by a separate healthcare professional or organization, generally not a primary care provider, when additional information or specialty care is required for either diagnosis or treatment.

Consumer   Defined in UCITA 102(a)(15) as an "individual who is a licensee of information or informational rights that the individual at the time of contracting intended to be used primarily for personal, family, or household purposes. The term does not include an individual who is a licensee primarily for professional or commercial purposes, including agriculture, business management, and investment management other than management of the individual's personal or family investments."

Consumer Protection Law   A state or federal statute designed to protect consumers against unfair trade and/or credit practices that involve consumer goods, as well as to protect consumers against faulty and dangerous goods.

Contestation of Suit   In law, the point in a legal action when the defendant answers the plaintiff's complaint. Also known as the plea and joinder of an issue.

Contextualize   Using the surrounding text of a word to determine its meaning.

Contingent Liability   In law, the liability that occurs when a specific or uncertain event happens in the future.

Continued Stay Review   A review used to determine if current levels of medical care require the present location of care.

Continuing Course of Conduct   A concept under which the statute of limitations is tolled when a physician commits a wrong on the patient, owes a continuing duty to a patient that is related to the original wrong, and breaches that duty. In this instance, a breach can be defined either as misconduct or an act of omission.

Continuing Injury   An injury that does not occur in a single event, but occurs over time in repeated intervals.

Continuing Treatment Rule   A rule under which the statute of limitations does not begin to run until treatment is terminated when the injurious consequences arise from a course of treatment run continuously and is related to the same original condition or complaint.

Continuous Representation Doctrine   The legal principle that the statute of limitations period for bringing a legal-malpractice action is tolled as long as the lawyer continues the representation that is related to the negligent act or omission.

Continuum of Care   Clinical services provided to either an inpatient or outpatient across the entire spectrum of treatment and medical care.

Contract   An exchange of promises between established parties (may be oral or written) to perform or refrain from performing a certain activity that is legally recognized and binding in a court of law.

Contract of Adhesion   A contract built on essentially a take-it-or-leave-it basis. In such conditions, one party has enough bargaining power over the other that the weaker has no choice regarding contract terms.

Contractual Allowance   The difference between the amount a provider bills and the amount paid by the third party.

Contribution   The right, based on appointment of fault, of an entity required to pay more for a loss to later seek reimbursement from another also involved with the cause of the injury.

Contributory Negligence   The common law doctrine that operates on causation and holds if a person was harmed or injured in whole or part during an accident as a result of his/her own negligence, then the injured party is not entitled to collect monetary damages from the defendant.

Cookie   Data files written to a hard drive by a web server, containing specific information that identifies the user. Websites use cookies to recognize users who have previously visited them. The next time the user accesses that site, the information in the cookie is sent back to the user so the information displayed can vary depending on the user's preferences.

Coordination of Benefits   Refers to the process for determining the responsibilities of two or more health plans that bear some financial responsibility for a health claim.

Copayment   The amount an insured individual (and in some Medicare plans) must pay for each medical service received. In the Medicare program, a copayment is usually a set amount a beneficiary pays for a service—for example, $5 or $10 for a doctor visit.

Copeland Act   A federal anti-kickback law that makes it illegal for federal contractors and/or subcontractors to induce employed persons contracted for repair of public buildings or public works to give up any part of their compensation.

CORE   Committee on Operating Rules for Information Exchange—A Council for Affordable Quality Healthcare (CAQH) initiative endorsed by CMS and HIMSS, designed to give providers access to healthcare administrative information before or at the time of service using the electronic system of their choice for any patient or health plan.

Coroner's Inquest   A hearing conducted by the coroner's office into the cause and circumstances of a suspicious death. The inquest will make a determination as to the cause and circumstances of death through a combination of autopsy and police investigation.

Corporate Liability   In law, the doctrine that holds an organization responsible for the actions of those working within it or under contract to it.

Corporate Negligence   The hospital's duty to a patient independent of an individual physician's duty. These hospital duties include providing and maintaining safe and appropriate medical facilities and equipment, keeping premises in a safe condition, disallowing negligent termination of medical care, using reasonable care in adopting and enforcing rules, policies, and procedures to govern the medical staff and employees, exercising reasonable care in selecting and retaining the medical staff, and overseeing all people who practice medicine within the building.

Cost Allocation   The method for determining how costs associated with system development are shared across different programs or funding sources. Factors to consider when developing a cost allocation methodology include analyzing system data elements; evaluating the specific functions to be programmed into the system; examining the caseloads of the programs to be served; and projecting the level of effort in the design or programming activity.

Cost-Benefit Analysis   An analytical technique that measures the costs of a proposed decision against the expected advantages.

Cost Outlier   An entity, such as a patient, who is significantly more costly to treat than most such entities with the same condition.

Cost Sharing   The provision of a health plan that requires the insured to pay some part of the costs for services in the form of deductibles or copayments.

COT   Chain of Trust—A HIPAA term related to security NPRM for a pattern of agreements that extend the protection of healthcare data by requiring that each covered person who shares healthcare data with another require that person to provide protections comparable to those provided by the original covered person who, in turn, requires any other entities with whom he/she shares the data to satisfy the same requirements.

Counterclaim   A claim brought by the defendant against the plaintiff in the same suit asserting an independent cause of action.

Covenant   A promise.

Covered Benefit   A medically necessary service included under the terms of insurance coverage.

Covered Entity   The term used to describe a provider, healthcare clearinghouse, or health plan under HIPAA. The Title II Administrative Simplification regulations define a HIPAA-covered entity to be: 1. a healthcare provider that conducts certain transactions in electronic form (also known as a covered healthcare provider); 2. a healthcare clearinghouse; and 3. a health plan.

CPCA   Consumer Credit Protection Act—A federal wage garnishment law that limits the amount of an employee's earnings that may be garnished in any one week and protects employees from discharge because their wages have been garnished for any one debt.

CPG   Clinical Practice Guideline—A utilization review and quality management mechanism designed to aid payers and providers in making decisions about the most appropriate course of treatment for a specific clinical case.

CPOE   Computerized Provider Order Entry—A computer program that allows a doctor's orders for diagnostic and treatment services to be entered electronically rather than being recorded on prescription paper, and that warns the physician of conflicts, allergies, or drug interactions.

CPR   Computerized Patient Record—A computer-based, electronic record that resides in a system designed to support users by providing access to complete and accurate data, alerts, reminders, clinical-decision support systems, links to medical information, and other aids.

CPT4   Current Procedural Terminology, 4th Edition—An annual publication of the American Medical Association (AMA). CPT4 is used to assign code numbers to and classify data in medical and surgical procedures.

CPU   Central Processing Unit.

CQI   Continuous Quality Improvement—The ongoing assessment of processes to improve quality through feedback and education.

Credentialing   The process required by law to qualify licensed professionals or organizations through assessment of education, training, and experience.

Critical Incidents   Occurrences, as defined by Cooper, the author of a classic human factors study, that are pivotal close calls with potentially undesirable consequences that may harm a patient.

Critical Path   Treatment that includes only the most vital elements proven to affect a patient's outcome, by commission or omission, or by the timing of intervention.

CRT   Cathode-Ray Tube—A screen on which computers display text as it is entered on a keyboard. Also called a video display terminal.

Cryptanalysis   The data encryption science of turning encrypted data into unencrypted data.

Cryptanalyst   A person skilled in the decoding and analysis of codes and cryptograms.

CryptoExpert   A commercial Windows disk encryption package.

Cryptography   The mathematical manipulation of electronic data for the purpose of reversible or irreversible transformation. A piece of data, called cleartext or plaintext, is transformed into a piece of data called ciphertext or cyphertext. This process is called encryption. The reverse process is called decryption.

Cryptography Key   A variable value that applies an algorithm to a string or block of unencrypted text to produce encrypted text or to decrypt encrypted text. The length of the key is a factor in considering how difficult it will be to decrypt the text in a given message.

Cryptology   A science that incorporates both cryptography and cryptanalysis.

Cryptoloop   A Unix disk encryption methodology.

CSF   Critical Shortage Facility—A healthcare facility that the Secretary of Health and Human Services has determined has a critical shortage of nurses.

CTRDS   CERT Tracking and Reporting Database System—A Comprehensive Error Rate Testing (CERT) program database.

CT Summation   A commonly used litigation support software used by the legal profession to search, retrieve, and organize documents.

Culling   The process that refers to reducing a large population of documents into a smaller set. Data culling saves time and money by reducing the number of documents requiring legal review. Culling is also sometimes also known as harvesting.

Culture   An integrated pattern of human behavior, including thoughts, communications, actions, beliefs, customs, institutions of a racial, ethnic, religious, or social group, and values. In addition, culture may also include, but is not limited to, race, ethnicity, national origin, and migration background; sex, marital status, and sexual orientation; religion, age, and political beliefs; mental, physical, or cognitive disability; gender, gender identity, or gender expression.

Custodial Care   Care that is provided to help an individual meet the needs of daily living.

Custodian   The term used to refer to a person(s) or data location(s) (such as a network server) that is knowledgeable about, involved with, or maintains potentially relevant information that is responsive to threatened or impending litigation. The term custodian can be applied to three levels: 1. direct or primary custodians—those person(s) who work with the data directly or have direct involvement or knowledge of the events in the case; for example, a staff nurse who has made an entry into the medical record and is knowledgeable about the events of a case in litigation; 2. officially designated records custodians, such as HIM and IT professionals; and 3. third-party custodians that house and maintain a client organization's electronically stored information (ESI), such as IT vendors and other business associates.

CY Calendar Year—A 12-month period that commences on the effective date (January 1) and ends at midnight on the last day of the year (December 31).

Cyberattack   Any destructive electronic intrusion or attack that disrupts a computer system and affects national functioning.

Cyberlaw   A legal term used to denote the broad area of law that relates to the use of the Internet as well as computers, computer software, databases, and computer networks.

Cybernetics   A term coined by American mathematician Norbert Weiner, cybernetics is the analysis of the communication and control processes of biological organisms and their similarity to mechanical and electrical systems.

Cybernotary   An attorney admitted to practice in the United States who is qualified to act as a notary with a primary focus on international, computer-based transactions.

Cyberspace   A term used to refer to the Internet and a worldwide network of computer networks that use TCP/IP network protocols to facilitate data transfer.

Cybersquatting   A term used to describe a bad-faith intent to profit from the goodwill of a trademark belonging to someone else.

Cybertort   A civil wrong committed through the use of computers and/or the Internet. For example, the dissemination of threatening or defamatory e-mail or the use of the Internet to carry out a fraud.

Cypher Cryptainer LE   A 25MB disk encryption for Windows that implements the Blowfish algorithm.

D

DAMA Data Management Association—A not-for-profit organization composed of international technical, business, and records management professionals. DAMA is dedicated to advancing the concepts and practices of managing data and information. http://www.dama.org

Damages   In law, the term damages refers to the injury suffered by a party. Damages can be economic, psychological, or the result of personal injuries. It can also refer to an award of damages. Damages can include, for example, punitive damages intended to punish a wrongdoer for certain actions.

DARN **Dollars at Risk of No Documentation**—An acronym used to refer to Medicare's documentation requirements, which if not met will result in a denial of a healthcare claim.

DAT **Digital Audio Tape**—A storage medium contained in some backup systems.

Data A representation of information for which meaning or instruction might be assigned in a computer system.

Database Foreign Key In the context of a database table, the foreign key is a key from another table that refers to (or targets) a specific key, usually the primary key, in the table being used.

Database Key In the context of a database, the database key is a field that is selected for sorting. The primary key is a key unique to each record and is, as such, is used to access that record. A foreign key is one that targets a primary key in another table.

Database Primary Key In the context of a database, the primary key is a key in a relational database that is unique for each record. It is a unique identifier, such as a medical record number. A relational database must always have one and only one primary key. Primary keys typically appear as columns in relational database tables.

Data Compilation Information in a format that cannot be read without being converted.

Data Compression The automated process in which data are compressed and wrapped by removing trailing blanks and spaces from segments, groups, and/ or transactions. Data compression is used to reduce data field information to its minimum for cost effectiveness.

Data Condition The circumstances in which data are required.

Data Content A term used under HIPAA that refers to all the data elements and code sets inherent to a transaction and not related to the format of the transaction.

Data Corruption Unintended change to data in storage or in transit that makes the data undecipherable or unreliable.

Data Council A coordinating body that has high-level responsibility for overseeing the implementation of the A/S (Administrative Simplification) provisions under HIPAA.

Data Custodian   A term used within some healthcare organizations to describe the person or persons responsible for maintaining the server or set of servers in which electronic data are stored.

Data Element   A term used under HIPAA that refers to the smallest named unit of information in an electronic data transaction set. A data element may be single-character codes, literal descriptions, or numeric values.

Data Encryption   The practice and study of hiding information, primarily for security purposes, by converting plaintext into gibberish by means of a code.

Data Integrity   The assurance that the data regardless of their form or location are consistent and correct during any operation.

Data Mapping   Under HIPAA, the process of matching one set of data elements to their closest equivalents in another set.

Data Mart   A small, single-subject data warehouse, generally confined to a department or other unit within an organization.

Data Mining   A term used to describe the process of finding correlations or patterns among dozens of fields in large relational databases. Data mining software is often one of a number of analytical tools used to analyze information extracted from a database. The process of data mining is a critical component to measure the quality and improvement of EHRs.

Data Model   Under HIPAA, a conceptual model of the necessary information to support a business function.

Data Owner   A term used within some healthcare organizations to describe the person or device that originates data.

Data Repository   A term often used synonymously with data warehouse, a data repository differs from a data warehouse in that it has data query function capabilities. See Data Warehouse.

Data Resource Manager   An individual who uses tools such as computer-based health record systems to ensure that the organization's information systems meet the needs of those who provide and manage patient services.

Data Rights   A term usually applied to medical and scientific research projects that denotes the level of ownership and stewardship of the data and records.

Data Security   The physical and electronic protection of computer-based information and the resources used to manipulate it.

Data Steward   A term used within some healthcare organizations that refers to the person responsible for managing the data in a corporation in terms of integrated, consistent definitions, structures, calculations, and derivations. The data steward role is common in health information exchanges (HIE).

Data Stewardship   The requirement to protect the integrity and security of data.

Data Warehouse   An information infrastructure that functions as a central repository for the significant parts of data collected by the organization. A data warehouse is generally a database that integrates data from the various operational systems and is typically uploaded from the organization's information systems at regular intervals. A data warehouse can be useful in the review and analysis of the organization's historical business processes and performance over time. See Data Repository.

Davis-Bacon Act   A federal law that requires payment of prevailing wages and benefits to government construction project contractor employees.

DCC   Data Content Committee—A designated organization of the Department of Health and Human Services chosen for oversight of the business data content of HIPAA-mandated transaction standards.

DCN   Document Control Number—A term used to refer to the number assigned to a claim when received for processing, facilitating ease of search on the part of CMS.

DD   Data Dictionary—According to HIPAA, a document that characterizes the data content of a system.

DDE   Direct Data Entry—The direct entry of data that are immediately transmitted to a health plan's computer, according to HIPAA.

DDL   Data Definition Language—An SQL statement.

DEA   Drug Enforcement Administration—The federal agency responsible for enforcement of the Controlled Substances Act of 1970. The DEA brings to the criminal and civil justice system of the United States, or any other competent jurisdiction, organizations and/or principal members of organizations involved in the growth, manufacture, or distribution of controlled substances appearing in or destined for illicit traffic in the United States. It also recommends and supports nonenforcement programs aimed at reducing the availability of illicit controlled substances on the domestic and international markets.

DEA Number   Drug Enforcement Administration Number—A unique numerical identifier that is assigned to healthcare providers and/or providers licensed to write prescriptions for eyeglasses and contact lenses that allows them to write prescriptions for controlled substances, medications, and/or eyeglasses and contact lenses.

Decimal   The base-10 representation of data in a computer system.

Decision Support   A system used for advising or providing guidance about a clinical decision at the point of care.

Decision Support System   The computer tools and applications used to assist doctors in clinical decisions by providing evidence in the context of patient-specific data.

Decision Tree   A tool used in decision analysis that examines alternatives, options, and possible outcomes.

Declaratory Judgment   In law, a judgment that rules on a dispute without awarding damages. May lead to an injunction.

Decommissioned   A term used to refer to an obsolete information system or data set.

Decommissioning a System   A term used to refer to the process that must be undergone by the Information Technology Department to close down an obsolete information system or set of data.

Decryption   The mathematical manipulation of ciphertext data into cleartext or plaintext data. The transformation typically requires the use of an electronic key.

Deductible   The amount of expense that must be incurred and paid by a patient within a specified time period before a third-party healthcare plan pays.

Deduping   Refers to the process of matching different lists for the purpose of identifying and eliminating duplicative information.

De Facto   An obligation or a right established as a matter or custom or common conduct that is not founded upon common law or statute.

Defamation   A civil or criminal tort. The intentional telling of harmful untruths about another person, resulting in harm to that person and/or to his/her reputation. Defamation can occur either in written or broadcast form or orally. See also Libel and Slander.

Default   In law, the failure to fulfill a legal obligation such as payment of a debt, performance of a contract, or responding to a summons.

Default Judgment   When a defendant to a lawsuit fails to respond to a complaint in the time set by law, the plaintiff can request the failure be entered into the court record by the clerk, which gives the plaintiff right to a default judgment. If complaints are made for a specific amount of monies owed, or when the amounts due are easy to calculate, the clerk of the court can enter a default judgment. When proof of damages or other relief is necessary, a hearing will be held in which the judge determines terms of the default judgment. In either case, the defendant cannot speak for himself or herself. A defendant who fails to file an answer or other legal response when it is due can request that the default be set aside, but must show a legitimate excuse and a good defense to the lawsuit.

Defendant   Refers to the person against whom a lawsuit is filed. The defendant is also known as the respondent.

Defensible Record   A health record that is created and maintained in a way that supports and protects its integrity and authenticity and can be used for medico-legal purposes.

Defensive Medicine   A term used to refer to medical practices designed to avert the possibility of a future medical malpractice lawsuit. In defensive medicine, doctors may order tests, procedures, or visits, or avoid high-risk patients or procedures, primarily (but not necessarily solely) to reduce their exposure to malpractice liability.

Deidentified Information   A term used to refer to identifying information that has been stripped, blacked out, or removed from an individual's record for the purpose of protecting the individual's privacy rights.

De Jure   As a matter of law rather than as a matter of custom.

Delegated Utilization Review   Handling of utilization review by healthcare providers contracting with third-party entities.

Delete   To remove information or data from a computer. Most data, when initially deleted, remain in a separate storage area until further action is taken.

Deleted Data   Deleted data are data that have been deleted by the computer or through end-user activity. Deleted data may remain in storage in whole or in part until they are overwritten or wiped out.

Deleted File   A file with disk space that has been designated as available for reuse. A deleted file will remain intact until it is overwritten.

De Minimus   In law, the Latin term meaning of minimal importance or insignificant. Generally, the term refers to an injury or burden that is of little or no consequence. For example, in e-discovery, a party with a de minimus burden of production of electronically stored information (ESI) is unlikely to be relieved of that burden by a court.

Demographics   The statistics of a defined population.

Demurrer   A written response to a complaint filed in a lawsuit that, in effect, pleads for dismissal on the point that even if the facts alleged in the complaint were true, there is no legal basis for a lawsuit. A hearing before a judge (on the law and motion calendar) will then be held to determine the validity of the demurrer. A demurrer may defeat some causes of action while others may survive. Some demurrers contend that the complaint is unclear or omits an essential element of fact. If the judge finds these errors, he or she will usually sustain the demurrer (state it is valid), but with leave to amend in order to allow changes to make the original complaint good. An amendment to the complaint cannot always overcome a demurrer, as in a case filed after the time allowed by law to bring a suit. If after amendment the complaint is still not legally good, a demurrer will be sustained. In rare occasions, a demurrer can be used to attack an answer to a complaint. Some states have substituted a motion to dismiss for failure to state a cause of action for the demurrer.

Denial   The determination that certain care or services cannot be reimbursed.

De Novo   In law, the Latin term meaning anew or starting over. The term generally refers to a litigant's right to start over anew after an unfavorable ruling.

Deontological Theories   Theories of ethics that are based on the calculation of duties rather than outcomes.

Deposition   The pretrial legal process that refers to the taking and recording of testimony of a witness under oath before a court reporter away from the courtroom. An attorney sets up a deposition for one of the parties to a lawsuit demanding the sworn testimony of the opposing party, a witness to an event, or an expert intended to be called at trial by the opposition. If the deponent (person requested to testify) is a party to the lawsuit or someone who works for an involved party, notice of time and place of the deposition can be given to the other side's attorney. If the witness is an independent third party, a subpoena must be served on him or her if he or she is reluctant to testify. The deposition testimony is taken down by the court reporter, and typewritten into a transcript that may be used at trial.

Derivative Liability   In law, the liability that a person other than the wronged individual has the right to redress. For example, the liability owed to a widow in a wrongful-death action.

DES   **Data Encryption Standard**—A symmetric block cipher, defined in the Federal Information Processing Standard (FIPS) number 46 as the federal government–approved algorithm for sensitive, nonclassified information.

Descenders   Refers to the portion of a character that falls below the main part of the letter; for example: g, p, q, y.

Deshading   Refers to the process of removing shaded areas to render images more easily recognizable by optical character recognition. The software used for deshading generally searches for areas with a regular pattern of tiny dots.

Designated Record Set   The term as described by HIPAA as a group of records maintained by or for an organization consisting of:
1. An individual's medical and billing records maintained by or for those entities within the organization that provides care, services, or supplies related to the health of an individual; or
2. Enrollment, payment, claims adjudication, and case or medical management record systems maintained by or for those entities within the organization that are health plans; or
3. Records used, in whole or in part, by or for an organization to make decisions about an individual.

Deskewing   The process of removing skew. Errors that can occur in scanning due to poor camera angle or paper placement, from images.

Desktop   An individual user's desktop computer. Occasionally refers to the initial menu on a computer screen following boot up.

Deviation   The difference between the value of an observation and the average of the population values in either mathematics or statistics.

DGI   **Drummond Group International**—An interoperability testing laboratory located in Austin, TX, offering global testing services through the product life cycle. On August 30, 2010, CCHIT was officially designated as an Authorized Testing and Certification Body (ONC-ATCB) by the Office of the National Coordinator (ONC). Scope of ONC-ATCB authorization: Complete EHR and EHR Modules. http://www.drummondgroup.com

Diagnostic   Procedures used to discover the nature of or underlying causes of a particular illness.

DICOM   **Digital Imaging and Communications in Medicine**—The standard for communicating digital images such as x-rays. DICOM is managed by the Medical Imaging and Technology Alliance. http://medical.nema.org

Dicta   The commentary of a judge in a written opinion that expresses the judge's feelings on the matters under discussion but is not necessary to the decision in the case. Dicta are not binding on courts in subsequent cases. See Holding.

Dictionary Attack   A term used to denote an attempt of trying every word in the dictionary as a possible password for an encrypted message.

Digital   Electronic technology that generates, stores, and processes data in terms of two states: positive and nonpositive. Positive is expressed or represented by the number 1 and nonpositive by the number 0. Data transmitted or stored with digital technology are expressed as a string of zeros and ones.

Digital Certificate   An attachment to an electronic message that is attached for security purposes to prove the identity of the sender.

Digital Forensics   A term used to refer to the use of technology to retrieve things that appear to be permanently deleted from a system or database.

Digital Signature   The digital signature provides authentication of incoming data, such as in incoming e-mail messages. A digital signature will simulate the security properties of a signature in digital rather than in written form and normally provides for two algorithms. The first algorithm serves to sign the user's message through a user's private key. The second algorithm verifies the signature through the user's public key. The end result of this two-step signature process is the actual digital signature. A digital signature is different from an electronic signature in that a digital signature is a subset of the electronic signature and employs the cryptographic techniques that provide for the authentication and security of the signature. See Private Key, Public Key, and Electronic Signature.

Direct Evidence   Proof proffered that shows existence of a fact in question without the intervention of the proof of any other fact.

DISA   **Data Interchange Standards Association**—A HIPAA body that provides administrative services to X12 and related groups. http://www.disa.org

Disability   A condition that results in limitations that prevent usual activities.

Disaster Recovery   The processes related to the preparation for the recovery of technology and data critical to an organization following the events of a disaster.

Discharge Plan   A plan that identifies what a patient's healthcare needs will be after discharge from a hospital or nursing facility.

Disclose   To make known or public.

Disclosure   Under HIPAA, the release of information by a person to people or organizations outside of himself or herself.

Disclosure History   A list of any entities that have received personally identifiable healthcare information for uses unrelated to treatment or payment under HIPAA.

Discount Rate   An interest rate that a central bank will charge depository institutions that borrow from it. The discount rate is a key variable in the calculation of the net present value.

Discovery   The pretrial legal process by which parties secure relevant information from the other parties. Discovery can be conducted through interrogatories, requests to produce, requests to admit, depositions, subpoenas, and experts. The purpose of discovery is to ensure that neither party is subjected to surprise at trial.

Discrete Data   Quantitative data including category (type) data, binominal data (1/0), or count data (consecutive numbers).

Disease Management   Refers to the collection and assessment of a patient's clinical data from a series of coordinated healthcare interventions and communications for populations with conditions in which patient self-care efforts are important in reducing costs and improving quality of life, particularly in cases of chronic disease.

Dismissal without Prejudice   The termination of a lawsuit with preservation of the right to reinstitute the proceedings.

Dismissal with Prejudice   The termination of a lawsuit without the right to reinstitute the proceeding.

Disparate Systems   Information technology systems that are separate from one another, but that can be merged or integrated.

Dispute   A written objection regarding the accuracy of a report or the fact that a specific event was reported to another body.

Distributed Data   A business's data residing on backup media or nonlocal devices, such as personal computers or PDAs. Any data held by third parties also falls into this category.

DMERC   **Durable Medical Equipment Regional Carrier.**

DML Data Manipulation Language—An SQL statement.

DNFB Discharged Not Final Billed—A commonly used operational measure to report the number and dollar amount of uncoded or unbilled inpatient and outpatient claims. The DNFB number is a financial benchmark to measure and assess accounts receivable.

DNR Do Not Resuscitate.

Doctor/Patient Privilege A rule in a number of jurisdictions that precludes the disclosure of information obtained by the physician in the course of the doctor/patient relationship.

Doctrine of Alternative Liability A theory that holds that when more than one medical professional participates in an injurious procedure in which it is uncertain which one caused the harm, all individuals must prove their own nonculpability.

Doctrine of Therapeutic Privilege Refers to an exception to the informed consent doctrine that allows a physician to withhold information from the patient when disclosure of such information poses a significant detriment to the patient.

Document Blowback A term used in litigation support services to describe the process of printing massive amounts of document images and scanned files to hard copy.

Document Consumer The seller who receives information, views a document, imports, or stores the document for later viewing.

Document Imaging The process of replication of paper documents into a digital copy via a document scanner for storage on a computer or storage media along with indexes that identify the unique document. The electronic documents can then be accessed by document retrieval software. Document imaging allows for rapid retrieval of paper documents from desktop computers.

Document Management System An automated computer system designed to store electronically stored information (ESI) and scanned hard copy documents.

Document Retention Policy A presumably written policy that provides for the systematic review, retention, and destruction of all documents received or created in the course of business. The document retention policy will identify documents that need to be maintained and contain guidelines for how long certain documents should be kept and how they should be destroyed. HIM and IT professionals should work with legal counsel in the development and ongoing review and revision of the policy and ensure its compliance with electronic and paper document storage, retention, and legal requirements.

DOD   **Department of Defense**—A federal department responsible for coordinating all government agencies related to national security and the military. http://www.defenselink.mil

DOI   **Department of Insurance**—A series of state agencies charged with the task of protecting consumers by regulating insurance organizations.

DOL   **Department of Labor**—A cabinet department of the federal government responsible for occupational security, hour and wage standards, unemployment benefits, and employment services. http://www.dol.gov

Domain Name   A unique name that identifies an Internet site. Domain names consist of two or more parts separated by dots. For example: http://www.BCBSA.com or http://www.bcbsil.com.

Donut Hole   The gap phase of the Medicare Part D prescription drug coverage during which the beneficiary is responsible for paying 100 percent of the beneficiary's drug costs ($2,930 in 2012). Once the beneficiary reaches the maximum out-of-pocket expenses, he or she becomes eligible for Medicare Part D catastrophic coverage.

DOS   **Date of Service**—The date on which medical services are given.

Downcoding   A term used to describe the process by which third-party payers or other reviewers change a code on a claim to a less complex or lower-cost procedure than was originally reported.

Downgraded Data   In law, a term used to refer to electronically stored information (ESI) that has been changed from one format into a less reasonably searchable format.

Download   To transmit a file from one computer to another.

Draft   A report that is temporarily stored and may be revised before any distribution.

DRAW   **Direct Read, After Write.**

DRG   **Diagnosis-Related Group.**

DriveCrypt   A commercial disk encryption system that supports Windows and Pocket PCs.

Drug Categories   Prescription drugs in the same class that are used to treat a specific condition or illness such as high blood pressure, high cholesterol, heartburn, or depression.

DSG **Digital Signature Guidelines**—Guidelines developed by the American Bar Association for the use of digital signatures.

DSH **Disproportionate Share Hospital**—A nonprofit hospital that: 1. has a disproportionately large share of low-income patients, and 2. receives (a) an augmented payment from the state under Medicaid, or (b) a payment adjustment from Medicare. Hospital-based outpatient services are included under this definition.

DSMO **Designated Standard Maintenance Organization**—An organization designated by the Secretary of HHS to maintain standards for healthcare transactions.

DSS **Digital Signature Standard**—Promulgated in 1994 by the National Institute of Standards and Technology (NIST), DSS is the US government cryptographic standard for authenticating electronic documents.

DSS **Division of State Systems**—The federal agency that oversees the Advance Planning Document (APD) process and the approval of the State-wide Automated Child Welfare Information System (SACWIS).

DSTU **Draft Standard for Trial Use**—An HL7 standard used to denote a standard undergoing a period of evaluation and comment before incorporation into a fully balloted and accredited version of the standard. The DSTU directive was established by HL7 in 2003 to provide a means for development organizations to undergo adequate testing of infrastructure, data types, and message representation.

Dual Eligible An individual covered by both Medicare and Medicaid.

Due Care In law, the level of care that a reasonable person would exercise under a given set of conditions; used to indicate the standard of care one owes to others.

Due Diligence Review A review of all aspects of an organization to determine if it is adequate to meet expected health demands and community standards.

Due Process Clauses found in the Fifth and Fourteenth Amendments to the US Constitution and most state constitutions that provide the right of an individual to fundamental fairness in judicial proceedings.

Dump Transferring the contents of a memory store to another memory store or other output in order to save or study the data.

DUN **Dial-Up Networking**—Computer networking that relies on communication through ordinary telephone lines via modem.

DUPLEX   Refers to the mode of transmitting data through a modem.

Durable Power of Attorney for Healthcare   A legal document that can be composed by a patient to empower another agent to make important medical decisions should the patient be rendered unable.

Duty   In law, a legal obligation that, if breached, can result in liability. In a lawsuit, a plaintiff must allege and prove that there was a duty owed by the defendant to the plaintiff. For example, in e-discovery, a duty to preserve relevant electronically stored information (ESI) in which the failure to do so may result in the imposition of sanctions.

Duty of Care   A legal relationship arising from a standard of care that, when violated, subjects the actor to liability.

Duty to Notify   The obligation to notify a client (legal domain) or a patient (healthcare domain) of significant changes that will impact the client's case or care.

Duty to Preserve   The legal requirement that a person or entity maintain information relevant to actual or reasonably anticipated litigation. See Duty.

Duty to Warn   The obligation to release confidential information on a patient when it is necessary to warn another person who is in imminent danger, mandated by law in many states.

E

EAP   **Employee Assistance Program**—An employer-sponsored program designed to assist employees and employers in identifying solutions for workplace and personal problems.

Early Case Assessment   The pretrial process of discovery in which legal counsel reviews all potentially responsive information and/or data prior to trial.

ECM   **Enterprise Content Management**—The concept of electronic storage and management of all records within the organization. Examples of the types of records that might be found and managed through an ECM system include contracts, financial records, and other files, including but not limited to the management of e-HIM data and records. See also Enterprise Content Management.

E-Commerce   The transaction of business online. The linkage of the buyer's computer with a business information system. Examples of e-commerce vendors include Amazon.com, Orbitz.com, Priceline.com, and a host of other vendors that conduct retail business online.

Economic Damages   Injuries or losses that can easily be calculated in monetary amounts.

E-Copy   A term used to denote an electronic copy sent to someone other than the intended recipient.

ECPA   Electronic Communications Privacy Act of 1986 (Pub. L. 99-508)— Enacted by Congress on October 21, 1986, this legislation extends government restrictions on wire taps on telephone calls including the transmissions of electronic data by computer. This law prohibits unauthorized access to communications held by a service provider and imposes specific requirements on government entities seeking to obtain such communications. See also Stored Communications Act (SCA).

EDD   Electronic Data Discovery.

EDI   Electronic Data Interchange—1. A term used to denote computer-to-computer transmission of electronic data in a standard format, which replaces a traditional paper business document. 2. A term used to denote criteria that, if unmet, will cause an automated claims processing system to dismiss a claim.

EDIS   Electronic Document Information System—A central repository for all documents filed in relation to an investigation conducted by the United States International Trade Commission (USITC). EDIS provides the capability to file documents for an investigation as well as search for documents that have been submitted to the USITC.

e-Discovery   E-discovery is used to describe the collection, review, and production of electronically stored information (ESI). See Discovery.

EDI Translation   The conversion of application data to and from a specified format for the electronic exchange of data into a standard format.

EDI X12   Electronic Data Interchange—An electronic data format based on ASC X12 standards used for the electronic exchange of data between two or more trading partners, companies, or organizations. Every new release contains a new version number. Version number examples: 4010, 4020, 4030, 5010, 5030. Major new releases start with a new first number. 4010 and 5010 are major releases. Minor releases contain minor changes or improvements or major releases. 4020, 4030, and 5030 are minor releases.

EDRM   Electronic Discovery Reference Model—An e-discovery practice tool developed by George Socha Jr. and Tom Gelbmanan to help consumers and providers. The reference model divides the discovery process into six areas—information management, identification, preservation/collection, processing/review/analysis, production, and presentation—and identifies the functions associated with each area. http://edrm.net

EEOC **Equal Employment Opportunity Commission**—The federal agency charged with the enforcement of federal laws (described below) that prohibit job discrimination:

- Title VII of the Civil Rights Act of 1964 (Title VII)
- Equal Pay Act of 1963
- Age Discrimination Act of 1967 (ADEA)
- Title I and Title V of the Americans with Disabilities Act of 1990 (ADA)
- Sections 501 and 505 of the Rehabilitation Act of 1973
- The Civil Rights Act of 1991

The EEOC also provides oversight and coordination of employment opportunity regulations, practices, and policies.

EEOICPA **Energy Employees Occupational Illness Compensation Program Act**—A federal worker's compensation law that provides lump-sum payments and medical benefits to Department of Energy employees and subcontractors (or certain survivors) for cancer caused by radiation exposure.

EER **Equal Error Rate**—The point at which the probability of a false accept is equal to the probability of a false reject.

E-Evidence E-evidence is information that has met, among other things, authentication requirements and is admitted before the finder-of-fact. See also Evidence.

Effectiveness A measure of the degree to which a diagnosis or procedure leads to an expected outcome measure within a specific population.

Efficiency A measure of the degree to which costs of resources expended are met by benefits to a patient.

EFT **Electronic Funds Transfer.**

EH **Eligible Hospital** as defined in HITECH.

E-Health The use of the Internet to conduct health- and healthcare-related business transactions.

E-Health Initiative An independent nonprofit organization with the mission to drive improvement in the quality, safety, and efficiency of healthcare through information and information technology. An affiliate of the Foundation for E-Health Initiative.

E-HIM   A major strategic focus of the American Health Information Management Association (AHIMA), its goals are to: 1. promote the migration from paper to an electronic health information infrastructure; 2. reinvent how institutional and personal health information and records are managed; and 3. deliver measurable cost and quality results from improved information management.

EHR   Electronic Health Record—A system that stores and maintains patient health data. This includes clinical, administrative, and payment data.

EHR/IM   Electronic Health Record Interoperability Model—An HL7 draft standard for trial use published in March 2007 that is undergoing a period of trial review and evaluation. The EHR/IM describes characteristics of interoperable EHR records and is being reviewed and mapped against HL7 interoperability and CDAr2 functionality requirements.

EHRS   Electronic Health Record System—The healthcare industry's first ANSI-approved standard developed by HL7 that specifies the functional requirements for an electronic health record system (EHRS). See also EHRS/FM.

EHRS/FM   Electronic Health Record System—Functional Model—A normative HL7/ANSI standard published in March 2007 that describes the functions and functional characteristics of an EHR. An EHR conforms to the functional profiles of the EHRS/FM.

EHR Standards   The expectations or requirements for an EHR.

EIN   Employer Identification Number—The Internal Revenue Service (IRS) federal tax number of a healthcare business.

Election Periods   The time in which a Medicare beneficiary may choose to join or leave Original Medicare or a Medicare managed care plan. There are four periods during which a beneficiary may choose to join or leave Medicare managed care plans: annual election period, initial coverage election period, special election period, and open enrollment period.

Electronic Claim   A healthcare claim submitted by a provider or vendor via computer-to-computer transmission via modem or Internet connection. ANSI transaction standard 837 provides the standard for transmission of an electronic healthcare claim.

Electronic Envelope   The electronic equivalent of a paper envelope. A term used to denote an electronic address, communications transport protocols, and control information in a transaction. An electronic envelope is also sometimes called a communications package or simply an envelope.

Electronic Health Record   A system that stores and maintains patient health data; a system of electronically maintained information (clinical, administrative, and payment data) about an individual's lifetime health status and healthcare, stored such that it can be accessible to authorized users (for example, physicians, nurses, pharmacists, hospitals, and other providers) of record.

Electronic Image   An electronic representation of a document in the form of a bitmap, represented as a two-dimensional continuum of brightness values for pixels.

Electronic Key   A unique information system key that allows the authorized system user access to the system in accordance with his or her role, job function, and/or access parameters. Smart cards, tokens, and digital fingerprints are examples of electronic keys.

Electronic Record   A collection of data terms that are processed by a computer program. Multiple records are contained in a data set or a file. The programming language of the information system usually defines the organization of the record and/or the applications that process it. Typically, records can be of fixed length or be of variable length, with the length information contained within the record.

Electronic Records Management   The electronic management of digital and analog records contained in IT systems using computer equipment and software.

Electronic Remittance Advice   Under HIPAA, electronic formats for explaining the payments of healthcare claims. Sometimes referred to as ERA.

Electronic Search   The ability to access all documents pertinent to litigation in electronic form and use selected keywords to find applicable documents for further review.

Electronic Signature   The term electronic signature has several different meanings as defined by various United States and international laws. In 1999, the Uniform Electronic Transactions Act (UETA) defined the electronic signature as "an electronic sound, symbol, or process, attached to or logically associated with a record and executed or adopted by a person with the intent to sign the record." Enactment of the US E-Sign Act in 2000 incorporates most of the UETA definition for application in the United States at the federal level. The term electronic signature is often confused with and used interchangeably with digital signature. An electronic signature is different from a digital signature in that cryptographic techniques are not employed to verify the authenticity and security of the signature and incoming message. A digital signature is a subset of an electronic signature. See also Digital Signature, Private Key, and Public Key.

E-Mail   Electronic Mail—A message both created and received through an electronic mail system.

E-Mail String   A series of linked e-mails, responses, and forwards, often treated as a single document in litigation.

Emancipated Minor   The legal status of a minor when married or otherwise no longer subject to the control and regulation of parents.

Emotional Distress   Mental distress or anxiety suffered as a response to a sudden, severe, and saddening experience. In tort law, this can refer to both intentional and negligent infliction of emotional distress.

EMPI   Enterprise Master Patient Index—Merged listing of all master patient indices in an integrated delivery system.

Employer Identifier   A standard to identify employers in transactions, adopted by HHS.

Employers' Liability Insurance   An agreement between the organization and the insurer to indemnify an employer against an employee's claim not covered under the workers' compensation system, or an agreement to indemnify the employer for an employee's negligence that injures a third party.

Employment-Practices Liability Insurance   Insurance that provides coverage for claims arising from an insured's injury-causing employment practice, such as sexual harassment, defamation, or discrimination.

EMTALA   Emergency Medical Treatment and Active Labor Act—(42 USC. § 1395dd) An act of Congress that requires hospitals and ambulance services to provide care for anyone who needs emergency medical treatment, regardless of legal status or ability to pay.

Encoder   A hardware or software device that converts information from one format into another for viewing, editing, storage, security, or transmission. Many HIM departments utilize encoders for coding and DRG assignment.

Encoding   The process of converting analog electrical or optical signals into digital format for storage, manipulation, and display. Encoding also means transferring digital information from one format to another format for a specific purpose, such as space saving.

Encryption   The algorithmic scheme that encodes plain text into nonreadable form known as ciphertext, (also known as cyphertext) to prevent anyone except the intended recipient from reading that data. The receiver of the encrypted text uses a key to decrypt the message, returning it to its original plaintext form.

Endpoint   The end or final point in a process.

End-Stage Renal Disease   The point at which there is permanent kidney failure, and dialysis or transplant are the only two options of treatment left for a patient. On April 15, 2008, the Medicare ESRD Conditions Final Rule was updated to modernize Medicare's ESRD health and safety conditions for coverage and updated CMS standards for delivering safe, high-quality care to dialysis patients. The revised regulations are patient-centered, and reflect improvements in clinical standards of care, the use of more advanced technology, and, most notably, a framework to incorporate performance measures viewed by the scientific and medical community to be related to the quality of care provided to dialysis patients.

End-to-End Principle   The central design principle of Internet Protocol (IP) whose premise is communications protocol operations should be defined to occur at the endpoints of a communications system.

Enforcement Rule   HIPAA regulations that govern the procedures for enforcement of other regulations.

Enrollment   The number of members of a managed care plan or members assigned to a medical group under contract.

Enrollment   The process of initial collection of data (biometric or nonbiometric) from a user and then storage of it in a reference template for later comparison.

Enterprise Content Management   Refers to the utilization of technologies for the capture, management, storage, preservation, and delivery of content and documents that relate to the organization's business processes. ECM tools and strategies allow for easier management and utilization of an organization's unstructured information, wherever that information may exist.

Enterprise Liability   In law, liability that is imposed on each member of an enterprise of an industry responsible for the manufacture of a harmful or defective product, allotted by each manufacturer's market share of the industry. Also known as industry-wide liability or market-share liability.

Entry Errors   Small errors in transcription or larger mistakes involving test results, doctor orders, and inadvertently omitted information.

Environmental Health   A directed effort to minimize the risk of environmental damage or hazards by preventing the transmission of a potentially injurious agent into the environment and protecting the population from contaminated environments.

EOB **Explanation of Benefits**—A statement provided by an insurer summarizing covered and noncovered costs. Also called a remittance.

EOMB **Explanation of Medicare Benefits**—See Medicare Summary Notice.

EP **Eligible Professionals**—Under the Health Information Technology for Economic and Clinical Health Act (HITECH), for Medicare incentives an eligible professional is defined as a physician, as defined in section 1861(r) of the Social Security Act. This includes doctors, osteopaths, dentists, podiatrists, optometrists, and chiropractors. For Medicaid incentives, an eligible professional means a 1. physician, 2. dentist, 3. certified nurse midwife, 4. nurse practitioner, or 5. physician assistant practicing in a rural health clinic led by a physician assistant or practicing in a federally qualified health center led by a physician assistant.

EP **Eligible Provider** as defined in HITECH.

E-Paper The electronic version of a document.

Ephemeral Data A term used to describe data that are relatively short lived. RAM is one example of a type of ephemeral data. In e-discovery the retention of ephemeral data has become a controversial topic because, in one recent court opinion, the defendant was ordered to produce RAM data because they were uniquely relevant to proving the legal claims and could not be obtained through any other alternate means.

E-PHI **Electronic Protected Health Information.**

Epidemiology The study of factors affecting the health status of populations, which serves as the foundation of interventions made in the name of public health.

Episode of Care Medical services provided for a specific disorder in a defined period of time.

EPO **Exclusive Provider Organization.**

E-Prescribing A term used to describe the process of creating, ordering, and signing prescriptions through the use of online computerized tools and systems.

EPSDT **Early and Periodic Screening, Diagnosis, and Treatment**—A health program for Medicaid recipients designed to identify physical and mental defects and provide treatment to correct these conditions from birth through age 20.

Equal Protection Clause A clause of the Fourteenth Amendment that provides "no state shall . . . deny to any person within its jurisdiction the equal protection of the laws."

ERA **Electronic Research Administration**—The administrative process in which research is conducted through utilization of electronic resources such as the Internet and the World Wide Web from templates, databases, and other tools.

ERA **Electronic Remittance Advice**—Information on a healthcare claim form that provides an explanation of a payment from a healthcare payer. The requirements for the electronic interchange and translation of data are contained under ANSI transaction standard 835.

ERISA **Employee Retirement Income Security Act**—A federal statute that is intended to regulate employee benefits for most employees in the United States. Nearly any type of employee benefit can be covered by ERISA, including: pensions and 401K plans, health insurance, long-term disability insurance, life insurance, and accidental death and dismemberment insurance.

ER Modeling A term used in the context of information management and technology to describe a graphic technique used for the understanding and organization of data independent of actual implementation of a database.

Errata A listing of errors and the corrections to the errors.

Errata Sheet An attachment to the transcript of a deposition that contains the deponent's corrections upon reading of the transcript and the reasons for the corrections.

Errors and Omissions Insurance An agreement made between the insurer and the organization to indemnify for losses sustained because of a mistake or oversight by the insured, with the exception of losses incurred as a result of intentional wrongdoing by the insured party.

ERX **Electronic Prescribing**—A form of technology that allows doctors to use computer devices to review drug and formulary coverage to transmit prescriptions to a printer or pharmacy.

ESI **Electronically Stored Information**—A phrase introduced in the Federal Rules of Civil Procedure in amendments that became effective December 1, 2006. ESI includes information located on, for example, computers, file servers, disks, tapes, or other devices or media.

E-Sign **The Electronic Signatures in Global and National Commerce Act**—Federal legislation enacted in 2000 to protect consumers by requiring adequate consent to electronic transactions and to validate contracts executed by electronic signature.

ESMI **Electronically Stored Medical Information.**

ESRD   End-Stage Renal Disease—Kidney failure that is severe enough to require lifetime dialysis or a kidney transplant.

Estoppel   In law, a doctrine by which a party can be precluded from contesting a particular fact.

Et al.   And other persons.

Ethical Hacking   Refers to an information security assessment that may be undertaken by an organization to evaluate the organization's information security vulnerabilities through use of the same tools and techniques employed by hackers to map out an organization's information security vulnerabilities and threaten its information.

Ethics   A broad branch of philosophy that seeks to address questions about morality. In law, ethics are the standards of minimally acceptable conduct within the profession, related to the duties that members of the profession owe each other, their clients, and the courts.

ETI   Electronic Tool Integration.

ETL   Extraction, Transformation, and Loading—A data warehouse component and function.

Et Seq.   A Latin term that means and those that follow.

Evaluation and Management Service   A nonprocedural service provided by a doctor for diagnosis and treatment.

Evidence   In law, a word encompassing anything admitted at a hearing or a trial intended to prove or disprove a contested fact. Evidence includes oral testimony of laypeople and experts, documents, electronically stored information (ESI), objects, and photographs. Evidence can be direct, based on the actual observation of a witness, or circumstantial, which relies on an inference to establish a fact.

Evidence-Based Criteria   The guidelines for clinical practice that incorporate current and validated research findings.

Evidentiary Fact   A vital fact for the determination of an ultimate fact by furnishing evidence of this fact's existence.

Exabyte   A unit of information or computer storage equal to one quintillion bytes.

Excess Charge   The difference between the Medicare-approved amount and the actual charge for services or goods received. (Applies to people with Original Medicare plans only.) Nonparticipating doctors cannot charge more than 15 percent above the Medicare-approved amount.

Excess Insurance   An agreement that indemnifies the organization for losses that exceed the amount of coverage under another policy.

Exculpatory Clause   A clause in a written agreement that relieves once party from liability for any failure to perform.

Executive Committee   A committee whose sole purpose is to provide access to decision-making and confidential discussions for an organization's board.

Exhaustion of Remedies   In law, a doctrine that requires a plaintiff to exhaust all nonjudicial remedies before filing a suit.

Ex Parte   In law, the Latin term meaning for one party. The term is used to refer to motions, hearings, or orders granted on the request of one party and in the absence of another. An ex parte proceeding is an exception and is disfavored.

Ex Parte Communication   A taboo communication between counsel and court in the absence of opposing counsel.

Expedited Appeal   An appeal of a healthcare decision made by a health plan or provider where a medical service is at issue.

Experience Rating   In insurance, a method for determining the amount of the premium by analyzing the client's loss record over time to assess the risk that certain events will occur and the amount of probable damages such events will do.

Expert   A person who has developed skill or knowledge of a subject through education or experience so that he or she can form an opinion that will assist in litigation.

Expert Witness   A person with specialized education or experience who is able to provide information on a topic beyond that of an average person. Expert witnesses in medical malpractice are not limited to any one class of persons.

Explanation of Benefits or Coverage   A statement provided by an insurer summarizing covered and noncovered costs. Also called a remittance.

Extended Care Facility   A residential medical care setting that provides custodial care services.

External Counsel   An attorney who is not employed by his or her client but is retained by the client to represent him or her in a particular matter or matters. Outside counsel.

External Disclosure   The disclosure of information either in written or verbal form outside the walls of the organization. External disclosures may or may not be part of the legal process.

Extract   A summary or synopsis of a document or a portion of a document.

Extrapolation   The process of estimating an unknown on the basis of a known range of variables, such as another case.

F

FACA   Federal Advisory Committee Act (Pub. L. 92-463)—A federal law that governs the behavior of federal advisory committees.

Facebook   A social networking utility that connects people through school, city, and company networks.

Faceting   Several attributes that items have and that can be used for navigation in information retrieval.

Fact   An actual or alleged circumstance, independent of consequence and interpretation.

FACTA or FACT Act   Fair and Accurate Credit Transaction Act (Pub. L. 108-159)—A federal law, passed by Congress, that mandates the secure disposal of consumer information. FACTA also contains provisions to help reduce identity theft by providing individuals the ability to place alerts on their credit histories and obtain a free credit report once every year from each of the three national credit reporting agencies.

False Claims Act   A federal law that allows individuals to assert fraud claims against entities that receive federal funds. The individual who files a lawsuit under the False Claims Act is known as a whistleblower.

False Statement Act   A federal statute that covers any false, fictitious, or fraudulent statements or representations in any matter within the jurisdiction of any department or agency of the US government.

Family Relationship   In the information technology context, documents that have a connection because of common characteristics.

FBI   Federal Bureau of Investigation—A federal law enforcement agency that, among other things, investigates healthcare fraud and abuse as well as cybercrimes. http://www.fbi.gov

FCC   Federal Communications Commission—The federal agency that regulates interstate and foreign communications by radio, television, telephone,

and telegraph and oversees broadcasting standards, cable-television operations, two-way radio operators, and satellite communications.

FDA   Food and Drug Administration—The FDA is one of 11 federal agencies that make up the Department of Health and Human Services. "The FDA
is responsible for protecting the public health by assuring the safety, efficacy,
and security of human and veterinary drugs, biological products, medical
devices, our nation's food supply, cosmetics, and products that emit radiation. The FDA is also responsible for advancing the public health by helping
to speed innovations that make medicines and foods more effective, safer,
and more affordable; and helping the public get the accurate, science-based
information they need to use medicines and foods to improve their health."
http://www.fda.gov

Feasibility Study   An analysis of factors to determine whether an information
system will achieve the desired objectives. It is a preliminary study to determine whether it is sufficiently probable that effective and efficient use of automated equipment or systems can be made to warrant a substantial investment
of staff, time, and money requested and whether the plan is capable of being
accomplished successfully.

Feature Extraction   A term used to describe the automated process of locating
and encoding distinctive characteristics from a biometric sample in order to
generate a template.

FECA   Federal Employees' Compensation Act (5 USC. 8101 et seq.)—A
comprehensive and exclusive federal workers' compensation law that provides
for the compensation for the disability or death of a federal employee sustained in employment.

Federal Court   A generic term. It relates to courts created by Article III of the
Constitution and by federal statute. The term includes US bankruptcy courts,
US district courts, the courts of appeals, and the US Supreme Court. The
district courts are the trial-level courts. There are 93 separate district courts
across the United States, including the District of Columbia, Puerto Rico, Virgin Islands, Guam, and the Northern Mariana Islands.

Federal Court of Appeals   A federal court of appeals is also known as a circuit court. A total of 12 regional circuit courts make up the federal court of
appeals system. A circuit court will hear appeals from the 94 district courts,
as well as decisions of federal administrative agencies. The federal circuit also
has nationwide jurisdiction to hear appeals in specialized cases such as those
involving patent laws and/or cases decided by the Court of International
Trade and the Court of Federal Claims.

Federal Drug Abuse, Prevention, Treatment and Rehabilitation Act   A federal statute enacted in 1972, intended to provide substance abuse treatment research participants with additional rights of confidentiality and protection under the law.

Federal Employees Health Benefits Program   A health benefits program administered through the US Office of Personnel Management.

Federal Hospital   Any federal institution in a state that is primarily engaged in providing, by or under the supervision of physicians, to inpatients: (a) diagnostic and therapeutic services for medical diagnosis, treatment, and care of injured, disabled, or sick persons; or (b) rehabilitation of injured, disabled, or sick persons. Hospital-based outpatient services are included under this definition.

Federally Designated Health Center   A nonprofit entity that is receiving a grant, or funding from a grant, under section 330 of the Public Health Service Act, as amended, to provide primary health services and other related services to a population that is medically underserved. Federally Qualified Health Centers include community health centers, migrant health centers, healthcare for the homeless health centers, and public housing primary care health centers.

Federally Designated Health Center Look Alike   A nonprofit entity that is certified by the Secretary of HHS as meeting the requirements for receiving a grant under section 330 of the Public Health Service Act, but is not a grantee.

Federal Register   A daily publication in which administrative agencies of the US government publish their regulations, including proposed regulations for public comment.

Federal Rule of Evidence 502   Enacted in 2008, the rule is intended to address, among other things, the cost of privilege review in civil litigation. It is also intended to create uniform standards across the US courts for intentional and inadvertent disclosure of privileged materials, allow the issuance of nonwaiver orders by federal judges, and bind state courts in certain areas.

Federal Rules of Evidence   The rules that govern the admissibility, or lack thereof, of evidence at trials in federal court.

FED SPEC   Federal Specifications.

Felony-Reporting Statute   Statutes mandated by states that indicate the conditions under which an individual who is aware of a felon-level crime must report it to the authorities.

FERPA   **Family Educational Rights and Privacy Act**—The body of privacy law that provides for the availability of funds to educational agencies or institutions; inspection and review of education records; specific information to be made available; the procedure for access to education records; reasonableness of time for such access; and hearings and written explanations by parents.

FFP **Federal Financial Participation**—The federal government's share of an approved state cost.

FFY **Federal Fiscal Year**—The accounting period of the federal government. The FFY begins on October 1 and ends on September 30 of the next calendar year.

FHA **Federal Health Architecture**—A body composed of several collaborating departments and agencies, providing the framework for linking health business processes to technology solutions and standards while demonstrating how said solutions achieve improved health performance outcomes.

Fiber Optics Transmission technology using modulated infrared light sent through a glass fiber.

Fiduciary One who owes a duty of loyalty to safeguard the interests of another person or entity, such as a guardian, conservator, or trustee.

Fiduciary Relationship A term used to describe the responsibility one has for the management of monetary affairs for another and is therefore obligated to act in absolute good faith with regard to those affairs. This degree of duty has also been imposed on physicians and other providers in some jurisdictions with regard to the provider's responsibility to safeguard protected health information.

File A set of data maintained in computer memory or a program that has a specific name through which it can be accessed.

File Conversion Changing data or a file from one format to another.

File Extension The period and three- or four-letter tag at the end of a file's name that identifies its format or the application used to create it.

File Format A form of storage for electronic documents that varies in compression, file use, depth of color, and software compatibility.

Filtering A term used to describe software optimized for controlling what content is visible to a reader, especially when it is used to restrict material delivered over the World Wide Web.

Final Rule A regulation issued to amend the Code of Federal Regulations and that finalizes proposed rules (regulations) previously issued or takes final action without a prior proposed rule.

FINRA Financial Industry Regulatory Authority—FINRA is the largest non-governmental regulator for all securities firms doing business in the United States. http://www.finra.org

FIPS Federal Information Processing Standard.

Firewall A system designed to prevent unauthorized access to or from a private network. Firewalls can be implemented in both hardware and software, or a combination of both.

Firmware Software on a chip rather than on a disc or tape.

First Amendment The First Amendment to the Constitution, establishing freedom of speech, freedom of the press, freedom of religion, and freedom to petition.

Fiscal Intermediary An insurance company contracted by CMS for a region to determine and provide Medicare payments to providers. See also Carrier and Medicare Administrative Contractor (MAC).

FISMA Federal Information Security Management Act (Pub. L. 107-347)—A federal law enacted in 2002 that requires each agency of the federal government develop, document, and implement an agency-wide information security program for the information systems that support the operations and assets of the agency, including those provided or managed by another agency, governmental contractor, or other source.

Fixed Phrase A method of authentication in which a predefined sentence is spoken by the user.

Flat File A HIPAA term referring to a file that consists of a series of fixed-length records with some sort of record-type code.

Flickr A digital photo sharing website and service.

Floppy Disk A magnetic disk on which data can be stored.

Flow Chart A diagram used for the definition and analysis of a problem, which utilizes symbols.

FLSA Fair Labor Standards Act—The federal law that applies to most private and public organizations, which prescribes standards for wages and overtime pay.

FMLA Family Medical Leave Act—The federal law administered by the Wage and Hour Division of the Department of Labor (DOL) that requires employers of 50 or more employees to give up to 12 weeks of unpaid job-protected leave to eligible employees for the birth or adoption of a child or for the serious illness of the employee, spouse, parent, or child.

FMR **Focused Medical Review**—A program in which Medicare carriers provide a targeted medical review of items and services that present the greatest risk of inappropriate Medicare Part B program payment.

FOIA **Freedom of Information Act** (Pub. L. 89-554, 80 Stat. 383)—A federal act, amended in 1996, 2002, and 2007, that allows for disclosure of previously unreleased information and documents controlled by the government. It defines agency records subject to disclosure, outlines mandatory disclosure procedures, and grants nine exemptions to the statute.

Fons Juris In law, the Latin term for source of law. A document or custom that provides authority for legislation and for judicial decisions.

Forensic Copy An exact copy of a computer drive and unallocated computer space.

Forfeiture In Rem A term used to refer to the forfeiture of a property.

Form 35 Part of the Federal Rules of Civil Procedure. It is intended as a model for use by litigants to report to the court on the litigants' meet-and-confer pursuant to Federal Rule 26(f). The form is intended to report on the litigants' agreements and disagreements about e-discovery.

Format Under HIPAA, those data elements that provide the enveloping structure or assist in identifying data content of a transaction, under HIPAA.

Formulary The panel of drugs, when available, chosen by a hospital that is available for the treatment of members or patients.

FORTRAN **FORmula TRANslator**—A high computer language used primarily in math and science.

Foundation for E-Health An independent, nonprofit organization with the mission to drive improvement in the quality, safety, and efficiency of healthcare through information and information technology. An affiliate of the E-Health Initiative.

FQHC **Federally Qualified Health Center**—A US reimbursement designation that refers to a number of health programs, such as community health centers, migrant health centers, and healthcare for the homeless programs, funded by the Health Center Consolidation Act.

Fraud and Abuse A complex and expanding array of legislative restrictions on the way healthcare providers conduct business and structure their relationships. Provisions dictating conduct are found in the Medicare/Medicaid statute, Stark legislation, and the civil False Claims Act. Violations of these provisions include executing a scheme to defraud healthcare benefit programs, committing theft or embezzlement, and making false statements in obstruction of criminal investigations.

Fraudulent   An intentional deception made for either personal gain of one party or damage of another.

Fraudulent Concealment   In law, the affirmative hiding or suppression of a fact or event that one is legally bound to disclose, with the intent to deceive or defraud.

FRCP   Federal Rules of Civil Procedure—Governs how the US district courts conduct the business of federal civil litigation.

FRCP Rule 16   This rule addresses conferences before the US district courts. FRCP 16(b) describes what subjects scheduling orders should consider, including ones related to e-discovery.

FRCP Rule 26   This rule, generally speaking, governs discovery in the US district courts. Rule 26(b)(2)(B) established the concept of sources of electronically stored information (ESI) that are not reasonably accessible. Rule 26(b)(2)(C) addresses proportionality in discovery. Rule 26(f) requires that parties meet and confer before their Rule 16(b) initial conference.

FRCP Rule 34   This rule, among other things, governs the manner in which litigants request and produce electronically stored information (ESI).

FRCP Rule 45   This rule governs the issuance of subpoenas to nonparties and the not reasonably accessible concept of Rule 26(b)(2)(B).

FRE 803(18)—Medical Literature as Evidence   In law, the Federal Rule of Evidence 803(18), which holds that articles from medical periodicals are not admissible as evidence in a trial.

Freedom of Information Act   A law enacted in 1966 establishing the presumption that records in the possession of agencies and departments of the executive branch are accessible to the people.

Freedom of Speech   Rights established by the First Amendment and applied to the states by the Fourteenth Amendment.

Free OTFE   Open source disk encryption software for Windows that supports the Advanced Encryption Standard (AES) and Twofish.

FTC   Federal Trade Commission—An independent agency of the US government that investigates and eliminates unfair and deceptive trade practices. http://www.ftc.gov

FTCA **Federal Tort Claims Act**—A 1948 statute that permits private parties to sue the United States in federal court for most torts committed by individuals acting on behalf of the country.

FTE **Full-Time Equivalent**—A measure of a person's percentage of full-time employment or student's enrollment in school. An FTE is defined by the Government Accountability Office (GAO) as the number of total hours worked divided by the maximum number of compensable hours in a work year as defined by law. For example, if the a work year is defined as 2,080 hours then an individual working 1,500 hours in the year would be 0.72 of an FTE. The formula to calculate an FTE is as follows:

$$\frac{1,500 \text{ Hours Worked in a Year}}{2,080 \text{ Maximum Compensable Hours in a Year}} = 0.72 \text{ Full-Time Equivalent}$$

Functional Profile An HL7 standard that is a convention of the EHR system functional model standard. A functional profile identifies a subset of EHR system functions for a specific purpose; for example, records-management and evidentiary support, long-term care, public health reporting, clinical research, and vital records.

Future Damages The injury or loss expected to occur in the future for which the law allows recovery.

Fuzzy Search A search that returns results even when text is misspelled or corrupted.

FY **Fiscal Year**—A 12-month period used by many organizations for budgeting and/or financial reporting. An organization's fiscal year may or may not coincide with the calendar year.

G

Gaming Using improper means to evade the intent of a rule or law or contract to attempt to gain a financial advantage.

GAO **Government Accountability Office**—The legislative branch of the US government that serves as the investigative, evaluative, and audit arm of Congress. http://www.gao.gov

Gatekeeper The primary care provider who has economic and medical responsibility for managing all member medical services for a specialty.

GDP   Gross Domestic Product—The market of all final goods and services made within the borders of a nation over a year; it is a basic measure of economic performance.

GEM   General Equivalence Mapping—A program created to facilitate the translation between ICD-9-CM and ICD-10-CM/PCS.

General Accounting Office   The office that audits (including the NHB), oversees, and investigates the operations of other agencies.

General Damages   Damages that do not need to be specifically claimed or proven to have been sustained. The law presumes general damages to follow from the type of wrong complained of.

General-Disability Insurance   Disability insurance that provides benefits to a covered person who cannot perform any job that the person is qualified for.

Generic Drug   A prescription drug that is not protected by trademark, but is produced and sold under the chemical formulation name.

Genetic Information   Information derived from an individual or family's genes, gene products, or characteristics.

GHP   Group Health Plan—A health plan supported by an employer or employee organization that provides coverage to employees, former employees, and their families. GHP coverage is usually the primary and Medicare is secondary for people who are over age 65, eligible for Medicare, and work at a company with 20 or more employees.

GIF   Graphic Interchange Format—An acronym used to denote the computer compression format for images.

Gigabyte   A unit of information or computer storage equal to one billion bytes.

GIPSE   Geocoded Interoperable Population Summary Exchange—A data format created by the US Centers for Disease Control and Prevention (CDC) to allow the electronic exchange of health condition/syndrome summary data that have been stratified by a number of variables, including geography. GIPSE data will be utilized by public health agencies in the United States to conduct situational awareness, including early event detection and monitoring, for potential public health events.

Global Budget   A government-imposed limit on annual healthcare spending.

Global Fee   A total charge for a specific set of services.

Good Faith Operation   A phrase used in FRCP 37(e). Intended to preclude rule-based sanctions for the loss of data that occurs as a result of the routine, good faith operation of a computer system or the organization's information systems.

Good Samaritan Laws   Laws enacted that generally provide some form of immunity to those who, although without a duty to act, provide assistance in an emergency.

Google   A trademarked name of a commonly used search engine that uses text-matching techniques to find web pages that are important and relevant to a user's search.

Google Health   A free virtual online health application, developed by Google, that allows a user to collect, store, and manage his/her own personal health information in one central location.

Governance   The legal authority and responsibility for an organization.

GPEA   **Government Paperwork Elimination Act**—A body of law that requires, by October 21, 2003, when and where practical, federal agencies use electronic forms, electronic filing, and electronic signatures to conduct official business with the public. The law was specifically written to "preclude agencies or courts from systematically treating electronic documents and signatures less favorably than their paper counterparts."

GPG   Privacy guard software that allows the user to encrypt and sign a message utilizing a versatile key management structure and access modules for public key directories. Also known as GnuPG.

GPRA   **Government Performance and Results Act of 1993**—A federal law that requires agencies to engage in project management tasks such as setting goals, measuring results, and reporting progress. In order to comply with GPRA, agencies must produce strategic and performance plans and conduct gap analysis of projects.

Gramm-Leach-Bliley Act   (Pub. L. 106-102) An act to enhance competition in the financial services industry by providing a prudential framework for banks, security firms, insurance companies, and other financial service providers, and for other purposes.

Grant   A written agreement between the sponsor and an organization to carry out an approved activity for which a sum of money is awarded to the organization. A grant is used whenever the sponsor anticipates no substantial programmatic involvement in the activity during the performance of the activity.

Grayscale   A type of image that uses black, white, and shades of gray, with a better presentation the more gray used.

Gross Negligence   A common-knowledge instance in which there is such a gross want of care or skill as to give rise to an almost conclusive inference of negligence that the testimony of an expert is not necessary.

Group Practice   A collection of physicians who are affiliated with one another and operate as single unit. Each of the physicians in a group practice may cover for one another and/or sign or authenticate entries of another provider.

Guardian Ad Litem   In law, an individual appointed by the court with the authority and duty to represent the interests of a minor in a legal action.

Guidelines   Standards of practice that may or may not have the force and authority of law behind them.

H

Habeas Corpus   The procedure to challenge the legality of detention or custody.

Hacker   A criminal who breaks into computers.

Hard Disk   A nonflexible magnetic disk used for data storage on personal computers.

Hardware   The physical parts of a computer.

Harvesting   Refers to the process of the retrieval of electronic information from various computers, hard drives, file servers, CDs, DVDs, voice, backup tapes, and legacy and orphan systems. Harvesting is sometimes also known as culling.

Hash Value   The process by which a unique ID number is assigned to electronic data (no matter how small), and that is used to categorize and detect changes to the data. An algorithm is applied to each discrete piece of data to create what is known as a digital fingerprint of the data.

HCCA   Health Care Compliance Association—A professional membership organization that champions ethical practice and compliance standards and provides the necessary resources for ethics and compliance professionals and others who share these principles. http://www.hcca-info.org

HCERA   Health Care and Education Reconciliation Act of 2010 (P.L. 111-152)—A federal law enacted by Congress through reconciliation in order to make changes to the Patient Protection and Affordable Care Act. HCERA was signed into law by President Barack Obama on March 30, 2010. Also known as HR 4872.

HCFA-1450   A name for the institutional uniform claim form, according to the Centers for Medicare and Medicaid Services. Also known as a UB-92.

HCFA-1500   A name for the professional uniform claim form, according to the Centers for Medicare and Medicaid Services. Also known as a UCF-1500.

HCPCS   Healthcare Common Procedure Coding System—An annual publication of the American Medical Association (AMA). HCPCS is a coding classification system designed to organize and classify medical claims data.

HCQIA   Healthcare Quality Improvement Act—The HCQIA was enacted in 1986 to reduce medical errors and protect the public.

Header   The portion of the message that precedes the actual body and trailer of the business transaction.

Health 2.0   An indefinite term. Health 2.0 is focused on the user-generated aspects of Web 2.0 for the healthcare industry but does not directly interact with the mainstream healthcare system. Health 2.0 is sometimes referred to as user-generated healthcare or participatory medicine. Health 2.0 is a set of technologies that are interactive (search, communities, and tools for individual and group consumer use) and combine user-provided content with automated networking applications to create personalized but collaborative information for an individual or a provider.

Health and Human Services Agencies   Eleven total agencies make up the US Department of Health and Human Services (HHS), and are overseen by the Secretary of Health and Human Services. The federal agencies of the HHS are as follows:

- Administration for Children and Families (ACF)
- Administration on Aging (AoA)
- Agency for Healthcare Research and Quality (AHRQ)
- Agency for Toxic Substances and Disease Registry (ATSDR)
- Centers for Disease Control and Prevention (CDC)
- Centers for Medicare and Medicaid Services (CMS)
- Food and Drug Administration (FDA)
- Health Resources and Services Administration (HRSA)
- Indian Health Services (IHS)
- National Institutes of Health (NIH)
- Substance Abuse and Mental Health Services Administration (SAMHSA)

Health Care Claim Submission   The ANSI 837 transaction standard for electronic claims submissions that outlines the requirements for submission of healthcare claims for professional, institutional, and dental services to payers for payment.

Healthcare Clearinghouse   An entity that processes information (usually claims data) received in nonstandard format or containing nonstandard data into standard elements. A healthcare clearinghouse can also function in the reverse.

Healthcare Reform   A term used to refer to the concept of making changes to governmental policy that affects healthcare delivery within the United States. Generally, the emphasis of US healthcare reform is to improve the quality and safety of healthcare, improve access, and provide consumers with more choices at affordable prices while decreasing the overall costs of healthcare.

Health Care Request for Review and Response   The ANSI 278 transaction standard for electronic claims submission that outlines the requirements for a batch request for claims review.

HealthDataRights.Org   A virtual initiative launched in June 2009 that seeks rights for individuals to take responsibility for their own information and healthcare.

Health Informatics   A term is used to describe a specialized body of science and knowledge. Health informatics is an intersection of science, medicine, and healthcare.

Many subdomains of health informatics exist including bioengineering and healthcare clinical informatics, which includes: nursing informatics, imaging informatics, consumer health informatics, public health informatics, dental informatics, clinical research informatics, bioinformatics, and pharmacy informatics. Health informatics is also known as medical informatics (MI) or clinical informatics (CI).

Health Information Management Director   Oversees the operation of the Health Information Management (HIM) Department and is often named as the official custodian of the record. Also plays a key role in the security and legal use of protected health information by establishing appropriate procedures for the handling, disclosure, and dissemination of individually identifiable data.

Health Information Technology Extension Program   A federally funded program established under the HITECH Act to provide implementation and technical assistance to providers seeking to select and successfully implement certified electronic health records (EHRs) and utilize technology.

Health Insurance   Insurance that covers the medical expenses that result from illness or an injury.

Health Insurance Portability and Accountability Act of 1996   (Pub. L. 104-191) An amendment to the Internal Revenue Code of 1986, this legislation was signed into law on August 21, 1996, and was enacted to improve portability and continuity of health insurance coverage in the group and individual markets; to combat waste, fraud, and abuse in health insurance and healthcare delivery; to promote the use of medical savings accounts; to improve access to long-term care services and coverage; to simplify the administration of health insurance; and for other purposes. See also HIPAA.

Health IT Policy Committee   A federal advisory committee that makes recommendations to the National Coordinator for Health Information Technology (HIT) on a policy framework for the development and adoption of a nationwide health information infrastructure, including standards for the exchange of patient medical information.

Health Outcomes   Changes in the current or future health status of communities or individuals that can be attributed to antecedent actions or measures.

Health Plan   A covered entity under HIPAA. A health plan is a legal entity that functions as a group health plan or health insurance issuer, and provides for, or pays for, the cost of medical care. Health plans include Medicare, Medicaid, employer self-insurance, commercial carriers such as PPO, or managed care plans such as HMOs.

Health Savings Account   A tax-deferred plan available to taxpayers in the United States to cover current and future medical expenses. Money is placed in an account before tax is paid on it. Money from this account can be used tax free for qualified medical expenses. Health savings accounts (HSAs) were enacted in 2003 by the Medicare bill and are designed to help individuals save for future qualified medical and retiree health expenses on a tax-free basis.

HealthVault   A free virtual online health application developed by Microsoft that allows a user to collect, store, and manage his/her personal health information in one central location.

Hearsay   An out-of-court statement offered to prove the truth of the matter asserted in that statement.

HEAT   Health Care Fraud Prevention and Enforcement Action Team—A joint initiative between the US Department of Justice and HHS to reduce and prevent Medicare and Medicaid fraud through enhanced cooperation. The HEAT is composed of top-level law enforcement agents, prosecutors, and staff from both departments and their operating divisions.

HEDIS   Health Plan Employer Data and Information Set—A set of managed care performance measures that are reported and measured annually. Participation is mostly voluntary with the exception of Medicare and Medicaid that are usually required to submit reports to the state.

Hertz   A unit of frequency that measures the number of cycles per second of a periodic phenomenon. Hertz is generally used to measure the clock speed of a computer's CPU.

Heuristic   A rule of thumb generally stated in if/then terms that cannot be proven logical, but are nevertheless useful in problem solving.

Hexadecimal   A base-16 numbering system in which the numbers 0 to 9 denote their typical digits and the letters A through F denote the numbers 10 through 15.

HHA   Home Health Agency—An organization that provides healthcare services in the home, like skilled nursing care, physical therapy, occupational therapy, speech therapy, and care by home health aides.

HHS   Department of Health and Human Services—The US government's principal agency that protects the health of Americans and provides essential human services. http://www.hhs.gov

HIAA   Health Insurance Association of America—An industry association that represents the interests of commercial healthcare insurers and participates in the maintenance of some code sets, under HIPAA. http://www.ahip.org

HICN   Health Insurance Claim Number—An identification number assigned to Medicare beneficiaries by the Social Security administration, usually consisting of the individual's social security number, preceded by an alpha prefix.

HIE   Health Information Exchange—The provision of healthcare information electronically across organizations within a region or community, with the goal of assisting access to and retrieval of clinical data to provide safer, more timely, efficient, effective, equitable, patient-centered care.

HIEM   Health Information Event Messaging—An extension of OASIS Web Services that initiates subscriptions for information from other participants in the Nationwide Health Information Network.

High Availability   A system design protocol and associated implementation that ensures a certain degree of operational continuity during a given measurement period. Availability refers to the ability of the user community to access the system, whether to submit new work, update or alter existing work, or collect the results of previous work.

High-Level Language   A type of computer language in which the language is removed from the machine dependence imposed by assembly programming.

HIM Health Information Management—A management discipline that focuses on healthcare data and the management of healthcare information, regardless of the medium and format.

HIMSS Health Information Management Systems Society—A member organization composed of 20,000 individuals and 300 corporate members focused on providing leadership for the optimal use of healthcare information technology and management systems for the betterment of healthcare. http:// www.himss.org/ASP/index.asp

HIMSS EHRA Health Information Management Systems Society Electronic Health Record Association—A trade association of electronic health record (EHR) companies and industry experts addressing national efforts to create interoperable EHRs in hospital and ambulatory care settings. The association operates on the premise that the rapid, widespread adoption of EHRs will help improve the quality of patient care as well as the productivity and sustainability of the healthcare system. http://www.himssehra.org/ASP/index.asp

HIO Health Information Organization—Regional organization responsible for motivating and causing integration and information exchange in the nation's revamped healthcare system.

HIPAA Health Insurance Portability and Accountability Act of 1996 (Pub. L. 104-191)—A federal body of law enacted by Congress in 1996 and effective on July 1, 1997. HIPAA is a two-part body of law that works to improve the effectiveness and efficiency of the healthcare system and combat fraud, waste, and abuse.

Title I protects the health insurance coverage for people who lose or change jobs.

Title II, also known as Administrative Simplification (AS), mandates the standards and requirements for the electronic transmission and exchange of certain healthcare information and requires that organizations exchanging information for healthcare transactions follow national implementation guidelines. Key components of Title II include:

1. Establishes the HIPAA Privacy and Security Rules that protect any information related to a person's health status, their use of healthcare, and payment made for healthcare, and requires that any health information in a covered entity's possession be safeguarded from improper use

2. Requires use of standard electronic transactions and data for certain administrative functions

3. Standardizes the medical codes that providers use to report services to insurers
4. Creates specific identification numbers for employers (standard unique employer identifier [EIN]) and for providers (National Provider Identifier [NPI])

HIPAA 2   The term used to denote industry adoption of and transition to new sets of transactions and code sets under HIPAA. January 1, 2012, was the target date for implementation of X12 5010 for HIPAA transactions. In addition, October 1, 2013, was established as the target date for adoption of ICD-10 code sets.

HIPAA 25010 X12 HIPAA Transaction Standards   The HIPAA electronic data interchange (EDI) standard mandated by the Department of Health and Human Services in January 2009 for the electronic processing of healthcare claims. As of January 1, 2012, providers, payers, and clearinghouses must be using the new HIPAA 5010 standards for electronic claims processing. See also EDI X12.

HIPAA Amendments and Corrections   The final privacy rule under HIPAA establishes that an amendment to a record is an indication that the data are in dispute, while retaining the original information. A correction to a record alters or replaces the original record.

HIPAA Breach   The impermissible use or disclosure under the HIPAA Privacy Rule that compromises the security or privacy of the protected health information, such that the use or disclosure poses a significant risk of financial, reputational, or other harm to the affected individual. Effective September 23, 2009, HIPAA-covered entities and their business associates are required to provide notice of the breach of the individual's protected health information to the individual and provide notice of the breach to the Secretary of Health and Human Services (HHS) and, in some instances, to the media.

HIPAA—PHI   Health Insurance Portability Accountability Act—Protected Health Information—Protected health information under HIPAA is defined as "any information in any form or medium created or received by a health provider, health plan, public health authority, employer, life insurer, school or university, or healthcare clearinghouse" and involves the health or condition or payment for provision of an individual's healthcare.

HIPAA Privacy Rule   A rule finalized in 2003 that establishes guidelines for the application of technologies for controlling access to health information.

HIPAA Security Standard   The final rule of administrative simplification provisions of the Health Insurance Portability and Accountability Act (Title II of

HIPAA) specifies a series of administrative, technical, and physical security procedures for covered entities to use to assure the confidentiality of electronic protected health information. The standards are delineated into either required or addressable implementation specifications.

HIPAA Transaction   A term under Title II of HIPAA that refers to the exchange of information between two parties to carry out financial or administrative functions related to healthcare. Every HIPAA-covered entity doing business electronically must utilize the same healthcare transactions, code sets, and identifiers. Under HIPAA, transactions are defined as the transmission of healthcare information for specific purposes.

Hippocratic Oath   The pledge taken by many medical students upon graduation or upon entering into practice. The Hippocratic Oath is named after the Greek physician and teacher Hippocrates (c. 460–c. 377 BC), who practiced on the island of Kos. There are ancient and modern versions of the oath, and its text varies by translation. One important line reads, "I will prescribe regimen for the good of my patients according to my ability and my judgment and never do harm to anyone."

HIS   Health Information System—NCVHS describes an HIS as a "comprehensive, knowledge-based system capable of providing information to all who need it to make sound decisions about health. Such a system can help realize the public interest related to disease prevention, health promotion, and population health."

HISPC   Health Information Security and Privacy Collaboration—A multistate and territory initiative that aims to address the privacy and security challenges presented by electronic health information exchange and to develop common, replicable multistate solutions that have the potential to reduce variation in and harmonize privacy and security practices, policies, and laws. http://healthit.hhs.gov

HIT   Health Information Technology—The US Department of Health and Human Services defines HIT as the tangible technical aspects of a health information system, including network backbones such as the Internet in its present and future versions—the World Wide Web, wireless connections, hardware, Internet appliances, and handheld devices—as well as applications for information management, decision-support tools, and communication and transactional programs. Also involved are technical capabilities in areas such as bandwidth and latency.

HIT Certification   Healthcare IT Certification—A major HHS initiative designed to provide purchasers and other users of healthcare IT systems assurance that the information system technologies will: 1. provide needed capabilities; 2. securely manage information and confidentially; and 3. work with other systems without reprogramming.

HITECH Act   **Health Information Technology for Economic and Clinical Health Act**—The HITECH Act is a component of the American Recovery and Reinvestment Act of 2009. The purpose of the HITECH Act is to save US lives and lower costs through technology and the adoption of electronic health records.

HITEP   **Health Information Technology Expert Panel**—An appointed panel of 12 to 18 individuals who represent a wide range of EHR stakeholder perspectives. The role of the HITEP is to identify quality measures and establish a framework to evaluate the quality of electronic information required by performance measures through electronic health records (EHRs).

HITRC   **Health Information Technology Research Center**—One of two components of the Health Information Technology Extension Program established in Section 3012 of the Public Health Service Act and added through the HITECH Act. The HITRC is focused on conducting research into health information technology and assuring, among other things, that the unique needs of providers serving historically underserved populations such as American Indians, Alaska Natives, and non-English-speaking persons are being met.

HIT Regional Extension Center Program   A federal initiative established through the ARRA and HITECH Act to encourage adoption of electronic health records (EHRs), assist clinicians and healthcare organizations to become meaningful users of EHRs, and increase the likelihood that adopters of EHRs will become meaningful users of the technology.

HITSP   **Healthcare Information Technology Standards Panel**—An appointed panel composed of a diverse spectrum of healthcare industry stakeholders. Operating under the American National Standards Institute (ANSI), HITSP serves as a cooperative partnership between the public and private sectors for the purpose of achieving a widely accepted and useful set of standards specifically to enable and support interoperability among healthcare software applications. The panel interacts in a local, regional, and national health information network for the United States and will assist in the development of the US Nationwide Health Information Network (NHIN) by addressing issues such as privacy and security within a shared healthcare information system.

HL7   **Health Level Seven**—The ANSI-accredited standards to which healthcare application vendors adhere, when developing application interfaces, to exchange patient data. The HL7 standard defines the interoperability by which clinical data are exchanged between independent medical applications in near real time.

HL7 Ballot   The process in which HL7 obtains feedback and approval for standards.

HL7 EHR TC   **Health Level 7 Electronic Health Record Technical Committee—** An HL7 committee focused on standards applicable to EHR systems and EHR records.

HL7 RIM   **Health Level Seven Reference Information Model—**An HL7 conceptual model that is composed of six backbone classes of different specialized attributes that express data content needed in a specific clinical or administrative context and provides an explicit representation of the semantic and lexical connections that exist between the information in HL7 message fields.

HMO   **Health Maintenance Organization—**A specific type of health plan that offers many kinds of healthcare services to its members. In return, members (and their employers) pay a fixed cost each month for a member's healthcare services. HMOs are sometimes called health plans or managed care organizations.

Holding   The decision of the court on the specific question under consideration. Sometimes also referred to as a ruling made by the court.

Home Health Agency   A public agency or private nonprofit organization, certified under section 1861(o) of the Social Security Act that is primarily engaged in providing skilled nursing care and other therapeutic services.

Home Healthcare   Skilled nursing or therapeutic services provided in a home setting as an alternative to hospital confinement.

Home Organization   Refers to the home organization that registers, stores, and is able to authenticate information about its users.

Home Page   The first or top page in a collection of web pages that make up a website.

HOS   **Health Outcomes Survey—**The first health outcomes measure used in Medicare managed care and the largest survey effort ever undertaken by the Centers for Medicare and Medicaid Services (CMS). All Medicare Advantage contractors participate in the survey. The goal of the Medicare HOS program is to gather valid and reliable health status data in Medicare managed care for use in quality improvement activities, accountability planning, public reporting, and improving health.

Hospice   A public agency or private nonprofit organization, certified under section 1861(dd)(2) of the Social Security Act, that provides 24-hour care and treatment services (as needed) to terminally ill individuals and their families. This care is provided in individuals' homes, on an outpatient basis, and on a short-term inpatient basis, directly or under arrangements made by the agency or organization.

Hospice Care   Palliative care delivered in a holistic manner by a team, intent on relieving the suffering of patients with terminal illness who have elected to forego further treatment.

Hospital   An institution with an organized medical staff in a permanent facility that includes inpatient beds.

Hospital Compare   A search engine sponsored by the Department of Health and Human Services that allows users to search for hospitals by zip code and type. Users can compare up to three hospitals at a time according to various criteria including nurse response, doctor response, cleanliness, and recommendation. http://www.hospitalcompare.hhs.gov/hospital-search.aspx

Hotline   A compliance tool used by an organization by which an individual can report suspected occurrences of fraud, abuse, or noncompliance in an anonymous manner without fear of reprisal.

HPSA   Health Professional Shortage Area—A geographic area or location that the Department of Health and Human Services (HHS) designates as medically underserved.

HR 3590   Patient Protection and Affordable Care Act—The version of the healthcare reform bill introduced before the Senate on November 18, 2009, which passed on December 24, 2009, by a recorded vote of 60 to 39.

HR 3962   Affordable Health Care for America Act—The version of the healthcare reform bill introduced before the House on October 29, 2009, which passed on November 7, 2009, with a recorded vote of 220 to 215.

HRSA   Health Resources and Services Administration—One of 11 federal agencies that make up the Department of Health and Human Services. The HRSA is the principal federal agency charged with increasing access to basic healthcare for those who are medically underserved. http://www.hrsa.gov

HTS   Harmonized Tariff Schedule—A resource maintained and updated periodically by the International Trade Commission (ITC), used to determine tariff classifications for goods imported into the United States.

HTTP **Hypertext Transfer Protocol**—An application-level protocol for hypermedia information systems, which led to the establishment of the World Wide Web.

Human Research The use of human beings as research subjects, generally subjected to rigorous restriction and ethics.

Hybrid Entity An organization that uses or discloses protected health information for only a part of its business operations; for example, a pharmacy.

Hybrid Record A term used to describe a combination paper and electronic record. In healthcare today, the vast majority of organizations maintain some form of a hybrid medical record.

Hz Abbreviation for **Hertz**.

I

IAB **Internet Architecture Board**—Maintains responsibility for defining the overall architecture of the Internet, and provides guidance and broad direction to the Internet Engineering Task Force (IETF). The IAB also serves as the technology advisory group to the Internet Society, and oversees a number of critical activities in support of the Internet.

IACET **International Association for Continuing Education & Training**—A nonprofit, standard-setting organization dedicated to quality continuing education and training providers. In 2006, IACET was approved by the American National Standards Institute (ANSI) as a standards developer. http://www.iacet.org

IANA **Internet Assigned Numbers Authority**—Central coordinator for the assignment of unique parameter values for Internet protocols chartered by the Internet Society (ISOC) to act as the clearinghouse to assign and coordinate the use of numerous Internet protocol parameters. Each domain name is associated with a unique IP address, a numerical name consisting of four blocks of up to three digits each (for example, 204.146.46.8), which systems use to direct information through the network.

IAPD **Implementation Advanced Planning Document**—A document used by states to seek federal reimbursement for the costs of designing, developing, and implementing a system.

ICANN **Internet Corporation for Assigned Names and Numbers.**

ICD-9-CM **International Classification of Diseases, Ninth Revision, Clinical Modification**—A coding and classification system used in the United

States to report healthcare diagnoses, inpatient procedures and services, as well as morbidity and mortality information.

ICD-10-CM   International Classification of Diseases, Tenth Revision, Clinical Modification—The planned replacement for ICD-9-CM, volumes 1 and 2, developed to contain more codes and allow for greater flexibility.

ICEP   Initial Coverage Election Period—The period where individuals, newly eligible for Medicare, can join a Medicare Advantage plan. This period begins three months before the person is eligible for Medicare and ends the last day of the month the person's Medicare benefits begin.

ICH   Interoperability Clearinghouse—A not-for-profit collaboration of standards and industry groups, solution providers, testing/research organizations, and IT practitioners. ICH serves members and the general public by helping to advance the capability and integrity of information and communication infrastructures.

ICN   Internal Control Number—A systematically assigned, 13-digit number given to claims received by the EDS. This is used to track the case.

ICPC   Interstate Compact for the Placement of Children—A protocol that defines the conditions under which children from one state may be placed in a safe and suitable home in another state.

ICSA Labs   A vendor-neutral testing and certification laboratory located in Mechanicsburg, PA. On December 10, 2010, ICSA Labs was officially designated as an Authorized Testing and Certification Body (ONC-ATCB) by the Office of the National Coordinator. Scope of ONC-ATCB authorization: Complete EHR and EHR Modules. http://www.icsalabs.com

IDEA   International Data Encryption Algorithm—A commercial symmetric cipher developed in 1990 that uses 128-bit keys.

Identification   The procedure that allows the recognition of an entity by a system, usually by utilizing a unique machine-readable user name, with a digital ID.

Identify Theft   A criminal act that involves the theft of an individual's name and social security number and often results in financial and other losses to the victim.

IDN   Internationalized Domain Name—IDN provides the ability to use more characters in domain names besides letters and numbers, and specifically includes characters available in other alphabets.

IDS   Integrated Delivery System—A network of related healthcare organizations, many of which provide an HMO component.

IEC   International Electrotechnical Commission—An ANSI-accredited international standards body for all fields of electrotechnology focused on the development and promotion of international unification of standards or norms. http://www.iec.ch

IEEE   Institute of Electrical and Electronics Engineers—A professional membership organization that also functions as a publishing house and standards-making body. http://www.ieee.org

IEP   Initial Enrollment Period—A seven-month period for individuals who are turning age 65, which begins on the first day of the third month before the month in which they turn 65, includes the month of their 65th birthday, and ends on the last day of the third month after their 65th birthday. During this seven-month period, Medicare beneficiaries can enroll in Medicare Part A, Part B, and a Medicare drug plan (Part D).

IETF   Internet Engineering Task Force—Open to any interested individual, the IETF is a large international community of network designers, operators, vendors, and researchers concerned with the evolution of Internet architecture and the smooth operation of the Internet. The IETF defines the standard Internet operating protocols such as TCP/IP. http://www.ietf.org

IETF Standards Process   The process by which Internet operating protocol standards are developed.

IEWSA   Illinois Electronic Writing and Signature Act.

IFHIMA   International Federation of Health Information Management—Established in 1968 as a forum to bring together national organizations committed to improving the use of health records in their countries. IFHRO supports national associations and health records professionals in implementing and improving health records and the systems that support them. http://www.ifhro.org

IFIP   International Federation for Information Processing—A leading multinational, apolitical organization in information and communications technologies and sciences recognized by the United Nations and other world bodies. The IFIP represents IT societies from 56 countries or regions, covering all five continents. Total IFIP membership is over one half million. http://www.ifip.or.at

IG   Implementation Guide—A document created by an accredited standards organization such as HL7 or ANSI that explains the appropriate use of a standard for a specific business purpose under HIPAA.

IHE   Integrating the Healthcare Enterprise—An initiative by healthcare professionals and industry to improve the way computer systems in healthcare share information. IHE promotes the coordinated use of established standards such as DICOM, HL7, ISO, W3C, and others to address specific clinical needs in support of optimal patient care. http://www.ihe.net

IHE Domain Committees   A variety of committees of Integrating the Healthcare Enterprise (IHE) composed of clinical and technical users and experts who, on an annual basis, define critical-use cases and create detailed specifications for communication among systems by selecting and optimizing established standards, implementing specifications, and testing vendors' systems. The currently active IHE domain committees are summarized as follows:

- Cardiology
- Eye Care
- IT Infrastructure
- Laboratory
- Patient Care Coordination
- Patient Care Devices
- Quality, Research and Public Health
- Radiation Oncology
- Radiology, Mammography and Nuclear Medicine

IHE Profile   An integration profile described as the solution to a specific integration problem. A convenient way for implementers and users to be sure that all parties are discussing the same solution without having to restate the many technical details that ensure interoperability.

IHS   Indian Health Service—The IHS is one of 11 federal agencies that make up the Department of Health and Human Services.

IM   Information Management; also an abbreviation for **Instant Message**.

IMIA   International Medical Informatics Association—An independent organization established in 1989 under Swiss law. IMIA is the world body for health and biomedical informatics and plays a major role globally in the application of information science and technology in the fields of healthcare, research, and bio-informatics. IMIA maintains close working ties with the World Health Organization (WHO) and with the International Federation of Health Records Organizations (IFHRO). http://www.imia.org

Immunity   Any exemption from a duty, liability, or service of process, such as those granted to public officials.

Impact Rule   The requirement, abandoned in most jurisdictions, that physical contact must have occurred to allow damages for the negligent infliction of emotional distress.

Implementation Guide   A document prepared by an accredited standards organization that explains the proper use of a standard for a specific business purpose. The *ASC X12N HIPAA Implementation Guide* is an example of an implementation guide. See also TR3.

Implementation Specification   The specific instructions, under HIPAA, for implementing a standard.

Implicit Criteria   The establishment of standards based on knowledge, as opposed to written standards.

Implied Authority   A focus on the relationship between an HMO and its participating physicians in which these physicians are viewed as independent contractors. Factors that need to be considered include the HMO's right to terminate a doctor/patient relationship, the manner in which the HMO directs the physician, and the character of the HMO's supervision of medical work done by the physician.

Implied Consent   A consent inferred by a patient through the patient's statement, actions, or conduct in an emergent situation.

Implied Warranty   A warranty arising by the operation of law because of the circumstances of a sale rather than due to a seller's express promise.

IM Standard   A standard established by the Joint Commission on Accreditation of Healthcare Organizations (JCAHO) for the management of information within healthcare organizations.

INA   Immigration and Nationality Act—The federal law that applies to most private and public organizations that requires employers to obtain nonimmigrant visas for aliens authorized to work in the United States.

Inactive Record   Records related to completed activities that are no longer used routinely, but are still retained in long-term storage for purposes of audit, analysis, or reporting.

Inadvertent Production of Privileged Information   In law, a phrase referring to the accidental or unintentional production of a document or information protected from disclosure by attorney-client privilege or attorney-client work product doctrine.

In Camera   A Latin term for in chambers, or in private. A legal proceeding that is heard before the judge in his or her private chambers or when all spectators are excluded from the courtroom.

Incidence Rate   The number of new cases of a disease per population in a given time period.

Incident Report   A document generally considered to be privileged and not a subject of discovery. The incident report is an administrative record of an adverse event(s) that occurs within a healthcare organization. An incident report is used to assist in the identification of problems, occurrences, and trends within the organization.

Incident-to Services   Those professional services provided by the staff of a physician under his immediate supervision. Such services are billed as though performed by the physician himself.

Incurred But Not Reported Claims   An accounting term representing the potential or estimated liabilities due to the delivery of services that have not been reported or invoiced by the date of a financial report.

Indemnify   To promise to make good with a potential loss.

Indemnity   A promise in which one person agrees to secure another against certain anticipated losses.

Indemnity Insurance   An insurance policy that applies to an individual or one's own property, such as health insurance, life insurance, disability insurance, or fire insurance. Also known as first-party insurance.

Indian Health Service Center   A nonprofit healthcare facility (whether operated directly by the Indian Health Service or operated by a tribe or tribal organization, contractor, or grantee under the Indian Self-Determination Act, as described in 42 CFR Part 136, Subparts C and H, or by an urban, Indian organization receiving funds under Title V of the Indian Health Care Improvement Act) that is physically separated from a hospital, and that provides clinical treatment services on an outpatient basis to persons of Indian or Alaskan Native descent.

Indicator   Specific measures of factors or results of an action that can be used to gauge performance.

Indictment   A written accusation presented to a grand jury in a criminal court.

Indirect Costs   Costs that are incurred for a project in which the project shares common or multiple objectives with other initiatives, therefore preventing the costs of the project to be identified specifically and readily.

Individually Identifiable Data   Data associated with a specific individual, such as a name or address.

Individually Identifiable Health Information   Information, such as health data, that identifies a patient or is specific enough that an individual can be identified from it.

Infectious Diseases Society of America   A professional membership organization representing physicians, scientists, and other healthcare professionals who specialize in infectious diseases. IDSA's purpose is to improve the health of individuals, communities, and society by promoting excellence in patient care, education, research, public health, and prevention relating to infectious diseases. http://www.idsociety.org

Inferior Court   A court from which appeals may be taken to a higher court within the same judicial system.

InfoGard Laboratories Inc.   An independent, accredited IT security laboratory located in San Luis Obispo, CA, that provides accredited IT security assurance services and is focused solely on product and system evaluations and validations. On September 24, 2010, InfoGard Laboratories was officially designated as an Authorized Testing and Certification Body (ONC-ATCB) by the Office of the National Coordinator. Scope of ONC-ATCB authorization: Complete EHR and EHR Modules. http://www.infogard.com

Information Governance   The organizational policies that govern organizational practices related to creation, maintenance, retention, archiving, and destruction of information and records.

Information Management Plan   A document that exists in most JCAHO-accredited healthcare organizations that describes how information is managed and used within the organization. It is also known as the IM plan. US healthcare organizations established information management plans in the mid-1990s after the Joint Commission on Accreditation of Healthcare Organizations (JCAHO) established a new set of standards to assess organizational policies and process relating to the management of information. The information management plan is a tool that still exists in many healthcare organizations today. The information management plan describes how the organization complies with the JCAHO IM standards and should describe the infrastructure of the organization's electronic records systems.

Information Science   Informatics, or the study of information; a branch of computer science related to database, ontology, and software engineering. This is generally concerned with the structure and management of information, as well as its creation and storage.

Information Technology Director   Oversees the operation and management of the organization's information systems. The IT director is knowledgeable about the technical aspects of the organization's information system architecture (hardware and software).

Informed Consent   The consent (usually written) that is given by the patient or legal representative after receiving a sufficient explanation of the nature, risks, costs, and benefits of a proposed course of treatment. In the absence of such information, a patient's consent may not be legally valid; for example, a surgeon who performs surgery without a patient consent could be held liable under tort of battery.

Injunction   In law, a temporary prohibition that requires a party to refrain from participating in some specific activity prior to a trial. An injunction may become permanent following judgment.

Injury   Harm or damage of another's legal right, for which the law provides protection or remedy.

In Litem   A Latin term meaning for a suit or to the suit.

In Loco Parentis   Latin for in place of the parents. A legal doctrine that allows a "stand-in" to exercise the legal rights, duties, and responsibilities of a parent toward a child.

INET   An acronym, often used interchangeably to mean Internet, Intranet, and/or International Networking.

In-Network   The use of providers who participate in a health plan's provider network.

Inpatient   An individual who is admitted to a hospital or other health facility overnight for the purpose of receiving a diagnosis, treatment, or other health services.

Inpatient Care   Service provided after a patient is admitted to a hospital.

Inquest   A legal, fact-finding proceeding, such as a request for default judgment, or a coroner's inquest. See also Coroner's Inquest.

Inquiry—Legal   A writ to assess damages. Fact finding.

Inquiry—Insurance   An oral and written request that does not request reexamination or response to a previous determination.

In Re   In law, the Latin term that means in the matter of. It is used to refer to certain civil actions.

In Rem   In law, the Latin term that means against a property or thing. A term used to describe legal action involving a *res* (or property) rather than a person.

ISOC   **Internet Society**—A nonprofit international organization founded in 1992 to provide leadership in Internet-related Internet standards, education, and policy. Dedicated to ensuring the open development, evolution, and use of the Internet for the benefit of people throughout the world. http://www.isoc.org

Insurance   An agreement in which one party (the insurer) assumes a risk faced by another party (the insured) in return for a premium payment. The written contractual agreement between the parties specifies the amount for which someone or something is covered by the agreement.

Insurance Certificate   A document issued by an insurer as evidence of insurance coverage or membership in a health or pension plan.

Insurance Eligibility and Verification   The process by which a healthcare provider can access a patient's eligibility and benefit information. Most insurance eligibility can be done online in real time. Electronic insurance eligibility verification allows for instant verification of eligibility at the time patients are seen by the provider. In addition to online, real-time access, eligibility verification can also be accomplished through ANSI batch 270/271 transactions.

Instant Message   A form of real-time communication between two or more people based on typed text and generally conveyed by devices connected over the Internet.

Integrative Medicine   A term used to describe combining conventional Western medicine with alternative or complementary treatments, such as herbal medicine, acupuncture, massage, biofeedback, yoga, and stress reduction techniques—all in the effort to treat the whole person. Proponents of this type of medicine may also use the word "complementary" to emphasize that such treatments are used with mainstream medicine, not as replacements or alternatives.

Intellectual Property   Intangible rights protecting the commercial value of products of human intellect, comprising primarily trademark, copyright, and patent rights.

Intensity of Service   The number and complexity of resources used to provide healthcare service requirements for a particular diagnosis or patient.

Interface   The place where computer systems meet and/or communicate.

Interim Final Rule   A regulation that is the prevailing rule or law until such time as a final rule or law is enacted.

Internal Counsel   An attorney who is employed by an organization.

Internal Disclosure   The exchange of protected or privileged information (verbally or written) within the walls of the firm or organization.

Internet   A loosely organized, international collaboration of autonomous, interconnected networks that supports host-to-host communication through voluntary adherence to open protocols and procedures defined by Internet standards. Numerous isolated, interconnected networks, which are not connected to the global Internet but use the Internet standards, also are part of the Internet.

Interoperability   The Interoperability Clearinghouse defines interoperability as "the ability of information systems to operate in conjunction with each other encompassing communication protocols, hardware, software, application, and data compatibility layers."

Interoperable   The ability of different systems, applications, and networks to communicate in an effective manner.

Interoperable Medical Record   An electronically stored and maintained medical record that contains an individual's most current medical information, and is available and accessible to clinicians for care and treatment of the individual wherever and whenever it is needed.

InterPARES   **International Research on Permanent Authentic Records in Electronic Systems**—A three-phased research project aimed at developing the knowledge essential to the long-term preservation of authentic records created and/or maintained in digital form and providing the basis for standards, policies, strategies, and plans of action capable of ensuring the longevity of such material and the ability of its users to trust its authenticity.

Interrogatories   Written questions served on the one party by another in civil litigation. See Discovery.

Interstate Compact Agreement   An agreement based upon constitutional law between two or more states that serves as a coordination mechanism between independent authorities in the member states. The Interstate Compact Agreement on Mental Health is one example.

Intervening Cause   In law, an independent act that occurs between the time of the original negligence or malpractice and the time of injury.

Intimidation   In law, unlawful coercion; extortion.

Intranet   A network made up of smaller, interconnected private networks, isolated from the public Internet.

Intra Vires A Latin term that means within the powers of; usually refers to the scope of authority or action taken by a person or corporation.

Introduce into Evidence In law, to have an object or a fact admitted into a trial record, thus allowing it to be considered in the jury's or the court's decision.

Invasion of Privacy The unjustified exploitation of one's personality or intrusion into one's personal activity.

I/O **Input/Output** (computers) or **Intake/Output** (care delivery).

IOM **Institute of Medicine**—A member of the National Academies, the IOM provides science-based advice on matters of biomedical science, medicine, and health. It is one of a number of committees of professional experts that research and address critical national issues and provide advice to the federal government and the public. http://www.iom.edu

IPA **Independent Physicians Association or Independent Practice Association**—An entity composed of independent physicians or other organizations that contracts with independent physicians, and provides services to managed care organizations on a negotiated per capita rate, flat retainer fee, or negotiated fee-for-service basis.

IP Address The identification number (a string of four-digit numbers separated by periods) assigned to devices in a computer network connected to the Internet.

IPIA **Improper Payment Information Act**—A 2002 law that requires agencies to annually identify programs and activities vulnerable to significant improper payments, to estimate the amount of overpayments or underpayments, and to report to Congress on steps being taken to reduce such payments.

IPPS **Inpatient Prospective Payment System**—The methodology by which hospitals are reimbursed for acute hospital inpatient stays under Medicare Part A. Section 1886(d) of the Social Security Act sets forth a system of payment for the operating costs of acute care hospital inpatient stays based on prospectively set rates. Under the IPPS, each case is categorized by a diagnosis-related group (DRG). Each DRG has a payment weight assigned to it, based on the average resources used to treat Medicare patients in that DRG.

IPSec **Internet Protocol Secure Standard**—The method by which networking devices such as servers and routers are verified.

IRB **Institutional Review Board**—A committee within an organization that reviews all proposed biomedical and behavioral research projects involving human subjects to ensure that the rights of such subjects are protected, that adequate and informed consent for their participation is obtained, and that any possible benefits of the research are commensurate with the risks involved.

IRC   Internal Revenue Code—The main body of US domestic statutory tax law organized topically, including laws covering the income tax, payroll taxes, estate taxes, and gift taxes.

IRODS   Integrated Rule-Oriented Data System—A data grid software system developed by Data Intensive Cyber Environments research group. http://www.irods.org

IRR   Internal Rate of Return—The rate at which the net present value (NPV) of a project equals 0. The IRR also provides the expected return rate of the project, assuming certain conditions are met. For example, if C(n) is the cash flow for each period then:

$$NPV = C(0) + C(1)/(1+r)+C(2)/(1+r)2+...+C(n)/(1+r)n$$

Irrebuttable Presumption   A legal proposition that allows the trier of fact (judge or jury) to accept a fact as true if other underlying facts are proven.

ISM   Information and Technology Solutions Management—An association of state, local, and federal government information systems professionals working in health and human services functions.

ISO   International Organization for Standardization—An organization established to develop standards to facilitate the international exchange of goods and services and to develop mutual cooperation in areas of intellectual, scientific, technological, and economic activity. Unlike ANSI, ISO does not create standards. http://www.iso.org

ISO 15489   International Organization for Standardization 15489—An ISO standard that provides a framework for the management of electronic records. ISO 15489 defines electronic records management as "the field of management responsible for the efficient and systematic control of the creation, receipt, maintenance, use and disposition of records, including the processes for capturing and maintaining evidence of and information about business activities and transactions in the form of records." ISO 15489 plays a crucial role in helping organizations meet their goals through best practice in the management of their information assets. The objective of ISO 15489 is the standardization of electronic records management policies and procedures.

ISO 23081-1   International Organization Standards Organization 23081-1—An ISO standard that provides a framework for understanding, implementing, and utilizing metadata in records management. ISO 23081-1 is an extension of ISO 15489 and addresses the relevance of metadata in records management and business processes and delineates the roles and types of metadata utilized.

ISOC **Internet Society**—A professional membership organization of Internet experts that comments on policies and practices and oversees a number of other boards and task forces dealing with network policy issues.

Issue of Law A legal determination made by a judge alone that requires the judge to apply legal principles to the facts for resolution of a matter.

IT **Information Technology.**

ITC **International Trade Commission**—The International Trade Commission is an independent, quasi-judicial federal agency with broad investigative responsibilities on matters of trade. The ITC also serves as a federal resource where trade data and other trade policy–related information are gathered and analyzed. Also known as the United States International Trade Commission or USITC.

ITU-T **Telecommunication Standardization Sector**—An international cooperative body that develops worldwide standards for telecommunications technologies.

J

JAMA **Journal of the American Medical Association**—The most widely cited and circulated international peer-reviewed medical journal in the world.

Java A scripting language with a simpler object model than C and C++ but derived from much of the same syntax.

JCAHO **Joint Commission on Accreditation of Healthcare Organizations**— Now known as The Joint Commission.

J-Codes A subset of the HCPCS Level II code set, used to identify certain drugs, with a high-order value of J.

JHITA **Joint Healthcare Information Technology Alliance**—According to HIPAA, a healthcare industry association that represents AHIMA, AMIA, CHIM, CHIME, and HIMSS on issues, both legislative and regulatory, affecting the use of health information technology.

Jigsaw A web server platform providing a sample HTTP 1.1 implementation and a variety of other features along with an advanced architecture implemented in Java. It is W3C's Java server.

Joinder The addition of another party to a pending civil action.

Joint and Several Liability   The rule of law that allows a person who has suffered loss or injury as a result of the actions of more than one party to collect from any one of those liable without regard to the individual at fault.

The Joint Commission   An independent not-for-profit organization that evaluates and accredits more than 16,000 healthcare organizations and programs in the United States. The Joint Commission is the nation's predominant healthcare standards-setting and accrediting body. Formerly known as **Joint Commission on Accreditation of Healthcare Organizations** or **JCAHO**. http://www.jointcommission.org

Joint Liability   In law, the liability that is shared by two or more parties.

Joint Tortfeasor   In law, a phrase meaning that the negligence or fault of more than one person injured another person. Depending on the jurisdiction, joint tortfeasors may be jointly and severally liable for injury to another.

Joint Venture   A business endeavor between two or more for a specific purpose, involving mutual control and risk sharing.

JPEG   **Joint Photographic Experts Group**—JPEG is a standardized image compression mechanism.

Judge   A public officer, almost always an attorney, empowered by the law of a particular jurisdiction to exercise judicial functions. Judges may be elected or appointed, depending on the jurisdiction.

Judgment   A conclusion of the court based on the claims of the parties submitted.

Judicial Conference Committee   One of the committees established by the Judicial Conference of the United States to monitor the effectiveness of the various federal rules and recommend proposed amendments. http://www.uscourts.gov/FederalCourts/JudicialConference.aspx

Judicial Confession   In law, a plea of guilty or some other direct manifestation of guilt in a court of law or judicial proceeding.

Jurisdiction   In law, the power of a court over certain people or properties in dispute.

Jurisprudence   The study of the general elements of a legal system, excluding practical elements or concrete elements.

Jury   A group of peers selected according to the law and given the authority to decide questions of fact and reach a verdict in the case.

Justice   The fair and proper administration of the laws.

K

K K stands for kilo, which is equal to 1,000. In computer system applications, the symbol, K, stands for 1,024 bytes. In healthcare delivery, K also stands for potassium.

Key Person An important individual who is generally responsible for an organization or business's success.

Keyword Search The process of using keywords to examine collections of electronic documents.

Known Plaintext Attack A term used to describe the process where a crypt-analyst only has access to encrypted ciphertext. Also known as a crib.

L

Laches In law, a term used in equity to name behaviors that neglect to assert one's rights or do what a person legally should have done to assert a right that will give equitable defense to another party.

LAN **Local Area Network**—A computer network covering a small area. LANs can be linked together into a larger network called a wide area network (WAN).

LCD **Local Coverage Determination**—A decision by a fiscal intermediary or carrier whether to cover a particular service on an intermediary-wide or carrier-wide basis in accordance with the Social Security Act.

LDD **Logical Document Determination**—The process of document grouping or separation used in some e-discovery litigation support processes.

LDR **Legal Document Repository**—An electronic system for retrieval of documents in connection with litigation.

Lead Date A litigation support term used to denote the date of the document or its parent document. The lead date is used in a database as an option to allow for the chronological sorting of documents by parent. Without a lead date field, attachments would generally be sorted out of sequence, since they were usually drafted earlier than their parent document.

Leapfrog Group A voluntary initiative composed of consumers, hospitals, employers, and vendors aimed at improving healthcare safety, quality, and customer value. Leapfrog works with its employer members to encourage transparency and easy access to healthcare information as well as rewards for hospitals that have a proven record of high-quality care. http://www.leapfroggroup.org/home

Legacy System   The term used to refer to an obsolete information system.

Legal Counsel   An alternate term for lawyer.

Legal Document Management   The management of legal documents within an organization, usually involving document imaging, workflow, and text retrieval.

Legal EHR   **Legal Electronic Health Record**—A concept originated by the American Health Information Management Association (AHIMA) to address the medico-legal aspects of the health record and electronic health record. The legal EHR documents the care provided and supports compliance with regulations and laws.

Legal Hold   In law, the obligation to preserve information relevant to actual or reasonably anticipated litigation. This obligation is communicated within an organization by a legal hold notice.

Length of Stay   The number of consecutive days that a patient is treated in a specific hospital or nursing facility.

LGHP   **Large Group Health Plan**—A health plan supported by an employer or employee organization with 100 or more employees that provides coverage to employees, former employees, and their families.

LHII   **Local Health Information Infrastructure**—A regional health information organization dedicated to the exchange of health information.

LHWCA   **Longshore and Harbor Workers' Compensation Act**—A federal worker's compensation law that provides for compensation and medical care for certain maritime employees who are disabled or die due to injuries that occur in the navigable waters of the United States or in adjoining areas and their qualified dependent survivors.

LI   **Line Item**—A term used to refer to an item or number in a budget.

Liability   In law, the legal responsibility to another or to society, enforceable in a civil proceeding or through criminal punishment. Also known as legal liability.

Liability Limit   The maximum amount of coverage that an insurance company will provide on a single claim under the insurance policy.

Libel   A civil tort. A defamatory statement about another person.

License   A revocable permission to commit some act that would otherwise be unlawful without the existence of the license that certifies or documents the evidence of such permission.

Licensure   The process involved in the granting of a professional license.

Lien   A legal right that a creditor has on another person's property as long as a debt has not been satisfied.

Life Expectancy   The length a person of a given age is expected to live, based on actuarial tables, taking into account individualized characteristics.

Limitation of Liability   A provision designed to protect the beneficiary from liability under certain conditions when services received are found not to be reasonable or necessary.

Limited Liability   In law, liability that is restricted by a contract or by law.

LinkedIn   An online social network targeting working professionals.

Linking   A litigation support term that describes the ability of an automated litigation support program to connect evidence, transcripts, notes, pleadings, websites, and other documents to each other with hypertext links.

Linux   An operating system based on the Linux kernel that handles process control, networking systems, and peripheral access, used in numerous embedded systems and supercomputers.

Liquidated Damages   Those damages that can be reduced to a sum. Certain stipulated damages are those agreed to by the parties.

Litigant   A party to a lawsuit. A litigant may be, for example, a plaintiff or a defendant. Witnesses and attorneys are not considered litigants.

Litigation   The process by which rights are adjudicated in the civil justice system.

Litigation Lifecycle   A process that describes the stages of litigation, from filing of a complaint to the end of litigation. The processes and practices commonly used to define a legal event, beginning when suit is filed and continuing all the way through posttrial events.

Litigation Software   Software to help lawyers prepare and present cases in court.

Litigation Support   All processes that assist a lawyer in the prosecution or defense of an action, including, for example, interviewing witnesses, document review, and trial preparation.

Living Will   A legal document providing directions concerning medical care if a person becomes incapacitated to the point of being unable to make decisions personally.

LMRP   **Local Medical Review Policy**—A coverage policy that is developed by Medicare insurance carriers and applies directly to claims made under

Medicare. LMRPs outline how local carriers will review claims to ensure that they meet Medicare coverage and coding requirements. In addition, LMRPs specify under what clinical circumstances a service is covered and correctly coded. An LMRP includes a description of the service, specific procedure codes, and, for each of these procedures, a list of covered and noncovered diagnostic codes.

Load File   A file that establishes links between records in a database and any image files to which each record pertains. In electronic discovery, the load file is a critical deliverable of any document scanning and coding job. Without a correctly structured load file, the documents will not properly link to their respective database records.

Local Codes   Code values that are defined for a political subdivision, such as a state, or for a specific payer. This HIPAA term is commonly used to describe HCPCS Level III Codes, but it also applies to state-assigned institutional revenue codes, condition codes, occurrence codes, and value codes.

Locality   The geographic areas defined by Medicare for determining payment amounts.

Locality Rule   In malpractice law, a test used to measure the required level of care for a patient, based on the level of care provided by similar providers in the community. These rules can be modified or abandoned in most states, leading to erosion of rule. A physician is held to a standard of care applicable to physicians in similar circumstances under a locality rule.

Local Rule   A rule, based on the physical conditions of a state and the customs, beliefs, and character of the people living in the state, dealing with matters such as requiring extra copies of motions or the prohibition of newspapers in courtrooms.

Locking   A term used in the information management and technology context to refer to the lock associated with each item in a database. A lock within a database can be shared or exclusive.

Locum Tenums   In law, the Latin term for placeholder. This generally refers to a person who fulfills the duties of another person.

Logical Observation Identifiers, Names, and Codes   A set of universal names or ID Codes, maintained by the Regenstrief Institute, used to identify laboratory observations, and expected to be used in HIPAA claim attachments standards. Commonly known as LOINC.

LOINC   Logical Observation Identifiers Names and Codes—The set of standard codes adopted by the Indian Health Service.

Longitudinal Record A term used to describe a patient's medical history since birth. Also referred to as a birth to death record.

Long-Term Care Services provided in a nursing home, intermediate care facility, or skilled nursing facility.

Loop A series of instructions that are repeated until a certain condition is met. Each passage of an instruction through the loop is called an iteration.

Loop-AES A Unix disk encryption system that utilizes the Advanced Encryption Standard (AES) algorithm to encrypt a loop file system.

Loopback A term used to describe methods or procedures of quickly routing electronic signals, digital data streams, or other flows of items from their originating source back to the same source entity without intentional processing or modification.

Loopback Device A device used to test the transmission or transportation infrastructure with an information system.

Loss of Chance A form of medical malpractice in which the actions of a physician, while not causing the underlying harm to the patient, cause the patient to miss the opportunity to cure the underlying harm.

Lost Chance of Cure The allowable damages when a patient's opportunity to be cured has been diminished due to negligence.

Lost Chance of Survival Damages that allow recovery if a patient's chances to survive a disease have been reduced by negligence.

Low-Level Language A series of binary notations (1 and 0) that operate the hardware of the computer in a long sequence of instructions.

LPET **Local Provider Education and Training**—A plan developed by individual hospitals that addresses the needs of staff, patients, family members, and visitors as different medical needs arise on a national level.

LTC **Long-Term Care**—The term used to denote a variety of health and personal needs, including medical and nonmedical care, provided to people who have a chronic illness or disability.

M

MA **Medicare Advantage**—A health plan option that is part of the Medicare program and includes: Medicare health maintenance organizations (HMOs), preferred provider organizations (PPOs), private fee-for-service plans, and Medicare special needs plans.

MAC   Medicare Administrative Contractor—A company under contract with the federal government to process claims for Medicare services. There are currently 23 MACs under contract: 15 to process Medicare Part A and B Claims (A/B MACs); 4 to process durable medical equipment claims (DME MACS); 4 to process home health and hospice claims (HH & H MACs). See also Carrier and Fiscal Intermediary.

Mac OS   Apple Inc.'s graphical user interface–based operating system.

Magistrate   In law, a title given to a particular category of judge. The definition varies by jurisdiction.

Magnetic Stripe   A strip of magnetic tape affixed to the back of a card that contains identifying data, such as account number and cardholder name.

Malpractice   In law, refers to a cause of action arising out of the failure of a professional to adhere to an appropriate standard of care.

Malpractice Insurance   An agreement to indemnify a professional person, such as a physician or a lawyer, against claims of negligence.

Managed Care   The term used to describe any method of healthcare delivery designed to reduce unnecessary utilization of services and provide for cost containment while improving healthcare quality.

Mapping   A term used to denote the electronic exchange and association of data field contents from one internal computer system to the field contents in the electronic data exchange standard to which they are being applied. The same mapping takes place in reverse during the receipt of an electronic document.

Marginal Cost   The cost to produce an additional unit of product or increasing the quantity of services provided. Marginal cost is a key consideration in pricing and a useful method for calculating the implications of business expansion or contraction.

Market Basket Index   The annual change in the aggregate price of goods and services to produce health services.

Master Patient Index   A database that contains a master listing of all patients known to the organization. The master patient index should be retained for the foreseeable future.

Maximum Defined Data Set   The term used under HIPAA to describe all of the required data elements for a particular standard based on implementation of a specification. Refers to the transmission of data sets between authorized entities.

MCM   Medicare Carrier Manual—A document outlining the benefits and policies under Medicare.

McNamara-O'Hara Service Contract   The federal labor standard that sets rates and other labor standards for the employees of federal government contractors.

MCO   Managed Care Organization—Any group conducting or implementing healthcare through managed care concepts of preauthorization, utilization review, and a fixed provider network.

MD5   A message digest algorithm that takes a variable length input and produces a 128-bit message digest.

M-Device   Mobile Device.

Mean   The mathematical average of a set of numbers.

Meaningful Use   A term defined by CMS that describes the use of HIT and furthers the goals of information exchange and adoption of electronic health records among healthcare professionals.

Measure of Damages   The extent of loss or injury for which the law allows recovery.

Median   The digit number that is in the middle of a set of numbers when arranged in consecutive order. If an odd number of digits are present, the median then becomes the mathematical average of the two digits closest to the middle.

Medicaid   A combined state- and federally funded health insurance program for certain low-income individuals and families. Many groups of people are covered under Medicaid after certain state requirements are met. Administration of Medicaid is done through the Centers for Medicare and Medicaid Services (CMS) at the state level.

Medical Code Sets   The administrative codes that characterize a medical condition and its treatment.

Medical Director   The doctor responsible for bridging healthcare delivery considerations between providers and administration, keeping a provider network for necessary services and offering direction of utilization, risk, and quality management programs.

Medical Group Practice   Provision of health services by at least three physicians engaged in a formally organized and legally recognized entity.

Medical Home   A model that provides continuous, coordinated, accessible, and comprehensive patient-centered care and is managed by a primary care physician, accompanied by active involvement of nonphysician practice staff. Medical homes may receive supplemental payments to support operations, and physician practices may be encouraged or required to improve practice structure and meet certain qualifications in order to meet eligibility.

Medical Identity Theft   The use of a person's name and other forms of personal information such as health insurance and medical history to obtain healthcare services to file false claims for healthcare services. Medical identity theft is a criminal form of healthcare fraud.

Medically Necessary   Services required to preserve and maintain the health of an individual according to national standards.

Medical Necessity and Appropriateness   A term used to refer to the evaluation of proven need for medical treatment, based upon an evaluation of intensity of service and severity of illness criteria.

Medical Record   A collection of information related to the medical services that a patient receives from a professional.

Medical Review   The review of medical records as it relates to services rendered and billed for payment.

Medical Studies Act   An Illinois law (735 ILCS 5/8-2101) that creates a privilege for documents and communications created as part of a peer-review process performed by a committee of medical or hospital staff.

Medical Underwriting   The process an insurance company uses to decide, based on an individual's medical history, whether to accept the individual's application for insurance, whether to add a waiting period for pre-existing conditions, and how much to charge the individual for health insurance. Also known as health screening.

Medicare   A federally funded health insurance program derived from the Social Security Act. Medicare provides health insurance for people age 65 or older, people under age 65 with certain disabilities, and people of all ages with end-stage renal disease (permanent kidney failure requiring dialysis or a kidney transplant). The Medicare program is administered by the Centers for Medicare and Medicaid Services (CMS).

Medicare Advantage Managed Care Plan   A single type of Medicare Advantage plan that is primarily a health maintenance organization (HMO) but also includes preferred provider organizations (PPOs) or any other health plan that requires an individual to use a certain group of doctors and hospitals, known as a network, to provide and coordinate the care they receive.

Medicare Advantage Plans   Medicare Advantage plans include: health maintenance organizations (HMOs), preferred provider organizations (PPOs), special needs plans (SNPs), private fee-for-service (PFFS) plans, and medical savings account (MSA) plans. The Medicare Advantage plans are available through private insurance companies. Medicare Advantage plans were formerly known as Medicare managed care or Medicare + Choice plans.

Medicare Appeals Council   The entity that performs the fourth review in all Medicare appeals processes. All appeal requests must be in writing and sent directly to the Medicare Appeals Council.

Medicare CfCs   **Medicare Conditions for Coverage**—The minimum health and safety standards that providers and suppliers must meet in order to be Medicare and Medicaid certified. These minimum health and safety standards are the foundation for improving quality and protecting the health and safety of beneficiaries. See also Medicare CoPs.

Medicare CoPs   **Medicare Conditions of Participation**—The minimum health and safety standards providers and suppliers must meet in order to begin and continue participating in the Medicare and Medicaid programs. These minimum health and safety standards are the foundation for improving quality and protecting the health and safety of beneficiaries. See also Medicare CfCs.

Medicare Part A   A federally funded health insurance program that provides Medicare coverage for hospice care, home healthcare, skilled nursing facilities, and inpatient hospital stays.

Medicare Part B   A federally funded health insurance program that provides Medicare coverage for outpatient hospital care, doctors' services, and other medical services that Part A does not cover such as physical and occupational therapy. Other examples include x-rays, medical equipment, or limited ambulance service.

Medicare Part C   The option provided to Medicare beneficiaries with both Parts A and B to elect to receive Medicare benefits through a Medicare Advantage program. A Medicare beneficiary may choose to utilize an area Medicare Advantage plan or other options such as private pay, medical savings accounts, or managed care plans, or may elect to join provider-sponsored plans.

Medicare Part D   A federally funded prescription drug program that provides that everyone with Medicare, regardless of income, health status, or prescription drugs used, can get prescription drug coverage.

Medicare Prescription Drug, Improvement, and Modernization Act of 2003
(Pub. L. 108-173)—A landmark piece of legislation signed into law on
December 8, 2003, that was enacted to provide seniors and individuals with
disabilities with a prescription drug benefit, more choices, and better benefits under Medicare.

Medicare Program Integrity Manual   A CMS manual that delineates the obligations of providers participating in the Medicare program. Fraud committed
against a Medicare or Medicaid program under various provisions of the
United States Code could result in the imposition of restitution, fines, and, in
some instances, imprisonment. In addition, there is also a range of administrative sanctions (such as exclusion from participation in the program) and
civil monetary penalties that may be imposed when facts and circumstances
warrant such action.

Medicare RAC Program   Under the Medicare Prescription Drug, Improvement
and Modernization Act of 2003, CMS is replacing the current Medicare fiscal
intermediaries with new administrative contractors. The Medicare RAC Program is a demonstration project utilizing recovery audit contractors (RACs)
for the identification of underpayments and overpayments and recoupment of
overpayments under the Medicare program for services for which payment is
made under part A or B of title XVIII of the Social Security Act.

Medicare Remittance Notice   A summarized statement including payment
information for one or more patients.

Medicare Summary Notice   A notice sent by the Medicare carrier to the Medicare beneficiary following a healthcare visit or hospital stay. The Medicare
Summary Notice provides information about how the doctor or other healthcare provider was paid. People enrolled in Medicare managed care plans do
not receive Medicare Summary Notices. The Medicare Summary Notice was
formerly called the Explanation of Medicare Benefits (EOMB).

Medigap   A private insurance that supplements Medicare by paying the
Medicare deductibles and coinsurance.

Meet and Confer   In law, an obligation imposed on parties by FRCP 26(f) to
address certain issues at the onset of litigation, including several related to
preservation, protection of privilege, and form of production of electronically
stored information (ESI).

Megabyte   1,024K bytes.

Member   A participant in a health plan.

MER **Managing Electronic Records**—An annual educational conference sponsored by Cohasset Associates composed of lawyers, information technology professionals, and records managers.

Message Digest A file number created algorithmically that represents the file uniquely. If the file changes, the message digest will change. A message digest can help to identify duplicate files.

Meta-Analysis The systematic method for combining information from multiple unrelated studies.

Metadata Structured data that describe, explain, locate, or otherwise make it easier to retrieve, use, or manage an electronic record. In a legal setting, metadata facilitates the discovery of relevant information and may be used to authenticate the evidentiary value of electronic information and/or describe contextual processing of a record. Often referred to as data about data or information about information, metadata can be very helpful in understanding the usability and integrity of information over time and can enable the management and understanding of electronic information. Metadata may be in physical, analog, or digital form. Metadata is often used in court to authenticate a document and/or determine the date a document was created.

Metadata Repository A central place where metadata definitions are stored and maintained.

Metalanguage The term used to describe language about language. Extensible Markup Language (XML) is an example of metalanguage.

Metarecord A record about the record.

Metatags Meta elements are HTML or XHTML elements used to provide structured metadata about a web page. A metatag is used to help search engines categorize pages. Metatags are invisible to the user.

MGMA **Medical Group Management Association**—A professional organization for the medical group practice profession with a mission to continually improve the performance of medical group practice professionals and the organizations they represent. http://www.mgma.com

M-Health **Mobile Health.**

M-Health Alliance An umbrella organization established in 2009 by the Rockefeller Foundation, United Nations Foundation, and Vodafone Foundation and created to draw together, complement, and expand upon the m-Health initiatives of multiple organizations around the world. The m-Health Alliance will cultivate cross-sector public and private collaboration in support of innovation and projects that address global health needs.

M-Health Community An Internet-based community open to healthcare professionals and developers and other healthcare industry stakeholders for the purpose of researching resources of vendors and applications as well as exchanging experiences with the implementation and use of mobile health (m-Health) applications.

mHI M-Health Initiative—Established in 2009 through the Medical Records Institute (MRI), an initiative open to vendors, individuals, and others. The m-Health Initiative aims to provide the healthcare community with information and resources about new and emerging cell phone, PDA, and other mobile technologies for use in healthcare. Both national and international workshops and seminars are planned for the exploration of mobile device (m-device) applications in healthcare.

MI Medical Informatics—A term used to describe a specialized body of science and knowledge. Informatics is an intersection of science, medicine, and healthcare.

Many subdomains of informatics exist including bioengineering and healthcare clinical informatics, which includes: nursing informatics, imaging informatics, consumer health informatics, public health informatics, dental informatics, clinical research informatics, bioinformatics, and pharmacy informatics. Medical informatics is also known as health informatics (HI) or clinical informatics (CI).

MICR Magnetic Ink Character Recognition—Electronic technology primarily used by financial services and the banking industry to facilitate the processing of checks.

Microblog A web-based service that allows the user to broadcast short messages, typically 140 to 200 characters, to other users of the service. The microblog can be delivered in real time, through SMS text messaging, or as an instant message.

Microchip The chip that serves as the CPU and controls the computer.

Micron One millionth of a meter.

Microsoft A United States–based computer technology corporation that develops and markets software and developer of the DOS and Windows operating systems.

Mimeograph A printed copy created by a rotary duplicator that passed ink through a stencil. A ubiquitous technique utilized until the 1990s for the reproduction of documents for offices, classrooms, and churches.

Minimum Metadata Set   A function identified in the HL7 RM-ES profile in which a minimum set of metadata is identified for health record content, which should be retained for the life of the record.

Minimum Necessary   The requirement, under the HIPAA Privacy Rule, in which a covered entity is required to limit the use of, disclosure of, and request for PHI to the amount needed to accomplish the intended purpose of use, disclosure, or request.

Minimum Scope of Disclosure   A HIPAA principle that individually identifiable health information should only be shared to the extent needed to support the purposes of disclosure.

MIPPA   Medicare Improvements for Patients and Providers Act of 2008—(Pub. L. 110-275) Enacted by Congress on July 15, 2008, to "amend titles XVIII and XIX of the Social Security Act to extend expiring provisions under the Medicare Program, to improve beneficiary access to preventive and mental health services, to enhance low-income benefit programs, and to maintain access to care in rural areas, including pharmacy access, and for other purposes." Among healthcare providers, MIPPA is well-known for blocking scheduled cuts in Medicare payments to physicians and extending the Physician Quality Reporting Initiative (PQRI) to December 31, 2010.

Mips   One million instructions per second. A way to measure computer speed.

Mirror Image   An exact copy (at the bit level) of a computer hard drive, used to ensure the system is not changed during a forensic investigation.

Misconduct in Science   A serious deviation (fabrication, plagiarism, fraudulent activity, or other activities) from commonly accepted scientific practices for the purpose of proposing, conducting, or reporting research.

MITA   Medicaid Information Technology Architecture—A CMS initiative designed to foster integrated business and IT transformation across the Medicaid enterprise to improve the administration of the Medicaid program.

Mixed Use   A term used to describe the utilization of electronic systems for both personal and professional use.

MLLP   Minimal Lower Layer Protocol—The HL7 messaging standard that defines how HL7 messages are wrapped in a header and footer so a user will know where a message starts and stops, and where the next message begins.

MMA   Medicare Modernization Act—See Medicare Prescription Drug, Improvement, and Modernization Act of 2003.

MMCO   Medicaid Managed Care Organization—A jointly funded (federal and state) managed care program to specifically address the needs of enrollees who are low income, have special cultural needs (such as language differences), or have special healthcare needs (such as chronic illnesses or disabilities).

MMIS   Medicaid Management Information Systems—An integrated group of procedures and computer processing operations (subsystems) developed at the general-design level to meet principal objectives. The objectives of this system and its enhancements include the Title XIX program to control administrative costs; service recipients, providers, and inquiries; operate claims control and computer capabilities; and management reporting for planning and control.

MMSEA   Medicare, Medicaid, and SCHIP Extension Act of 2007—(Pub. L. 110-275) Signed into law on December 29, 2007, by the president, MMSEA was enacted to continue to improve accountability in the Medicare program by improving the ability of the Secretary of HHS to identify beneficiaries for whom Medicare is the secondary payer by requiring group health plans and liability insurers to submit data to the Secretary of HHS. MMSEA requires that insurers report the identity of Medicare beneficiaries and other information the Secretary deems necessary to make determinations concerning coordination of benefits including any applicable recovery of claims.

Mode   The most frequently occurring statistic in a data set.

Model Rules of Professional Conduct   Published by the American Bar Association (ABA), a set of 52 rules, some mandatory and some discretionary, that serves as a set of ethical guidelines for lawyers.

Model Rules of Professional Responsibility   Promulgated by the American Bar Association, the Model Rules describe the ethical obligations of lawyers. States may adopt the Model Rules.

MODEM   Modulator-Demodulator—An electronic device that converts sound waves into electronic signals and electronic signals into sound waves.

Modifiers   Two-digit codes that indicate services that have been altered by some specific circumstance, but do not change the definition of the reported procedure codes.

Moral Awareness   A concept used to refer to an individual's ability to recognize a situation as having a moral implication.

Moral Hazard   A form of financial risk resulting from dishonesty, carelessness, or poor judgment.

Morbidity A term for the statistical incidence or severity of a medical abnormality such as a complication from a disease; a state of disease, injury, or illness.

Mortality Costs The costs related to a premature death due to any factor, estimated as the current monetary value of future lost output.

Motion In law, a procedure by which a litigant makes a formal request to a judge for a ruling on a particular matter.

MOU **Memorandum of Understanding**—A HIPAA document providing a description of the responsibilities to be assumed by parties in their pursuit of a goal.

Mounting Making offline data available for online processing.

Mouse Handheld device used to move the cursor on the computer screen.

MRA **Magnetic Resonance Angiography.**

MRI **Magnetic Resonance Imaging.**

MSA **Medical Savings Account**—A tax-exempt trust or custodial account established for the payment of medical expenses in conjunction with a high-deductible healthcare plan. Also known as a health savings account.

MS-DOS **Microsoft Disk Operating System**—Disk operating system for 16-bit microcomputers developed by Microsoft.

MS-DRGs **Medical Severity—Diagnosis-Related Groups**—The Medicare inpatient prospective payment classification scheme that became effective on October 1, 2007. A total of 538 DRGs were replaced with 745 Medicare Severity DRGs. The weights of the MS-DRGs were adjusted based on the severity of a patient's condition and are part of CMS plans to phase in a new system that would base payments on cost rather than charges and better reflect the patient's state of health.

MSO **Management Services Organization**—The MSO provides administrative services, usually including contracts, claims management, quality management, and utilization review, through an umbrella organization. Participants or shareholders may be hospitals, individual physicians, independent practice associations (IPAs), or other providers.

MSP **Medicare Secondary Payer**—A situation in which there is another insurance company that is primary to Medicare and pays first.

MU The concept that providers must show they're using certified EHR technology in ways that can be measured significantly in quantity and quality.

Multifactor Authentication   A system in which multiple factors (pieces of information and processes used to authenticate a person's identity) are used to authenticate an individual's identity for the purpose of delivering a higher level of authentication assurance than use of a single authentication factor. Multifactor authentication is often said to retrieve something you have with something you are. The term is sometimes used interchangeably with strong authentication.

Municipal Hospital   Hospitals owned by the city and operated by its health and hospitals corporation.

MySpace   A free social networking site originally created by eUniverse employees in 2003. Users are able to connect with friends, family, or coworkers to share thoughts, emotions, media, and other types of personal information. In addition, users can join groups of people with common interests. A social networking utility.

N

NAHDO   National Association of Health Data Organizations—A HIPAA-related group that promotes the development and improvement of health information systems at both the state and national level. http://www.nahdo.org

NAIC   National Association of Insurance Commissioners—A 501(c)(3) organization dedicated to organizing the regulatory and supervisory efforts of the various state insurance commissioners across the country. http://www.naic.org

Nanosecond   One-billionth of a second.

NAPHIT   National Association for Public Health Technology—A member organization of leaders in public health IT whose purpose is to facilitate communication between those who are developing, administering, and maintaining public health information technology and integrate the public health technologies into a system that works together across local, state, and federal programs. http://www.naphit.org/default.asp

NARA   National Archives and Records Administration—A government agency dedicated to preserving historical records and increasing public access to those documents.

NASMD   National Association of State Medicaid Directors—A collective of state Medicaid directors, affiliated with the American Public Health Human Services Association. http://www.nasmd.org/Home/home_news.asp

National Drug Code　A medical code set maintained by the FDA containing codes for drugs that have been approved for use.

National Institute of Diabetes and Digestive and Kidney Diseases　Funded by the National Institutes of Health (NIH), the National Institute of Diabetes and Digestive and Kidney Diseases supports research on many of the most serious diseases affecting public health. The Institute supports much of the clinical research on the diseases of internal medicine and related subspecialty fields, as well as many basic science disciplines. http://www2.niddk.nih.gov

National Institutes of Health　One of 11 federal agencies that make up the Department of Health and Human Services. The National Institutes of Health (NIH) is the primary federal agency for conducting and supporting medical research. Composed of 27 institutes and centers, the NIH provides leadership and financial support to researchers in every state in the United States and throughout the world. http://www.nih.gov

National Library of Medicine　Located on the campus of the National Institutes of Health (NIH) in Bethesda, MD, the National Library of Medicine (NLM) collects materials and provides information and research services in all areas of biomedicine and healthcare. It is the largest medical library in the world. http://www.nlm.nih.gov

National Pancreas Foundation　A charitable foundation that supports research of diseases of the pancreas and provides information and humanitarian services to those people who are suffering from such illnesses. http://www. pancreasfoundation.org

National Patient ID　A HIPAA system that uniquely identifies all recipients of healthcare services.

National Payer ID　A system for uniquely identifying all organizations that pay for healthcare services. Also known as Health Plan ID, or Plan ID.

National Standard Rule　A standard for measuring the required level of care based on the level of care provided by similar practitioners throughout the United States.

Native File Format　A form in which electronically stored information (ESI) is maintained and used and may be produced in discovery.

Natural Death Acts　Laws that establish procedures by which an individual can make provision for the withholding or withdrawing of medical treatment at the time when he or she loses the capacity to make such decisions.

Natural Language Processing   A subset of artificial intelligence and linguistics, natural language processing is the use of technology to manipulate and interpret free text words as part of a language. Computational techniques are applied to one or more levels of linguistic analysis (for example, morphological, syntactic, semantic, and pragmatic analysis).

NBS   National Bureau of Standards—A federal physical science research laboratory in operation from 1901 to 1988 that was dedicated to promoting US innovation and industrial competitiveness by advancing measurement science, standards, and technology in ways that improve quality of life and economic security. In 1988, NBS became the National Institute of Standards and Technology (NIST), and operates under the US Department of Commerce. http://www.nist.gov

NCANDS   National Child Abuse and Neglect Data System—A voluntary national data collection and analysis system that is the repository for data required by the Child Abuse Prevention and Treatment Act (CAPTA).

NCCA   National Commission for Certifying Agencies—An agency created in 1987 by the National Organization for Competency Assurance (NOCA) to help ensure the health, welfare, and safety of the public through the accreditation of a variety of certification programs and organizations that assess professional competence. http://www.noca.org

NCCUSL   National Conference of Commissioners on Uniform State Laws—A nonprofit organization with the purpose of discussing and debating in which areas of law there should be uniformity among the states and drafting acts accordingly. http://www.nccusl.org

NCCUSL Uniform Rules   A set of rules for electronic discovery promulgated by the National Conference of Commissioners on Uniform State Laws in 2007 as an appropriate act for those states desiring to adopt the specific substantive law suggested therein.

NCH   National Claims History—A database in the CMS Office of Information Services that houses all Common Working File (CWF)–processed Part A and Part B Medicare claims transaction records (includes initial, interim, debit/credit adjustments), beginning with service year 1991.

NCHC   National Coalition on Health Care—A large and broadly represented alliance established in 1990 to improve US healthcare. NCHC is composed of large and small businesses, the nation's largest labor, consumer, religious, and primary care provider groups, and the largest health and pension funds. http://nchc.org

NCHS   National Center for Health Statistics—The federal agency responsible for use of the International Statistical Classification of Diseases and Related Health Problems. http://www.cdc.gov/nchs

NCI   National Cancer Institute—One of 11 agencies that are part of the Department of Health and Human Services (HHS), the NCI is part of the National Institutes of Health and was established under the National Cancer Institute Act of 1937. NCI is the federal government's principal agency for cancer research and training. http://www.cancer.gov

NCPDP   National Council for Prescription Drug Programs—An American National Standards Institute (ANSI) accredited organization that maintains a number of standard formats for use by the retail pharmacy industry, some of which are included in the HIPAA mandates.

NCPDP Provider ID   A seven-digit number assigned to every pharmacy and qualified nonpharmacy dispensing site (NPSD) in the United States.

NCPDP Telecommunication Standard   An NCPDP standard mandated under HIPAA for use by high-volume dispensers of pharmaceuticals, such as retail pharmacies.

NCPHI   National Center for Public Health Informatics—A center within the CDC responsible for protecting the public's health, promoting health equity, and transforming public health practices through the advancement of informatics and information systems. http://www.cdc.gov/nchs

NCQA   National Committee on Quality Assurance—A nonprofit accreditation organization that examines healthcare effectiveness data in order to improve healthcare quality. http://www.ncqa.org

NCSC   National Center for State Courts—The NCSC is an independent nonprofit 501(c)(3) organization that serves as a national voice for state courts and provides knowledge and information about judicial administration. The NCSC helps state courts by exploring issues such as pro se litigation, judicial selection, and race, ethnic, and gender bias. http://www.ncsconline.org/index.html

NCVHS   National Committee on Vital and Health Statistics—The public advisory body to the Secretary of Health and Human Services. http://www.ncvhs.hhs.gov

Near Miss   A term used to refer to an event or situation that did not produce harm or injury, but only because of chance.

Needs Assessment   A systematic evaluation of current information system and programmatic operations and projected needs. This evaluation is performed as part of the system development life cycle prior to design and implementation.

Negligence   An unintentional failure to conform to a standard of care recognized by the law. To be actionable, an act of negligence must be accompanied by an injury to another individual.

Negligence Per Se   Negligence that is recognized as such without proof as to the circumstances because it is so obviously contrary to accepted standards of prudence.

Negligent Infliction of Emotional Distress   The accidental failure to exercise reasonable care to avoid causing emotional distress to another individual.

Negotiation   A process of bargaining with another.

NeHC   National e-Health Collaborative—A private-sector entity, established to encourage broad-based participation from the public and private sectors to further advance the use of common standards and policies. NeHC is the successor to American Health Information Community (AHIC). http://www.nationalehealth.org

NEMA   National Electrical Manufacturers Association—A trade association founded in 1926 for the electrical manufacturing industry. NEMA's 450 member companies manufacture products used in the generation, transmission and distribution, control, and end-use of electricity, including medical imaging products. http://www.nema.org

Network   Healthcare providers who contract with a health plan to participate in health benefits plans.

NHB   National Health Board—An oversight board that regulates all aspects of the health industry and oversees government healthcare agencies.

NHIE   National Health Information Exchange—A summit for support of national, state, and local healthcare leaders working with challenges in building health information across a continuum of practices and institutions.

NHII   National Health Information Infrastructure—The physical and national network needed for interoperability to occur, established prior to the NHIN.

NHIN   Nationwide Health Information Network—The NHIN is an Internet-based architecture that links disparate healthcare information systems to allow patients, physicians, hospitals, community health centers, and public health agencies across the country to share clinical information securely. The NHIN is a critical portion of the HHS health IT agenda intended to provide a secure nationwide, interoperable health information infrastructure that will connect providers, consumers, and others involved in supporting health and healthcare. The NHIN will enable health information to follow the consumer, be available for clinical decision making, and support appropriate use of healthcare information beyond direct patient care so as to improve the nation's health. http://www.hhs.gov/healthit/healthnetwork/background

NIAAA National Institute on Alcohol Abuse and Alcoholism—An agency that operates as part of the National Institutes of Health (NIH), the NIAAA provides leadership in the national effort to reduce alcohol-related problems by conducting and supporting research; coordinating and collaborating with other research institutes and federal programs on alcohol-related issues; collaborating with international, national, state, and local institutions, organizations, agencies, and programs engaged in alcohol-related work; and translating and disseminating research findings to healthcare providers, researchers, policymakers, and the public. http://www.niaaa.nih.gov

NIH National Institutes of Health—One of 11 federal agencies that make up the Department of Health and Human Services. The NIH is the primary federal agency for conducting and supporting medical research. Composed of 27 institutes and centers, the NIH provides leadership and financial support to researchers in every state in the United States and throughout the world. http://www.nih.gov

NIST National Institute of Standards and Technology—Founded in 1901, NIST is a nonregulatory federal agency whose mission is to promote standardization of measurements by working with industry to develop and apply technology, measurements, and standards.

NLM National Library of Medicine—A collection of resources and databases maintained by the National Institutes of Health. http://www.nlm.nih.gov

NLRB National Labor Relations Board—A federal agency that administers the primary law (the National Labor Relations Act) governing relations between unions and employers in the private sector. http://www.nlrb.gov

NOCA National Organization for Competency Assurance—An organization that represents the credentialing community and strives to provide leading-edge information to certification organizations, licensing bodies, regulatory bodies, those seeking quality credentialing services, and consumers. http://www.noca.org

NOI Notice of Intent—A legal document that describes a subject area for which the federal government is considering developing regulations and the presumably relevant considerations, inviting comments from interested parties.

Nominal Damages   An award that is of insignificant value, reflecting an invasion rather than actual damages.

Noncovered Services   Services that the patient pays for instead of Medicare.

Nondelegable Duty   An obligation imposed by law or contract that cannot be passed on or delegated to another.

Noneconomic Damages   In law, a term used to describe those elements of injury or loss that cannot be accurately calculated in terms of money, such as pain and suffering.

Nonfederal Nondisproportionate Share Hospital   Any public or private nonprofit institution in a state that is primarily engaged in providing, by or under the supervision of physicians, to inpatients: (a) diagnostic and therapeutic services for medical diagnosis, treatment, and care of injured, disabled, or sick persons, or (b) rehabilitation of injured, disabled, or sick persons. Hospital-based outpatient services are included under this definition.

Nonrepudiation   The inability to deny the origin of an electronic document or the fact that an electronic document has been received. Nonrepudiation is the strong and substantial evidence of the identity of the signer of a message and of message integrity, sufficient to prevent a party from successfully denying the origin, submission, or delivery of the message and the integrity of its contents.

Normalization of Data   The refinement of data in a step-by-step process into a simple and stable data structure.

Notice   In law, the term used to refer to the legal notification required by law or agreement, or imparted by the operation of law. Examples of legal notices are complaints, subpoenas, depositions, and such.

Notice of Motion   A written form that a party in a suit has filed a motion or that a motion will be heard by the court at a particular time.

Notice of Orders or Judgments   A written notice of the entry of an order provided by the court clerk or a party in the suit.

Notice of Privacy Practices   A legal notice under HIPAA provided to patients that informs patients that the entity and its staff, employees, and volunteers will use and disclose protected health information for purposes of treatment, payment, and healthcare operations, and for other purposes that are permitted or required by law. See also Privacy Rule.

Notice to Appear   A summons in which a person is notified to appear in court.

NPDB **National Practitioner Data Bank**—Created by the Healthcare Quality Improvement Act of 1986, the NPDB is a federal repository of information on selected disciplinary actions and malpractice claim histories for all US practitioners.

NPDS **Nonpharmacy Dispensing Site.**

NPF **National Provider File**—Under HIPAA, a database envisioned for use in maintaining a national provider registry, which assigns national provider IDs.

NPI **National Provider Identification**—A unique identifier for a provider of healthcare services.

NPI Rule The HIPAA regulation establishing and governing national provider identifiers, found at 69 Fed. Reg. 3434, issued January 23, 2004.

NPIOI **National Provider Identifier Outreach Initiative**—An initiative of the Workgroup for Electronic Data Interchange (WEDI). The WEDI NPIOI serves as the focal point for the industry for information related to the planning, transition, and implementation of the national provider identifier (NPI). The primary roles of the NPIOI are to: 1. develop and implement a national coordinated NPI outreach plan; 2. act as a central repository for NPI resources; and 3. disseminate industry consensus information on policy and operational issues regarding the deployment and use of the NPI. The outreach plan will be targeted to providers, payers, clearinghouses, vendors, and other industry participants affected by the new NPI.

NPRM **Notice of Proposed Rulemaking**—A document that describes and explains regulations that the federal government proposes to adopt in the future, inviting interested parties to submit comments that will be used in developing the final regulation.

NPS **National Provider System**—The HIPAA administrative system envisioned for supporting a national provider registry.

NPV **Net Present Value**—A calculation performed to determine whether to invest in a project by looking at the projected cash inflows and outflows. The formula to calculate the NPV is as follows:

$$\frac{Rt}{(1 + i)t}$$

t = The time of the cash flow
i = The discount rate (the rate of return that could be earned on an investment in the financial market with similar risk)
Rt = The net cash flow (the amount of cash inflow, minus cash outflow) at time, t

NQF National Quality Forum.

NRA Not Reasonably Accessible—In law, a concept by which a party or sub-poenaed nonparty declines to produce electronically stored information (ESI) from a source by reason of alleged burden or cost.

NSF National Standard Format—Any nationally standardized data format; more specifically, the Professional EMC NSF flat file record format used to submit professional claims.

NUBC National Uniform Billing Committee—A HIPAA organization that maintains the UB-92 hardcopy institutional billing form and the data element specifications for both hardcopy and electronic flat file EMC format.

NUCC National Uniform Claim Committee—A HIPAA organization that maintains the HCFA-1500 claim form, the Professional EMC NSF, the Provider Taxonomy Codes, and the X12 837. It also consults on all trans-actions affecting nondental and noninstitutional professional healthcare services.

Nursing Home A public or private institution (or a distinct part of an insti-tution), certified under section 1919(a) of the Social Security Act, that is primarily engaged in providing, on a regular basis, health-related care and service to individuals who, because of their mental or physical condition, require care and service (above the level of room and board) that can be made available to them only through institutional facilities. A nursing home is not primarily for the care and treatment of mental diseases.

O

OASAM Office of the Assistant Secretary for Administration and Manage-ment's Civil Rights Center—Administers and enforces equal opportunity civil rights laws for recipients who receive federal financial assistance from the Department of Labor (DOL). OASAM also provides guidance to the Secretary of the Department of Labor in the areas of budget, human resources, informa-tion technology, safety and health, facilities management, and administration to ensure that the DOL maintains the necessary resources (financial, staff, and technology) to perform its programs mission and maintain compliance with DOL statutes.

OASIS Organization for the Advancement of Structured Information Standards—A not-for-profit consortium founded in 1993, composed of more than 5,000 participants representing over 600 organizations and individual members in 100 countries. OASIS drives the development, convergence, and adoption of open standards for the global information society and produces more web services standards than any other organization, along with standards for security, e-business, and standardization efforts in the public sector and for application-specific markets.

OASIS   A Medicare-certified home health outcomes and assessment information data set that contains data items that were developed for measuring patient outcomes for the purpose of performance improvement in home healthcare. Only Medicare- and/or Medicaid-certified home care agencies are required to conduct patient-specific comprehensive assessments at specified time points. The data are collected at start of care, 60-day follow-ups, and discharge. OASIS data items address sociodemographic, environmental, support system, health status, functional status, and health service utilization characteristics of the patient.

Objection   A formal statement by legal counsel in opposition to something that was said or has occurred in court, which seeks the judge's immediate ruling.

Obligatory Action   An obligation that someone is required by law to undertake.

OCR—Office of Civil Rights   The OCR promotes and ensures that people have equal access and opportunity to participate in and receive services from all HHS programs without facing unlawful discrimination, and that the privacy of their health information is protected while ensuring access to care. Through prevention and elimination of unlawful discrimination and by protecting the privacy of individually identifiable health information, OCR helps HHS carry out its overall mission of improving the health and well-being of all people affected by its many programs. The administrative agency responsible for HIPAA enforcement. http://www.hhs.gov/ocr

OCR—Official Court Reporter   Official Court Reporter.

OCR—Optical Character Reader/Recognition   A computerized process that generates a searchable text file from a digital image or picture file. It cannot recognize handwriting. Software compares the shape of letters in the picture with a library of fonts and then generates the appropriate letter. Depending on the quality of the original document, OCR can be more or less accurate.

OCSP   Online Certificate Status Protocol—A protocol that provides the ability to verify the validity of certificates for the secure exchange of information.

Octal   The base-8 number system, which can easily be read by humans and translated into binary format.

OEM   Original Equipment Manufacturer.

OEP Open Enrollment Period—The time period between January 1 and March 31 that provides a Medicare beneficiary with the opportunity to enroll in, disenroll from, or change a Medicare Advantage plan. In order to make a change, the Medicare beneficiary must have both Medicare Parts A and B and live in the Medicare Advantage plan's service area.

OFCCP Office of Federal Contract Compliance Programs—Responsible for the administration and enforcement of federal contract-based civil rights laws that require federally assisted contractors and subcontractors provide equal opportunity in employment.

Of Counsel In law, a category of lawyer within a firm. May also refer to an attorney who assists another attorney in litigation.

Offer of Proof In legal procedure, a presentation of evidence for the record, made after a judge has sustained an objection to the admissibility of evidence so that the evidence can be preserved on the record for an appeal of the judge's ruling.

Office of Personnel Management An agency administering and directing the federal employees' health benefits.

Offline Not connected to a network.

OIG Office of Inspector General—The role of the OIG is to provide independent, objective oversight of the Department of Health and Human Services (HHS) to carry out the mission of promoting economy, efficiency, and effectiveness through the elimination of waste, fraud, and abuse. The OIG is empowered to conduct independent audits and investigations, identify systemic weaknesses that permit fraud, coordinate efforts to detect fraud, and keep the HHS informed of problems related to the administration of its programs. http://oig.hhs.gov

OLAP Online Analytical Processing—A system that facilitates the ability of the operating system to analyze data (through views and reports) and make intelligent decisions that potentially affect its future.

OLDIIS Orphaned, Legacy, and/or Dormant Inactive Information Stores—A term used to refer to inactive data that may be unidentified or orphaned (that is, no one within the organization has knowledge of or responsibility for the data) that are stored on media that may be deteriorating, inaccessible, and/or stored on obsolete software or hardware.

OLTP Online Transaction Processing.

OMB Office of Management and Budget—The OMB's predominant mission is to assist the US president in overseeing the preparation of the federal budget and to supervise its administration in executive branch agencies. In addition, the OMB oversees and coordinates the administration's procurement, financial management, information, and regulatory policies.

Ombudsman   A patient representative, often providing representation during conflicts with health plans.

OMSPH   **Office of Medicine, Science and Public Health**—An office of the Assistant Secretary for Preparedness and Response (ASPR) responsible for providing expert medical, scientific, and public health advice on domestic and international medical preparedness policies, programs, initiatives, and activities. http://www.hhs.gov/aspr/omsph/index.html

ONC   **Office of the National Coordinator**—The ONC provides counsel to the Secretary of HHS and departmental leadership for the development and nationwide implementation of an interoperable health information technology infrastructure. It also provides management of and logistical support for the American Health Information Community (AHIC). http://www.hhs.gov/healthit/onc/mission

ONC—ATCB   **Office of the National Coordinator—Authorized Testing and Certification Body**—An organization that has been designated by the ONC to test and certify health information technology.

ONCHIT   **Office of National Coordinator for Health Information Technology**—Now known as the Office of the National Coordinator (ONC).

One-Time Pad   A private key or symmetric cipher where the key size is equal to the plaintext size. The key is never reutilized; therefore, there is no basis for mathematical cryptanalysis. The one-time pad is theoretically the only unbreakable cipher.

Online Social Networking   The grouping of individuals into specific groups through use of the Internet and websites. Examples of online social networks include Facebook and LinkedIn.

OOA   **Out of Area**—Healthcare services received while outside the geographic service area of a managed care plan. Typically, prior approval is needed from the primary care provider before the plan will pay for out-of-area care, except in emergencies.

OODBMS   **Object-Oriented Database Management System.**

OORDBMS   **Object-Oriented Relational Database Management System.**

OPEO   **Office of Preparedness and Emergency Operations**—An office of the Assistant Secretary for Preparedness and Response (ASPR) responsible for developing operational plans and participating in training and exercises to ensure the preparedness of the ASPR Office, the Department of Health and Human Services, the federal government, and the public to respond to domestic and international, public health, and medical threats and emergencies.

Operating System   A program that organizes the activities of a computer and its attachments.

Operations and Maintenance   Activities associated with the ongoing support of information systems. This term includes the use of supplies, software, hardware, and personnel directly associated with the functioning of the mechanized information system. Examples of operational activities include: providing routine maintenance; updating commercial software used in the system; updating changes to tables; creating new reports, edits, alerts, and data elements; reformatting screens; and/or other minor system changes.

OPSP   Office of Policy and Strategic Planning—An office of the Assistant Secretary for Preparedness and Response (ASPR) responsible for policy formulation and coordination for preparedness and response strategic planning. In coordination with other ASPR and departmental offices, OPSP analyzes proposed policies and presidential directives and regulations, and develops short- and long-term policies and strategic objectives.

Oracle   In the context of information management and technology, Oracle is a leading supplier of information management software and relational database products, such as RDBMS, a relational database management system.

Oral Confession   In law, a confession that is not made in writing. Oral confessions are admissible, though as a practical matter, it is preferable for a police interrogator to take a written or recorded confession from a suspect.

Ordinary Care   The degree of care that a reasonable person of ordinary intelligence and prudence would exercise given the circumstances. This is the standard of care expected of everyone at all times; a failure to exercise ordinary care is negligence. Also known as standard of care.

Original Medicare   The federal health insurance program that covers most people age 65 or older, some people under age 65 who are disabled, and people with end-stage renal disease. Original Medicare is divided into two parts: Part A, which is hospital insurance, and Part B, which is medical insurance. Medicare Parts C and Part D are both offered by private insurance companies. Original Medicare (Parts A and B) is provided by the government. Original

Medicare also refers to an individual who is not enrolled in a Medicare Advantage plan, but maintains a fee-for-service Medicare policy, and possibly Medicare supplement insurance such as Medigap.

Originator   Author of a document.

Orphan Records   Records of data that no longer have connections to other data. Orphan records are created when the source data with referential integrity is deleted.

OS   Operating System—Software that relies on other system software to make the system function. Examples of operating systems include Windows, Unix, Linux, and Mac OS.

OS DHSS   Office of the Secretary of the Department of Health and Human Services.

OSHA   Occupational Safety and Health Act (P.L. 91-596)—A federal law enacted on December 29, 1970, to assure the safe and healthful working conditions for men and women.

OSI   Open System Interconnection—A multilayer ISO data communications standard. HL7 is responsible for specifying the level seven OSI standards for the healthcare industry.

Ostensible Agency   The legal doctrine based on Section 429 of the Second Restatement of Torts of 1965 that provides: "One who employs an independent contractor to perform services for another which are accepted in the reasonable belief that the services are being rendered by the employer or by his servants, is subject to liability for physical harm caused by the negligence of the contractor in supplying such services, to the same extent as though the employer were supplying them himself or by his servants. Also known as apparent authority.

OST File Format   A file format saved on the local computer and used by Microsoft Outlook as an offline folder file to allow the user to work offline and then to synchronize changes with the exchange server at another time.

Outcome   Changes in a patient's health status. The result of treatment.

Outcomes Measurement   The measurement of the changes in a patient's health status due to treatment.

Outliers   Data outside the expected norm.

Outlook Express   A Microsoft e-mail client that has been included with a number of versions of Microsoft Windows.

Out-of-Network Providers Doctors and other healthcare providers who are not contracted to offer services with a specific HMO or PPO plan. Also referred to as nonpreferred providers.

Outpatient An individual who receives treatment at a hospital or clinic but does not require an overnight stay.

Outpatient Surgery Surgical procedures that do not require an overnight stay in the hospital. Also known as ambulatory surgery.

Overutilization Unnecessary services offered by providers or demanded by members.

OWCP Office of Workers' Compensation Programs—A branch of the Department of Labor (DOL) responsible for the administration of the four major disability compensation programs providing wage replacement benefits, medical treatment, vocational rehabilitation, and other benefits to certain workers or their dependents who experience work-related injury or occupational disease. The OWCP administers the following disability compensation programs:

> DFEC—Division of Federal Employees Compensation
> DEEOIC—Division of Energy Employees Illness Compensation
> DLHWC—Division of Longshore and Harbor Workers' Compensation
> DCMWC—Division of Coal Mine Workers' Compensation

OWR Optical Word Recognition—Software that interprets document images using several OCR engines at the same time and compares the results to a built-in dictionary. OWR is generally more accurate than OCR, especially on poor-quality or older originals.

P

PAC Post-Acute Care—The care provided to a patient postdischarge from a hospital. Examples of post-acute care include skilled nursing and home healthcare.

PACS Picture Archival Communication System—A medical imaging system created to provide storage, rapid retrieval, and access to images acquired with multiple modalities, simultaneously, at multiple sites without the need for physical files or film jackets.

PACS System Picture Archiving and Communications System—A system that enables images such as x-rays and scans to be stored electronically and viewed on screens.

PA DSS **Payment Application Data Security Standards**—A set of worldwide information security standards designed to help vendors and others develop secure payment applications that do not store prohibited data. See also PCI SSC.

PAG **Policy Advisory Group**—A generic term used to describe healthcare workgroups such as Workgroup for Electronic Data Interchange (WEDI).

PAHP **Prepaid Ambulatory Health Plan**—A prepaid ambulatory health plan that provides less than comprehensive services on an at-risk or other than state plan reimbursement basis, and provides, arranges for, or otherwise has responsibility for the provision of any ambulatory health service.

PAHPA **Pandemic and All-Hazards Preparedness Act**—A public health interoperability initiative aimed at the development of a near real-time, electronic nationwide public health situational awareness capability through an interoperable network of systems and inventory of telehealth initiatives.

Pain and Suffering The allowance of recovery for physical pain that one has had to endure and its subsequent mental sequelae, or mental torment.

Palliative Care Any form of medical care or treatment that concentrates on reducing the severity of disease symptoms rather than seeking a cure.

PAPD **Planning Advanced Planning Document**—A document prepared by a state agency that is used to obtain approval and funding commitments for planning costs associated with major system development projects.

Paper-Based Discovery Discovery using information that can be read without the aid of a device, such as a computer. Discovery that is not electronically stored information (ESI).

Paragon Encrypted Disk A commercial Windows disk encryption package.

Parens Patriae In law, the Latin term for father of the people. It refers to the power of a state to intercede in, among other things, parental decision making under certain circumstances.

Parent-Child Functional Profile The parent-child functional profile is an HL7 numbering scheme used to describe parent-child functional relationships and dependencies.

Parent Document The term used to refer to the first document in a group that has been bundled together by the author; a cover document that has others attached to it. See also Child Document.

Parity—Health Insurance   A term used to refer to the Mental Health Parity Act of 1996 (MHPA). A federal law that applies to two different types of coverage:

1. Large-group, self-funded group health plans; CMS has jurisdiction over self-funded public-sector (nonfederal governmental) plans, while the Department of Labor has jurisdiction over self-funded private-sector group health plans.
2. Large-group, fully insured group health plans.

Parity—Information Systems   A method of error checking through adding 1s and 0s to a word.

Part A Hospital Insurance   Premium-free coverage that helps pay for inpatient hospital care and some skilled nursing care, with a deductible per benefit period.

Part B Medical Insurance   Coverage with premiums and deductibles that helps pay for medical and surgical services by healthcare providers as well as benefits such as ambulance rides, durable medical equipment, outpatient services, and laboratory services.

Participating Provider   A doctor or supplier who agrees to accept assignment on all Medicare claims for people with Original Medicare. These doctors and suppliers may bill the beneficiary for Medicare deductibles and/or coinsurance amounts only.

Party   The person, legal entity, or organization that files a lawsuit or defends against a lawsuit. See also Plaintiff, Defendant, and Respondent.

Passive Concealment   In law, the concealment of words or acts by maintaining silence when one is legally bound to disclose such information.

Password Reset   The process of resetting a password that is lost, stolen, or forgotten, which typically involves first authenticating the individual requesting a password reset, then provisioning a new password, and finally notifying the requestor of the new password.

Patient-Centered Focus   A term used to describe the vision of health and healthcare transformed with respect to the directives of the American Recovery and Reinvestment Act (ARRA) of 2009.

Patient Perception   A type of outcome measure related to how the patient feels following treatment.

Patient Safety   The healthcare discipline that emphasizes the reporting, analysis, and prevention of errors.

Patient's Bill of Rights A statement of the rights to which patients are entitled as recipients of medical care in the United States. The Patient's Bill of Rights typically grants autonomy to healthcare providers.

Payer In healthcare, the term is used to denote the entity that assumes the risk of paying for medical treatments. This can be an uninsured patient, a self-insured employer, a health plan, or an HMO.

PBM **Pharmacy Benefit Manager**—An organization that provides administrative services in processing and analyzing prescription claims for pharmacy benefits and coverage programs. PBM services can include: contracting with a network of pharmacies; establishing payment levels for provider pharmacies; negotiating rebate arrangements; developing and managing formularies, preferred drug lists, and prior authorization programs; maintaining patient compliance programs; performing drug utilization review; and operating disease management programs.

PC **Personal Computer**—Refers to both desktops and laptops.

PCI **Peripheral Component Interconnect.**

PCI DSS **Payment Card Industry Data Security Standard**—A worldwide information security standard designed to prevent credit card fraud, applicable to all organizations that hold, process, or pass cardholder information from any card containing the logo of one of the card brands. See also PCI SSC.

PCI PED **Payment Card Industry PIN Entry Device.**

PCI SSC **Payment Card Industry Security Standards Council**—An independent council of credit card companies engaged in the management and evolution of the Payment Card Industry Data Security Standards. See also PCI DSS.

PCMH **Patient Centered Medical Home**—An approach to providing comprehensive primary care for children, youth, and adults. The PCMH is a healthcare setting that facilitates partnerships between individual patients and their personal physicians, and, when appropriate, the patient's family.

PDA **Personal Digital Assistant**—A handheld digital device. Examples include the Blackberry and the Palm.

PDF **Portable Document Format**—Developed by Adobe Systems, Inc., PDF is the de facto standard for the exchange of electronic documents. A PDF file preserves the fonts, images, graphics, and layout of any source document, regardless of how the original document was created. PDF files can be shared, viewed, and printed with Adobe Reader, a free viewer application. Documents can be converted to a PDF using software products created by Adobe and other providers. PDF files are also searchable by either retaining text from the source document or by having a source image file converted by OCR. Depending on the capture methodology, PDF files may retain some metadata.

PDPs   Prescription Drug Plans—Plans offered by commercial companies for Medicare Part D prescription drug coverage. Plans differ in monthly premiums, drugs covered, cost-sharing amounts, and participating pharmacies.

Peer Review   A process in which medical staff members review other staff members and applicants to determine eligibility to practice in a hospital or office.

Peer-Review Privilege   Information that is not discoverable because it was obtained in the course of a healthcare institution's quality of care review.

Penalty   An amount of money agreed upon in advance when payment or performance is not made on time; for example, fines paid by a vendor for the inability to install an information system on time. In criminal law, a penalty is the fine or forfeiture of property as ordered by the judge after a person is convicted of a crime.

Pended   A claims term when a case has been set aside for review that indicates that it is not known whether authorization has or will be issued for delivery of a healthcare service.

Per Diem   A daily negotiated rate for the provision of all or selected hospital services and supplies regardless of the actual type or volume of services provided.

Performance Measure   An assessment or ranking as to whether performance meets the specified goal.

Performance Measurement   The regular collection and reporting of data in order to track the work produced and its results.

Periodic Payment   A term used to describe the periodic interim payments made biweekly to a hospital on the Periodic Interim Payment (PIP) program that are based on the hospital's estimate of Medicare reimbursement for the current cost-report period.

Period of Records Retention   Denotes the length of time a series of records must be kept for regulatory, legal, and/or business purposes or a combination thereof.

Peripheral   A device used as an accessory to a computer.

Per Se Violation   Violations, such as price fixing, that are so anticompetitive that no study is necessary to establish their illegality.

Personal Health Information Technology   Technology that enables documentation of a person's complete health and medical history in a secure format that he or she controls, but is still accessible to healthcare providers from any location.

Personal Health Record   A personal health record that is maintained by the patient and ideally contains a detailed profile of the patient's medical history since birth. The vision of healthcare providers is such that the patient's personal health history can be securely exchanged between the patient and the provider's EHR system for care coordination and treatment.

Personal Injury   Any harm or loss suffered by an individual.

Petabyte   A unit of information equal to 1,000 terabytes or 10^{15} bytes.

Petitioner   An alternative title for a plaintiff. Use is dependent on the jurisdiction and the nature of the action.

PET Scan   Positron Emission Tomography—A technique in nuclear imaging that creates a three-dimensional picture of functional processes in a patient's body with directed gamma rays.

PFFS Plan   Private Fee-for-Service Plan—A type of Medicare Advantage plan. The PFFS plan differs from other Medicare Advantage HMO or PPO plans in that the beneficiary is not required to use a network of providers. Under a PFFS plan, a beneficiary can see any provider who accepts Medicare and agrees to accept payment from the PFFS plan. Medicare is not billed for services under a PFFS plan; instead the provider must bill the PFFS plan. Services covered by the plan usually require a copayment, and in some cases require the beneficiary to pay a percentage of the Medicare-approved amount, at times up to 35 percent.

PGPdisk   A commercial disk encryption package that supports both Windows and Mac OS.

PGP   A public key encryption methodology used to protect e-mail and data files that contains a sophisticated key management digital signature and data compression. PGM allows for secure communication with unknown persons and without the need for secure channels for prior exchange of keys.

PHI   Protected Health Information—Under HIPAA, PHI is individually identifiable health information that is maintained or transmitted in any form or medium about an individual's health status, provision of healthcare, or payment for healthcare.

PHIN   Public Health Information Network—A network run by the Centers for Disease Control and Prevention that seeks to improve the capacity of public health to use and exchange information electronically by promoting the use of standards and defining functional and technical requirements. http://www.cdc.gov/PHIN

Phishing   The technique used to obtain personal information for identify theft or other illegitimate purpose. E-mails are sent pretending to be from a legitimate source with intent to obtain personal information from an unknowing victim.

PHO   Physician Hospital Organization—A managed care organization of providers and one or more hospitals that contracts with HMOs and PPOs to provide care.

PHR   Personal Health Record—A PHR combines data knowledge and software tools to help consumers and patients take an active role in the management of their care. When the PHR is integrated with an electronic health record (EHR) it becomes a powerful tool for both provider and consumer. The PHR is accessed by an individual through the Internet, using state-of-the-art security and privacy controls, at any time and from any location. In a crisis, emergency room staff can access and retrieve vital information from the PHR, and physicians, family members, and school nurses can see portions of a PHR when necessary.

PHS   Public Health Service—The primary division of the US Department of Health and Human Services. The PHS comprises all agency divisions of the Department of Health and Human Services.

PHSA   Public Health Service Act—A federal law enacted in 1944 that has been amended many times, most recently in 2010 through enactment of the Patient Protection and Affordable Care Act. The full text of the Public Health Service Act is found under Title 42 of the United States Code, the Public Health and Welfare Chapter 6A Public Health Service.

Physical Attachments   Documents that are clipped or stapled or otherwise bound together. Unlike a true attachment, there may be no express indication by the author or custodian that the documents were intended to be grouped together other than the fact of their physical connection. See also True Attachments.

Physician-Patient Relationship   A relationship that arises when a physician renders professional services, thereby incurring responsibilities to the patient. Among the responsibilities is the physician-patient privilege, prohibiting the physician from violating patient confidentiality or revealing information without the patient's approval.

PICS **Platform for Internet Content Selection**—PICS is W3C specification that enables metadata to be associated with Internet content.

PIHP **Prepaid Inpatient Health Plan**—A prepaid inpatient health plan that provides less than comprehensive services on an at-risk or other than state plan reimbursement basis; it provides, arranges for, or otherwise has responsibility for the provision of any inpatient hospital or institutional services.

PIP **Periodic Interim Payment**—A payment made to a hospital that participates in the Medicare PIP Program.

PIP **Program Improvement Plan**—A plan completed by the state to address areas of noncompliance identified through a federal review.

Pixel **Picture Element**—Any of the small discrete elements that together form an image; the greater number of pixels, the higher the resolution, and the more detailed the graphics.

PKI **Public Key Infrastructure**—A cryptography arrangement that facilitates third-party examination of and vouching for user identities.

PKI Authorities Three different authorities that make up the public key infrastructure system. The three authorities are the Registration Authority, Certification Authority, and Certificate Directory.

PKIX Public Key X.509 Certificate as defined by the Internet Engineering Task Force (IETF).

PL, P.L., or Pub. L. **Public Law**—As in Pub. L. 111-5, the American Recovery and Reinvestment Act of 2009 (ARRA).

Plaintext Plaintext data are usable data before encryption or after successful decryption. See also Cleartext.

Plaintiff Also known as a petitioner. This term is commonly used to refer to the person(s) or organization or that initiated a lawsuit. A plaintiff is also known as a party.

Plan Sponsor The sponsor of a health plan, such as an employer, union, or some other legal entity.

Plausible Deniability A data security term that means to avoid being coerced into decrypting one's own data for an attacker.

Playback Protection A feature that increases security by preventing use of prerecorded phrases. Following authentication, the user is asked to repeat several sets of random digits of which the number of digits in each set is configurable.

Pleading   In law, a term used to describe certain documents that are filed with a court, including the complaint and the answer.

PM/PM   Per Member Per Month—A common term used in managed care to describe the revenue or cost for each enrolled employee each month. PM/PM is calculated by dividing the number of units of something into member months. Often used to describe premiums or capitated payments to providers, but can also refer to the revenue or cost for each enrolled employee each month.

Pointer   An index entry in the directory of some form of storage media that is used to identify the space on the media where an electronic document resides, preventing that space from being overwritten.

Point of Service   Refers to the location where a transaction, point of care, or treatment occurs.

Police Power   The authority of a state to act in the public interest.

Port   A connection through which signals flow into and out of a computer.

POS Code   Place of Service or Point of Service Code—A two-digit code placed on provider claims to indicate the setting in which a service was provided.

Power of Attorney   A document granting an individual the right to perform acts on behalf of another, generally the person executing the document.

PPAC   Practicing Providers Advisory Council—A discontinued advisory council created by the CMS that provided channels by which physicians could stay current with CMS and its practices.

PPACA   Patient Protection and Affordable Care Act (P.L. 111-148)—A federal law signed into law on March 23, 2010, by President Barack Obama. PPACA will be implemented over a four-year period beginning in 2010 and contains a large number of health-related provisions, which include the expansion of Medicaid, the establishment of health insurance exchanges, and support for medical research. Also known as HR 3590.

PPDD   Practical Privacy Disc Driver—A Linux disk encryption methodology that creates a device that looks like a disk partition. It utilizes a Blowfish algorithm.

PPO   Preferred Provider Organization—A group of healthcare providers that agree to provide medical services at a discount to covered persons in a given geographic area.

PQRI **Physician Quality Reporting Initiative**—A CMS initiative that establishes financial incentives for eligible professionals to participate in a voluntary quality reporting program. In 2011, the program name was changed to Physician Quality Reporting System.

Practice Guidelines An agreed-upon strategy of specific options for patient management that is considered appropriate practice, based on current information.

Practitioner A person who provides healthcare services.

Preauthorization or Preadmission Certification Terms commonly used in managed care to denote a need for prior review and approval before a healthcare service can be rendered. These terms are often used to refer to a decision made by the payer, HMO, or insurance company prior to admission. The payer determines whether the payer will pay for the service. Most managed care plans require pre-certification. This is a method of controlling and monitoring utilization by evaluating the need for service prior to the service being rendered. The practice of reviewing claims for inpatient admission prior to the patient entering the hospital in order to assure that the admission is medically necessary. An administrative procedure whereby a health provider submits a treatment plan to a third party before treatment is initiated. The third party usually reviews the treatment plan, monitoring one or more of the following: patient's eligibility, covered service, amounts payable, application of appropriate deductibles, copayment factors, and maximums. Similar processes: preauthorization, pre-certification, preestimate of cost, pretreatment estimate, prior authorization.

Precedent An earlier judicial decision that may be binding on lower courts.

Predictive Modeling The process of mapping relationships among elements of data that have a commonality. Through this process, data are examined with software to recognize patterns and trends, which can then potentially predict clinical and cost outcomes.

Pre-Existing Condition A health problem discovered and treated before health insurance is bought. Usually, treatment must have been received sometime during the last six months for the condition to be considered pre-existing.

Premium A periodic or monthly payment made to Medicare, an insurance company, or a healthcare plan for healthcare coverage.

Preservation Notice, Preservation Order A form of legal hold.

Presumption A legal assumption that a fact exists, based on the proven existence of other such facts or groups of facts.

Pretrial Conference   In law, a meeting between the judge and the attorneys in a particular case to discuss issues and move the action toward disposition.

Prevalence   The total number of cases of a disease in a population at a given time or else the total number of cases, divided by the number of individuals in the population.

Prima Facie Argument   A principle that is assumed to be true unless there is sufficient argument offered to rebut it.

Prima Facie Case   A case that seems to have enough evidence to prevail in a suit if it is not contradicted by evidence to the contrary.

Primary Care Physician   A patient's designated physician for basic medical care, such as a family practitioner, pediatrician, or internist.

Primary Insurance   Insurance that attaches immediately on the happening of a loss; insurance that is not contingent on the exhaustion of an underlying policy.

Primary Liability   In law, the liability for which one is personally responsible and for which a wronged party can seek redress out of the wrongdoer's personal assets.

Primary Payer   An insurance policy, plan, or program that pays first on a claim for medical care.

Privacy   The right of an individual, created by the Constitution or other law, to have personal information protected from disclosure.

Privacy Act of 1974 5 USC. § 552a   (P.L. 93-579) A body of federal law that has been in effect since September 27, 1975. The Privacy Act of 1974 is located under 5 USC. Section 552a. It is generally characterized as an omnibus "code of fair information practices" that attempts to regulate the collection, maintenance, use, and dissemination of personal information by federal executive branch agencies. The act's imprecise language, limited legislative history, and somewhat outdated regulatory guidelines have rendered it a difficult statute to decipher and apply. Moreover, even after more than 25 years of administrative and judicial analysis, numerous Privacy Act issues remain unresolved or unexplored. Adding to these interpretational difficulties is the fact that many Privacy Act cases are unpublished district court decisions.

Privacy Factors   Refers to those restrictions to information and data that may or may not result in added time, expense, and burden in the discovery of electronically stored information (ESI). Most restrictions are the result of HIPAA privacy and security regulations.

Privacy Rule Title I of HIPAA. This legislation was enacted to protect the privacy of individuals' protected health information. Title I of HIPAA requires that a covered entity and its staff, employees, and volunteers use and disclose protected health information for purposes of treatment, payment, and health-care operations, and for other purposes that are permitted or required by law, and provide the patient with a legal notice that outlines the organization's privacy practices. See also Notice of Privacy Practices.

Private Key One of two keys used in public key cryptography. The private key is known only to the owner and is used to sign and decrypt messages. This key is used to electronically sign outgoing messages, and is used to decrypt incoming messages.

Private Network A network that is connected to the Internet, but isolated from it by certain privacy measures, such as passwords.

Privilege In law, a protection afforded to a particular relationship from disclosure of information. See also Attorney-Client Privilege, Patient-Physician Relationship, and Psychotherapist-Patient Privilege.

Privilege Review A litigation support term that describes the combination of keyword searching and reading of documents by counsel to flag privileged documents that will be excluded from production. In cases with large volumes of electronic documents, counsel sometimes agrees to a nonwaiver simply because a document-by-document review can be too time consuming. When a nonwaiver is in place, if privileged documents are produced inadvertently, the receiving party cannot use them.

PRO **Peer Review Organization**—Established in the Tax Equity and Fiscal Responsibility Act of 1982, the PRO monitors the medical necessity and quality of services provided to Medicare and Medicaid beneficiaries to reduce inappropriate and unnecessary admissions and validate provider coding assignments under the Medicare prospective payment system.

Pro Bono Latin, for the public good. Generally, uncompensated legal services.

Procedural Due Process Rights that ensure a fair consideration of an issue, generally provided for by the US and state constitutions.

Procedure Code An HCPCS code used by physicians to describe the procedure rendered to the patient.

Proceeding A unique event in the course of litigation, such as a hearing or deposition, or the entire course of the litigation.

Process Evaluation   An examination of the procedures and tasks between initiation and completion of a given protocol or program.

Process Quality   The assessment of interactions between clinicians and patients.

Professional Component   The physician work of a diagnostic test, such as interpretation.

Professional Review Action   An action of a healthcare entity that is taken in the course of professional review activity.

Program Instruction   A federal issuance that clarifies and explains procedures and methods for the establishment of program policies. It adds details to program regulations or policy requirements, and conveys to grantees program guidance or information about actions they are expected or required to take. Program instructions may also be used to transmit state plan preprints, financial reports, program allotment tables, nonregulatory materials on which comments are solicited, and other materials.

Project Management   The coordination of tools, activities, and techniques required to ensure that a project can be completed in a timely and fiscally responsible fashion without sacrificing quality.

Prolog   **Programming Logic**—A high-level language used for programming logical processes and making deductions automatically.

PROM   **Programmable Read-Only Memory.**

Proportionality   In law, this is a concept by which discovery of information from the opposition is measured against, among other things, a cost-benefit analysis. It appears in FRCP 26(b)(2)(C).

Proportionality Test   Generally, proportionality is a term used by a judge to assess the reasonableness of an approach or course of action. For example, the discovery, testing, and sampling of data in a $20 million case versus a $100,000 case. An e-discovery costs-versus-needs analysis should be undertaken early to determine what e-discovery efforts are appropriate. See also Cost-Needs Analysis.

Proprietary   Owned, copyrighted, or for which exclusive legal rights are held.

Prospective Review   A prior authorization process to verify the medical necessity for the proposed service and location.

Protective Order   In law, an order intended to limit or bar the disclosure of certain information. A common example would be a request for health information that is not relevant to a plaintiff's injuries.

Protocol A standard for communicating data and graphics. It is the general methodology by which two systems pass control information and data back and forth.

Provider Licensed healthcare facility or professional who provides care under a contract.

Provider Taxonomy Codes An administrative code set, used in the X12 278 Referral Certification and Authorization and the X12 837 Claim transactions under HIPAA, for identifying the provider type and area of specialization for healthcare providers.

Proximate Cause In law, a term used to describe the relationship between a person's wrongful conduct and injuries sustained by another.

Prudent Patient Rule A rule under which a physician must disclose to the patient in lay terms all the material information that an individual would consider significant in making an informed decision about treatment.

PSC **Program Safeguard Contractor**—A CMS contractor who detects and deters fraud and abuse and maintains the integrity of the programs provided by the CMS.

PSDA **Patient Self-Determination Act**—An act requiring Medicare and Medicaid providers to grant patients information about their right to direct and participate in their own healthcare decisions (including writing an advance directive) and to accept or refuse medical treatment.

PSO **Provider-Sponsored Organization**—A type of managed care plan in which a group of doctors, hospitals, and other healthcare providers agree to give healthcare to people with Medicare for a set amount of money from Medicare every month. These plans are run by the doctors and providers themselves, and not by an insurance company.

PST File Format The file format used by the Microsoft Outlook personal information management (PIM) program, which includes programs for e-mail, task management, and calendar maintenance.

Psychotherapist-Patient Privilege A privilege that a person can invoke to prevent the sharing of a confidential communication made in the course of mental or emotional treatment.

Public Bill A bill that proposes a public law. A public law is one that applies to the general public.

Public Domain That which belongs to the community at large; unprotected by copyright.

Public Health   The science of preventing disease, prolonging life, and promoting health through the organized efforts and informed choices of society, public and private organizations, public and private communities, and individuals.

Public Health Service Act   Enacted in 1946 as the Public Health and Welfare Act, 42 CFR Ch.6. The Public Health Service Act replaced the US Public Health Service (PHS) as the primary division of the Department of Health, Education, and Welfare (HEW), which later became the US Department of Health and Human Services (HHS). The law has been amended many times, most recently with the addition of Section 3012, as added by the HITECH Act.

Public Interest and Benefit Activities   Activities performed in the interest of public health.

Public Key   One of two keys in public key cryptology. A key transforms cleartext data into cyphertext. This is called a public key. The key used to decrypt the data is called the private key. The two keys are related, and a mathematical operation is used to generate them. The two keys are called a key pair.

Public Network   A network both connected to and part of the public Internet.

Punitive Damages   Monies awarded to a plaintiff in excess of actual damages. Punitive damages are awarded to punish a defendant and to deter others from engaging in certain similar conduct.

PWBA   **Pension Welfare and Benefits Administration**—The administrator of the Employee Retirement Income Security Act.

Q

QALY   **Quality-Adjusted Life Year.**

QDS   **Quality Data Set.**

QI   **Qualified Individual**—An assistance program that pays a portion of Medicare Part B premiums for individuals who have a low monthly income and have Medicare Part A.

QIC   **Qualified Independent Contractor**—The entity that performs the second review in the Medicare Part A and B appeals process. The request for it must be in writing and sent directly to the Qualified Independent Contractor.

QIO   **Quality Improvement Organization**—A group of practicing doctors and other healthcare experts who have a contract with the federal government to check and improve the care given to Medicare beneficiaries. They must review the individual's complaints about the quality of care given by inpatient hospitals, hospital outpatient departments, hospital emergency rooms, skilled nursing facilities, home health agencies, private fee-for-service plans, and ambulatory surgical centers.

QRPH   Quality, Research and Public Health—An IHE domain committee responsible for the development of standards-based profiles and the technical framework for sharing information within care sites and across networks.

Qualified EHR   As defined in HITECH, a qualified EHR is one that includes patient and demographic health information such as medical histories and problem lists and has the capacity to provide decision support; support order entry; capture and query information related to healthcare quality; and exchange information with and integrate such information from other sources.

Qualifying Event   An event, such as loss of job or divorce, that triggers an individual's legal right to continue employer group health benefits when it might otherwise end. This continuation coverage is referred to as the Consolidated Omnibus Reconciliation Act (COBRA).

Quality   As defined by the Institute of Medicine, "The degree to which health services for individuals and populations increase the likelihood of desired health outcomes and are consistent with current professional knowledge." Quality is generally evaluated in three dimensions: 1. structure, 2. process, and 3. outcome.

Quality-Adjusted Life Year   A concept used in malpractice claims and insurance settlements. A QALY is a unit of measure designed to quantify outcomes as a result of an intervention. A value assigned to determine the number of years at full health versus the number of years of life experienced at a lesser level. For example, the number of years of life experienced as a quadriplegic versus with normal ambulation.

Quality Assurance   A term used to refer to the programs and activities aimed at improving the quality of patient care. The concept is based upon assessing and evaluating care, identifying problems, and designing mechanisms to overcome identified deficiencies, as well as following-up to measure and ensure effectiveness. The term is sometimes used interchangeably with quality management or quality improvement.

Quality Improvement   A theory of management engineering for obtaining continuous and incremental improvements in healthcare delivery. The term is sometimes used interchangeably with quality assurance or quality management.

Quality Indicator   Description of a process of care that should occur for a particular type of patient or clinical circumstance through evaluation of whether the patient's care or clinical circumstance is consistent with the indicator.

Quality Management   Measures put in place to maintain consistent, acceptable service in healthcare. Also may be a separate operating department within the healthcare organization. The term is sometimes used interchangeably with quality assurance or quality improvement.

Qui Tam   In law, an action brought against a private party by a whistleblower under the False Claims Act on behalf of the United States or by the United States to recover the use of public funds.

Qui Tam Statutes   Laws that permit private individuals to bring lawsuits against the government alleging individual or organizational fraudulent behavior.

R

RAC   **Recovery Audit Contractor**—See Medicare RAC Program.

RAM   **Random Access Memory**—The main working memory in a computer. When the computer is turned off, the contents of the computer's RAM are extinguished.

Rate   A number derived by dividing the numerator (for example, cases that meet a clinical criterion for quality or substandard care) by the denominator (for example, all cases to which the criterion applies) within a given time frame. Occurrence or existence of a particular condition expressed as a proportion of units in the population; for example, live births per 100,000.

Rating   The method used to determine the cost of healthcare premiums; may be community-based on the actuarial statistics for a population, group-based using experience rating for a specific group's medical cost experience, or related to an individual's history.

Ratio   The relationship between two counted sets of data, which may have a value of zero or greater. In a ratio, the numerator is not necessarily a subset of the denominator. For example, the ratio of the number of hospital-acquired infections to the number of patients discharged.

Rationale   An explanation and justification for a given position. The rationale may include supportive evidence such as published literature, quality studies, focus studies, and other bases.

RBRVS **Resource-Based Relative Value Scale**—A fee schedule and service documentation system established by Medicare in 1992 to provide for equitable and balanced compensation to providers. The RBRVS is adjusted annually and is composed of three additive components plus a conversion factor or multiplier for primary and specialty physicians.

RCB **Recognized Certification Body**—A body recognized by the Secretary of HHS to help accelerate the adoption of health information technology functionality, interoperability, and security.

RDBMS **Relational Database Management System**—A computer program that helps the user create, update, and administer a relational database. Most RDBMS systems utilize Structured Query Language (SQL) to access the database.

RDE **Pharmacy/Treatment Encoded Message**—An HL7 clinical application messaging term used to send an order to the pharmacy and/or dispensing systems. It may be sent as either an order containing a single pharmacy, a treatment order for a patient, or as an order containing multiple pharmacy or treatment orders for a patient.

Reasonable In law, a standard of conduct.

Reasonable Anticipation of Litigation In law, a time when a punitive party becomes aware that it is likely to become involved in litigation.

Reasonable Degree of Medical Certainty In law, a standard employed to determine whether an expert is qualified to offer an opinion.

Reasonable Patient Standard A standard whereby a doctor's duty to provide information is determined by the information needs of the patient rather than the physician.

Reasonable Person In law, a hypothetical person of ordinary intelligence and prudence against which the conduct of an actual person is measured to determine whether the person was negligent.

Reasonable Physician Standard A standard that requires a physician to provide the information that a reasonable doctor would provide under the same circumstances.

Rebundling A comprehensive, standardized package of computerized data edits to identify and prevent reporting (using billing and coding data) on a national level.

Rebuttable Presumption In law, a presumption that the party opposing the presumed fact is allowed to offer evidence to contradict it.

Reckless Disregard   In law, acting without regard to the possible consequences of one's actions.

Recollection   In law, the act of recalling something to memory through concerted effort.

Reconsideration   The second step in the appeals process for denied Medicare Part A, B, C, and D claims. This step is reviewed by the Qualified Independent Contractor (QIC) for Part A and B claims, and by the Independent Review Entity (IRE) for Part C and D claims.

Record   Data that have value to an organization.

Record Lifecycle   The time period from creation to disposal of a record.

Records Committee   Refers to a committee (usually a Medical Staff Committee) within the healthcare organization that reviews the quality, timeliness, and appropriateness of medical record documentation practices within the organization. The records committee may take an active role in the organization's preservation practices and policies and procedures for retention and destruction of health and business records.

Records Management   The field of management responsible for the efficient and systematic control of the creation, receipt, maintenance, use, and disposition of analog and digital records, including processes for capturing and maintaining evidence of and information about business activities and transactions in the form of records.

Records Retention Schedule   A schedule for the management of records, establishing how long they are kept before being disposed of.

Recredentialing   A retrospective review and determination of credentials and clinical privileges for a provider. Usually occurs every two years following conclusion of the initial credentialing process.

Recycling of Backup Tapes   The process of overwriting backup tapes with new backup data. Recycling of backup tapes generally occurs on a fixed, regular schedule.

Redaction   Redaction is the process of obscuring or removing from view the data in an EHR report or document to prevent the receiver from seeing the data. This may be necessary in responding to requests or litigation requests in which a portion of report must be disclosed, but some data elements may not disclosed.

Redaction   A litigation support term used to refer to a blacking out of confidential information from a document. When an automated litigation support program is used for electronic discovery, a redaction is usually done by way of an overlay (so the original document image is not actually altered). When producing documents in an electronic production, the redactions are permanently burned into the version of the image produced.

Redetermination The first step in the appeals process for denied Medicare Part A, B, or D claims. The process is afforded to Medicare beneficiaries who don't agree with Medicare's initial determination on their claim (stated on the Medicare Summary Notice). To request a redetermination, the beneficiary must submit a written, signed request to appeal within 120 days of the determination.

Referral Refers to the term used to describe a primary care provider's determination that a patient is suffering from a clinical condition that requires evaluation and/or care by an appropriately qualified specialist.

Referral Authorization Refers to the process of review of a request for a member of a health plan to receive services by a provider outside of the capitated medical group.

Reinsurance Insurance purchased by an insurance company or health plan from another insurance company to protect against losses. The term is also used to describe the limiting of risk a provider or managed care organization assumes through the purchased insurance that becomes effective after a set amount of healthcare services have been provided. This insurance is intended to protect a provider from the extraordinary healthcare costs that just a few beneficiaries with extremely extensive healthcare needs may incur. Also known as a contract by which an insurer procures a third party to insure it against loss or liability by reason of such original insurance. Also known as stop-loss insurance.

Regional Extension Center Mandated by the American Recovery and Reinvestment Act (ARRA). The centers that provide technical assistance to providers to adopt or enhance electronic health records systems.

Rejected or Returned Claim Refers to the process where a claim was returned or rejected because essential information is missing from the claim. Examples of reasons for rejection of claims include missing ICD9 Codes or a missing Unique Provider Identification Number (UPIN).

Relational Database A database that groups data using common attributes found in the data set, creating families of information. One of the advantages of a relational database is that duplication of entries is reduced or even eliminated, allowing for the efficient management of larger databases.

Release A mechanism by which a party relinquishes the right to maintain a claim or cause of action.

Relevancy Screening   A litigation support term that describes the review of documents prior to scanning to minimize processing of irrelevant documents. In electronic discovery, relevancy screening can be facilitated with good search tools that can filter out irrelevant files by date range, custodian, folder, or, in the case of e-mails, by date, author, or recipient.

Reliance Damages   Damages awarded for losses the plaintiff suffers in reliance on a contract.

Remittance   A statement sent to a medical provider from the insurer to show the payment that was issued to the provider. Also called an explanation of benefits (EOB).

Remuneration   The term used to describe a reward or payment. The act of payment for goods or services or to compensate for loss.

Reportable Diseases and Conditions   Diseases and conditions that are mandated by law to be reported by healthcare providers to a local health officer.

Report Card   A term used within the healthcare industry to refer to a set of performance measures applied uniformly.

Repository   A storage space for records and all associated data.

Repudiation   To deny the origin of an electronic document or the fact that an electronic document has been received.

Request for Proposal   A document that provides a template that can be followed to outline the requirements for a service, to evaluate potential vendors, and ultimately to make an informed decision.

Requests   Protected health information that is asked for by a covered individual.

Requirements Specification   The term used to describe the identification and documentation of the detailed functional and nonfunctional requirements for an information system.

Residual Data   Data that are not active on a computer system, found in ambient data allocation areas of a drive.

Res Ipsa Loquitur   In law, the Latin term meaning the thing speaks for itself. A rule of evidence that allows a fact finder to assume negligence when the instrument causing the injury to the plaintiff was in the control of the defendant and when the same incident does not normally occur without some form of negligence.

Res Judicata   In law, the Latin term meaning the thing that has been judged. Refers to a prior decision that is binding on parties to pending litigation.

Resource Management   The planning, directing, organizing, and controlling of a healthcare product in a fiscally responsible manner without sacrificing the quality of patient care.

Respondeat Superior   In law, the Latin term meaning let the master answer. A key doctrine in tort law by which an employer may be held liable for the negligent acts of an employee.

Respondent   The party against whom an appeal is taken and who answers legal charges.

Responsive Pleading   A written answer to charges set out in a pleading filed by another party.

REST   **Representational State Transfer**—An architectural style of large-scale networked software that allows for distributed hypermedia systems and takes advantage of the technologies and protocols of the World Wide Web. REST describes how distributed data objects, or resources, can be defined and addressed, stressing the easy exchange of information and scalability.

Restitution Damages   A legal term that refers to the restoration or compensation for loss or injury for something that was taken away, lost, or surrendered.

Restore   To move data from a backup medium to an active, online system for purposes of recovery.

Restraint of Trade   Federal antitrust statutes that regulate the degree to which a business entity or individual can be shut off from a particular area of economic enterprise.

Retention Schedule   The practice (preferably written) that outlines the organization's policies and practices for retention and destruction of records, both paper and electronic.

Retraction   The process of removing a document from view that was inappropriately or incorrectly placed in a patient's EHR. For example, removal of the wrong patient's lab result.

Retrieval   In e-discovery, this term refers to the act of locating and securing electronically stored information (ESI) for review and possible production.

RFA   **Regulatory Flexibility Act**—A comprhrehensive federal effort to balance the social goals of federal regulations with the needs and capabilities of small businesses, first passed in 1980. The law requires federal agencies to analyze the impact of their regulatory actions on small businesses and seek less burdensome alternatives when the impact is deemed significant and significant to a large number of businesses.

RFI   **Request for Information**—A commonly accepted business practice that shares most of the same characteristics as a request for proposal (RFP), and is used as a means to collect basic data in preparation for deciding which vendors will be selected to receive an invitation to submit a formal proposal.

RFP   **Request for Proposal**—An invitation to vendors and suppliers to bid on providing a specific service or commodity to an organization. The RFP shares many of the same characteristics as a Request for Information (RFI) but will usually go beyond a request for basic information and ask that additional data and more detailed information be provided, including pricing of a product or a service and timing involved with installation or implementation.

RHC   **Rural Health Clinic**—A public or private nonprofit entity that the Centers for Medicare and Medicaid Services has certified as a rural health clinic under section 1861(a)(2) of the Social Security Act. A rural health clinic provides outpatient services to a nonurban area with an insufficient number of healthcare practitioners.

RHHI   **Regional Home Health Intermediary**—A Medicare fiscal intermediary to which home health agencies are assigned for medical review issues.

RHIO   **Regional Health Information Organization**—Regional organizations responsible for motivating and causing integration and information exchange in the nation's revamped healthcare system through establishment of mechanisms for the secure exchange of health information for the promotion and improvement of health quality, safety, and efficiency.

RHQDAPU   **Reporting Hospital Quality Data for Annual Payment Update**—A Medicare initiative that was initially developed as a result of the Medicare Prescription Drug, Improvement, and Modernization Act (MMA) of 2003. The intent of this initiative is to equip consumers with quality of care information to make more informed decisions about their healthcare, while encouraging hospitals and clinicians to improve the quality of inpatient care provided to all patients. The hospital quality of care information gathered through the initiative is available to consumers on the Hospital Compare website. RHQDAPU requires hospitals classified as Subsection (d) to submit data for specific quality measures for health conditions common among people with Medicare, and which typically result in hospitalization.

Rider   A legal addendum or provision that modifies, by either expanding or decreasing, the covered services of a health plan.

Right of Privacy   The right, implied in the zones of privacy defined by the Supreme Court, to personal autonomy.

Rijndael The algorithm selected by the US National Standards of Technology (NIST) as the basis for the Advanced Encryption Standard (AES). Rijndael is a new generation symmetric block cipher that supports key sizes of 128, 192, and 256 bits, with data handled in 128-bit blocks that will supplant the Data Encryption Standard (DES) and the later Triple DES over the next few years in many cryptography applications. Rijndael is also known as Federal Information Processing Standard (FIPS) Number 197.

Risk The likelihood or probability of loss.

Risk Adjustment The statistical adjustment of outcomes measured to account for risk factors that are separate from the quality of care provided, such as gender or age.

Risk Analysis A formal technique used to identify and assess factors that may jeopardize the success of an objective or an outcome.

Risk Assessment An assessment done immediately following a trigger or adverse advent to determine the nature, scope, and probability of liability to the organization.

Risk Bands Utilization data analyzed to fix changes in capitation payments for very high or low utilization.

Risk Management Generally refers to a four-step process to identify, evaluate, and resolve the actual and possible sources of loss. The four steps of risk management are: 1. risk identification, 2. risk evaluation, 3. risk handling, and 4. risk monitoring. Also may be a separate department within the healthcare organization.

Risk Manager A professional, who may or may not be an attorney, responsible for the protection of the assets of the organization. The risk manager may be a potential 30(b)(6) witness for the organization and ideally should be a part of the organization's litigation response team.

Risk Retention Financial liability kept by one of the parties to a risk contract.

Risk Sharing Any arrangement where separate parties share risk for the costs of services to a specific group or population.

Risk Stratification The process of classifying people and populations by their likelihood to experience adverse outcomes.

RM-ES Profile **Records Management and Evidentiary Support Profile—** An HL7 standard based on the EHR-S Functional Model Standard in which a framework of electronic record functions and conformance criteria were identified to support EHR records management and the use of those records for evidentiary purposes.

Robust Computer Systems   Computer systems that are trustworthy under changing circumstances.

ROI   Return on Investment—An estimate of the amount of money that will be generated as a result of an investment; often used to evaluate management of a service or product line or in the purchase of a piece of equipment (such as an EHR system).

ROM   Read Only Memory—A type of computer and electronic device memory that normally can only be read, as opposed to random access memory (RAM), which can be both read and written.

Root Certificate   The most common commercial type of root certificates is based on the ISO X.509 standard. It is a self-signed certificate or an unsigned public key certificate, which forms an important part of the public key infrastructure. It usually carries the digital signature of a certification authority.

ROT-13   A simple substitution cipher used to obfuscate Usenet posts; it is not meant for use as a data encryption cipher.

Router   Hardware that directs data from the local network between all other devices connected to that network.

RPE   Office of Resources, Planning, and Evaluation—An office of the Assistant Secretary for Preparedness and Response (ASPR) responsible for providing expertise and analysis in the formulation and implementation of policies, procedures, and operational strategies, which ensure efficient and effective allocation and utilization of program resources in support of ASPR's mission.

RPPO   Regional Preferred Provider Organization—A type of Medicare Advantage managed healthcare plan. An RPPO must maintain and monitor a network of appropriate providers that is supported by written agreements and is sufficient to provide adequate access to covered services to meet the needs of all enrollees in its entire service area.

RRE   Responsible Reporting Entity—As of July 1, 2009, an entity defined under MMSEA (Pub. L. 110-275) that requires that all responsible insurers (liability insurer, self-insurer, no-fault insurer, and workers' compensation carriers) determine whether a claimant is a Medicare beneficiary and, if so, provide certain information to the Secretary of HHS when the claim is resolved.

RTP   Return to Provider—The many processes utilized today for notifying medical providers or suppliers of service that their claims cannot be processed and that they must be corrected or resubmitted.

Rubber Hose Cryptanalysis   A term to describe the process of extracting encryption from a user through the motivating use of a rubber hose.

Rule 502   An FRE rule intended to reduce the risk of forfeiture of attorney-client privilege or work product protection "so that parties need not scrutinize production of documents to the same extent as they do now." The intent of FRE 502 is to opt for middle ground in determining whether inadvertent disclosure of attorney-client privileged or work product material is a waiver, in accord with the majority view. Under FRE 502, the inadvertent disclosure of privileged or protected information during discovery would constitute a waiver only when the party did not take reasonable precautions to prevent disclosure and/or did not make reasonable and prompt efforts to return or destroy privileged information.

S

SAA   Society of American Archivists—A professional organization dedicated to ensuring the identification, preservation, and use of records of historical value. http://www2.archivists.org

SaaS   Software-as-a-Service—A software application delivery model in which an enterprise vendor develops a web-based software application, and then hosts and operates that application over the Internet for use by its customers.

SACWIS   Statewide Automated Child Welfare Information System—A single statewide system that automates the collection of federally mandated child welfare data and provides support for the delivery and management of child welfare services.

Safe Harbor   In law, a concept embodied in FRCP 37(e) that precludes the imposition of sanctions for the loss of electronically stored information (ESI) by reason of the routine, good-faith operation of a computer system.

Safe Workplace   A place of employment that is clear of all dangers that should reasonably be removed, given the nature of the work performed.

SAMHSA   Substance Abuse and Mental Health Services Administration— One of 11 federal agencies that make up the Department of Health and Human Services. The vision and mission of SAMHSA is to build resilience and facilitate recovery for people of all ages with or at risk for mental or substance use disorders.

Sampling   Statistically testing information to check for likelihood of relevant information.

Sanction   In law, a penalty imposed on a litigant and/or its attorney by a court for failure to comply with a legal obligation and/or order.

Sandbox Network   A network not connected to other networks.

SAP   Systems, Applications and Products in Data Processing—Changed in the 1980s from its original name in German, Systeme, Anwendungen und Produkte in der Datenverarbeitung, SAP is a protocol for NetWare.

SAS   Statistical Analysis System—An integrated suite of software for organization-wide information delivery, built around the four data-driven tasks common to virtually any application (access, management, analysis, and presentation).

SCA   Stored Communications Act (18 USC. §§ 2701 to 2712)—An act that addresses voluntary and compelled disclosure of "stored wire and electronic communications and transactional records" held by a third-party.

Scanning   Converting a hard copy document into a digital image.

Scan Resolution   A scan setting that refers to the number of dots per inch (dpi) that are stored, where the greater the dpi, the greater the amount of detail on the scan.

SCHIP   State Children's Health Insurance Program—The SCHIP program is administered by the Centers for Medicare and Medicaid Services (CMS) at the state level and is jointly financed by the federal and state governments.

Scienter   In law, refers to knowledge of intent of wrongdoing.

SCO   Standards Charter Organization—The SCO is a formal collaboration among US healthcare standards development organizations (SDO) to support industry-wide standardization and interoperability. http://www.scosummit.com

Scope of Practice   A term used by state licensing boards for various professions that defines the procedures, actions, and processes permitted for the licensed individual. The scope of practice is limited to that which the law allows for specific education, experience, and demonstrated competency.

Scrolling   Causing the text on a computer screen to move, allowing portions to appear while other portions disappear.

SDLC   System Development Life Cycle—An approach to develop an information system or software product that is characterized by a linear sequence of steps that progress from start to finish. The SDLC model is one of the oldest systems development models and is still probably the most commonly used. The six general steps are: 1. evaluate existing system; 2. define new system requirements; 3. design system; 4. develop new system; 5. implement the system; and 6. maintain the system.

SDO Standards Development Organization—Any organization involved in the development of standards. ANSI and ISO are examples of SDOs.

Searchable PDF A PDF file that has either been created from an existing electronic document containing text, or a scanned or image-based file that has had the document image or bitmap converted to readable text by OCR.

Search Engine A tool used to search the Internet.

Secondary Payer An insurance policy, plan, or program that pays after the primary payer on a claim for medical care.

Second Life Account A 3D-virtual and social networking world where users connect, socialize, and create using voice and text chat.

Section 504 of the Rehabilitation Act of 1973 A national law that applies to organizations and employers that receive financial assistance from any federal department or agency, including the Department of Health and Human Services (DHSS), many hospitals, nursing homes, mental health centers, and human service programs. Section 504 protects qualified individuals with disabilities from discrimination based upon their disability and forbids excluding or denying individuals with disabilities an equal opportunity to receive program benefits and services.

Secure Payment Gateway A company that helps processors of payment information to conduct secure business on the Internet using Secure Socket Layer (SSL) technology.

Security Audit A manual or automated systematic and technical assessment of a system or application.

Security Rule Refers to the HIPAA regulations governing the security of protected health information. The HIPAA security rule is found under 45 CFR Sections 164.302 et seq.

The Sedona Conference A 501(c)(3) research and educational institute composed of academics, industry experts, lawyers, and judges dedicated to the advancement of law and policy in the areas of antitrust law, intellectual property rights, and complex litigation. Publisher of *The Sedona Principles, Second Edition, Best Practices for Addressing Electronic Document Production.* http://www.thesedonaconference.org

Self-Insured An entity that assumes the financial risk of paying for healthcare.

SEM Security Event Management—A log management tool used to pick up information from across the organization using rule-based algorithmic correlation to detect probable threats and policy violations (unauthorized access)

that demand attention and might require immediate remediation. See also Security Information Management (SIM).

Sentencing Guidelines   In law, a series of standards established by federal law to guide judges in the imposition of criminal sentences.

Sentinel Effect   The change or alteration of a clinical or administrative practice as a result of knowing that a focused review or monitoring of the practice is occurring.

Sentinel Event   An adverse health event that triggers the case for review and investigation by quality improvement and/or risk management.

Serious Bodily Injury   Significant physical impairment to the human body that creates a significant risk of death or permanent disfigurement of a body's function or organ.

Serious Illness   A disease, sometimes curable, with the potential to impair a person's functioning, leading to terminal illness or causing death.

Server   A computer on a network that contains data or programs shared by the other computers on the network.

Service Area   The geographic area in which a health plan accepts members. For plans that require an individual to use their doctors and hospitals, it is also the area in which services are provided.

Service of Process   Delivery regarding the procedural rules of the jurisdiction of a document authorized by the law of said jurisdiction that commands an entity to act or refrain from acting in a particular manner.

SET   **Secure Electronic Transaction**—A system for ensuring secure financial transactions over the Internet.

Settlement   The conveyance of a property to provide for beneficiaries in a way that differs from what they would receive as heirs, usually ending a lawsuit.

Sexual Harassment   Unwelcome sexual advances on the job that create a hostile working environment.

SGML   **Standard Generalized Markup Language**—Developed by the International Standards Organization (ISO), SGML is both a language and a standard to describe information embedded within a document. Hypertext Markup Language is based on SGML.

SHA-1   **Secure Hash Algorithm**—SHA-1 is the most commonly used of five hash functions designed by the National Security Agency (NSA) and published by the National Institute of Standards and Technology (NIST). The five algorithms are SHA-1, SHA-224, SHA-256, SHA-384, and SHA-512.

Shared Risk   An agreement to share risk for the cost of delivering specific services.

Sherman Act   An antitrust act passed in 1890 aimed at preserving free and unfettered competition by prohibiting monopolies and conspiracies that restrain trade.

Sibling Document   A document sharing a common parent with another document.

SIM   Security Information Management—A log management tool used to collect, store, and protect ever-larger volumes of raw security information of hosts systems and applications for long periods of time, as increasingly required for information systems management compliance activities. A SIM is the keeper of the security date for forensic purposes. See also Security Event Management (SEM).

Slack Space   The term used to describe unused space between the end of a file and the last sector of cluster of data used by that file.

Slander   A defamatory statement expressed in speech or other transitory form, which the plaintiff must prove caused damage.

SLI Global Solutions   A testing and certification laboratory located in Denver, CO, SLI Global's focus has been helping customers build quality and innovation into their products and system implementations, while minimizing technology risk. On December 10, 2010, SLI Global Solutions was officially designated as an Authorized Testing and Certification Body (ONC-ATCB) by the Office of the National Coordinator. Scope of ONC-ATCB authorization: Complete EHR and EHR Modules. http://www.sliglobalsolutions.com

Smart Card   A plastic card containing a computer chip that can be used to identify its processor and can compare data to external information.

SMHP   State Medicaid Health Information Technology Plan—A plan developed by the state and reviewed and approved by CMS that provides for 100 percent recoupment of the administrative costs associated with state expenditures for healthcare provider incentive payments. Implemented to encourage the purchase, implementation, and operation of electronic health record (EHR) technology.

S/MIME   Secure Multipurpose Internet Mail Extensions Protocol—The basic standard for secure e-mail and electronic data interchange (EDI).

SMS   Short Message Service—A standardized communications protocol for the interchange of short text messages between electronic mobile devices. See also Texting.

SMTP   Simple Mail Transfer Protocol—The standard Internet protocol used today for sending e-mail to mail servers. After an e-mail is sent using SMTP, e-mail messages can be retrieved from the server using an email client. Radio Frequency Identification (RFID) anywhere allows XML reports generated by its application-level events (ALE) and Report Engine MP, or custom business module output, to be sent using the SMTP messaging connector.

SNF   Skilled Nursing Facility—A public or private nonprofit institution (or a distinct part of an institution), certified under section 1819(a) of the Social Security Act, that is primarily engaged in providing skilled nursing care and related services to residents requiring medical, rehabilitation, or nursing care and is not primarily for the care and treatment of mental diseases. A less expensive alternative to such care in a hospital.

SNIP   Standard National Implementation Process—An initiative of the Workgroup for Electronic Data Interchange (WEDI), the WEDI SNIP: 1. facilitates a collaborative, industry-wide approach and readiness for health information technology (HIT), clinical initiatives, and standards including those for security, privacy, electronic data interchange (EDI) transactions, code sets, and identifiers; and 2. fosters implementation of HIT, HIPAA, clinical initiatives, and standards in a manner that preserves the confidentiality, integrity, and availability of health information, while enabling efficient business processing.

SNMP   Simple Network Management Protocol—A networking management protocol used to monitor network-attached devices. SNMP allows messages (called protocol data units) to be sent to various parts of a network. Upon receiving these messages, SNMP-compatible devices (called agents) return data stored in their management information bases. These data contain the device's configuration, status, and statistical information.

SNOBOL   String Oriented Symbolic Language—A high-level computer language designed for pattern matching and list processing.

SNODO   Standard Nomenclature of Disease and Operations—An early publication of the American Medical Association (AMA). SNODO is a coding classification system that utilizes a code for the topography (site), a hyphen, and a code for the etiology (cause) of the condition.

SNOMED CT   Systematized Nomenclature of Medicine Clinical Terms—A comprehensive clinical terminology, in both English and Spanish, developed in 2007 and distributed, cost-free, by the International Health Terminology

Standards Development Organisation. SNOMED can codify all the activities within the patient medical record, including medical diagnoses and procedures, nursing diagnoses and procedures, patient signs and symptoms, occupational history, and the many causes and etiologies of diseases including such things as infectious conditions, genetic and congenital conditions, and the physical causes of injury.

SNOP **Systematized Nomenclature of Pathology**—A coding and classification terminology developed in the 1950s by the College of American Pathology (CAP) and the precursor to the SNOMED CT coding system.

SNP **Special Needs Plan**—A type of Medicare Advantage plan designed for certain populations. The goal of an SNP is to provide healthcare and services to those who can benefit the most from the expertise of the plans' providers and focused-care management.

SOAP **Simple Object Access Protocol**—An XML-based message protocol that allows messages to be sent and received over a network. HTTP is usually used as the application layer protocol for transferring the messages.

SOAP **Subjective Objective Assessment Plan**—A medical-record documentation methodology used by some clinicians and healthcare organizations for the documentation of patient admission and progress notes.

SOC **Standard of Care**—A term used to refer to the duty, care, caution, and/or prudence that should be expected of a reasonable person given the situation and circumstances. Failure to meet the standard of care is negligence, and any resulting damages may be claimed in a lawsuit by an injured party. Standards of care are often a subjective issue upon which reasonable people can differ.

Social Security Program (42 USC. 301 et seq.) A federal program enacted in 1935 to provide old age, survivors, and disability insurance benefits to workers and their families.

Software The programming and instructions that make the intelligence of a computer.

Software Development Life Cycle The planning, selection, implementation, and maintenance processes of software development.

Source Code The original version of a program, as understood by human intelligence, that must be translated for a computer.

SOX **Sarbanes-Oxley Act**—Legislation that sets enhanced standards for public company boards, management, and accounting.

Special Damages In law, damages that must be described in a pleading.

Special Election Period   A set time period, triggered by certain events, when a beneficiary can change health plans or return to Original Medicare. These events include a move by an individual outside the service area, a violation by the Medicare managed care plan with the subscriber, a nonrenewal of the health plan's contract with the federal government, or other exceptional conditions. The special election period is different from the special enrollment period.

Special Enrollment Period   A set time when an individual can sign up for Medicare Part B if he or she did not take Part B during the initial enrollment period because the individual or his or her spouse was currently working and had group health plan coverage through an employer or union. An individual can sign up for Medicare Part B at any time while he or she is covered under the group plan. If the employment or group health coverage ends, the individual has eight months to sign up. The eight-month special enrollment period starts the month after the employment ends or the group health coverage ends, whichever comes first. The special enrollment period is different from the special election period.

Specialists   Providers who have training, credentials, and privileges to provide expertise in the diagnosis and treatment of specific diseases, parts of the body, age groups, or procedures.

Special Master   In law, a person appointed by the court to assist in the resolution of one or more disputes or issues raised in a proceeding. See FRCP 53.

Special Purpose Equipment   Equipment that is used exclusively for medical, scientific, research, or other technical activities.

Specials   In law, jargon that describes elements of damages that are expressed in monetary terms, such as lost wages, medical expenses, and earning capacity.

Spoliation   In law, a term for the loss or destruction of relevant information. Spoliation can have both civil and criminal consequences.

Spoofing   Refers to the forgery of an e-mail header so that it appears as if the message originated from someone or somewhere other than the actual source of the message.

SPSS   Statistical Package for the Social Sciences—Software for data management and analysis that can perform a variety of functions.

SQL   Structured Query Language—A method for retrieving records or parts of records in databases and performing calculations before the results are displayed.

SSA   Social Security Administration—The administrative branch of the Department of Health and Human Services that operates the various programs funded under the Social Security Act. The SSA also determines beneficiary eligibility for Medicare.

SSDI   Social Security Disability Insurance—A federally sponsored income support program administered for disabled US citizens that provides monthly payments based on the individual's previous work or contributions.

SSI   Supplemental Security Income—A federally sponsored income support program for low-income, disabled US citizens that provides monthly payments based on the individual's current status without regard to previous work or contributions.

SSL   Secure Socket Layer—A well-established industry standard that encrypts the channel between a web browser and web server to ensure the privacy and reliability of data transmitted over this channel.

SSO   Secure Sign-On—A term used to denote that the user sign-on to the system is secure.

SSO   Single Sign-On—An SSO enables a user to gain access to multiple resources through one time authentication.

SSPS   Statistical Package for the Social Sciences—SSPS software utilizes predictive analytics to anticipate change and manage both daily operations and special initiatives more effectively.

Stakeholder   Any individual, group of people, or organization involved in or affected by policy development, implementation, management, or outcome. Examples of healthcare stakeholders include the patients, providers, payers, consumers, public health, and employers.

Standard Benefit Package   A term used to describe a set of standard benefits provided by several insurers for purposes of comparison of price by the consumer.

Standardized Measure   A performance measure with precisely defined specifications and standardized data collection protocols that meets established criteria for evaluation that can be uniformly adopted for use.

Standard of Care   A legal term that describes the degree of prudence and caution required of an individual who is under an obligation to another individual.

Standard of Proof   The level of proof demanded in a case. Associated with the burden of persuasion.

Standards   A set of accepted measures that establishes a basis for quantitative and qualitative comparison.

Standards of Ethical Coding   An American Health Information Management Association code of conduct created to provide a basis for ethical decision making in coding practice.

Standing   Refers to the right(s) a party has to file a petition or lawsuit given the circumstances.

Stare Decisis   In law, the Latin phrase meaning stand by things decided, which is a doctrine of precedent under which it is necessary for the court to follow earlier decisions when the same points arise again.

Stark Law   A federal law that prohibits physicians from referring Medicare patients to an entity for the provision of designated health services if the physician and/or an immediate member of his or her family has a direct or indirect financial relationship with the entity. Also known as the Self-Referral Act.

State Court   In law, a court whose authority is derived from the law of a particular state rather than federal law. State courts may be of general or specialized jurisdiction, presiding over, for example, family or traffic matters.

State Law   A statutory action having the force and effect of law, such as a constitution, statute, regulation, rule, or common law. A law passed by the state legislature and signed into law by the state governor. State law exists in parallel and sometimes conflicts with US federal law. Disputes arising out of conflicts between state and federal law are resolved in district courts.

State or Local Public Health Department   The state, county, parish, or district entity in a state that is responsible for providing population-focused health services, which include health promotion, disease prevention, and intervention services provided in clinics that are operated by the health department. This includes public health clinics within the public health department.

Static Data   A term used to describe data that are relatively long-lived and have a longer period of validity compared to ephemeral data, which are shorter-lived.

Statute of Frauds   In law, a requirement that certain contracts must be made in writing and cannot be enforced if they are simply oral agreements.

Statute of Limitations   In law, the measure of time in which a civil or criminal action may be commenced. Statutes of limitations vary by nature of the claim.

Statutory Counter-Reformation   The statutory rejection of the application of a general or national standard of care, in some states, as part of a program to reduce medical malpractice insurance costs.

Statutory Law   A law created by state and federal legislative bodies.

Steganography   The art and science of hiding messages inside of another file, such as an MP3 or a picture file. It is often combined with cryptography. In e-discovery, special computer forensic tools are utilized to discover such files.

Stewardship   The responsible and financially considerate management of resources.

Stipulation   An agreement by the attorneys on opposing sides of a case to any matter regarding the proceedings.

Stop-Loss Insurance   Insurance that provides excess coverage for a self-insured organization from catastrophic losses or unusually large health costs of covered employees. The organization and the insurance carrier agree to the amount the organization will cover, and the stop-loss insurance will cover claims exceeding that amount.

Stored Communications Act   Passed in 1986 as part of the Electronic Privacy Communications Act (EPCA), the act prohibits unauthorized access to records or other information pertaining to a subscriber to or to a customer of the provider by government officials and entities seeking to obtain such information. See also Electronic Privacy Communications Act of 1986.

Stream Cipher   One of two interdependent categories of cipher used in classical cryptography. The other cipher category is known as a block cipher. Block and stream ciphers differ in how large a piece of the message is processed in an encryption.

Strict Liability   In law, liability that does not depend on actual negligence or intent to harm, but that is based on the breach of an absolute duty to make something safe. Strict liability is most often applied in products-liability cases or in cases involving ultrahazardous activities.

Strict Products Liability   The liability of all parties involved in the manufacture of a product for all damages caused by this product.

Strong Authentication   A two-factor authentication (T-FA) or multifactor sign-on authentication to create a higher level of security for granting privileges to an application. Strong authentication combines two or more independent factors of identification, such as a password (something you know), a token (something you have), voice verification (something you are), or a fingerprint. Also sometimes called strong security.

Structural Quality   The evaluation of the capacities of a health system.

Structured Data   Data that reside within fixed fields in a record or file. Relational databases and spreadsheets are examples of structured data. The opposite of unstructured data.

Structured Settlement   A method of paying an agreed amount that allows predetermined periodic payments.

STS   Society of Thoracic Surgeons—A professional membership organization founded in 1964, with a mission to enhance the ability of cardiothoracic surgeons to provide the highest quality patient care through education, research, and advocacy. The STS represents more than 6,000 surgeons, researchers, and allied healthcare professionals worldwide who are dedicated to ensuring the best possible outcomes for surgeries of the heart, lung, and esophagus, as well as other surgical procedures within the chest. http://www.sts.org

STTT   Software Tools for Technology Transfer.

Subacute Care   The term used to refer to a distinct phase of patient care between inpatient hospital care and a nursing home (custodial care). Subacute care is a level of care provided by skilled nursing facilities (SNFs), transitional care units (TCUs), or rehabilitation hospitals.

SUBC   State Uniform Billing Committee—A state-specific affiliate of NUBC.

Subpoena   In law, a document issued by a court that commands the presence of a person and/or the production of documents, including electronically stored information (ESI). See FRCP 45.

Subpoena *Duces Tecum*   This form of subpoena commands the production of documents. See also Subpoena.

Subrogation   The assumption of an obligation for which another is primarily liable. Through subrogation, parties seek reimbursement from other entities or persons primarily responsible for defined areas of medical expense such as workers' compensation, third-party liability, or no-fault auto insurance coverage.

Subsidiary   An organization that is owned or controlled by another.

Substantive Due Process   Those rights that spring from the Constitution, specifically found in the Fifth and Fourteenth Amendments, that guarantee that no person may be deprived of life, liberty, or property without the due process of law.

Substitution Cipher   One of two interdependent categories of cipher used in classical cryptography. The other cipher category is known as a transition cipher. Substitution and transposition differ in how chunks of the message are handled by the encryption process.

Summary Judgment   In law, a ruling that establishes the rights and liabilities of parties when there is no genuine issue of material fact.

Summons   A form of process that directs the individual upon whom it is served to act within a set time limit.

Supererogatory Actions   Actions that go beyond the requirements of common morality.

Suppliers   Individuals or agencies (aside from doctors or hospitals) that provide medical equipment or services. Some examples are ambulance companies, medical equipment rental businesses, and laboratories.

Supra   Latin for above. A signal to refer to a previously mentioned or cited individual.

Surescripts LLC   An e-prescription network located in Arlington, VA, that certifies software used by prescribers, pharmacies, payers, and pharmacy benefit managers. On December 23, 2010, Surescripts LLC was officially designated as an Authorized Testing and Certification Body (ONC-ATCB) by the Office of the National Coordinator. Scope of ONC-ATCB authorization: EHR Modules: E-Prescribing, Privacy and Security. http://www.surescripts.com

Surveillance   The monitoring of the behavior of a person or group of people or an outcome. Surveillance is also an activity that routinely occurs within a healthcare organization; for example, infection control.

SyBase   An enterprise software and services company.

Synchronization   The ability of a system to merge two or more copies of a database together, preserving rather than overwriting the latest changes made in any copy.

Syntax   The rules and conventions that one needs to know or follow in order to validly record information, or interpret previously recorded information, for a specific purpose. The rules and conventions may be either explicit or implicit.

Sysadmin   System Administrator—The person responsible for keeping the systems and the network operational. Sometimes used interchangeably with sysop.

System Administrator   The person in charge of network operations. Sometimes used interchangeably with sysop.

System Alert and Reminder Features   The functions of an electronic health record system that alert providers to important facts and help them remember to take action.

System Alert and Reminders   Automated messages provided to the user pertaining to important updates, changes in software, or deviations from a standard of care or practice.

System Security   A process in which a system functions in a defined operational environment, serves a defined set of users, contains prescribed data, defines network connections, and incorporates safeguards to protect the system against threats.

Systems Software   Programs that control the internal operations of a computer.

T

Tagging   Designating a keyword or term associated with or assigned to a piece of information stored electronically.

Taking   In tort law, the act of securing an article with an implicit transfer of possession, regardless of physical removal.

TANF   **Temporary Assistance to Needy Families**—The federal financial assistance program that provides assistance and work opportunities to needy families by granting states the federal funds and wide flexibility to develop and implement their own welfare programs.

Targeted Review   A term used to refer to a focused review of specific diagnoses, services, hospitals, or practitioners rather than all services. Targeted reviews are performance evaluations used in utilization review and quality management activities as well as by health plans.

Taxonomy   The practice and science of classification.

TCP/IP   **Transmission Control Protocol/Internet Protocol**—A standard protocol developed by the Internet Engineering Task Force (IETF) that defines the basic working language and features of the Internet.

TDC   **Total Direct Costs**—The total of all direct costs in the performance of a project, such as the total costs to procure an EHR system.

TDD   **Telephone Device for the Deaf.**

Team Surgery   A term used to refer to the performance of a single surgical procedure that requires the skills of two or more surgeons of different specialties.

Technical Bulletin   Documents issued by the Department of Health and Human Services (HHS) to supplement official guidance, providing clarification or additional information to previously released documentation.

Telecommunications   The process of transmitting electronic information over a long distance.

Telehealth   The administration of health-related services and information over distances via telecommunications technologies. Also known as telemedicine.

Telemedicine   A longstanding term used to describe the use of electronic information and other communication technologies to connect primary care physicians, providers, and specialists to the patient. Telemedicine provides for the remote evaluation, monitoring, and management of patients.

Teleprocessing   Processing data via telecommunications technologies.

Telework   A term used to describe work at a location other than an individual's official place of work through the use of portable computers, high-speed telecommunications links, mobile devices, and networking technologies.

Temporary Restraining Order   A court order of a very limited duration to do or refrain from doing some action in order to maintain the status quo while information is being gathered.

TEPR   **Towards the Electronic Patient Record**—A 25-year research and consultancy conference established with a vision of every doctor having the capability to store and transfer patient records electronically. In 2009, the TEPR conference was renamed the M-Health Conference.

Terabyte   A trillion bytes.

Terminable at Will   A contract that can be terminated at any time without cause.

Terminal Illness   A disease that limits life expectancy.

Termination Provision   A provider contract clause that describes how and under what circumstances the parties may end the contract.

Termination with Cause   A contract provision that allows the provider to terminate the contract when the patient does not live up to its his or her obligations.

Termination without Cause   A contract provision that allows the provider to terminate the contract without proving any breach or providing any reasons.

Tertiary Care   Refers to highly specialized medical care offered by specialists at major academic medical centers or large referral hospitals.

Testing and Sampling   The term used to refer to the process of selecting a subset of data for review. Testing and sampling will occur when the size of the collection of data is too large to permit individual examination of each piece of information. Testing and sampling measures determine the confidence intervals and confidence levels of a subset of data and determine its statistical significance. Statistical sampling techniques are widely employed in healthcare, business, and government. Data testing and sampling activities are used in quality improvement studies, public health research, ICD9CM and CPT4 data integrity audits, financial audits, and organizational compliance monitoring activities as well as a host of other uses in business analysis and within the government. As stated in the *Federal Judicial Center Reference Manual on Scientific Evidence: Reference Guide on Statistics,* "Sampling has long been considered an acceptable method for determining the characteristics of a large universe."

Text Dependent   A term used to denote a biometric system requirement that the individual say a specific set of numbers or words.

Text Independent   A term used to denote a biometric system requirement that does not require the individual to say a specific set of numbers or words. Voiceprints are created from unconstrained speech.

Texting   A term used to describe the common practice of sending short or abbreviated (160 characters or less, including spaces) text messages from mobile devices using the Short Message Service technology. Texting is the most widely used data application on the planet.

Text Retrieval Conference, Legal Track   A leading research effort established in 2006 that is composed of lawyers and scientists who are working to improve the process of information retrieval in e-discovery. See TREC. http://trec.nist.gov

T-FA   Two-Factor Authentication—A mechanism for strong authentication.

Third-Party Administrator   A term used to refer to the claims payer responsible for administering health benefit plans as a fiscal intermediary without assuming financial risk.

Third-Party Liability   In law, when a third party assumes responsibility or is held responsible for the actions of another.

Third-Party Payer   Any organization (for example, Medicare, Medicaid, PPOs, HMOs, and other commercial insurance) that insures or pays the health or medical expenses on behalf of beneficiaries or recipients. The third-party payer is an organization that pays bills on the patient's behalf after the individual or employer has paid a premium for such healthcare coverage. Such payments are called third-party payments, and are distinguished by the separation between the individual receiving the service (the first party), the individual or institution providing the service (the second party), and the organization paying for it (the third party).

Third-Party Service   A term used to describe electronic applications and services provided by someone other than the organization or agent. Examples of third-party services include Yahoo, Google, and America Online.

Threat   A risk to an organization or to system security, in the form of a hacker or virus. A threat placed to the organization would require intervention and investigation from the risk management department. An electronic threat to the information system or system security will require intervention and investigation from the information technology department.

Thumb Drive   A portable memory storage unit.

TIFF   **Tagged Image File Format**—A TIFF file is an electronic copy of a paper document in the form of an image, and as such contains no embedded text, fonts, images, or graphics. TIFFs are compatible with a wide range of hardware and software platforms, and future development is not tied to any single company. TIFF files do not retain the metadata from the source electronic document.

Time Limit   The period of time during which a notice of claim or proof of loss must be filed.

Time-Stamping   A digitally signed notation indicating the date and time the notation was appended or attached, and the identity of the person appending or attaching the notation. Metadata may contain time-stamp data.

TIN   **Tax Identification Number**—A unique identifying number used for tax purposes in the United States.

Title VII of the Civil Rights Act of 1964   A federal law that prohibits employment discrimination or harassment, and employer retaliation in legal complaint, on the basis of race, sex, religion, national origin, and pregnancy.

Title XIX   The title of the Social Security Act that established a federal-state health insurance program for low-income families, the blind, and disabled individuals, known as Medicaid. Also known as Grants to States Medical Assistance Program.

Title XVIII   The title of the Social Security Act that contains the primary legislative authority for the Medicare program. Also known as Title II—SSDI.

Tolling of Statute   In law, refers to circumstances by which a statute of limitations can be extended. For example, a minor's right to bring an action for injuries when he or she turns 18.

Tort   A French term that means wrong. Also known as wrongful act or a civil wrong. Tort law is one of the four major areas of law. Contract, real property, and criminal are the other areas of law. Tort theory forms the basis for all negligence cases and results in more civil litigation than any of the other three categories of law. Some intentional torts, such as assault, battery, wrongful death, fraud, theft, defamation, libel, slander, and property trespass are criminal.

Tortfeasor   A person or entity that has committed a civil wrong resulting in loss or injury.

Tortious   That which constitutes a tort.

Tortious Interference   In law, an intentional and damaging intrusion on another's potential business, contract, or employment.

Tort Reform   In law, a term referring to attempts to change existing law that establishes the liability of parties.

Tort Tax   A term arising out of the findings of a Tillinghast-Towers Perrin study, *US Tort Costs: 2003 Update,* which examines the costs of the US tort system.

TPA   **Third-Party Administrator**—A legal entity that makes, or is responsible for making, payments on behalf of a group health plan.

TPO   **Treatment, Payment, and Operations.**

TQM   **Total Quality Management**—An organizational management practice focused on consistently meeting or exceeding customer requirements by establishing controls and process measurements as a means of continuous improvement.

TR3   **Technical Report Type 3**—An HL7 document that explains the proper use of a standard for a specific business purpose. The *ASC X12N HIPAA Implementation Guide* is an example of a TR3. The TR3 serves as the primary reference document used by those implementing the associated transactions, and is incorporated into the HIPAA regulations by reference. A TR3 is also called an implementation guide.

Traceability   A term used to describe the ability of an electronic information system to interrelate uniquely identifiable entities in a chronological and verifiable way.

Transdisciplinary   A term used to describe a strategy that crosses many disciplinary boundaries to create a holistic approach. It applies to research efforts focused on problems that cross the boundaries of two or more disciplines or professions, such as physicians, nurses, HIM professionals, IT professionals, and clinicians.

Transfer   As defined in the UCITA 102(a)(60), "(A) with respect to a contractual interest, includes an assignment of the contract, but does not include an agreement merely to perform a contractual obligation or to exercise contractual rights through a delegate or sub licensee; and (B) with respect to computer information, includes a sale, license, or lease of a copy of the computer information and a license or assignment of informational rights in computer information."

Transferable Record   Defined in the UETA 16(a) as, an "electronic record that 1. would be a note under Article 3 of the Uniform Commercial Code or a document under Article 7 of the Uniform Commercial Code if the electronic record were in writing; and 2. the issuer of the electronic record has expressly agreed is a transferable record."

Transition Cipher   One of two interdependent categories of cipher used in classical cryptography. The other cipher category is known as a substitution cipher. Substitution and transposition differ in how chunks of the message are handled by the encryption process.

Transitions of Care   The transfer of patients from one healthcare practitioner or setting to another as needs and conditions change.

Traverse   A formal denial of an allegation made in the pleadings of an opposing party.

Treble Damages   In law, an award of damages equal to three times the actual damages. Treble damages are awarded under statutes that specifically provide for such an award, such as fraud and abuse.

TREC   **Text Retrieval Conference**—The TREC series of conferences, cosponsored by the National Institute of Standards and Technology (NIST) and the US Department of Defense. TREC is a workgroup composed of distinguished scientists and academics who are working to support research within the information retrieval community by providing the infrastructure necessary for large-scale evaluation of text retrieval methodologies.

TRHCA   **Tax Relief and Health Care Act of 2006** (P.L. 109-432)—Signed into law by the president on December 20, 2006, TRHCA established the Physician Quality Reporting System (PQRI), which provides for incentive payments for eligible professionals who satisfactorily report on quality measures for covered professional services furnished to Medicare beneficiaries during the second half of 2007. TRHCA also amends the Harmonized Tariff Schedule (HTS) of the United States to temporarily modify certain rates of duty, makes technical amendments to certain trade laws, extends certain trade preference programs, and includes other provisions.

Trial Court   A court in which evidence is presented to either a judge or jury.

Trial Graphics   In law, the animations, diagrams, visuals, or other graphics used by lawyers to better explain complex technology, issues, and situations to finders of fact.

Tribunal   Any court, administrative agency, judicial body, or board that has quasi-judicial functions.

TRICARE   A three-option healthcare plan available to military personnel, and their families.

Trier of Fact   A fact-finder who hears testimony and reviews evidence.

Trigger   In law, the event that requires parties to implement a litigation hold. Triggers can include: receipt of a legal notice (summons, subpoena, deposition, and such) and/or the occurrence of an adverse event that results in an injury or harm.

Trojan Horse   A category of computer virus in which a subprogram is embedded in a larger program or file that then destroys data or programs.

True Attachments   The term used to describe the attachments created by an author or custodian that are explicitly referred to in a cover or parent document. Documents are meant to be bound together. For example, a report that follows a letter referencing the report. See also Physical Attachments.

TrueCrypt   The Microsoft Windows open source disk encryption package that supports AES-256, Blowfish, CAST5, Serpent, Triple DES, and Twofish.

Trustworthy System   An automated information system that consists of computer hardware and software that:

1. are reasonably secure from intrusion and misuse
2. provide a reasonable level of availability, reliability, and correct operation
3. are reasonably suited to performing their intended functions.

TSC Rule   Refers to the HIPAA regulations that govern the standards for electronic transactions and code sets. TSC can be found at 45 CFR Section 162.100 et seq.

Tweet   A post to the Twitter social networking and blogging service; a microblog.

Twitter   A social-networking and blogging service that allows users to type up to 140 characters of information about their current status.

Two-Factor Authentication   A specific form of multifactor authentication. A typical two-factor authentication could be a password (something you know) combined with voice verification (something you are). In two-factor authentication, exactly two independent factors of identification are utilized together to create a stronger authentication than the use of a single factor, such as a password.

TwoFish   A block-ciphering algorithm based on Blowfish that uses a single key of any length up to 256 bits. It is efficient both for software that runs in smaller processors such as those in Smart Cards and for embedding in hardware.

Two-Tiered Discovery   In law and in the context of e-discovery, a process by which parties agree or are ordered to limit discovery to active sources of electronically stored information (ESI) rather than seek discovery of ESI from sources that are not reasonably accessible.

U

UB-82   A uniform institutional claim form developed by the NUBC that was in general use under HIPAA from 1983 to 1993.

UB-92   A uniform institutional claim form developed by the NUBC that has been in general use under HIPAA since 1993.

UCC   Uniform Commercial Code—A series of laws enacted by the states that regulate commercial transactions.

UCF   Uniform Claim Form.

UCITA   Uniform Computer Information Transactions Act—A substantive statute of contract law that provides a comprehensive set of rules for the licensing of computer software or other clearly identified forms of electronic information. UCITA applies to contracts for the licensing and/or purchase of software, software development contracts, and Internet database access contracts.

UCR   Usual, Customary, and Reasonable—A fee-for-service payment screen based on the usual charge by the provider, customary charges by other area providers, and a determination of a reasonable cost(s) for the service(s) provided.

UCTF   Uniform Claim Task Force—An organization, under HIPAA, that developed the initial HCFA-1500 Professional Claim Form before maintenance responsibilities were assumed by the NUCC.

UCUM   Unified Codes for Units of Measure—A system of codes for the unambiguous measurement of machines and humans.

UETA   Uniform Electronic Transactions Act—Enacted by the National Conference of Commissioners of Uniform State Laws (NCCUSL) in 1999 to make electronic transactions as enforceable in a court of law as manual signatures. UETA applies only to voluntary agreements involving electronic records and signatures on a transaction.

UHI   Unique Health Identifier.

UIACP   Uniform International Authentication and Certification Practices.

ULC   Uniform Law Commission—Lawyers with the National Conference of Commissioners on Uniform State Laws who have been appointed by state governments to research, draft, and promote enactment of uniform state laws in areas where uniformity is desirable and practical. http://www.nccusl.org

Ultimaco Safeguard   A commercial Windows disk encryption package.

Umbrella Insurance   Supplemental insurance that provides coverage that exceeds the basic or usual limits of liability.

UML   Unified Modeling Language—An industry-standard, graphic notation system for the specification, visualization, construction, and documentation of the components of software systems.

UMLS   Unified Medical Language System—A multipurpose database developed by the National Library of Medicine (NLM) for use by information system developers in building or enhancing electronic systems that create, process, retrieve, integrate, and/or aggregate biomedical and health data and information, as well as in informatics research.

Unavailability   The condition of not being available as recognized under the Federal Rules of Evidence as an exclusion to the hearsay rule.

Unbundling   The separation of the charge for a product from that made for related services.

UN/CEFACT   United Nations Centre for Facilitation of Procedures and Practices for Administration, Commerce, and Transport—An international organization dedicated to simplifying procedural barriers to international commerce.

Unclean Hands   A legal doctrine that prevents a plaintiff who has acted unethically in relation to a suit from winning said suit or from recovering as much money as would have been awarded for honorable behavior.

UN/EDIFACT   **United Nations Rules for Electronic Data Interchange for Administration, Commerce, and Transport**—A series of syntax rules for international EDI format.

Uniform Determination of Death Act   An act, adopted in most states, that provides a medically sound basis for determining death as applying to an individual who has sustained either irreversible cessation of circulatory and respiratory functions, or irreversible cessation of all functions of the entire brain.

Uniform Rules Relating to the Discovery of Electronically Stored Information   An independent set of rules for e-discovery to provide the states with a set of rules regarding mandatory conferences and reporting, rules governing scope and form of discovery, rules describing limitations on sanctions, rules covering claims of privilege, and rules for discovery directed at third parties.

UNII   **Unique Ingredient Identifier**—A core component of the joint FDA/USP Substance Registration System (SRS) used to support health information technology initiatives by generating unique ingredient identifiers (UNIIs) for substances in drugs, biologics, foods, and devices. The UNII is a nonproprietary, free, unique, unambiguous, nonsemantic, alphanumeric identifier based on a substance's molecular structure and/or descriptive information.

UNII   **Unlicensed National Information Infrastructure**—A three-range radio band frequency spectrum utilized by IEEE-802.11a devices and many wireless Internet service providers (ISPs).

Unitization   A litigation support term that describes the identification of document boundaries in an automated litigation support program. Unitization also refers to the identification and linking in an automated litigation support program of cover documents and their attachments (parent and children documents). Unitization decisions will play a critical role in discovery, given that digital files do not contain staples, binders, tabs, or file folder labels. It is important for a litigation support professional to work closely with a document management specialist during the scanning process to appropriately determine where breaks occur in the document database.

Universal Access   The concept of access to health insurance coverage for all US citizens.

Unix   A computer operating system that enables computers to share data.

UNL   Universal Networking Language.

UNML   United Nations Model Law on Electronic Commerce.

UNSM   United Nations Standard Messages.

Unstructured Data   Data that are represented as free-form text that do not reside in a fixed location. Documents, e-mail, images, graphics, and video are examples of unstructured data. The opposite of structured data.

UP   Universal Parser.

Upcoding   A term used to describe the assignment of a code (CPT or ICD) or a DRG classification to a higher level of services for the purpose of indicating a greater level of resource intensity for the purpose of obtaining a higher level of reimbursement.

UPIN   Unique Provider Identification Number—UPINs are six-place alpha-numeric identifiers assigned to all Medicare physicians for the purpose of identification.

Upload   To transmit a file from a central system to a remote location, usually via the Internet or mobile storage device, with the intent that the remote system save a copy of the file. Many online file hosting services practice remote uploading, which transfers data from one remote storage space to another.

URAC   Utilization Review Assessment Commission—A nonprofit health-care organization that promotes healthcare quality through quality bench-marking programs and a voluntary review and accreditation process.

Urgent Care   Services rendered for an unexpected illness or injury that is not life threatening, but requires immediate outpatient care and cannot be postponed.

URI   Uniform Resource Identifiers—A string of characters used to identify a name or a resource on the Internet. A URI enables interaction with represen-tations of the resource over a network (typically the World Wide Web) using specific protocols.

URL   Uniform Resource Locator—A URL is a short-cut method for the loca-tion of an Internet file.

USB   Universal Serial Bus—A port designed to connect external hardware to a central computer.

USC   United States Code.

US Constitution   Establishes the general organization of the federal government and grants certain powers to the federal government and places limits on what the federal and state governments may do.

Use and Disclosure   The two limited mechanisms—access and release—by which health information may be handled, according to the HIPAA privacy rule.

User   A registered or authenticated member of a home organization. Users are generally given access to information systems based upon their role and job functions.

US Supreme Court   The highest court in the United States, created by the Constitution.

US TAG   United States Technical Advisory Group—Each US TAG is accredited by the American National Standards Institute (ANSI).

Usual, Customary, and Reasonable   Fees that are commonly charged for healthcare services within a certain area. Also used to denote the use of fee screens to determine the lowest value of provider reimbursement based on: 1. the provider's usual charge for a given procedure; 2. the amount customarily charged for the service by other providers in the area (often defined as a specific percentile of all charges in the community); and 3. the reasonable cost of services for a given patient after medical review of the case. Most health plans provide reimbursement for usual and customary charges, although no universal formula has been established for these rates.

Utilitarianism   A theory arguing that ethical decisions must be based on a requirement of efficiency and consideration for what is good for the greatest number of individuals.

Utilization Review   Refers to the process by which nonemergent care is evaluated for necessity and appropriateness.

V

VA   Veterans Affairs—The VA administers an independent healthcare system for American military veterans.

Vacate   When a court sets aside a previously entered order or decision.

Validation   A litigation support term that describes the various automated processes utilized by an outside service bureau to ensure the accuracy of scanned images and coded data. Validation is also used to verify the accuracy of attachment ranges and dates.

Valid Certificate   An electronic certificate that 1. a licensed certification authority issued; 2. the subscriber listed in it has accepted; and 3. has not been revoked or suspended; and 4. has not expired.

Value   A standard, quality, or principle that is considered desirable.

Variance Management   The establishment of thresholds or standards and measures of outliers.

Venue   The location in which a court may hear cases.

Verdict   The final decision on the matter presented in court for consideration.

VETS   **Veterans' Employment and Training Service**—A division of the Department of Labor (DOL) that investigates claims of federal labor employment violations. Veterans and other eligible persons are afforded with special federal employment rights such as preference in hiring and protection in reductions in force.

Vicarious Liability   In law, a concept by which an entity is responsible for the negligent acts of another. Often referred to as passive or secondary negligence.

Virtual Storage   Memory space provided by a secondary storage device.

Virtue-Based Ethics   An ethical approach that stresses how an action expresses the character of the person performing it.

Virus   A malignant computer program that replicates itself and infects other computer programs, often causing damage to memory and function.

Visual Integration Tools   Electronic information management tools used for extracting, transforming, and loading data from one data source to any data source to support enterprise integration of data and systems.

VMS   Voice Messaging System.

Voicemail   Also known as V-Mail or Voice Messaging System (VMS), a voicemail is a telephone message that digitizes analog voice files and stores the file onto a disk or flash memory in a central computer. Voicemail messages can be stored and retrieved by a user by logging into a server or forwarding the message to another user's voice mailbox.

VOIP   Voice Over Internet Protocol—Refers to the use of technology to transmit voice files over a data network using the Internet or a corporate intranet.

Voir Dire   In law, the Latin term for meaning to speak the truth. The procedure whereby possible jurors are questioned before determining who will sit in judgment on the case.

Voluntary Disclosure Protocol A procedure in which providers may self-disclose any claims presented to the government that are found to be fraudulent.

VPN **Virtual Private Network**—A computer network that resides on top of another computer network and is set up for use by a limited number of individuals, such as employees of an organization who operate over a large area. A VPN typically uses encryption to keep information secure

Vulnerability A gap in policy or in safeguards, both physical and electronic.

W

W3C **World Wide Web Consortium.**

Wage Loss Damages The amount of money a victim or plaintiff loses by not being able to work.

Walsh-Healey Public Contracts Act The federal labor standard that requires payment of minimum wages and adherence to other labor standards by contractors who provide materials and supplies to the federal government.

WAN **Wide Area Network**—A term used to describe a collection of local area networks (LANs) that spans a large geographical area; a larger network.

WARN **Worker Adjustment and Retraining Notification Act**—A federal labor standard that requires employers with 100 or more employees provide 60 days advance notice of plant closings and mass layoffs. WARN actions are enforced through private actions in the federal courts.

Warranties The issuance of a certificate by a certification authority gives certain warranties to its subscriber by operation of law "and makes a certification to all those who rely on the certificate." Utah Code 46-3-303 states, "By issuing a certificate, a licensed certification authority warrants to the subscriber named in the certificate that:

1. the certificate contains no information known to the certification authority to be false
2. the certificate satisfies all material requirements of [the statute]
3. the certification authority has not exceeded any limits of its license in issuing the certificate
4. the certification authority may not disclaim or limit the warranties of this subsection."

Warranty of Merchantability Under the Uniform Commercial Code, an implied promise to a buyer that goods purchased conform to ordinary standards of care and that they are of the same average grade, quality, and value as similar goods sold under similar circumstances.

Web 2.0   An indefinite term. Web 2.0 may be defined as a set of technologies that are interactive, combining user-provided content with automated networking applications to create personalized but collaborative information. See also Cloud Computing.

WebMD   A public Internet site with information on health and healthcare.

Website   A collection of URLs and Uniform Resource Identifiers (URIs) under the control of one entity.

WEDI   Workgroup for Electronic Data Interchange—An open, government-sponsored organization through the Centers for Medicare and Medicaid Services member workgroup whose core purpose is to "improve the quality of healthcare through effective and efficient information exchange and management." http://www.wedi.org

WHO   World Health Organization—The directing and coordinating authority for health within the United Nations system. The WHO owns and publishes the ICD coding classification systems. http://www.who.int/en

Wikipedia   A free online multilingual encyclopedia that allows users to share, access, and modify the content of the website.

Winchester Drive   A hard drive permanently installed on a computer.

Wireless Life Sciences Alliance   A member organization focused solely on the application of wireless cellular technology to enable new business models and business process improvements in all sectors of the life sciences industries, including the healthcare services, healthcare information technology, biopharmaceutical, and medical device sectors. http://www.wirelesslifesciences.org

Wordlist   A text file containing a collection of words for use in a dictionary attack.

Workers' Compensation   Providing benefits to an employee for injuries occurring in the scope of employment.

Work-Product Privilege   A rule that provides for qualified immunity of a lawyer's work product from discovery and/or disclosure.

World Privacy Forum   An independent 501(c)(3) public interest research group focused on conducting in-depth research, analysis, and consumer education in the area of privacy. http://www.worldprivacyforum.org

WORM **Write Once, Read Many Times**—A form in which electronic information can be maintained for security purposes.

Worm Term used to describe bits of code placed by a programmer into an operating system program that duplicates itself repeatedly. A worm is different than a virus. A worm will destroy data and adversely affect any program while the operating system is running. A virus will alter or destroy the program it infects in a directed versus a repeated manner.

WPC **Washington Publishing Company**—A company that publishes the X12N HIPAA implementation guides, developed the X12N HIPAA data directory, and hosts the EHNAC STFCS testing program. http://www.wpc-edi.com

Wrongful Death A cause of action for the recovery of losses caused by the death of a person by civil wrong.

WWW **World Wide Web**—A network, often used synonymously with the Internet, made up of all computers on the Internet that use HTML software to share data and information, characterized by graphical interfaces, links, images, video, and sound.

X

X.509 Certificate The ITU-T standard format for public key cryptography certificates that defines specific formats for public key certificates. It is also an algorithm that verifies a given certificate path is valid under the public key infrastructure (PKI) known as the certification path validation algorithm. See also Certification Path Algorithm.

X12 An ANSI-accredited group that defines electronic data interchange (EDI) standards for many industries, including healthcare insurance. The majority of electronic transaction standards under HIPAA are X12.

X12 148 A standard not included in the HIPAA mandate. The X12 First Report of Injury, Illness, or Incident transaction.

X12 270 The X12 Health Care Eligibility and Benefit Inquiry transaction, a version of which has been included in HIPAA mandates.

X12 271 The X12 Health Care Eligibility and Benefit Response transaction, a version of which has been included in HIPAA mandates.

X12 274 The X12 Provider Information transaction.

X12 275 The X12 Patient Information transaction.

X12 276 The X12 Health Care Claims Status Inquiry transaction, a version of which is included in HIPAA mandates.

X12 277 The X12 Health Care Claims Status Response transaction, a version of which is included in HIPAA mandates.

X12 278 The X13 Referral Certification and Authorization transaction, a version of which has been included in HIPAA mandates.

X12 811 The X12 Consolidated Service Invoice and Statement transaction.

X12 820 The X12 Payment Order and Remittance Advice transaction, a version of which is included in HIPAA mandates.

X12 831 The X12 Application Control Totals transaction.

X12 834 The X12 Benefit Enrollment and Maintenance transaction, a version of which has been included in the HIPAA mandates.

X12 835 The X12 Health Care Claim Payment and Remittance Advice transaction, a version of which has been included in HIPAA mandates.

X12 837 The X12 Health Care Claim or Encounter transaction, a version of which has been included in HIPAA mandates. This transaction is used for institutional, professional, dental, and/or drug claims.

X12 997 The X12 Functional Acknowledgement transaction.

X12 5010 TR3S The new standard under HIPAA for claims transactions.

X12F A subcommittee of X12 that defines electronic data interchange (EDI) standards for the financial industry and maintains several transactions.

X12 IHCEBI & IHCEBR The X12 Interactive Healthcare Eligibility and Benefits Inquiry and Response transactions, which are being combined with UN/EDIFACT.

X12 IHCLME The X12 Interactive Healthcare Claim transaction.

X12J A subcommittee of X12 that reviews work productions for compliance with the design rules of X12.

X12N A subcommittee of X12 that defines electronic data interchange (EDI) standards for the insurance industry.

X12N/SPTG4 The HIPAA Liaison Special Task Group of the Insurance Subcommittee of X12, which has rendered its responsibilities to another working group, X2N/TG2/WG3.

X12N/TG1 The Property and Casualty Task Group of the Insurance Subcommittee of X12.

X12N/TG2 The Health Care Task Group of the Insurance Subcommittee of X12.

X12N/TG2/WG1 The Health Care Eligibility Work Group of the Health Care Task Group, which maintains the X12 270 and X12 271 as well as the IHCEB and IHCEBR transactions.

X12N/TG2/WG2 The Health Care Claims Work Group of the Health Care Task Group, which maintains the X12 837 transaction.

X12N/TG2/WG3 The Health Care Claim Payments Work Group of the Health Care Task Group, which maintains the X12 835 transaction.

X12N/TG2/WG4 The Health Care Enrollments Work Group of the Health Care Task Group, which maintains the X12 834 transaction.

X12N/TG2/WG5 The Health Care Claims Status Work Group of the Health Care Task Group, which maintains the X12 276 transaction.

X12N/TG2/WG9 The Health Care Patient Information Work Group of the Health Care Task Group, which maintains the X12 275 transaction.

X12N/TG2/WG10 The Health Care Services Review Work Group of the Health Care Task Group, which maintains the X12 278 transaction.

X12N/TG2/WG12 The Interactive Health Care Claims Work Group of the Health Care Task Group, which maintains the IHCLME Interactive Claims transaction.

X12N/TG2/WG15 The Health Care Services Provider Information Work Group of the Health Care Task Group, which maintains the X12 274 transaction.

X12N/TG2/WG19 The Health Care Implementation Coordination Work Group of the Health Care Task Group, which has become X12N/TG3/WG3.

X12N/TG3 The Business Transaction Coordination and Modeling Task Group of the Insurance Subcommittee, which maintains the X12N Business and Data Models and the HIPAA data dictionary.

X12N/TG3/WG1 The Property and Casualty Work Group of the Business Transaction Coordination and Modeling Task Group.

X12N/TG3/WG2 The Healthcare Business and Information Modeling Work Group of the Business Transaction Coordination and Modeling Task Group.

X12N/TG3/WG3   The HIPAA Implementation Coordination Work Group of the Business Transaction Coordination and Modeling Task Group.

X12N/TG3/WG4   The Object-Oriented Modeling and XML Liaison Work Group of the Business Transaction Coordination and Modeling Task Group.

X12N/TG4   The Implementation Guide Task Group of the Insurance Sub-committee of X12, which supports the development and maintenance of X12 implementation guides.

X12N/TG8   The Architecture Task Group of the Insurance Subcommittee of X12.

X12/PRB   The X12 Procedures Review Board.

X12 Standards   A term used to describe the set of standards developed by the ASC X12 Committee. See also ASC X12.

XHTML   **Extensible HyperText Markup Language**—XHTML is a partial merge of XML and HTML standards and very similar to HTML.

XML   **Extensible Markup Language**—XML is the World Wide Web Consortium standard for creating markup languages, which describe the structure of data. Unlike HTML, it is not a fixed set of elements but is a language for describing languages.

XML Integration   A term used to describe the process of using an XML standards-based approach to integrate and retrieve data from mainframe applications and other systems through connectors and adapters.

XOR   **Exclusive OR**—A Boolean-associative operation of two logical values. It returns a "True" when only one of the operands is "True" and returns a "False" when both of the operands are either "True" or "False."

XPD   **Cross Polarization Discrimination**—A ratio that quantifies the separation between two transmission channels that use different polarization orientations.

X-Ray   **Energetic High-Frequency Electromagnetic Radiation**—One of the oldest forms of medical imaging; it utilizes electromagnetic radiation to make pictorial images of bones, teeth, and the internal organs.

Y

Yahoo!   A public corporation providing Internet services, including a search engine, social media service, and e-mail service.

Yammer   An enterprise microblogging service used by business, organizations, and groups to facilitate workplace communications and collaboration.

Yelp   A Web 2.0 site that operates as a social networking, user review, and local search engine. The Yelp site features forums in which to review restaurants, shopping, health and medical services, beauty services, nightlife, home services, event planning, arts, and other institutions.

YouTube   A free video-sharing website owned by Google in which MPEG-4 video clips are uploaded and shared.

Z

Zettabyte   One sextillion bytes.

Zip   An open standard for both the compression and decompression used for PC download archives, under the file extension .zip.

Zone of Danger Rule   The zone of danger rule requires that the person claiming negligent infliction of emotional distress must have been in the zone of danger and be in fear for his or her own physical safety before recovery is allowed for the negligence of the defendant.

ZPIC   **Zone Program Integrity Contractor**—An independent organization or contractor hired to perform a wide range of medical review, data analysis, and Medicare evidence-based policy auditing activities. Unlike other types of audits, the focus of the ZPIC audits is to identify and address potential Medicare fraud implications.

e-Discovery
Glossary of Websites

http://www.aaaai.org
American Academy of Allergy, Asthma & Immunology—A database of information about allergies, asthma, and immunology, including a virtual allergist application.

http://www.aap.org
American Academy of Pediatrics—A comprehensive website dedicated to children's health.

http://www.abanet.org/tech/ltrc/lawlink/home.html
American Bar Association: Legal Technology Center—An online legal research hub which provides resources including surveys, electronic discussion forums, publications, and legal comparative studies selected and evaluated by the American Bar Association staff of lawyers and librarians.

http://www.ada.org
American Dental Association—A dental and oral health website with professional resources, public resources, job listings, and advocacy information.

http://www.ahima.org
American Health Information Management Association—The premier professional member organization of more than 61,000 health information management (HIM) professionals dedicated to the effective management of personal health information required to deliver quality healthcare to the public.

http://www.aha.org
American Hospital Association—A national organization that provides advocacy for 5,000 hospitals, healthcare systems, networks, and 37,000 individual members and provides education for healthcare workers as a source of information on healthcare issues and trends.

http://www.ahd.com
American Hospital Directory—A directory of over 6,000 public and private hospitals in the United States.

http://www.ahrq.gov
Agency for Healthcare Research and Quality—A website sponsored by the US Department of Health & Human Services, whose mission is to improve the quality, safety, efficiency, and effectiveness of health care for all Americans.

http://www.behavenet.com
BehaveNet—An Internet database of behavioral healthcare resources, publications, and terminology.

http://biotech.icmb.utexas.edu
BioTech—An online database of life sciences resources and reference tools suitable for high school students up through college professors and researchers. Includes a listing of biomedical links.

http://www.bcbs.com
Blue Cross/Blue Shield Association—The homepage for Blue Cross/Blue Shield health insurance, featuring resources on health and wellness and cost studies.

http://www.caredata.com
CareData—A privately owned company offering a host of solutions in the areas of medical practice management, electronic health records, e-prescribing, personal health records, advanced patient tracking, and risk management.

http://www.cdc.gov/az/a.html
Centers for Disease Control and Prevention: A to Z Health Index—A comprehensive index of health conditions and concerns recognized by the US Centers for Disease Control and Prevention.

http://www.cms.hhs.gov
Centers for Medicare & Medicaid Services—The Medicare/Medicaid homepage with information on coverage, research, statistics, systems, and data.

http://clinicalevidence.bmj.com/ceweb/index.jsp
Clinical Evidence—An authoritative resource for informed treatment decisions and improving patient care, featuring a comprehensive glossary of conditions and a selection of commissioned papers.

http://www.cochrane.org
The Cochrane Collaboration—An international network of people helping healthcare providers and policy makers as well as patients, their advocates, and their carers make well-informed decisions about human health care by preparing, updating, and promoting the accessibility of the Cochrane Reviews, which are sets of systematic reviews of primary research in human healthcare and health policy.

http://www.law.cornell.edu
Cornell Law School, Legal Information Institute—A database of collections of research and publications from the Cornell Law School including directories, court opinions, constitutions, and codes.

http://www.dentaldictionary.net
Dental Dictionary—A comprehensive glossary of dental terms, offered in numerous languages including English, Spanish, French, and Arabic.

http://www.discoveryresources.org
Discovery Resources—A database of information, resources, and news about electronic discovery aimed at legal professionals.

http://dynamed.ebscohost.com
DynaMed—A point-of-care reference tool for physicians with clinically organized, evidence-based summaries for more than 3,000 topics. DynaMed monitors the content of over 500 medical journals for daily updates.

http://www.ehealthinitiative.org
eHealth Initiative—An online, nonprofit organization focused on improving the quality, safety, and efficiency of healthcare through information and the implementation of information technology, including electronic prescribing.

http://www.fiercehealthit.com
Fierce Health IT—A website offering weekly news updates, interactive webinars, and resources on health IT.

http://www.findlaw.com
FindLaw—A website that provides lawyer profiles and legal information to the general public, in an effort to achieve the best legal decisions possible.

http://www.guidelines.gov
Guidelines.gov—A website sponsored by the Agency for Healthcare Research and Quality (AHRQ) that is designed to be a public resource for evidence-based clinical practice guidelines.

http://www.lib.uiowa.edu/hardin/md/
Hardin MetaDirectory of Internet Health Sources—A University of Iowa–sponsored site with a medical picture gallery and disease database.

http://www.healthdatamanagement.com
Health Data Management—An industry website offering web seminars and news related to electronic health records and medical imaging.

http://healthit.hhs.gov/portal/server.pt
Health Information Technology—An organization dedicated to improving healthcare quality, preventing medical errors, reducing costs, increasing efficiency, decreasing paperwork, and expanding affordable care through implementation of new technology.

http://histalk2.com
HIStalk—A useful EHR industry blog by an anonymous professional with several years of experience as a clinical department head. The HIStalk website is updated regularly and contains highly relevant news and useful information about healthcare IT and the status of events within the industry.

http://www.hl7.org
Health Level Seven—An American National Standards Institute (ANSI) in the nonprofit sector that provides standards for interoperability that improve healthcare delivery, optimize workflow, reduce ambiguity, and enhance knowledge transfer to healthcare providers and government agencies.

http://www.hrsa.gov/healthit
Health Resources and Services Administration—The US Department of Health and Human Services' promotion of the widespread availability and use of digital networks to improve access to healthcare services, particularly for those without adequate coverage, through communication technology.

http://www.healthcareitnews.com
Healthcare IT News—An integrated media company that publishes articles about IT and finance in the medical fields and provides research resources.

http://www.health-infosys-dir.com/yp_hc.asp
Healthcare IT Yellow Pages—A database of healthcare links from a variety of companies.

http://www.hmstn.com
Healthcare Management Systems, Inc.—A healthcare organization that provides information technology systems that integrate clinical and financial applications on a single PC platform to over 600 hospitals in the country.

http://www.hospitalconnect.com
Hospital Connect Search—A search engine that goes only to assigned health websites and is designed to provide information on hospital management.

http://infomine.ucr.edu/cgi-bin/search?category=bioag/
InfoMine—A collection of scholarly resources in biological, agricultural, and medical sciences, sponsored by the Regents of the University of California.

http://information-security-resources.com
Information Security Resources—An organization with the mission of helping industry stakeholders, government regulators, and the public better comprehend and address information security threats from an increasingly digital world.

http://www.iom.edu
Institute of Medicine—A detailed database of health topics, researched by the National Academies, including healthcare, quality, mental health, public policy, and treatment.

http://www.ietf.org
Internet Engineering Task Force—An international community, open to any interested individuals, of network designers, operators, vendors, and researchers devoted to the enhancement of Internet architecture and the continued, smooth operation of the Internet.

http://www.ilrg.com
Internet Legal Research Group—A resource of information for both lawyers and the general public concerning law and the legal profession, including over 2,000 legal forms and documents.

http://www.isoc.org
Internet Society—An independent international non-profit organization founded in 1992 to provide leadership on Internet-related standards, education, and policy around the world.

ftp://ftp.rfc-editor.org/in-notes/bcp/bcp9.txt
Internet Standards Best Practices—A public document that specifies best current practices for the Internet and the Internet community, and requests discussion and suggestions for improvements.

http://dictionary.law.com
Law.com Legal Dictionary—An online dictionary of legal words and phrases, featuring an alphabetical listing as well as a search engine.

http://www.refdesk.com/factlaw.html
Law/Legal Resources—A dictionary of legal terms accessible by search engine, accompanied by a listing of valuable links to sites containing additional legal information and statistics.

http://www.lectlaw.com/def.htm
The 'Lectric Law Library's Legal Lexicon's Lyceum—A dictionary of both legal phrases and legal concepts, accompanied by definitions and explanations.

http://www.online-dictionary.net/law/index.htm
Legal Dictionaries Online—A brief listing of available law dictionaries accessible through the Internet by both lawyers and the public.

http://www.medterms.com/script/main/hp.asp
MedicineNet.com—A dictionary of medical terms accessible by search engine or alphabetical listings.

http://www.pharma-lexicon.com
MediLexicon—A database of medical abbreviations and their meanings as well as a medical dictionary.

http://www.nlm.nih.gov/medlineplus/encyclopedia.html
MedlinePlus—A healthcare information website featuring the A.D.A.M. Encyclopedia with over 4,000 entries on diseases, tests, symptoms, injuries, and surgeries. Includes some illustrations and photographs.

http://www.lib.umich.edu/government-documents-center/
MLibrary—A database of legal sources, organized by state, including bills, constitutions, newspapers, attorneys general, and regulations.

http://www.modernhealthcare.com
ModernHealthcare.com—A news site with breaking news on medical care, videos, podcasts, and webinars, as well as healthcare related lists.

http://health.msn.com
MSN Health & Fitness—A site hosted by MSN featuring a medical encyclopedia and over 25,000 medical links. The site also covers medical news, including information on outbreaks and epidemics.

http://www.myphr.com
myPHR—A web resource that allows individuals to create and maintain their own personal health records and clearly spells out their health information rights.

http://www.archives.gov
National Archives and Records Administration—NARA holds documents deemed necessary to be maintained forever for legal or historical purposes for both the nation as a whole and private citizens.

http://www.ncbi.nlm.nih.gov/pubmed/
National Center for Biotechnology Information—A national resource for molecular biology information, featuring the PubMed search engine for topics, authors, and journals about medicine.

http://www.ncsconline.org/wc/CourTopics/ResourceGuide.asp?topic=EIDisc
National Center for State Courts—A library with both hardcopy and digital resources and publications regarding the practice of law, along with job descriptions, judicial salaries, court websites, and an overview of e-discovery.

http://csrc.nist.gov
National Institute of Standards and Technology: Computer Security Division—A computer-security resource center with an archive of publications.

http://www.nih.gov
National Institutes of Health—A national medical research agency providing training, grants, and a glossary of health topics for healthcare professionals.

http://www.nlm.nih.gov
National Library of Medicine—A collection of resources and databases maintained by the National Institutes of Health.

http://www.womenshealth.gov
National Women's Health Information Center—A page with medical tools, publications, and links regarding campaigns and activities, focused on women's health.

http://www.nhinwatch.com
NHINWatch—A website covering the creation of the nation's health information network, sponsored by the editors of Healthcare IT News.

http://www.nolo.com/glossary.cfm
Nolo—A law dictionary aimed at the layperson, with plain English definitions of legal terms not generally used in everyday language.

http://oig.hhs.gov
Office of Inspector General—An organization designed to protect the integrity of the Department of Health and Human Services programs as well as the health of the public, featuring publications and articles about healthcare fraud and the prevention of fraud.

http://healthit.hhs.gov
Office of the National Coordinator—The principal federal entity charged with coordination of nationwide efforts to implement and use the most advanced health information technology and the electronic exchange of health information.

http://healthit.hhs.gov/portal/server.pt?open=512&mode=2&objID=3120

ONC-Authorized Testing and Certification Bodies Directory—A current directory of organizations that have been selected by the Office of the National Coordinator (ONC) to test and certify EHRs to the applicable certification criteria adopted by the Secretary under subpart C of Part 170 Part II and Part III as stipulated in the Standards and Certification Final Rule.

http://www.pohly.com/terms.shtml

Pam Pohly's Net Guide—A management resources website for medical and healthcare professionals with a glossary of managed healthcare terms, job search resources, a directory of healthcare recruiters, tools for managers, and more.

http://www.pharmainfo.net

Pharmainfo.net—A resource page for pharmaceutical and healthcare professionals that features information, news, blogs, profile pages, videos, reviews, and articles.

http://www.romingerlegal.com

Rominger Legal—A comprehensive database of links to legal resources, professional directories, and federal institutions, as well as state and federal court links.

http://searchfinancialsecurity.techtarget.com/sDefinition/0,,sid185_gci1150017,00.html

Search Financial Security—A detailed definition of e-discovery from a comprehensive glossary of tech terms and management strategies.

http://www.thesedonaconference.org

The Sedona Conference—A 501(c)(3) research and educational institute comprised of academics, industry experts, lawyers, and judges dedicated to the advancement of law and policy in the areas of antitrust law, intellectual property rights, and complex litigation.

http://www.law.stetson.edu

Stetson University College of Law—The website for Stetson University College of Law, a three-year law program in Gulfport, FL, featuring a law library of databases.

http://www.trizetto.com/index.asp

TriZetto—A technology solutions corporation driving integrated healthcare management and offering both healthcare solutions and services.

http://lib.law.washington.edu

University of Washington, School of Law, Library—The Marian Gould Gallagher Law Library, a website that features case law, articles and legislation, databases and free legal resources.

http://www.uscourts.gov

US Courts—A guide to state and federal courts, including a court locator, online database of commonly used court forms, and a comprehensive list of web resources.

http://www.hhs.gov

US Department of Health and Human Services—The federal government's primary agency for protecting the health of US citizens and providing essential human services, with an emphasis on those with difficulties taking care of themselves.

http://www.usdoj.gov

US Department of Justice—A government department with a mission "to enforce the law and defend the interests of the United States according to the law; to ensure public safety against threats foreign and domestic; to provide federal leadership in preventing and controlling crime; to seek just punishment for those guilty of unlawful behavior; and to ensure fair and impartial administration of justice for all Americans." The website features many medical and legal headlines.

http://www.webmd.com

WebMD—A public Internet site with information on health and healthcare.

http://whatis.techtarget.com

WhatIs.com—A glossary of computer terminology, including programming, security, hardware, and Internet terms.

http://www.worldhealthnews.harvard.edu

World Health News—Harvard's School of Public Health news digest page from the Center for Health Communication, featuring articles and public health links.

http://www.yourdictionary.com/diction5.html

YourDictionary.com—Specialty dictionaries organized by institution, including law, medicine, computing, and the Internet.

Bibliography

Books

Adams, K., and J.M. Corrigan, eds. *Priority Areas for National Action: Transforming Health Care Quality*, Washington, DC: The National Academies Press (2003).

Allman, T.Y., P.M. Robertson, and G. Howard. *Electronic Discovery and Retention Guidance for Corporate Counsel*. New York, NY: Practising Law Institute (2006).

Bennett, Barbara, Bureau of National Affairs (Arlington, Va.) and American Bar Association. Health Law Section. *E-health Business and Transactional Law*. Washington, DC: Bureau of National Affairs (2002).

Boumil, M.M., and D.J. Sharpe. *Liability in Medicine and Public Health*. St. Paul, MN. West Group (2004).

Brecher, A., and S. Childress. *eDiscovery Plain & Simple*. Bloomington, IN: AuthorHouse (2009).

Center for Medicaid and State Operations/Survey and Certification Group. *Clinical Laboratory Improvement Amendments of 1988 (CLIA)*. Baltimore, MD: Centers for Medicare & Medicaid Services (2010).

Daschle, T., S.S. Greenberger, and J.M. Lambrew. *Critical: What We Can Do about the Health-care Crisis*. New York, NY: Thomas Dunne Books (2008).

Donabedian, A. *An Introduction to Quality Assurance in Health Care*. New York, NY: Oxford University Press, Inc. (2003).

Garner, B.A., ed. *Black's Law Dictionary*. Abridged 7th ed. St. Paul, MN: West Publishing Co. (2000).

Haydock, R.S., D.F. Herr, and J.W. Stempel. *Fundamentals of Pretrial Litigation*. 7th ed. St. Paul, MN: Thomson/West (2008).

Hedges, R.J. *Discovery of Electronically Stored Information: Surveying the Legal Landscape*. Washington, DC: BNA Books (2007).

Institute of Medicine, Committee on Quality of Health Care in America. *Crossing the Quality Chasm: A New Health System for the 21st Century*. Washington, DC: National Academy Press (2001).

Kidwell, B., M. Neumeier, and B. Hansen. *Electronic Discovery*. 7th ed. New York, NY: Law Journal Press (2009).

Kole, J.S. *Chasing Paper: The Keys to Learning about and Loving Discovery*. Chicago, IL: American Bar Association (2009).

Lange, M.C.S., and K.M. Nimsger. *Electronic Evidence and Discovery: What Every Lawyer Should Know*. 2nd ed. Chicago, IL: American Bar Association (2009).

Losey, R.C. *e-Discovery: Current Trends and Cases*. Chicago, IL: American Bar Association (2008).

Nelson, S.D., B.A. Olson, and J.W. Simek. *The Electronic Evidence and Discovery Handbook: Forms, Checklists, and Guidelines*. Chicago, IL: American Bar Association (2006).

Paul, George L., and Bruce H. Nearon. *The discovery revolution: E-discovery amendments to the Federal Rules of Civil Procedure*. Chicago, IL: American Bar Association (2006).

Paul, G.L. *Foundations of Digital Evidence*. Chicago, IL: American Bar Association (2008).

Quinn, Campion: *The medical record as a forensic resource*. Sudbury, MA: Jones and Bartlett Publishers (2005).

Roach, W.H. Jr., R.G. Hoban, B.M. Broccolo, A.B. Roth, and T.P. Blanchard. *Medical Records and the Law*. 4th ed. Sudbury, MA: Jones and Bartlett Publishers, Inc. (2006).

Rogers, M. *Litigation Technology: Becoming a High-Tech Trial Lawyer*. New York, NY: Aspen Publishers, Inc. (2006).

Rothstein, Barbara J., Ronald J. Hedges, Elizabeth Corinne Wiggins, and Federal Judicial Center. *Managing discovery of electronic information: A pocket guide for judges*. Washington, DC: Federal Judicial Center (2007).

Scheindlin, S.A., and D.J. Capra. *Electronic Discovery and Digital Evidence in a Nut Shell*. St. Paul, MN: Thomson Reuters (2009).

Schuler, K. *E-Discovery: Creating and Managing an Enterprisewide Program: A Technical Guide to Digital Investigation and Litigation Support*. Burlington, MA: Syngress Publishing, Inc. (2009).

The Sedona Working Group. *The Sedona Principles: Best Practices Recommendations & Principles for Addressing Electronic Document Production*. 2nd ed (annotated). Arlington, VA: BNA Books (2007).

Shandel, R.E., and P. Smith. *The Preparation Trial of Medical Malpractice Cases.* 38th ed. New York, NY: Law Journal Press (2009).

Wager, Karen A., Frances Wickham Lee, and John Glaser. *Managing Health Care Information Systems: A Practical Approach for Health Care Executives.* San Francisco, CA: Jossey-Bass (2005).

Cases Cited

Aguilar v. ICE Div., 2008 WL 5062700 (S.D.N.Y. 2008).

Ak-Chin Indian Community v. United States, 85 Fed. Cl. 397 (2009).

American Society for the Prevention of Cruelty to Animals v. Ringling Bros. and Barnum & Bailey Circus, civil action no. 03-2006 (D.D.C. 2008).

Arista Records, LLC v. Usenet.com Inc., 2009 WL 185992 (S.D.N.Y. 2009).

Board of Regents v. BASF Corp., 2007 WL 3342423 (D. Neb. 2007).

Bray & Gillespie Management LLC v. Lexington Ins. Co., civil action no. 07-222-Orl-35KRS (M.D. Fl. 2009).

Cache La Poudre Feed, LLC v. Land O' Lakes Inc., 244 F.R.D. 614 (D. Colo. 2007).

Capitol Records, Inc. et al. v. MP3tunes, LLC, 2009 WL 2568431 (S.D.N.Y. 2009).

Cason-Merenda v. Detroit Med. Ctr., 2008 WL 2714239 (E.D. Mich. 2008).

In re Classicstar Mare Lease Litigation, 2009 WL 250954 (E.D. Kan. 2009).

Columbia Pictures, Indus. v. Bunnell, 2007 U.S. Dist. LEXIS 63620 (C.D. Cal. 2007).

Compl., Plumbers & Pipefitters Local Union No. 630 Pension-Annuity trust Fund v. Allscripts-Misys Healthcare Solutions, Inc., No. 09-4726 (N.D. Ill. Aug. 4, 2009) [DKT #1].

Convolve, Inc. v. Compaq Computer Corp., 223 F.R.D. 162 (S.D.N.Y. 2004).

Crawford-El v. Britton, 523 U.S. 574, 598 (1996).

Cumberland Truck Equip. v. Detroit Diesel Corp., 2008 WL 511194 (E.D. Mich. 2008).

D.N.J. L. Civ. R. 26.1(d)(3)(a).

In re Ebay Seller Antitrust Litigation, 2007 WL 2852364 (N.D. Ca. 2007).

ex rel. Edmondson v. Tyson Foods, Inc., 2007 WL 1498973 (N.D. Okla. 2007).

Equity Analytics LLC v. Lundin, 248 F.R.D. 331 (D.D.C. 2008).

In re Fannie Mae Securities Litigation, 2009 WL 21528 (D.C. Cir. 2009).

Fox Cable Networks, Inc. v. Goen Technologies Corp., 2008 WL 2165179 (D.N.J. 2008).

Haka v. Lincoln County, 246 F.R.D. 577 (W.D. Wisc. 2007).

Hawaiian Airlines, Inc. v. Mesa Air Group, Inc., 2007 WL 3172642 (Bankr.D. Haw. 2007).

In re: Honeywell Int'l Inc. Sec. Litig., 230 F.R.D. 293 (S.D.N.Y. 2003).

Hopson v. City of Baltimore, 232 F.R.D. 228 (D. Md. 2005).

John B. v. Goetz, 531 F.3d 448 (6th Cir. 2008).

Knifesource LLC v. Wachovia Bank, N.A., 2007 U.S. Dist. LEXIS 58829 (D.S.C. 2007).

Lorraine v. Markle American Ins. Co., 241 F.R.D. 534, 538 (D. Md. 2007).

Mancia v. Mayflower Textile Services Co., 253 F.R.D. 354 (D. Md. 2008).

McPeek v. Ashcroft, 202 F.R.D. 31 (D.D.C. 2001).

Muro v. Target Corp., 2007 WL 3254463 (N.D. Ill. 2007).

In re Napster Inc. Copyright Litigation, 2006 WL 3050864, *9 (N.D. Ca. 2006).

Newman v. Borders, 257 F.R.D. 1, 3 (D.D.C. 2009). Memorandum Opinion.

Palgut v. City of Colorado Springs, 2007 WL 4277564 (D. Colo. 2007).

Pension Comm. v. Banc of America Securities, LLC, 2010 WL 184312 (S.D.N.Y. 2010).

Peskoff v. Faber, 240 F.R.D. 26 (D.D.C. 2007).

Regan-Touhy v. Walgreen Co., 526 F.3d 641 (10th Cir. 2008).

Rhoads Industries, Inc. v. Building Materials Corp., 2008 WL 96404 (E.D. Pa. 2008).

Rimkus Consulting Grp. v. Cammarata, 2010 U.S. Dist. LEXIS (S.D. Tex. 2010).

Rhoads Industries, Inc. v. Building Materials Corp., 2008 WL 4916026 (E.D. Pa. 2008).

Rhoads Industries, Inc. v. Building Materials Corp., 2008 WL 96404 (E.D. Pa. 2008).

Rush Univ. Med. Ctr. v. Minnesota Mining and Manuf. Co., No. 04-C-6878 (N.D. Ill. Nov. 21, 2007).

SEC v. Collins & Aikman Corp., 2009 U.S. Dist. LEXIS 3367 (S.D.N.Y. 2009).

Spieker v. Quest Cherokee, LLC, 2008 WL 4758604 (D. Kan. 2008).

State of Texas v. City of Frisco, 2008 WL 828055 (E.D. Tex. 2008).

SubAir Systems, LLC v. PrecisionAire Systems, Inc., civil action no. 06-2620 (D.S.C. 2009).

Tomlinson v. El Paso Corp., 254 F.R.D. 474 (D. Colo. 2007).

United States v. O'Keefe, 2008 WL 44972 (D.D.C. 2008).

In re Vee Vinhnee, Debtor American Express Travel Related Services Company Inc. v. Vee Vinhnee, 336 B.R. 437 (9th Cir. BAP 2005).

Victor Stanley, Inc. v. CreativePipe, Inc., 250 F.R.D. 251 (D. Md. 2008).

Wachtel v. Health Net, Inc., 239 F.R.D. 81 (D.N.J. 2006).

Youle v. Raymond Ryan, MD and Sarah Bush Lincoln Health Center and Kevin M., Ill. App. 3d 377, 380, 811 N.E.2d 1281, 1283 (2004).

Zubulake v. UBS Warburg LLC, 220 F.R.D. 212 (S.D.N.Y. 2003).

Journals

Addison, K., J.H. Braden, J.E. Cupp, D. Emmert, L.A. Hall, T. Hall, B. Hess, et al. 2005. Update: Guidelines for defining the legal health record for-disclosure purposes. *Journal of AHIMA/American Health Information Management Association* 76, (8) (Sep): 64A–G.

AHIMA e-Discovery e-HIM Workgroup. 2006. The new electronic discovery civil rule. *Journal of AHIMA/American Health Information Management Association* 77, (8) (Sep): 68A–H.

AHIMA e-Discovery Task Force. 2008. Litigation response planning and policies for E-discovery. *Journal of AHIMA/American Health Information Management Association* 79, (2) (Feb): 69–75.

Amarasingham, R., L. Plantinga, M. Diener-West, D.J. Gaskin, and N.R. Powe. 2009. Clinical information technologies and inpatient outcomes: A multiple hospital study. *Archives of Internal Medicine* 169, (2) (Jan 26): 108–14.

Amarasingham, R., M. Diener-West, M. Weiner, H. Lehmann, J.E. Herbers, and N.R. Powe. 2006. Clinical information technology capabilities in four U.S. hospitals: Testing a new structural performance measure. *Medical Care* 44, (3) (Mar): 216–24.

Amatayakul, M., M. Brandt, and M. Dougherty. 2003. Working smart. Cut, copy, paste: EHR guidelines. *Journal of AHIMA/American Health Information Management Association* 74, (9) (Oct): 72, 74.

American Health Lawyers Association. 2004. Sarbanes-Oxley and corporate governance issues.

Annas, George J. 2006. The patient's right to safety—improving the quality of care through litigation against hospitals. *The New England Journal of Medicine* 354, (19) (May 11): 2063–6.

Ash, J.S., D.F. Sittig, E.M. Campbell, K.P. Guappone, and R.H. Dykstra. 2007. Some unintended consequences of clinical decision support systems. *AMIA . . . Annual Symposium Proceedings/AMIA Symposium. AMIA Symposium*: 26–30.

Ash, J.S., D.F. Sittig, E.G. Poon, K. Guappone, E. Campbell, and R.H. Dykstra. 2007. The extent and importance of unintended consequences related to computerized provider order entry. *Journal of the American Medical Informatics Association: JAMIA* 14, (4) (Jul-Aug): 415–23.

Baldwin-Stried, Kim. E-discovery and HIM: How amendments to the Federal Rules of Civil Procedure will affect HIM professionals. *Journal of AHIMA* 77, (9) (October 2006): 58–60.

Ball, Craig. 2006. Understanding metadata: Knowing metadata's different forms and evidentiary significance is now an essential skill for litigators. *Law Technology News* 36: 36.

Ball, Katherine. 2008. *Organizational Approaches to Early Litigation Readiness for Electronic Discovery of Electronic Health Records: A Modified Delphi Study.* Master of Science, Health Informatics., Johns Hopkins University, School of Medicine.

Ball, Katherine, G.E. DeLoss, E.F. Shay, and E. Zych. *EHRs and e-discovery: The readiness is all.* Paper presented at The American Health Lawyers Associations, Health Information Technology Practice Group, Webinar. May 22, 2008.

Ball, Marion J., Samuel Bierstock. 2007. Clinical Use of Enabling Technology: Creating a new healthcare system though the use of enabling technologies requires changes on a profound scale. *JHIM.* 21(3): 68–71.

Ball, M.J., C. Smith, and R. S. Bakalar. 2007. Personal health records: Empowering consumers. *Journal of Healthcare Information Management: JHIM* 21, (1) (Winter): 76–86.

Baron, J., and P. Thompson. 2007. *The search problem posed by large heterogeneous data sets in litigation: Possible future approaches to research.* Paper presented at The Proceedings of the 11th international conference on artificial intelligence and law. © 2007 Association for Computing Machinery.

Bartschat, W., A. Blevins, L. Burnette, K. Costa, M. D'Ambrosio, G. Glowacki, K.B. Griffin, et al. 2005. The legal process and electronic health records. *Journal of AHIMA/American Health Information Management Association* 76, (9) (Oct): 96A–D.

Baughman, John F., and H. Christopher Boehning. 2006. Benefits of transparency: Discussing what will be produced with your adversary. *New York Law Journal* (April 25, 2006).

Baxter, C., R. Dell, S. Publ, and R. Race. 2007. Assessing and improving EHR data quality. *Journal of AHIMA/American Health Information Management Association* 78, (3) (Mar): 69–72.

Bernstam, Elmer V., Jack W. Smith, and Todd R. Johnson. 2010. What is biomedical informatics? *Journal of Biomedical Informatics* 43, (1) (2): 104–10.

Bierman, E., and M. Buenafe. 2009. FDA and health IT—As role of health IT gains new significance, regulators will be keeping. *Health Lawyers News, American Health Lawyers Association* 13, (5) (May): 30–32.

Blakley, Alan, and Keith L. Altman. 2007. Sharpen your discovery from nonparties. *Trial (Boston, Mass.)* 43, (4) (Apr): 34.

Bodenheimer, Thomas. 2008. Coordinating care—A perilous journey through the health care system. *The New England Journal of Medicine* 358, (10) (March 6): 1064–71.

Brady, Kevin. 2007. Admissibility with ESI? The answer just might be in a 'Grimm' fairy tale. *Digital Discovery and E-Evidence: BNA* 7, (6) (June 1, 2007): 96.

Brady, Kevin, Katherine Ball, Ronald J. Hedges, and A. Estaban. 2008. E-discovery in healthcare litigation: What is ahead for ESI, PHI and EHR? *The Sedona Conference Journal* (Fall, 2008).

Brady, Kevin, and Paul Grimm. 2007. *Admissibility of electronic evidence.* Booklet presented by Capital Legal Solutions, LLC, Falls Church, VA.

Campbell, E.M., K.P. Guappone, D.F. Sittig, R.H. Dykstra, and J.S. Ash. 2009. Computerized provider order entry adoption: Implications for clinical workflow. *Journal of General Internal Medicine* 24, (1) (Jan): 21–6.

Campbell, E.M., D.F. Sittig, J.S. Ash, K.P. Guappone, and R.H. Dykstra. 2006. Types of unintended consequences related to computerized provider order entry. *Journal of the American Medical Informatics Association: JAMIA* 13, (5) (Sep–Oct): 547–56.

Campbell, Emily M., Dean F. Sittig, Joan S. Ash, Kenneth P. Guappone, and Richard H. Dykstra. 2007. In reply to: "e-iatrogenesis: The most critical consequence of CPOE and other HIT." *Journal of the American Medical Informatics Association* 14, (3) (May 1): 389.

Chaudhry, Basit, Jerome Wang, Shinyi Wu, Margaret Maglione, Walter Mojica, Elizabeth Roth, Sally C. Morton, and Paul G. Shekelle. 2006. Systematic review: Impact of health information technology on quality, efficiency, and costs of medical care. *Annals of Internal Medicine* 144, (10) (May 16): 742–52.

Coots, C., K. Joerling, M. Dougherty, W. Edwards, M.M. Foley, D. Kohn, A. Nicklas, et al. 2008. Enterprise content and record management for healthcare. *Journal of AHIMA/American Health Information Management Association* 79, (10) (Oct): 91–8.

Cottrell CM. 2006. On the road to the EHR, keep sight of the legal health record. *Health Management Technology* 27, (11).

Crowley, Conor. March, 2010. *Mapping your Client's Data*. Paper presented at 4th Annual Sedona Conference Institute: Program on Getting Ahead of the eDiscovery Curve, Philadelphia, PA.

Davidson, S.J., F.L. Zwemer Jr, L.A. Nathanson, K.N. Sable, and A.N. Khan. 2004. Where's the beef? The promise and the reality of clinical documentation. *Academic Emergency Medicine: Official Journal of the Society for Academic Emergency Medicine* 11, (11) (Nov): 1127–34.

DeLoss, G.E., and E.F. Shay. 2007. Electronic discovery and electronic health records: The impact of "e-discovery" involving "EHR" upon healthcare entities. *Health Lawyers News, American Health Lawyers Association* 11, (5) (May 2007): 4.

Dimick, C. 2007. Charting the legal health record. *JOURNAL-AHIMA* 78, (5): 30.

Dougherty, M. 2009. A new EHR standard for behavioral health. Stakeholders publish profile for use in behavioral health EHRs. *Journal of AHIMA/American Health Information Management Association* 80, (6) (Jun): 52–3.

Dougherty, M. How legal is your EHR? Identifying key functions that support a legal record. *Journal of AHIMA/American Health Information Management Association* 79, (2) (Feb 2008): 24,8, 30.

Dougherty, M. Linking anti-fraud and legal EHR functions. *Journal of AHIMA/ American Health Information Management Association* 78, (3) (Mar 2007): 60–1.

Dougherty, M., H. Rhodes, and M. O'Neill. 2007. Portrait of a legal EHR. Developing a legal EHR conformance profile. *Journal of AHIMA/American Health Information Management Association* 78, (6) (Jun): 66–7.

Dougherty M., and L. Washington. 2008. Defining and disclosing the designated record set and the legal health record. *The Journal of the American Health Information Medical Association* 79, (4) (April 2008): 65, 65–8.

Eslami, Saeid, Ameen Abu-Hanna, and Nicolette F. de Keizer. 2007. Evaluation of outpatient computerized physician medication order entry systems: A systematic review. *Journal of the American Medical Informatics Association* 14, (4) (July 1): 400–6.

Facciola, The Hon. John M, United States Magistrate Judge, District of the District of Columbia. (March, 2010) *Ethical Considerations Pertaining to Counsel's Entering Into Agreements that Particular Procedures: Do Not Waive Attorney-Client or Work Product Privileges*, Paper presented at 4th Annual Sedona Conference® Institute: Program on Getting Ahead of the eDiscovery Curve, Philadelphia, PA.

Foundation of Research and Education of AHIMA. 2005. Update: Maintaining a legally sound health record—paper and electronic. *Journal of AHIMA/American Health Information Management Association* 76, (10) (Nov-Dec): 64A–L.

Franks, Pat, and N. Kunde. Why metadata matters. *The Information Management Journal* (September/October 2006).

Fried B.M., and Zuckerman J.M. FDA regulation of medical software. *Journal of Health Law* 33, (1) (2006): 129–40.

Gelzer, R.D. 2008. Metadata, law, and the real world. *Journal of AHIMA/American Health Information Management Association* 79, (2) (Feb): 56,7, 64; quiz 65–6.

Ginn, Mary L., Brett Dietrich, Association of Records Managers and Administrators, and American National Standards Institute. 2004. *Records management responsibility in litigation support.* Lenexa, KS: ARMA International.

Hall, M.A., and K.A. Schulman. Ownership of medical information. *JAMA: The Journal of the American Medical Association* 301, (12) (Mar 25, 2009): 1282–4.

Harrison, M.I., R. Koppel, and S. Bar-Lev. Unintended consequences of information technologies in health care—an interactive sociotechnical analysis. *Journal of the American Medical Informatics Association: JAMIA* 14, (5) (Sep–Oct 2007): 542–9.

Hedges, Ronald J. Rule 702 and discovery of electronically stored information. *Digital Discovery and E-Evidence* 8, (5) (April 11, 2008).

Hedges, Ronald J. *Discovery of electronically stored information: Surveying the legal landscape.* Washington, DC: BNA Books (2007).

Herrin, B.S. Professional practice solutions. releasing records from other providers. *Journal of AHIMA/American Health Information Management Association* 79, (11) (Nov-Dec 2008): 55.

Herrin, B.S. Unsolicited medical information: Use it or lose it? *Legal HIMformation* 4, (5) (May/June 2008): 1–2.

Herrin, B.S. Identity proofing—just a fancy name for verification? *Journal of AHIMA/American Health Information Management Association* 78, (5) (May 2007): 54,5, 60.

Herrin, B.S., and J.D. Baxter. Outsourcing HIM functions to Europe. A perilous Atlantic crossing. *Journal of AHIMA/American Health Information Management Association* 79, (9) (Sep 2008): 56,7, 62.

Hersh, William R. *Information retrieval: A health and biomedical perspective.* New York, NY: Springer (2009).

HHS, Office National Coordinator, HIT Policy Committee. Meeting, July 16, 2009.

Hirschtick, Robert E. Copy-and-paste. *JAMA: The Journal of the American Medical Association* 295, (20) (May 24, 2006): 2335–6.

Hoffman, S., and A. Podgurski. Finding a cure: The case for regulation and over-sight of electronic health record systems. *Harvard Journal Law and Technolology* 22, (1): 1 (2008), 1–63.

Hoffman, S., and A. Podgurski. E-Health Hazards: Provider Liability and Electronic Health Record Systems. Forthcoming; Case Legal Studies Research Paper no. 09-25. *Berkeley Technology Law Journal.* (pre-press publication)., http://ssrn.com/abstract=1463671

Isaza, John. E-discovery compels: A seat for RIM at the counsel table. *Information Management Journal* 41, (1) (Jan/Feb 2007): 46.

Jenders, R.A., J.A. Osheroff, D.F. Sittig, E.A. Pifer, and J.M. Teich. Recommendations for clinical decision support deployment: Synthesis of a roundtable of medical directors of information systems. *American Medical Informatics Association. Annual Symposium Proceedings 2007*: 359–63.

Jha, Ashish K., Catherine M. DesRoches, Eric G. Campbell, Karen Donelan, Sowmya R. Rao, Timothy G. Ferris, Alexandra Shields, Sara Rosenbaum, and David Blumenthal. Use of electronic health records in U.S. hospitals. *The New England Journal of Medicine* 360, (16) (April 16, 2009): 1628–38.

Kahn R.A. Beyond HIPAA: The complexities of electronic record management. *Journal of AHIMA/American Health Information Management Association* 74, (4) (2003): 31–6.

Koppel, R. Defending computerized physician order entry from its supporters. *The American Journal of Managed Care* 12, (7) (Jul 2006): 369–70.

Koppel, R., and D. Kreda. Health care information technology vendors' "hold harmless" clause: Implications for patients and clinicians. *JAMA: The Journal of the American Medical Association* 301, (12) (Mar 25, 2009): 1276–8.

Koppel, R., C.E. Leonard, A.R. Localio, A. Cohen, R. Auten, and B.L. Strom. Identifying and quantifying medication errors: Evaluation of rapidly discontinued medication orders submitted to a computerized physician order entry system. *Journal of the American Medical Informatics Association: JAMIA* 15, (4) (Jul–Aug 2008): 461–5.

Koppel, R., J.P. Metlay, A. Cohen, B. Abaluck, A.R. Localio, S.E. Kimmel, and B.L. Strom. Role of computerized physician order entry systems in facilitating medication errors. *JAMA: The Journal of the American Medical Association* 293, (10) (Mar 9, 2005): 1197–203.

Koppel, R., T. Wetterneck, J.L. Telles, and B.T. Karsh. Workarounds to barcode medication administration systems: Their occurrences, causes, and threats to patient safety. *Journal of the American Medical Informatics Association: JAMIA* 15, (4) (Jul–Aug 2008): 408–23.

Korin, J.B., and M.S. Quattrone. Litigation in the decade of electronic health records. *New Jersey Law Journal* 188, (11 (183)) (June 11, 2007).

Lender, D. Duty to preserve: Should your client clam up when you make a mistake and hope it all goes away? *The Federal Lawyer* (Aug. 2007).

Levine, Ronald H., Jennifer A. Short, Stuart I. Silverman, Douglas K. Anning, and American Health Lawyers Association. *A new day for healthcare organizations: Sarbanes-Oxley certification requirements, compliance, and exposures.* Washington, DC: American Health Lawyers Association. 2004

Logan, D., J. Bace, and M. Gilbert. *Understanding e-discovery technology.* Gartner Research, Id. No. G00133224, 2005.

Mattox, A. Solving the unmanaged content conundrum. *Information Management Journal* 41, (6) (Nov/Dec 2007): 60.

McGowan, J.J., C.M. Cusack, and Eric G. Poon. Formative evaluation: A critical component in EHR implementation. *Journal of the American Medical Informatics Association* (February 28, 2008).

McLean, T.R., L. Burton, C.C. Haller, and P.B. McLean. Electronic medical record metadata: Uses and liability. *Journal of the American College of Surgeons,* 206, (3) (3): 405–11, 2008.

Miller, Randolph A., and Reed M. Gardner. Recommendations for responsible monitoring and regulation of clinical software systems. *Journal of the American Medical Informatics Association* 4, (6) (November 1997): 442–57.

Mitchell, J. Data source mapping workshop, CGOC conference, Data source synchronization for preservation and discovery and retention. New York. 2007

Munier, William. *Hearing on health information technology safety,* ed. The Adoption and Certification Working Group. Trans. Health and Human Services, ed. Office National Coordinator HIT Policy Committee. 2010

Okamoto, C. Legal medical record redefinition in a multimedia environment. *Journal of AHIMA/American Health Information Management Association* 69, (9) (Oct 1998): 70,2, 74, 76.

Paterno, M.D., S.M. Maviglia, P.N. Gorman, D.L. Seger, E. Yoshida, A.C. Seger, D.W. Bates, and T.K. Gandhi. Tiering drug-drug interaction alerts by severity increases compliance rates. *Journal of the American Medical Informatics Association: JAMIA* 16, (1) (Jan–Feb 2009): 40–6.

Quinsey, C.A. Digital disclosure and discovery. *Journal of AHIMA/American Health Information Management Association* 78, (8) (Sep 2007): 56–7.

Ragan, Charles R., and Lori Ann Wagner. Competence and credibility in e-discovery. *Trial (Boston, Mass.)* 43, (4) (Apr 2007): 40.

Roach, William H., and American Health Information Management Association. *Medical records and the law*. Sudbury, Mass.: Jones and Bartlett Publishers (2006).

Rodwin, M.A. The case for public ownership of patient data. *JAMA: The Journal of the American Medical Association* 302, (1) (Jul 1, 2009): 86–8.

Rollins, G. Printing electronic records. Managing the hassle and the risk. *Journal of AHIMA/American Health Information Management Association* 78, (5) (May 2007): 36,8, 40.

Rollins, G. The Prompt, the alert, and the legal record: Documenting Clinical decision support systems. *Journal of AHIMA/American Health Information Management Association* 76, (2) (Feb 2005): 24, 8; quiz 31–2.

RTI International. Requirements for enhancing data quality in electronic health records, prepared for the office of the national coordinator for health information technology. (May, 2007).

Schnipper, J.L., J.A. Linder, M.B. Palchuk, J.S. Einbinder, Q. Li, A. Postilnik, and B. Middleton. "Smart forms" in an electronic medical record: Documentation-based clinical decision support to improve disease management. *Journal of the American Medical Informatics Association: JAMIA* 15, (4) (Jul–Aug 2008): 513–23.

The Sedona Principles, Second Edition: Best Practices, Recommendations & Principles for Addressing Electronic Document Production (The Sedona Conference Working Group Series, 2007).

Shortliffe, Edward Hance, and James J. Cimino. *Biomedical informatics: Computer applications in health care and biomedicine*. Health informatics series. 3rd ed. New York, NY: Springer 2006.

Shuren, Jeffrey. *Hearing on health information technology safety*, edited by The Adoption and Certification Working Group. Trans. Health and Human Services and Office National Coordinator HIT Policy Committee.

Silverstein, S. The syndrome of inappropriate overconfidence in computing: An invasion of medicine by the information technology industry? *The Journal of American Physicians and Surgeons* 14, (2) (Summer 2009).

Sittig, Dean F., and David C. Classen. Safe electronic health record use requires a comprehensive monitoring and evaluation framework. *JAMA: The Journal of the American Medical Association* 303, (5) (February 3, 2010): 450–1.

Sittig, Dean F., and Hardeep Singh, Eight rights of safe electronic health record use. *JAMA: The Journal of the American Medical Association* 302, (10) (September 9, 2009): 1111–3.

Starren, Justin, *Hearing on health information technology safety*, edited by The Adoption and Certification Working Group. Trans. Health and Human Servicesand Office National Coordinator HIT Policy Committee.

State of California-Health and Human Services Agency, Public Records Act Inspection Request. (January, 2005).

Steinbrook R, Health care and the American Rrecovery and Reinvestment Act. *The New England Journal of Medicine* 360, (11) (2009): 1057–60.

Vigoda, M., J.C. Dennis, and M. Dougherty. E-record, e-liability. Addressing medico-legal issues in electronic records. *Journal of AHIMA/American Health Information Management Association* 79, (10) (Oct 2008): 48, 52; quiz 55–6.

Wachter, R.M. Expected and unanticipated consequences of the quality and information technology revolutions. *JAMA: The Journal of the American Medical Association* 295, (23) (Jun 21, 2006): 2780–3.

Wagner, L., and C. Kenreigh. CPOE: Fallible, not foolproof: Clinical decision support for E-prescribing. *Medscape Pharmacists* 6, (2) (November 17, 2005), http://www.medscape.com/viewarticle/516367_2.

Walker, J.M., P. Carayon, N. Leveson, R.A. Paulus, J. Tooker, H. Chin, A. Bothe Jr., and W.F. Stewart. EHR safety: The way forward to safe and effective systems. *Journal of the American Medical Informatics Association: JAMIA* 15, (3) (May–Jun 2008): 272–7.

Weiner, J.P., T. Kfuri, K. Chan, and J.B. Fowles. "e-iatrogenesis": The most critical unintended consequence of CPOE and other HIT. *Journal of the American Medical Informatics Association: JAMIA* 14, (3) (May–Jun 2008): 387,8; discussion 389.

Withers, Kenneth J. NJTP. Electronically stored information: The December 2006 amendments to the Federal Rules of Civil Procedure. *Northwestern Journal of Technology and Intellectual Property* 4, (2) (Spring, 2006): 171, 171–211.

Wright, A., and D. F. Sittig. SANDS: An architecture for clinical decision support in a national health information network. *AMIA . . . Annual Symposium Proceedings/ AMIA Symposium. AMIA Symposium 2007*: 816–20.

Other Resources

Advisory Committee Note to 1983 Amendment to FED. R. CIV. P. 26(b).

Advisory Committee Notes to 1993 Amendments FED. R. CIV. P. 26(b).

Advisory Committee Notes to 2006 amendment to FED. R. CIV. P. 26(b)(5).

Dougherty, M. Opening remarks, AHIMA Legal EHR Conference, Philadelphia, PA. October 6, 2007.

Fischer, Thomas G. Medical malpractice: Presumption or inference from failure of hospital or doctor to produce relevant medical records. *American Law Reports* 69 A.L.R. 4th 906 (1990).

Grossman, Joy M. 2007. *Physicians' use of electronic medical records for quality reporting.* Paper presented at Division of Health Sciences Informatics Grand Rounds, Johns Hopkins University, School of Medicine, Baltimore, MD.

Health and Human Services. *Health Information Technology: Initial Set of Standards, Implementation Specifications, and Certification Criteria for Electronic Health Record Technology. 45 CFR 170* (2010).

Herrin, B.S. Adapted from *American Health Information Management Association* presentation, August 18, 2008: The legal EHR: Beyond definition.

King, P., and Teresa Bunsen. E-Discovery, Case presentation, Risk Management and Legal Affairs NorthShore University Health System. AHIMA Legal EHR Conference Chicago. August 17, 2009.

Marchand, L. *Discovery of electronic medical records.* Paper presented at American Trial Lawyers Association Annual Convention Reference Materials.

The Sedona Conference. The Sedona Conference Commentary on Legal Holds. August 2007.

The Sedona Conference. The Sedona Conference Commentary on ESI Evidence & Admissibility. March 2008.

The Sedona Conference. The Sedona Conference Cooperation Proclamation. July 2008.

Shay, E.F. Ensuring health record integrity. Paper presented at *American Health Information Management Association* Annual Convention, Philadelphia, PA. (October 2007.

Web sites

Healthcare IT Failure and Difficulties Case Examples: Medical Informatics Perspectives on Clinical Information Technology. http://www.ischool.drexel.edu/faculty/ssilverstein/failurecases/

AHIMA. AHIMA mobilizes to meet the e-HIM call. [cited 8/5/2009 2009]. Available from http://library.ahima.org/xpedio/groups/public/documents/ahima/bok1_017431.hcsp?dDocName=bok1_017431

Appeal from Circuit Court of Coles County No. 02L75. No. 4-03-1025, Youle v. Ryan. [cited 8/5/2009 2009]. Available from http://www.state.il.us/court/opinions/appellatecourt/2004/4thdistrict/june/html/4031025.htm.

Baron, J. TREC legal track overview. [cited 8/5/2009 2009]. Available from http://trec-legal.umiacs.umd.edu/.

Cepelewicz, Barry B., and Denlea, James R. Electronic health records: A discovery landmine for physicians and counsel—give your practice a checkup, and treat it accordingly. [cited 3/27/2008 2008]. Available from http://www.lawjournalnewsletters.com/issues/ljn_ediscovery/3_8/news/147773-1.html.

Certification Commission for Health Information Technology. CCHIT criteria proposed final: Ambulatory 2009. [cited June, 17 2009]. Available from http://www.cchit.org/files/comment/09/03/CCHITCriteriaProposedFinal AMBULATORY09.pdf.

Civil Action No. C94-1023. U.S. v. Mercy Health Services: United States' third request for document production. [cited 8/5/2009 2009]. Available from http://www.justice.gov/atr/cases/f0100/0194.htm.

CLIA - subpart K. Available from http://wwwn.cdc.gov/clia/regs/subpart_k.aspx#493.1283.

Clinical & Risk Management Perspectives. 2009 (October). Electronic Health Records: Recognizing and Managing the Risks. http://www.norcalmutual.com/publications/claimsrx/oct_09.pdf.

CMS proposes requirements for the electronic health records (EHR) medicare incentive program. Available from http://www. cms.hhs.gov/apps/media/press/factsheet.asp?Counter= 3563 (accessed 2/12/2010).

DOD directive 5015.2, records management. [cited 4/27/2008 2008]. Available from http://www.dtic.mil/whs/directives/corres/writing/process_index.html#fr (accessed 4/27/2008).

Has your organization had a patient safety issue directly resulting from an electronic system? - iHealthBeat. [cited 2/12/2010 2010]. Available from http://www.ihealthbeat.org/data-points/2010/has-your-organization-had-a-patient-safety-issue-directly-resulting-from-an-electronic-system.aspx.

HHS, Office National Coordinator, HIT Policy Committee. Meeting, April 21, 2010. 2010. http://healthit.hhs.gov/portal/server.pt?open=512&objID=1473&&PageID=17117&mode=2&in_hi_userid=11673&cached=true

HHS/CMS. CMS guidance document: Survey and certification policy letter, hospitals–revised state operations manual (SOM) appendix A. March 17, 2008 [June 18, 2009]. Available from http://www.cms.hhs.gov/EOG/downloads/EO%200307.pdf.

HL7 RM-ES. HL7 EHR Records Management and Evidentiary Support Functional Profile Release 1. [cited 9/14/2010]. Available from https://www.hl7.org/store/index.cfm?ref=nav.

HL7 RMES. HL7 EHR-S records management and evidentiary support functional profile. [cited 8/2/2009 2009]. Available from http://www.hl7.org/index.cfm (accessed 8/2/2009).

Interpretive guidelines for laboratories clinical laboratory improvement amendments (CLIA). Available from http://www.cms.hhs.gov/clia/03_Interpretive_Guidelines_for_Laboratories.asp.

Issue 42: Safely implementing health information and converging technologies. The Joint Commission. Available from http://www.jointcommission.org/Sentinel Events/SentinelEventAlert/sea_42. 2008.

K&L Gates (December 15, 2004). Court directs production in native electronic form notwithstanding prior hard copy production: Electronic discovery law. Available from http://www.ediscoverylaw.com/2004/12/articles/case-summaries/court-directs-production-in-native-electronic-form-notwithstanding-prior-hard-copy-production/.

Kerr, Orin S. 2001. *Computer records and federal rules of evidence*, www.usdoj.gov/criminal/cybercrime/usamarch2001_4.htm.

Lynn, Cecil. 2007. Litigation preparedness: A checklist for corporate counsel. *The Metropolitan Corporate Counsel* (37) (July, 2007), http://www.metrocorpcounsel.com/pdf/2007/July/37.pdf.

McLean, T.R., Metadata: An Orwellian big brother within electronic medical records. (September 16, 2008). Available from http://www.hcplive.com/mdnglive/articles/Metadata_within_EMRs.

The Medical Products Agency: Working Group on Medical Information Systems. Proposal for guidelines regarding classification of software based information systems used in health care. 2009. Sweden: http://www.lakemedelsverket.se/upload/foretag/medicinteknik/en/Medical-Information-Systems-Report_2009-06-18.pdf.

Monegain, Bernie. Allscripts shareholders file class action suit. Healthcare IT news. (August 5, 2009). Available from http://www.healthcareitnews.com/news/allscripts-shareholders-file-class-action-suit.

Reynolds, H. 2009. *National Committee on Vital and Health Statistics Report of Hearing on "Meaningful Use" of Health Information Technology, April 28–29, 2009*, http://www.ncvhs.hhs.gov/090518rpt.pdf (accessed June 17, 2009).

Sinrod, E. E-discovery: Can't we all just get along? *Find Law*.

Index